SYNOPSIS OF CRITICAL CARE

Third Edition

SYNOPSIS OF CRITICAL CARE

Third Edition

Edited by

WILLIAM J. SIBBALD, M.D.

Coordinator, The Richard Ivey Critical Care Trauma Centre, Victoria Hospital,
Clinical Professor of Medicine
The University of Western Ontario, London, Canada

Illustrated by CATHERINE FARLEY

WILLIAMS & WILKINS
Baltimore • Hong Kong • London • Sydney

SYNOPSIS OF CRITICAL CARE

Third Edition

Editor: Timothy R. Grayson
Associate Editor: Carol Eckhart
Copy Editor: Gail Naron Chalew
Design: JoAnne Janowiak
Illustration Planning: Lorraine Wrzosek
Production: Anne G. Seitz

Williams & Wilkins
428 East Preston Street
Baltimore, MD 21202, U.S.A.

Accurate indications, adverse reactions, and dosage schedules for drugs are provided in this book, but it is possible that they may change. The reader is urged to review the package information data of the manufacturers of the medications mentioned.

Printed in the United States of America

First Edition, 1984

Library of Congress Cataloging in Publication Data

Synopsis of critical care.

Includes bibliographies and index.
1. Critical care medicine—Outlines, syllabi,
etc. I. Sibbald, William J. [DNLM: 1. Critical
Care. WX 218 S993]
RC86.7.S96 1988 616′.028 87-16133
ISBN 0-683-07709-0

Main entry under title:

88, 89, 90, 91, 92, 93
10 9 8 7 6 5 4 3 2 1

To my family . . .
for accepting with love
the unique frailties of a critical care physician

Preface

The growth of critical care medicine as a recognized discipline over the last decade has paralleled major changes in the care that can be provided for acutely ill patients. Because concepts of pathophysiology and treatment of life-threatening diseases are constantly changing, individuals working as the health care team in critical care are particularly cognizant of the importance of maintaining competence relating to the comprehensive management of such patients. For those who work within critical care or trauma units as a full-time avocation, this proves to be difficult at the best of times. Therefore, it is easily understood how difficult it must then be for the practitioner in a community hospital, practicing within an intensive care unit but not necessarily as a primary specialty, to attempt to maintain the required data base and perspective on changes in this rapidly evolving field of medicine.

With the major advances in therapeutic modalities available for the care of critically ill patients has come an increase in the number of "critical care" hospital beds and their concomitant life support monitoring and therapeutic tools, all of which provide the clinician with an ability to keep even the most desperately ill patient alive. The introduction of flow-directed catheters for continuous pressure recording, a better appreciation of the use of mechanical ventilators, and development of the intra-aortic balloon pump are but a few examples of the diagnostic and therapeutic modalities now available to the "team" caring for critically ill patients. The result of such advancements in knowledge and life support equipment is that patients are resuscitated more efficaciously, and kept alive longer; in the majority of circumstances this may be honestly appreciated as being in the patients' best interests. However, we are now faced with the realization that technological advancements occasionally exceed our ability to maintain the most appropriate perspective on the goals of patient care. Not infrequently, elderly and debilitated patients are admitted to critical care only to become "slaves" to life support systems and monitoring treatment devices and to eventually succumb after a prolonged period of caring from multiple organ failure. As one of my colleagues has so aptly put it, "The job of an intensive care unit is resuscitation, not resurrection!"

As a group those of us with an active interest in the future of critical care must be prepared to address the necessary decisions about who should be offered such expensive, time-consuming, and, at times, dehumanizing therapy. The expense of providing for critical care services is exponential and open-ended. If the health care team working within the field cannot discuss openly some of the very real problems that face our discipline, it can only be expected that major decisions about its future will be taken from us as a group, and commitments will be made on our behalf by individuals not necessarily as well prepared for such decisions as we would be. Our wish as a group could never be to discourage an attitude toward aggressive, yet appropriate, life support care. Rather, we must be prepared to accept a word of caution about some of the very real moral issues that will face physicians and allied health care workers alike in critical care. We must be prepared to discuss openly the issues with our colleagues, with those responsible for the financing of health care, and most importantly, with families of the patients for whom we care.

To provide rationalization in the provision of life support systems in a critical care environment, our institution has promoted the concept of a multidisciplinary critical care and trauma center. This philosophy is easily understood by appreciating that any critically ill or traumatized patient has multisystem disease from the outset and will therefore benefit from the advice and knowledge of consultants from all disciplines of the medical sciences. The establishment of one special care unit providing all major life support and monitoring systems for any critically ill or injured patient, regardless of the primary service under which the patient may have been admitted to the hospital, creates a multidisciplinary environment that has enabled the physical amalgamation of physicians, as well as the essential paramedical support services, in one area of the hospital to provide a degree of care and understanding that we believe would not be possible without such centralization.

This text illustrates some of the principles we have understood from this multidisciplinary approach to the care of critically ill patients. It grew out of an attempt to provide an educational data base for physicians who had not been previously involved in the care of critically ill patients. In this third edition, we have attempted to review some of the more important clinical problems that critical care physicians and other senior nursing and paramedical staff are faced with on a daily basis in order to provide a practical and reasonable approach toward a specific diagnostic or treatment goal. We have reviewed major topic headings under organ-based systems and have provided a section on specific syndromes where individual problems are more concisely reviewed. We have not attempted to provide a comprehensive review nor document basic literature that is available elsewhere. Rather we have attempted to present an approach to certain patient care problems that are particularly frequent in a critical care environment. Some of the concepts presented are controversial, and some of the subject areas stress only a few of the aspects of the total clinical problem, reflecting in part our bias, particular interests, and experience in what we believe is most important to emphasize for the clinician who is becoming newly acquainted with a critical care environment. However, the editor believes that the topics selected are ones commonly seen and has attempted to maintain the style of this text in such a way that you, the reader, are initially stimulated with a brief section on pathophysiology and are then provided with a more didactic presentation of necessary diagnostic and treatment modalities.

We updated this third edition where we felt a changing knowledge base demanded such revisions, and we added new sections that we hope will increase the value of this text to trainees and senior support staff in critical care. In so doing, we have strived to attain our goal of presenting information to meet the needs of the physician without much prior experience in critical care, as well as the needs of senior critical care nursing and paramedical personnel. As we found in the first two editions, there will always be shortcomings in any attempt of this sort. However, we sincerely hope that this review of our experience in current practice will be of benefit to all who work with critically ill or traumatized patients.

William J. Sibbald

Acknowledgments

The editor would like to thank all of the contributing authors to this *Synopsis of Critical Care,* without whose help and ongoing support this text on our experiences and views in managing critically ill and traumatized patients would not have been possible. Particular appreciation is expressed to David Girvan for his assistance in editing some of the chapters within this text. I sincerely appreciate the support of my associate coordinators in the Critical Care/Trauma Centre at Victoria Hospital—Ron Holliday, David Cunningham, and Frank Rutledge—for their efforts in demonstrating that a multidisciplinary approach to the management of the critically ill and traumatized patient is not only a very workable concept but also provides for excellence in patient care. The same appreciation must be extended to all of my colleagues who have diligently maintained the multidisciplinary flavor of the critical care environment within our hospital.

Our initial idea that we would be able to put together a book within a short time period turned out to be an extremely naive concept. As all of the authors became more involved, we became aware of how inadequate physicians are at expressing fluent ideas on paper. With the skillful assistance of Catherine Farley, this text has indeed finally come to fruition.

Contributors

A. Loren Amacher, M.D., F.R.C.S.(C). Director of Residency Training, Hartford Hospital. Professor of Neurosurgery, University of Connecticut, Hartford, Connecticut, U.S.A.

Thomas W. Austin, M.D., F.R.C.P.(C). Infectious Diseases Consultant, Victoria Hospital. Associate Professor of Medicine, The University of Western Ontario, London, Canada.

William C. Ballantyne, Senior Technical Assistant, Critical Care Trauma Centre, Victoria Hospital, London, Canada.

Kenneth A. Boyle, E.M.C.A., R.R.T., Program Coordinator, Critical Care Transport, Southwest Region, Victoria Hospital, London, Canada.

Gerald Bristow, M.D., Attending Staff, Invensive Care Unit, Health Sciences Centre, Associate Dean, Division of Post-Graduate Education, Professor of Anaesthesia, University of Manitoba, Winnipeg, Canada.

John D. Brown, M.D., B.Sc.(Med), Ph.D., F.R.C.P.(C). Neurologist, Victoria Hospital. Associate Professor, Department of Clinical Neurosciences, The University of Western Ontario, London, Canada.

James E. Calvin, M.D., F.R.C.P.(C). Cardiologist, University of Ottawa Heart Institute. Assistant Professor, The University of Ottawa, Ottawa, Canada.

Sandra G. Campbell, B.Sc. Phm. Liaison Pharmacist, Critical Care Trauma Centre, Victoria Hospital, London, Canada.

William F. Clark, M.D., F.R.C.P.(C). Director, Renal Out-Patient and Plasmaphoresis Services, Victoria Hospital. Professor of Medicine, The University of Western Ontario, London, Canada.

Robert G. Colcleugh, M.D., F.R.C.S.(C)., F.A.C.S. Active Staff, Division of Plastic and Reconstructive Surgery, Victoria Hospital. Clinical Associate Professor of Surgery, The University of Western Ontario, London, Canada.

David G. Cunningham, M.D., F.R.C.P.(C). Chief, Department of Anaesthesia, Victoria Hospital. Clinical Assistant Professor, Department of Anaesthesia, The University of Western Ontario, London, Canada.

Albert A. Driedger, M.D., Ph.D., F.R.C.P.(C)., F.A.C.P. Chief, Department of Nuclear Medicine, Victoria Hospital. Clinical Professor, Departments of Medicine, Nuclear Medicine, and Oncology, The University of Western Ontario, London, Canada.

John H. Duff, M.D., F.R.C.S.(C)., F.A.C.S. Chief of Surgery, University Hospital. Professor and Chairman, Department of Surgery, The University of Western Ontario, London, Canada.

Richard J. Finley, M.D., F.R.C.S.(C), F.A.C.S. Chief of Surgery, Victoria Hospital. Associate Professor of Surgery, The University of Western Ontario, London, Canada.

John H. Gallant, C.I.M., R.R.T. Clinical Instructor, Respiratory Therapy Program, Victoria Hospital. Associate Professor, Respiratory Therapy Program, Fanshawe College, London, Canada.

Adrian W. Gelb, M.B., Ch.B., F.R.C.P.(C). Assistant Medical Director, Intensive Care Unit, University Hospital. Associate Professor, Department of Anaesthesia, The University of Western Ontario, London Canada.

Alain Gilbert, M.D., F.R.C.S.(C). Fellow, Critical Care Medicine, The University of Western Ontario, London, Canada.

David P. Girvan, M.D., M.Cl.Sc., F.A.C.S., F.R.C.S.(C). Active Teaching Staff, Victoria Hospital. Associate Professor of Surgery and Paediatrics; Chairman, Division of Paediatric Surgery, The University of Western Ontario, London, Canada.

Martin M. Goldbach, M.D., F.R.C.S.(C)., F.A.C.S. Staff, Division of Cardiovascular and Thoracic Surgery, Victoria Hospital. Clinical Assistant Professor of Surgery, Division of Cardiovascular and Thoracic Surgery, The University of Western Ontario, London, Canada.

Patrick J. Gullane, M.D., F.R.C.S.(C)., F.A.C.S. Staff Otolaryngologist and Deputy Chief, Toronto General Hospital. Associate Professor, Department of Otolaryngology, The University of Toronto, Toronto, Canada.

M. J. Halls, M.D., F.R.C.S.(C). Staff, Division of Plastic Surgery, Victoria Hospital Corporation, London, Canada.

Thomas E. Havas, M.D. Senior Fellow, Department of Otolaryngology, University of Toronto, Toronto, Canada.

Ronald L. Holliday, M.D., F.R.C.S.(C)., F.A.C.S. Staff, Department of Surgery, Victoria Hospital. Associate Professor of Surgery, The University of Western Ontario, London, Canada.

John G. Kelton, M.D., F.R.C.P.(C). Professor of Medicine and Pathology, McMaster Medical Centre, Hamilton, Canada.

E. Garner King, M.D., F.R.C.P.(C)., F.A.C.P., F.C.C.P. Director, Intensive Care Unit, Health Sciences Centre. Professor and Chairman, Department of Medicine, University of Alberta, Edmonton, Canada.

Bryan W. Kirk, M.D., F.R.C.P.(C). Attending Staff, Medical Intensive Care Unit, Health Sciences Centre. Associate Dean (Academic), University of Manitoba, Winnipeg, Canada.

David Leasa, M.D., F.R.C.P.(C). Director, Intensive Care Unit, St. Joseph's Hospital. Assistant Professor, The University of Western Ontario, London, Canada.

Michael S. Lefcoe, M.D., F.R.C.P.(C). Associate Radiologist, Victoria Hospital. Clinical Associate Professor of Radiology, The University of Western Ontario, London, Canada.

Adam L. Linton, M.D., Ch.B., F.R.C.P.(G)., F.R.C.P.(C). Professor of Medicine, The University of Western Ontario, London, Canada.

Trevor R. Lobb, M.D., F.R.C.P.(C). Clinical Associate Professor of Anaesthesia, The University of Western Ontario, London, Canada.

Adel G. Matter, M.D. Staff Physician, Department of Nuclear Medicine, London, Canada.

John A. McCredie, M.B., M.Ch., F.R.C.S. (E & Edin.), F.R.C.S.(C)., F.A.C.S. Staff, Department of Surgery and Cancer Clinic, Victoria Hospital. Professor of Surgery and Therapeutic Radiology, The University of Western Ontario, London, Canada.

Lee J. Melendez, M.D., F.R.C.P.(C). Director of Cardiology, Victoria Hospital. Professor of Medicine, The University of Western Ontario, London, Canada.

John D. Moffat, M.D., F.R.C.S.(C). Staff Surgeon, Grey-Bruce Regional Health Centre, Owen Sound, Canada.

Nigel A. M. Paterson, M.B., B.S., B.Med. Sc. (Hons), F.R.C.P.(C). Chief, Department of Medicine, Victoria Hospital. Professor of Medicine, The University of Western Ontario, London, Canada.

Frank Stuart Rutledge, M.D., F.R.C.P.(C). Associate Coordinator, Critical Care Trauma Centre, Victoria Hospital. Associate Professor of Medicine, The University of Western Ontario, London, Canada.

Robert Roderick Shepherd, M.D., M.Sc., F.R.C.S.(C). Consultant Staff, Victoria Hospital. Clinical Assistant Professor of Surgery (Urology), The University of Western Ontario, London, Canada.

William J. Sibbald, M.D., F.R.C.P.(C)., F.A.C.P., F.C.C.P. Coordinator, Critical Care Trauma Centre, Victoria Hospital. Clinical Associate Professor of Medicine, The University of Western Ontario, London, Canada.

Stephen M. Sullivan, M.D., M.R.C.P.(UK), F.R.C.P.(C). Consultant (Internal Medicine, Gastroenterology, Hepatology), Victoria Hosptial. Associate Professor, The University of Western Ontario, London, Canada.

Bryan Taylor, M.D., F.R.C.S.(C). Staff, General Surgical, St. Joseph's Hospital. Assistant Professor of Surgery, The University of Western Ontario, London, Canada.

Irene Tiegs, B.Sc., M.S.W. Social Worker, Critical Care Trauma Centre, Victoria Hospital, London, Canada.

H. Ronald Wexler, M.D., F.R.C.P.(C). Medical Director, Intensive Care Unit, University Hospital. Associate Professor, Department of Anaesthesia, The University of Western Ontario, London, Canada.

R. Baxter Willis, M.D., F.R.C.S.(C). Consultant in Orthopaedic Surgery, Victoria Hospital. Clinical Assistant Professor, Division of Orthopaedic Surgery, The University of Western Ontario, London, Canada.

Contents

SPECIFIC SYNDROMES

APPENDICES

CHAPTER

1 A Philosophy of Critical Care Medicine

E. Garner King, M.D.

What makes a specialty in medicine? Most importantly, there must be a definable body of knowledge and skills that are not necessarily exclusive to the specialty but are viewed from a unique perspective. Further, there must be an identifiable group of people who possess the appropriate knowledge and skills and who develop their own systems of communication through meetings and ceremonies, journals, and texts. Finally, the identifiably cohesive group must develop a tradition with a recognizable history and an evolution of rules by which members interact and by which outsiders may join the group. Human beings are not unique among the animals in establishing a definable territory in which they can hold sway, feel comfortable and unthreatened, and seemingly control their destiny. They are unique, however, in investing such territorial behavior with a rationalized altruistic philosophy that guides and directs the group in activities toward a greater good for those beyond the group confines. By these criteria, critical care medicine has come of age: from gestation in the polio epidemics of 1953 and 1957, to birth in modified postanesthetic recovery rooms, to progressive sophistication and early maturity in monitoring and support of the critically ill in the late 1980s.

Critical care medicine now has its formalized societies (e.g., Society of Critical Care Medicine (SCCM), Canadian Critical Care Society (CCCS), Australian Society of Intensive Care), mounts major meetings (e.g., SCCM Annual Scientific Programs, the CCCS Royal College meetings, and International Congresses—London, Paris and Washington), maintains scientific journals (e.g., *Critical Care Medicine, Australian Journal of Anaesthesiology and Intensive Care, Journal of Critical Care, European Journal of Intensive Care*), and is currently in the process of defining the insider-outsider boundary through educational programs and codified specialty qualifications (e.g., the development of specialty examinations in critical care in the United States, the established existence of such examinations in Australia, and the accreditation process in Canada). Critical care medicine as a specialty activity achieves legitimacy not because of the associated complexity of patient monitoring and support equipment (although that certainly promotes the "'mystique"!) but because every critically ill patient ends up on a final common pathway of organ system failure in which respiratory, renal, nutritional, and other vital organ system support, alone or in combination, are required (Fig. 1.1). To the patient in hypoxemic respiratory failure, it matters little whether the lung was "hit" by a steering wheel, gastric juice, or a virus, the end result and supportive management are essentially the same and represent an example of the "definable body of knowledge" utilized by the specialty. In this regard, critical care medicine may be thought of as a horizontal specialty cutting across the traditional vertical specialties of medicine, surgery, pediatrics, and anesthesiology (Fig. 1.2). As such, it joins the other relative newcomers on the specialty scene, such as infectious disease, clinical pharmacology, and oncology.

That the use of specific systems support apparatus and techniques represents a real and definable body of knowledge can hardly be debated; what is less apparent is that critical care medicine represents a different and aggressive philosophy of patient care in which there is an attempt to coordinate properly *all* aspects of multidisciplinary management in the seriously ill. A common bit of gallows humor in days gone by was that when a patient had nine tubes and five consultants who were writing all over the chart, he or she was dead—the message being that fragmented care in the critically ill was not in the patient's best interests. Not only is the uncoordinated application of multispecialty care not in the patient's best interests but nurses and members of other caring professions generally find it very difficult to work in completely "open" intensive care units where there is neither direction nor unitary philosophy.

Who should look after an ICU? In truth, it matters little whether it is an internist, surgeon (although it is difficult to be actively engaged in an operating theater with any regularity and still provide the onsite ICU patient care required for the seriously ill), pediatrician, or anesthetist so long as the individual brings to his or her activities the knowledge, skills, and time commitment required to care comprehensively for the multisystem failure patient. It is not a hobby nor is it a part-time casual occupation. Despite speculation to the contrary, ICU physicians are not a pantheon of gods—it is impossible to be all things to all people—and there are great areas from which other consultants' expertise and knowledge must be drawn. However, a major role for the ICU physician is to act as an interlocutor (to borrow a term from the old minstrel shows) and bring together, coordinate, and filter all the available information from many different consultants for the potential benefit of the critically ill patient. In many ways the ICU physician of the late 1980s is comparable to our idealized images of the general

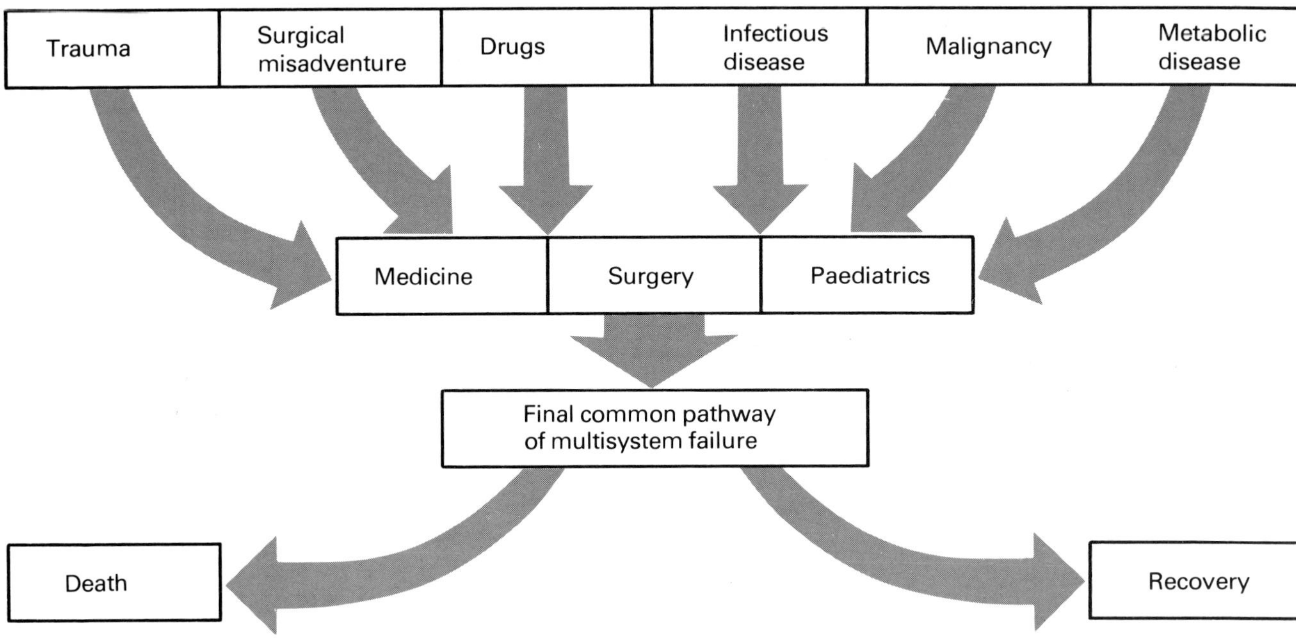

Figure 1.1. Philosophy of critical care.

practitioner of old, for critical care is a specialty that takes the ICU physician back to the bedside and into an intimate ongoing relationship with the patient, the patient's family, and the physician's many helping colleagues. Not only is the ICU physician the one who directly cares for critically ill patients when they are desperately ill and require constant use of life-support apparatus and techniques, but, by so doing, he or she also becomes the physician's physician extending, and at the same time focusing, the efforts of all the doctors looking after multifactorial problem patients. Whatever else the ICU physicians might be, they must above all be manager, diplomat, and teacher, for in order to apply and multiply their efforts, there must be an enormous pyramid of other caring, helping people—nurses, respiratory technologists, physiotherapists, physiologic support technicians, clerks, and others—without whom the ICU physicians' efforts would be puny indeed.

Who should be admitted to an ICU? To be admitted to a general systems failure ICU facility, a patient should have failure, impending or established, of one or more organ systems, requiring constant monitoring and/or

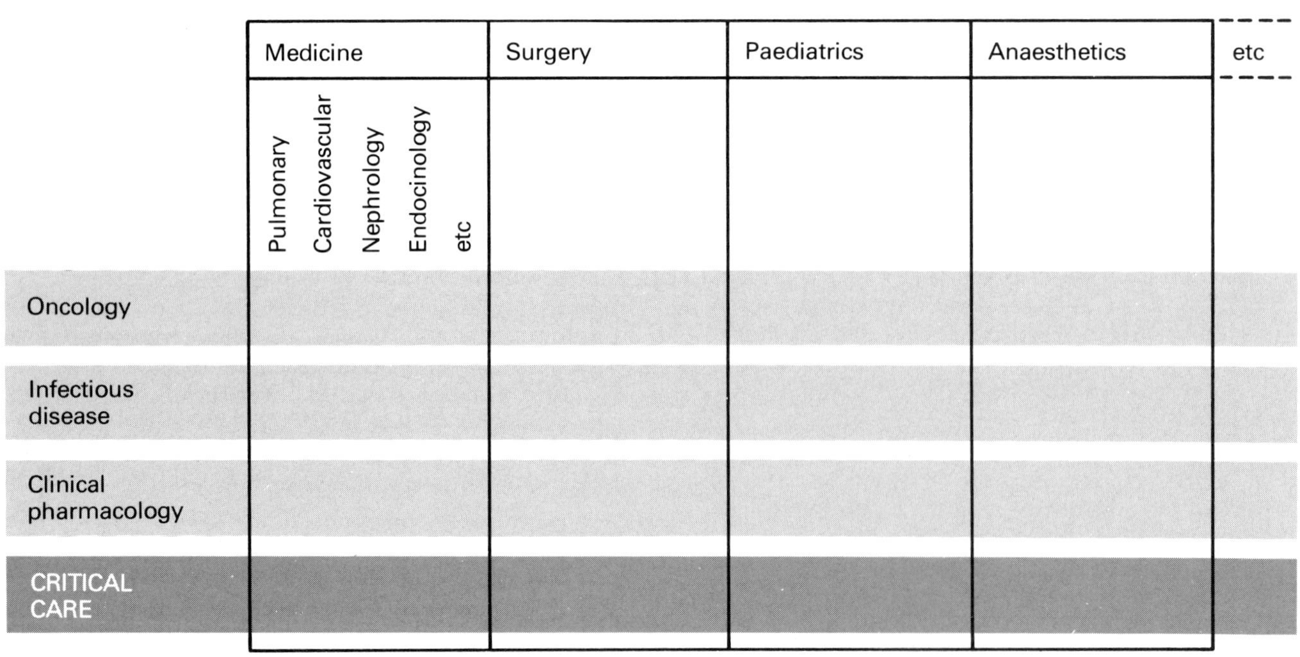

Figure 1.2. The horizontal nature of critical care medicine.

support. To this should be added the proviso that there should be a reasonable expectation of recovery with appropriate support and therapy. It is the major role of the ICU to provide whatever physiologic support is necessary until one of three things happens: the patient spontaneously recovers, specific therapy alleviates the basic problem, or the patient dies. It should be pointed out that the philosophy of coronary care is somewhat different from critical care in that the former essentially involves surveillance with only occasional active intervention and multiorgan system support: ICUs are places of active supportive and therapeutic intervention in which the usual activity and noise are inappropriate to the nonstress atmosphere of the ideal coronary care unit.

How should an ICU be run? Whether an ICU is run as a closed unit in which a full-time director and designees assume specific responsibility for all patient care and educational programs within the unit or as a semiclosed unit in which an ICU director is responsible for overall quality of patient care and staff education, good intensive care facilities require unitary direction. This is crucial, not only for adequate patient care but also for maintenance of staff morale and development of complex coordinated programs. Hospitals have realized that they have a major legal responsibility to establish and maintain properly functioning intensive care facilities and that this responsibility goes beyond the simple provision of space and equipment. Although each institution must wrestle with the problems of how to look after its own unique needs, there is an increasing trend in secondary and tertiary care hospitals toward the appointment of full-time ICU medical personnel, rather than relying on the laissez-faire practice of medicine or the "mandatory consultation" rule in the ICU.

What happens to patients admitted to this idealized kind of ICU? In 1976, Dr. David Fletcher completed a computerized survey of 850 patients admitted to the University of Alberta Hospital General Systems Failure ICU. This facility operates as a 10-bed closed unit in a 1200-bed tertiary referral and general hospital. An intensive follow-up on all patients demonstrated that about 25% died in the ICU and some 40% never left that hospital, and only 53% were alive at the end of the 3 years. This latter group, however, followed a life-table survival curve thereafter. Based on the New York Heart Physical Capabilities scale (out of 4), the mean self-assessment score of 1.4 on ICU admission changed to only 1.6 in all survivors, indicating that the quality of life preserved was certainly acceptable. The conclusion from this and other studies is that ICUs provide genuine salvage and the prospect of a return to a good quality of life.

A multitude of questions remain to be answered about the future development of critical care medicine. These relate to philosophies of patient care, such as development of precise prognostic profiles, philosophies of community organization, (the need for regionalization and stratification of services, as well as the development of appropriate transport systems), and philosophies of cost-effectiveness. This brief discussion is not intended to survey all aspects of the broad new specialty of critical care medicine but rather to draw to the reader's attention that such a specialty does indeed exist and that it is steadily moving toward an expanding and clearer definition of its identity. From the point of view of trainees in nursing, medicine, and the paramedical technologies, it presents the prospects of exciting career opportunities in both service and science. Critical care medicine has indeed come of age and, like a maturing adolescent, is in the process of defining and enlarging its roles in care of the seriously ill. It is clear that during the next 10 years there will be a continuation and refinement in the developmental process and that the chief beneficiaries will be those people unfortunate enough to be struck down by acute, life-threatening processes.

CARDIO-VASCULAR

CHAPTER

2 Acute Chest Pain

L.J. Melendez, M.D.

A patient presenting with acute chest pain may be affected by a life-threatening condition, such as myocardial infarction, dissection of the aorta, or pulmonary embolus. His or her survival may depend on a rapid and accurate assessment and management. The physician's intervention calls for a triple evaluation comprising, in order of priority: (1) functional assessment, the primary goal being to ensure the patient's immediate survival; (2) etiologic assessment, to determine the cause of the pain; and (3) therapeutic assessment, specific interventions required to change the natural course of the disease. Both diagnosis and management are facilitated by an understanding of the underlying pathophysiology of the commonest chest pain syndromes.

FUNCTIONAL ASSESSMENT

Regardless of the etiology of chest pain, the patient's immediate survival requires ensuring the adequacy of circulatory and respiratory functions and the institution of some precautionary measures (Table 2.1). The adequacy of circulation is assessed by determining the blood pressure, the heart rate, and observing the indicators of tissue perfusion (skin color and temperature, mental status, urinary output). Hypotension and severe cardiac arrhythmias may require immediate action (see Chapters 3 and 5). The adequacy of respiratory function may be grossly assessed by the rate and depth of respirations, lung auscultation, and inspection of the skin and mucous membranes for presence of cyanosis. A more reliable guide is provided by determination of blood gases. If acute respiratory insufficiency is evident, immediate measures must be instituted (see Chapter 7).

Some precautionary measures are advisable in all patients with sudden onset of acute chest pain. An intravenous infusion of 5% dextrose in water (D5W) should be established to provide an immediately available route for drugs or fluids that may be needed urgently. Oxygen should be administered (care to be taken in patients with chronic lung disease), and if available ECG monitoring should be instituted.

ETIOLOGIC ASSESSMENT

The differential diagnosis of acute chest pain includes myocardial ischemia (either acute coronary insufficiency or acute myocardial infarction), aortic dissection, pleuropericardial disease, and pulmonary embolus (Fig. 2.1). If these can be ruled out, disorders originating in the thoracic cage (musculoskeletal disease) or in extrathoracic structures may be considered.

Myocardial Ischemia

Cardiac work leads to a high oxygen extraction from the coronary circulation, even at rest. The increased myocardial metabolic demands imposed by exercise, hypertension, etc. must be met either through coronary vasodilation or through increased coronary perfusion pressure. In

Table 2.1
Functional Assessment of Acute Chest Pain

Object	Parameters	Possible findings	Further details
Adequacy of circulatory function	Blood pressure Heart rate Tissue perfusion	Marked tachycardia Marked bradycardia Hypotension, nausea, perspiration	Rate and rhythm disorders Shock and hypotension
Adequacy of respiratory function	Rate and depth of respiration Oxygenation	Cyanosis Abnormal respiratory dynamics and blood gases	Respiratory insufficiency
Precautionary measures	1. Establish IV route 2. Administer O_2 (caution: danger of hypercapnia in hypoventilators) 3. Set up ECG monitor		

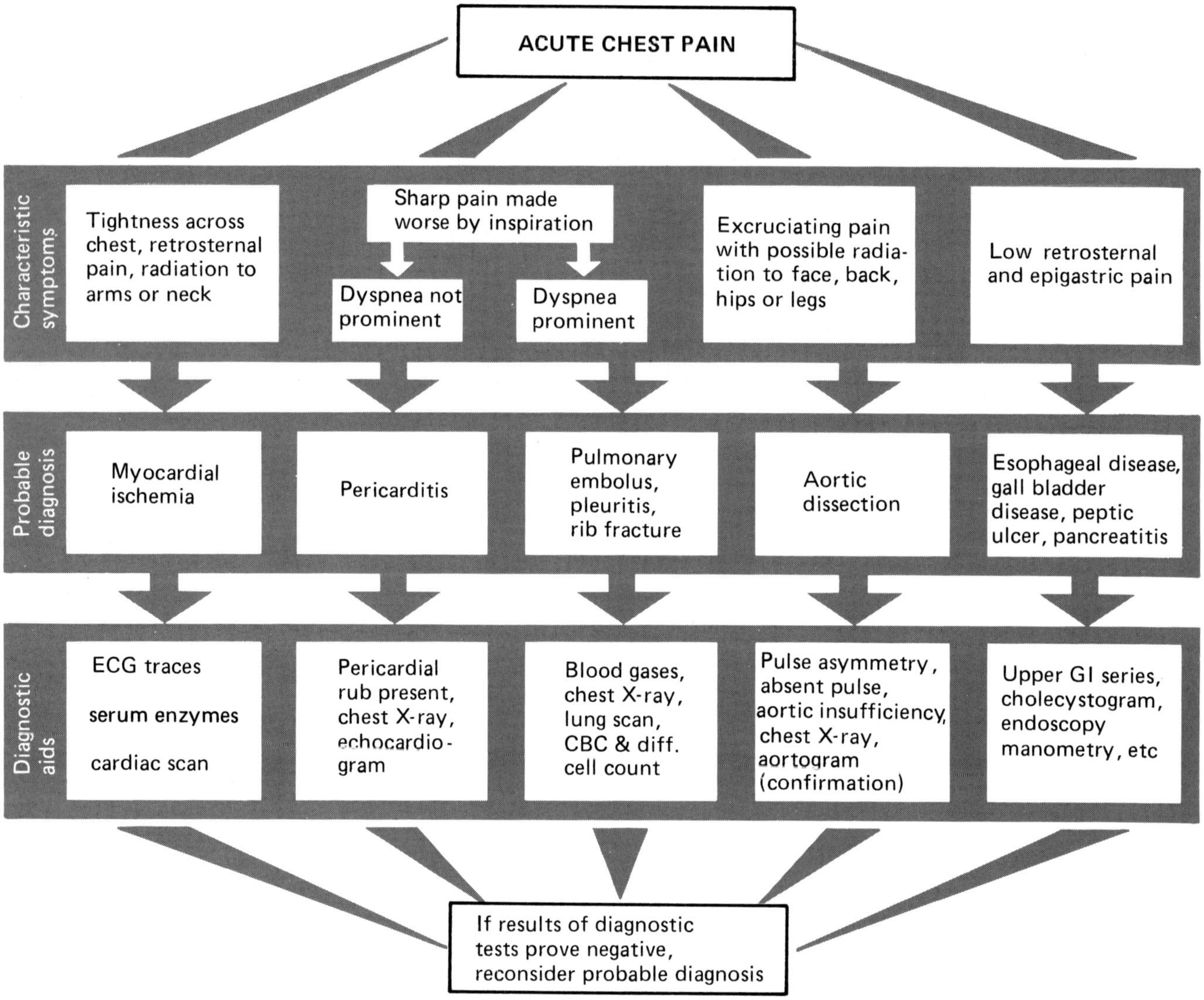

Figure 2.1. Diagnosis and management of acute chest pain.

the normal heart, a highly sensitive regulatory mechanism matches the coronary blood flow to the metabolic demands of the myocardium, mainly through coronary vasodilation. The extent to which coronary flow may be increased above that level at rest constitutes the coronary flow reserve. Reduction of coronary artery cross-sectional lumen by atherosclerosis, arterial spasm, or both, impinges upon the coronary flow reserve, and oxygen delivery to the myocardium becomes limited. As a result, the coronary circulation is unable to meet myocardial oxygen demands when they are increased by physical exercise, emotional distress, cardiac arrhythmias, or hypertensive crisis.

Coronary blood flow takes place mostly during diastole. Because diastole is shortened to a greater extent than systole as the heart rate increases, coronary vasodilation must occur in order for coronary flow to be maintained and/or increased. The compensatory vasodilation is limited or nonexistent in patients with atherosclerotic coronary artery disease. Equally important is the adequacy of diastolic blood pressure, particularly when coronary artery disease is present, because it results in greater impedance to coronary flow. A reduction in coronary blood flow leads to ischemic dysfunction of the left ventricle resulting in increased left ventricular end-diastolic pressure and systemic arterial hypotension, both of which lead to further coronary blood flow reduction.

Pain in the course of myocardial ischemia is probably related to the production of metabolites, such as lactic acid, by the ischemic myocardium when work is performed under relative oxygen deprivation. The characteristic location of the pain—retrosternal or across the chest with radiation to the arms and/or jaw—has been attributed to the anatomic relation of the sympathetic pathways conducting the afferent pain impulses, with neighboring somatic fibers originating in the regions where the pain is experienced or radiated.

The symptoms of myocardial ischemia may be referred to by the patient as either discomfort or pain. In either case, there is usually a connotation of tightness, constric-

Table 2.2
Electrocardiographic Signs of Myocardial Infarction

Characteristic changes	Site of infarction	Age of infarction
Abnormal Q waves Wider than 0.04 sec best criterion, exclude aVR and III. Deeper than one-third of accompanying R waves (except aVR and III) Any Q wave in V_1, V_2, or V_3, (LBBB and WPW excluded) Current of injury: convex ST segment elevation (early change, less specific than Q waves—seen also in pericarditis, variant angina, and ventricular aneurysm)	Shown by the leads reflecting characteristic changes V_1–V_2: septal V_3–V_4: anterior V_5–V_6: lateral V_7–V_8: true posterior I-aVL: high lateral II-aVF: inferior	Shown by repolarization changes (NB considerable individual variation) Acute: ST elevation Evolving: ST elevation and inverted T wave Recent: inverted T wave Old: flat or upright T wave

tion, or heaviness. In the vast majority of cases, the pain or discomfort is not located over the precordial area, but rather is found retrosternally or across the chest, often with characteristic radiation to the arms (more commonly the left) or the jaw. It is important to remember that, on occasions, there may be no pain or discomfort in the chest, but only in either or both arms, or in the neck/jaw region, or as an epigastric indigestion-like distress. A through-to-the-back radiation of ischemic pain is uncommon and should raise suspicion of a nonischemic mechanism, such as aortic dissection.

Angina pectoris is a term applied to transient episodes of ischemic pain that are generally related to circumstances that increase myocardial oxygen consumption, such as physical effort, anxiety, drugs, or paroxysmal tachyarrhythmias. Hypertension, hypotension, and hypoxia may also be identified as precipitating factors. The terms *acute coronary insufficiency* and *acute myocardial infarction* are applied to prolonged ischemic pain syndromes. In acute coronary insufficiency no evidence of permanent tissue damage is demonstrated, but acute myocardial infarction implies myocardial necrosis. Both may occur when the patient is at rest, even without an obvious precipitating factor.

The diagnosis of acute myocardial infarction may be confirmed by electrocardiographic changes (Table 2.2) and serial serum enzyme determinations. The characteristic electrocardiographic change in myocardial infarction is the appearance of abnormal Q waves (Fig. 2.2). However, Q waves may take several hours to appear, and in the very early stages only ST segment elevation (current of injury) may be noted. The age of the infarction is shown by the accompanying repolarization changes, as illustrated in Figure 2.2. Location is indicated by the lead showing the abnormality. It must be remembered that nontransmural (subendocardial or “non-Q”) infarction occurs without development of Q waves. A pre-existing left bundle branch block may obscure the classic ECG findings of infarction, or it may be the result of an acute infarction itself.

In cases where the electrocardiogram provides no help, the diagnosis must be based on the clinical picture and the serum enzyme determination. The most commonly used serum enzymes in the diagnosis of acute myocardial infarction are creatine phosphokinase (CPK), serum glutamic oxaloacetic transaminase (SGOT), and lactic dehydrogenase (LDH). If isoenzyme determination is feasible, better specificity is yielded by CPK fraction MB and by LDH fraction 1. The time sequence of serum enzyme rise in acute myocardial infarction is shown in Figure

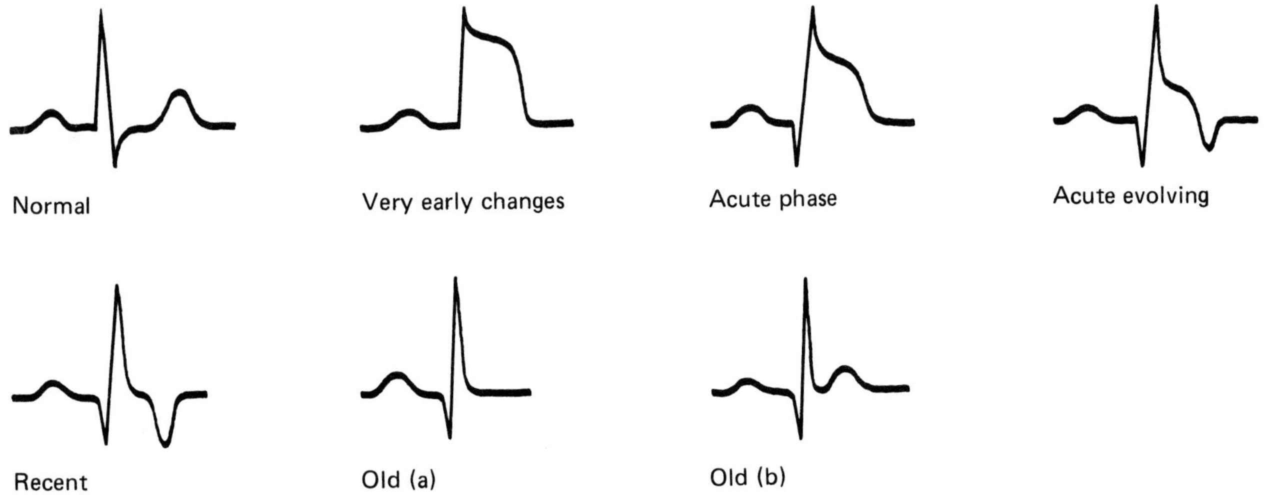

Figure 2.2. Typical ECG changes after myocardial infarction.

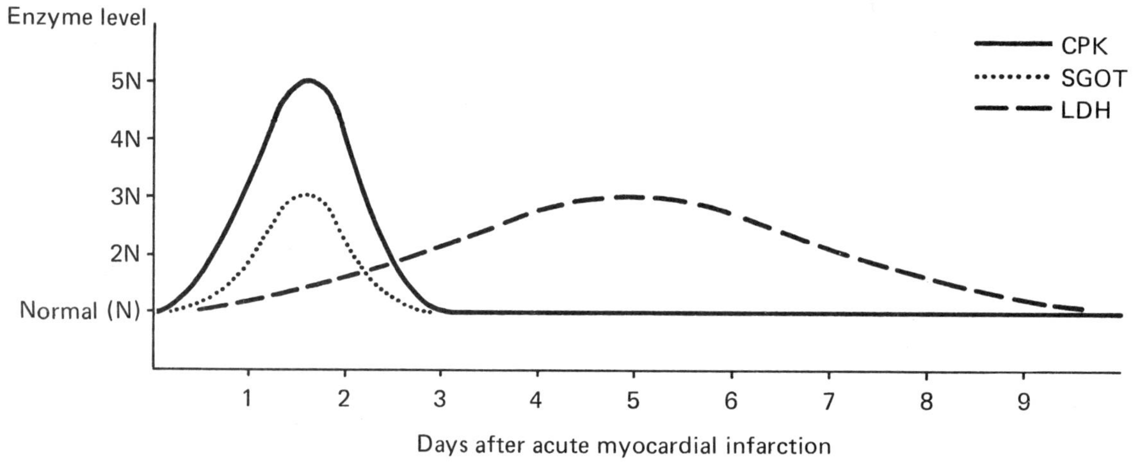

Figure 2.3. Enzyme changes after acute myocardial infarction.

2.3. It is evident that peak serum enzyme elevation may be missed by very early or very late blood sampling. Liver "congestion" and muscle disease or trauma (as in intramuscular injections) may make interpretation of enzyme results difficult, particularly if isoenzymes are not available. Small myocardial infarctions may cause only a mild and short-lived serum enzyme rise, which may be easily missed.

Radionuclide methods, particularly the ^{99m}TC-stannous pyrophosphate myocardial scan, may provide valuable information in cases where the electrocardiographic or enzyme changes are in doubt.

THERAPEUTIC ASSESSMENT

Relief of Pain

Chest pain associated with myocardial infarction, acute coronary insufficiency, aortic dissection, pulmonary embolus, and acute pericarditis usually requires the administration of an opiate for satisfactory relief. Morphine can be given subcutaneously or intravenously; intramuscular injections of any kind are to be avoided because they may alter serum enzymes and cause problems in interpretation of abnormal SGOT or CPK levels. Morphine has potent vagomimetic effects and may induce nausea, vomiting, bradycardia, or hypotension; we recommended that the first dose of morphine be given in combination with atropine, 0.6 mg subcutaneously (SC) or 0.4 mg IV.

The intravenous route for both morphine and atropine is preferred. The dose of morphine is 3–5 mg and may be repeated after 15 or 20 minutes. Special attention must be paid to heart rate, blood pressure, and respiratory function following morphine administration. Nausea and bradycardia occurring after morphine administration may be treated with atropine. Postmorphine hypotension may also respond to atropine, and it is helpful to have the patient in the horizontal or slight Trendelenburg position. If these measures are not effective, hypovolemia or pump failure may be present and require prompt specific action (see Chapter 5).

Recurrent pain in acute myocardial infarction may be treated with repeated injections of morphine. After the first 24–48 hours, recurrent pain may be due to reinfarction or pericardial reaction; the latter may respond to indomethacin 25 mg every 6 hours (q6h), aspirin 600 mg q6h, or ibuprofen 200–300 mg q6h.

Myocardial Infarction

Patients with acute myocardial infarction should be kept in the coronary care or intensive care unit until their stability is clearly shown. Arrhythmias are more likely to be a problem in the first 24 hours. There are at present two schools of thought regarding the prophylaxis of cardiac arrhythmias in the acute myocardial infarction patient. The traditional view recommends the use of a 75- to 100-mg bolus of lidocaine when rhythm disturbances are noted. This is followed by an intravenous drip of 3–4 mg/minute of lidocaine; a second bolus of 50–75 mg may be administered 5–10 minutes after the initial one to avoid the hiatus in therapeutic plasma concentration caused by the slow ascent of plasma concentrations from the intravenous drip once the initial bolus effect has faded away (Fig. 2.4). This dose of lidocaine requires downward adjustment in patients with acute or chronic liver dysfunction.

Other routine measures for acute myocardial infarction include a light diet (preferably fluids only during the first 48 hours) with no salt added and a gradual mobilization program that may be started after the first 48 hours in uncomplicated cases. Table 2.3 shows the mobilization program presently used at Victoria Hospital. Some patients may benefit from mild sedation for which diazepam 5 mg q8h may be appropriate.

Some investigators have shown that potentially fatal arrhythmias, specifically primary ventricular fibrillation, may not be preceded by "warning" rhythm changes, such as ventricular premature contractions (VPCs), and that VPCs do not necessarily herald more serious arrhythmias. They advocate the routine prophylactic administration of lidocaine during the first 24–48 hours after an acute myocardial infarction. In either case, caution must be exercised to avoid inducing lidocaine toxicity, which is manifested by mental confusion, muscle twitching, or convulsions.

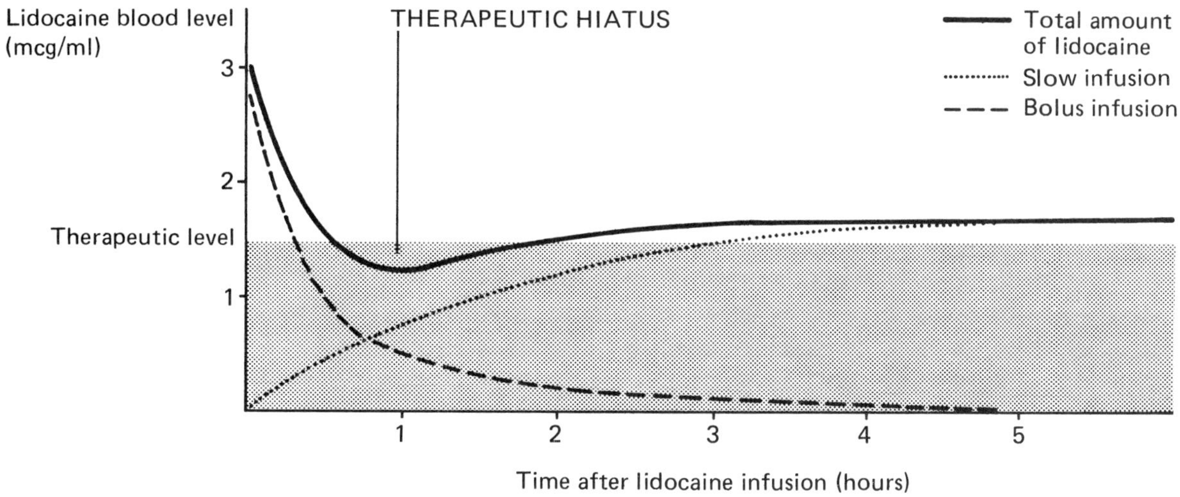

Figure 2.4. Therapeutic hiatus following bolus and slow infusion of lidocaine.

Aortic Dissection

Aortic dissection begins as a tear within the aortic intima in the setting of hypertension and atherosclerosis, or degenerative disease of the aortic wall (cystic medial necrosis). A high blood pressure forces the diversion of blood into the false lumen and extends the dissecting process. The false lumen may break distally into the true lumen (forming a double-barrel vessel) or into the aortic adventitia and periaortic tissues (Fig. 2.5*A*).

Involvement of the aortic root may disrupt the aortic valve, causing acute aortic insufficiency and left ventricular failure. Myocardial ischemia or infarction may be caused by coronary artery involvement. As the dissection progresses along the aorta, the innominate, carotid, and subclavian arteries may be occluded (Fig. 2.5*B*), leading to a constellation of manifestations, including stroke, disappearance of peripheral arterial pulses, bowel ischemia, and renal failure (Fig. 2.5*C*).

The excruciating features of pain caused by dissection of the aorta are related to the tearing of the aortic wall, and its location bears some relation to the level of the dissection. It may be experienced in the higher retrosternal area, sometimes with radiation to the face or through to the back, and not uncommonly to the hips and legs when the dissection involves the distal aorta and its branches. The features of ischemic pain may be associated if there is involvement of coronary circulation. Extension of the dissection into the neck vessels may produce neurologic manifestations (hemiplegia, aphasia, coma).

Aortic root dissection involving the aortic valve apparatus may cause acute valvular insufficiency; its presence is indicated by an immediate diastolic decrescendo murmur heard over the left sternal edge with manifestations of left ventricular failure. As the dissection progresses along the peripheral vessels (neck, arms, legs) the accumulation of blood or clot in the false lumen impinges upon the flow through the true lumen, and arterial pulsations become weakened or disappear altogether. Back or hip pain may become prominent. Abdominal pain, bloody diarrhea, and oliguria indicate involvement of splanchnic and renal circulation.

The diagnosis of dissection of the aorta may be strongly suggested by the characteristic features of the pain and the findings of pulse asymmetry or absence, aortic insufficiency, or a wide mediastinal shadow on the chest x-ray. Confirmation of the diagnosis is achieved only by performing an aortogram. If aortic dissection is strongly suspected, an aortogram must be performed.

Early consultation with a cardiovascular surgeon is advisable. Cases showing mechanical complications, such

Table 2.3
Mobilization Plan for Myocardial Infarction

The purpose of this exercise program is to increase gradually the amount of activity the patient is able to perform in accordance with the rate at which the heart is healing. The doctor should determine how fast the patient can progress from one stage to another.

Phase I	Complete bed rest for 24 hours—use of commode at bedside.
Phrase II	Complete bed rest, but patient may sit at the side of bed with back and legs supported—use bedside commode.
Phase III	Patient remains in bed, still being bathed by nurse—but may sit in a chair three times a day for 10 minutes, with nurse's supervision.
Phrase IV	Patient in bed, sitting in chair three times a day for 20 minutes—may wash hands, face and shave (in bed only) and use bedside commode.
Phase V	Patient bathes him- or herself in bed only—but may have bathroom privileges and start to walk in room. Rest for 1½ hours after each meal.
Phase VI	All self-care in bathroom, walk in room, rest after meals.
Phase VII	All self-care, walk in hall once the length only three times a day.
Phase VIII	Self-care, increase walk in hall three times a day for 5 minutes.
Phase IX	Increase hall walks to 10–20 minutes three times a day, all self-care.
Phase X	Patient may now shower. Walking is now unlimited. If pain or rapid heart rate occurs, patient should notify nurse immediately. Heart rate should not exceed 110 after any exercise. No stair climbing unless ordered by doctor and accompanied by nurse.

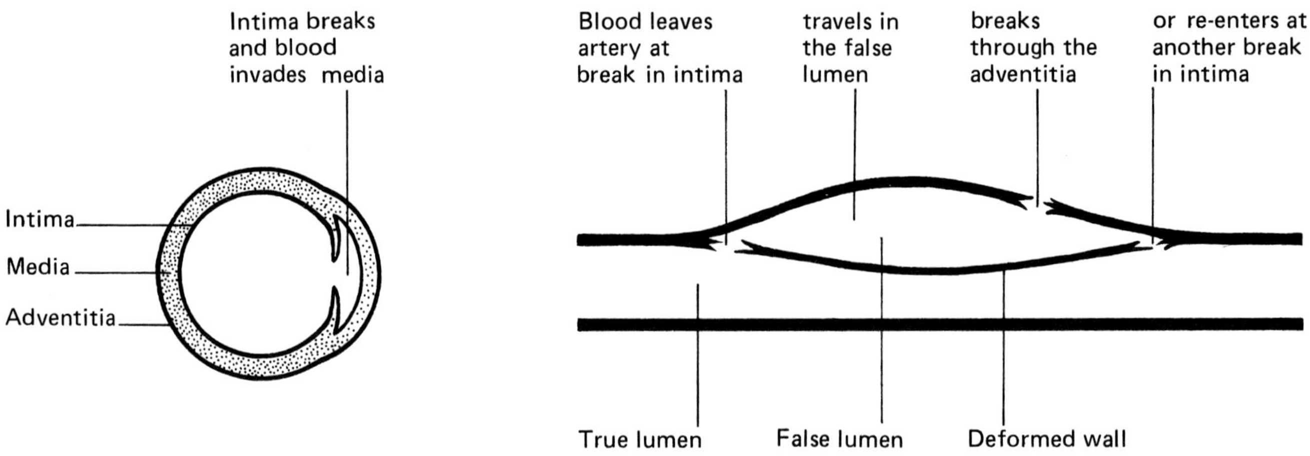

Figure 2.5*A*. Aortic dissection: formulation of the double lumen.

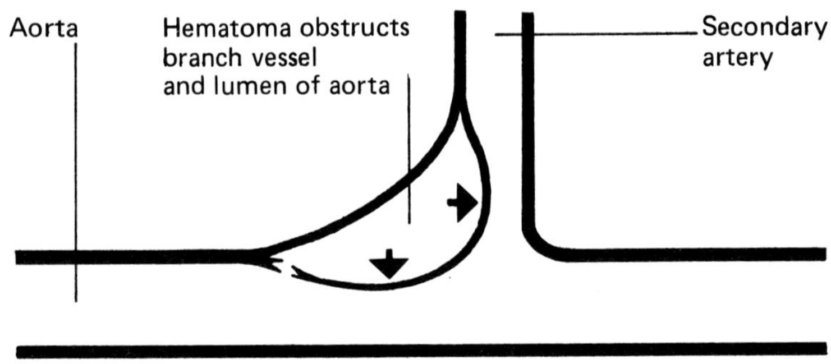

Figure 2.5*B*. Aortic dissection: occlusion of secondary artery.

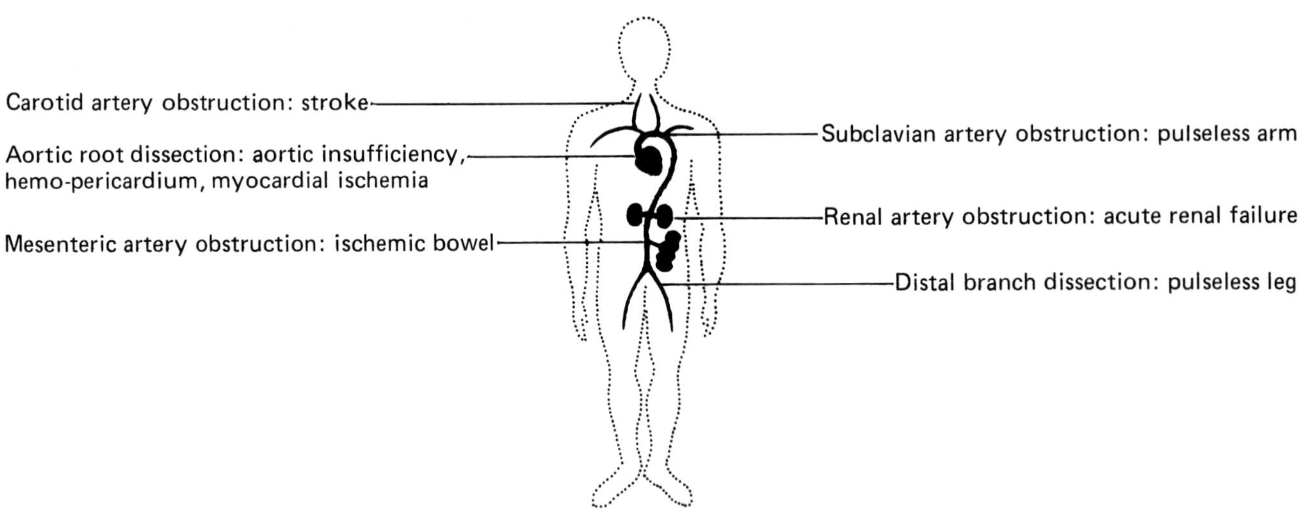

Figure 2.5*C*. Consequences of occlusion of secondary arteries.

as aortic insufficiency or vascular obstruction, may need urgent surgical intervention. Cases managed medically require antihypertensive medication if high blood pressure is present. Prompt response is desirable and is usually obtained by use of an agent that may be given intravenously, such as propranolol or sodium nitroprusside. Some authors emphasize the use of propranolol to reduce the rate of ejection, which is suspected of playing a role in aggravating dissection. Some hypotensive agents, such as nitroprusside and hydralazine, may increase the rate of ejection and should be used only in combination with propranolol.

Pleuropericardial Disease

Inflammatory processes of the pleura and pericardium give rise to pain described as sharp or knife-like, well localized, and typically aggravated by inspiration and changes in body position (pleuritic-type). If clearly described by the patient, these features are highly specific for pleural or pericardial origin and are often confirmed by the detection of a pericardial or pleural rub on auscultation.

The diagnosis of pericarditis is based on the typical features of the pain plus the presence of a pericardial friction rub. Pericardial effusion causes an increased cardiac size on the chest x-ray and a typical echocardiographic pattern. In such cases, careful attention must be paid to signs of cardiac tamponade: increased central venous pressure, hypotension, pulsus paradoxus, and oliguria.

Pain arising from the pleura may be due to a primary disorder of this structure (pleurodynia, pleural metastases, lupus pleuritis) or to extension of processes affecting neighboring structures, such as the lung (pulmonary embolus, pneumonia) or the thoracic cage (rib fraction). Pulmonary embolism, infection, and metabolic causes (uremia) may be involved, as well as immunologic mechanisms, as in systemic lupus erythematosus and certain drug reactions (hydralazine, procainamide). These and other causes of chest pain are shown on Figure 2.1.

Disease processes affecting the gallbladder, duodenum, stomach, and gastroesophageal sphincter may become extrathoracic causes of chest pain and mimic pain caused by myocardial ischemia. Hepatic pain due to distension of a "congested" or inflamed liver may be experienced in the epigastric and low retrosternal areas, causing confusion with ischemic cardiac pain. The same may be true of pain due to peptic ulcer, gastroesophageal reflux, and hiatus hernia where gastric acid irritation and smooth muscle spasm are involved.

The pain of acute pericarditis may be severe enough to require opiates, particularly in the early stages. It may also respond well to indomethacin (25 mg q6h or q8h) alone or in combination with codeine (15–30 mg q6h or q8h).

Pericardial effusion causing tamponade is manifested by central venous hypertension, a low blood pressure with a small amplitude of the arterial pulse, and "pulsus paradoxicus." The patient is usually dyspneic and restless. Oliguria is an ominous sign. Echocardiography is a highly reliable aid to document the presence of intrapericardial fluid, which should then be removed by pericardiocentesis or surgical drainage.

Musculoskeletal Disease

Trauma, particularly if it causes rib fracture, is the commonest musculoskeletal mechanism of chest pain. Less commonly encountered are inflammation of the costochondral joint, which produces pain on the anterior chest wall that is usually aggravated by local pressure, and disease of the cervical spine, producing nerve compression and pain with the characteristic radicular distribution.

Pulmonary Embolus

In pulmonary embolus, pain relief with opiates may be necessary, but close attention must be paid to physical and laboratory signs of respiratory function. If shock is imminent or present, embolectomy may be considered. This procedure, however, requires facilities and expertise that may not be available in all hospitals (see Chapter 12).

Suggested Readings

Hurst JW (ed): *The Heart,* ed 6. Philadelphia, McGraw Hill, 1986.
Braunwald E: *Heart Disease,* ed 2. Philadelphia, WB Saunders, 1987.

CHAPTER

3 Cardiac Arrhythmias

L.J. Melendez, M.D.

Each cardiac contraction is triggered by the spread of an electrical stimulus (the activation wave) throughout the myocardium. The stimulus originates in the sinus node, spreads throughout the atria, and enters the ventricle by means of the atrioventricular conduction system. The biophysical nature of this stimulus is the movement of electrically charged particles (ions) across the cell membrane.

Under resting conditions, each myocardial cell exhibits a transmembrane potential difference, with the inside of the cell being negatively charged in relation to the outside. The potential difference between the two sides of the membrane, which is approximately 90 mV, is thought to be due to ionic gradients and has specifically been attributed to the difference in potassium concentration between the intracellular and extracellular milieu. Pacemaker cells have the property of spontaneously losing this resting potential and initiating a depolarization wave that spreads over all neighboring and excitable myocardial cells. As this activation wave reaches the contractile cells, calcium ions are released from the sarcoplasmic reticulum to activate the contractile proteins and determine myocardial contraction.

The normal pacemaker site is the sinus node, which has a resting intrinsic rate of around 60–75/minute. The activation wave spreads throughout the atria causing atrial contraction, which is recorded on the ECG as the P wave (see Fig. 3.2*A*, overleaf). There is no histologic continuity between the atrial and ventricular myocardium. Because the fibrous skeleton of the heart cannot conduct the activation wave, the wave can only reach the ventricles through the conducting system, which consists of the atrioventricular node, the bundle of His, and its branches (Fig. 3.1).

The intraventricular conduction system (bundle branches and Purkinje system) distributes the activation wave very rapidly and simultaneously to both ventricles. This usually takes about 0.08–0.11 seconds and may be recorded as a narrow QRS complex. Should there be a bundle branch block, the activation wave reaches the affected ventricle through the slow-conducting contractile myocardium; the longer ventricular activation time (usually 0.12 seconds or more) is reflected electrocardiographically by an increased width of the QRS complex (see Fig. 3.2*B*). Ectopic activity originating in the ventricles also spreads through the contractile myocardium, inscribing a wide QRS complex.

PATHOPHYSIOLOGY

Ventricular arrhythmias are characterized by wide QRS complexes, whereas supraventricular arrhythmias typically have narrow QRS complexes. There are two exceptions to this rule: (1) a pre-existing bundle branch block and (2) the development of rate-related bundle branch block during a rapid supraventricular arrhythmia. The latter is due to the longer refractory period of one of the bundle branches (usually the right): supraventricular

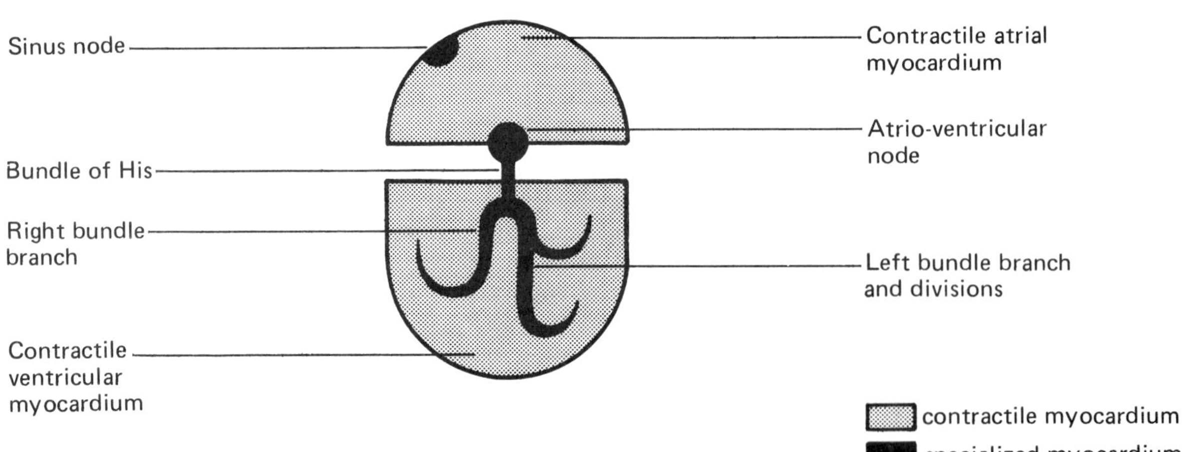

Figure 3.1. Conduction system of the heart.

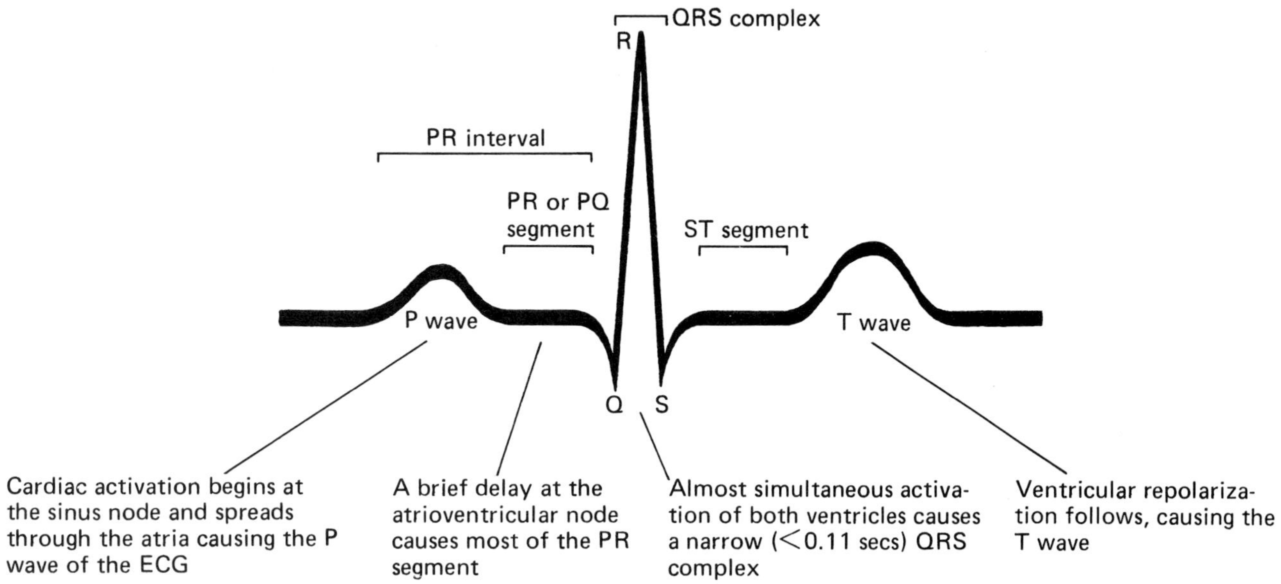

Figure 3.2*A*. Sequence of cardiac activation.

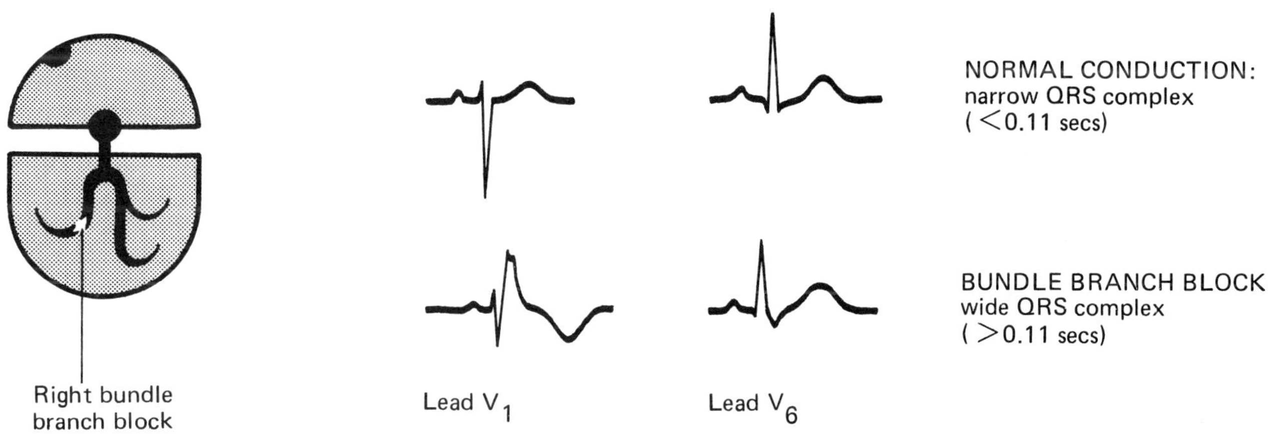

Figure 3.2*B*. Intraventricular conduction disturbance.

impulses can only conduct along the other branch, and they later spread to the affected ventricle through the contractile myocardium.

Some cardiac arrhythmias are caused by a disturbance in impulse conduction through diseased areas of the myocardium; this disturbance leads to slow activation of some cells from which the impulse re-enters previously activated myocardium that has already recovered (re-entry mechanism). In other cases, arrhythmias may be due to the ectopic production of impulses from areas that are not normally pacemaker sites (enhanced automaticity). It is likely that some arrhythmias are initiated by enhanced automaticity and sustained by re-entry, but in the clinical setting it is often impossible to ascertain the exact mechanisms involved.

Erratic atrial activity (Fig. 3.3*A*) with multiple sites of activation wave re-entry causes atrial fibrillation. Impulses reach the AV node in an equally erratic fashion and are transmitted to the ventricles, which respond with an irregularly irregular rhythm. AV nodal block induced by drugs or carotid sinus massage will not affect the atrial fibrillation itself, but will slow the rate of ventricular response.

A circular re-entrant pathway away from the AV node (Fig. 3.3*B*) causes atrial flutter; the re-entry circuit is generally completed at a rate of 300 ± 20/min. Ventricular rate depends on the ability of the AV node to conduct the impulses to the ventricles. With 1 to 1 (1:1) conduction, the ventricular rate is around 300/min; with 2:1 or 3:1 conduction, the ventricular rate is around 150 or 100/min, respectively. AV nodal block induced by drugs or carotid sinus massage will not affect the atrial flutter itself, but will decrease the rate of ventricular response, which makes the flutter waves apparent on the ECG tracing.

Most paroxysmal supraventricular tachycardias have the AV node as part of the re-entry circuit pathway (Fig. 3.3*C*). If AV nodal block is induced by drugs or carotid sinus massage, as AV block occurs, the pathway is interrupted and the arrhythmia stops.

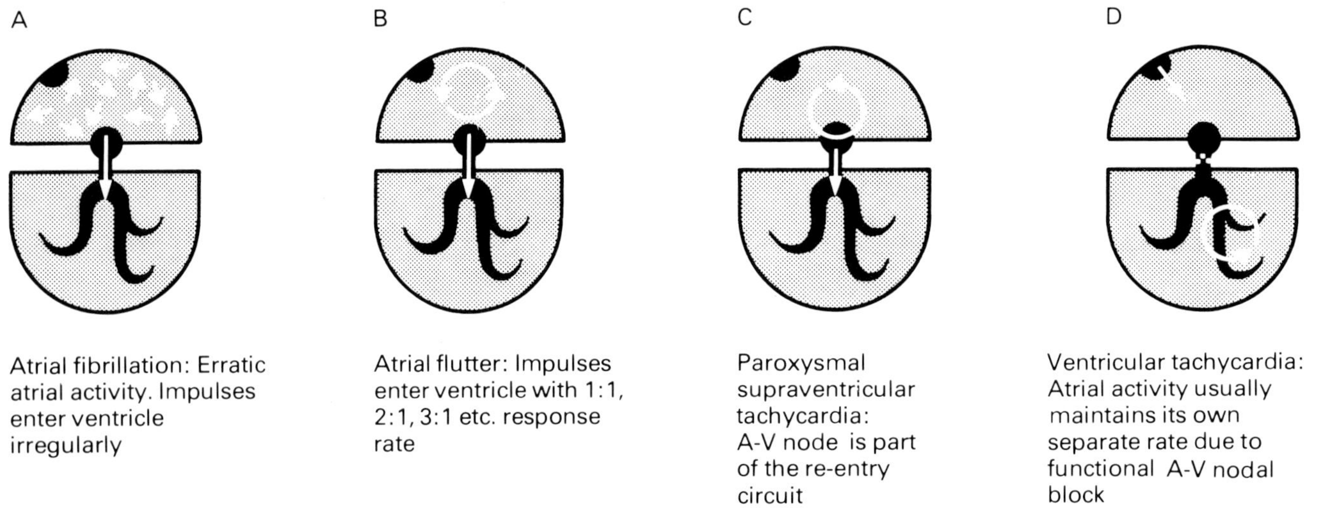

Figure 3.3. Re-entry mechanisms in paroxysmal dysrhythmias.

In ventricular tachycardia the re-entry path is limited to the ventricles (Fig. 3.3*D*). Atrial activity is not affected in the majority of cases, so maneuvers that produce AV nodal block will not affect ventricular rate and will not interrupt the arrhythmia.

Re-entry is usually caused by structural or functional derangement of a portion of the myocardium, which leads to slow conduction or unidirectional block in the affected area. However, in the Wolff-Parkinson-White syndrome, there is an anomalous myocardial bridge connecting the atria and the ventricles and providing a separate pathway for the impulse to enter the ventricles. The resulting ventricular activation is, therefore, a fusion of two front waves and is shown on the electrocardiogram as a QRS complex with a characteristically slurred onset, the latter referred to as delta wave (Fig. 3.4*A*). A critically timed and located ectopic atrial or ventricular extrasystole may, under this circumstance, initiate an atrioventricular reentry, with the impulse conducting back into the atria, either through the anomalous pathway or through the AV junction, and causing a paroxysmal reciprocating AV tachycardia (Fig. 3.4*B* and *C*).

Changes in the concentration of serum ions and the effect of ischemia, hypoxia, and acid-base balance on the cell membrane and the transmembrane potential difference may facilitate or precipitate cardiac arrhythmias (Table 3.1). Drugs and autonomically mediated reflexes may have a profound effect on cardiac rate and rhythm. The same may be said of psychodynamic influences. Cardiac arrhythmias may cause a wide spectrum of derangement of cardiocirculatory function. Arrhythmias that do not significantly change the overall cardiac rate per minute may have little or no hemodynamic effects; extreme changes in rate (either marked bradycardia or marked

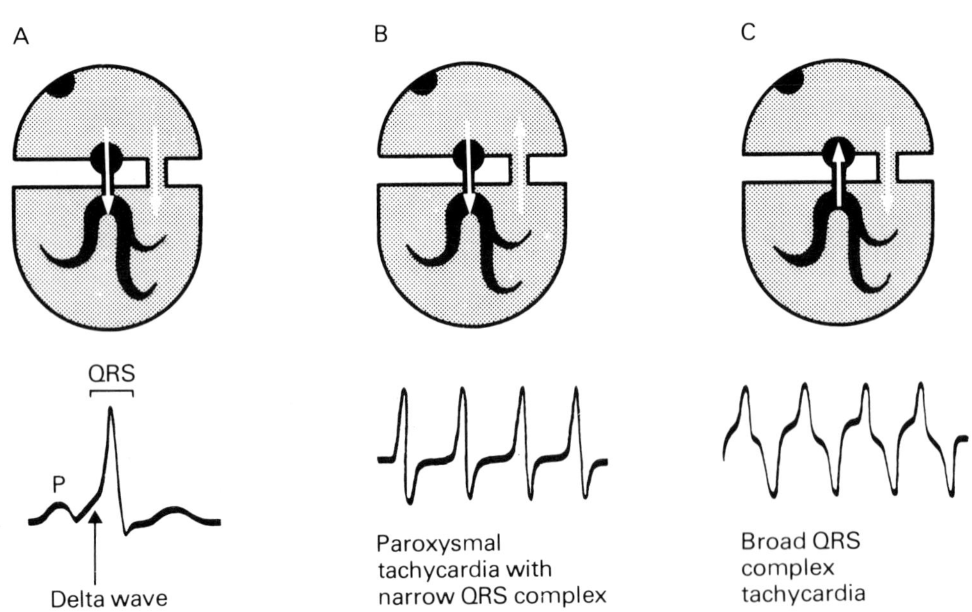

Figure 3.4. Atrioventricular reciprocating tachycardias.

Table 3.1
Factors Affecting the Incidence of Cardiac Arrhythmias

Acute myocardial injury or infarction
Hypoxia
Acidosis
Alkalosis
Electrolyte imbalance
Congestive cardiac failure
Shock
Side effects of drugs: digitalis, theophylline, beta-mimetic agents, antiarrhythmic drugs in toxic doses, tricyclic antidepressants
Autonomic responses: blood pressure changes, blood volume changes, pain, fear, anxiety, mechanical stimulation or irritation

tachycardia) will decrease cardiac output and tissue perfusion. Severe disorganization of the ventricular activation process (ventricular fibrillation) or lack of activation (ventricular asystole) is fatal if untreated.

The sudden decrease in cardiac output produced by ventricular tachyarrhythmias or bradyarrhythmias may lead to syncope or near syncope syndrome, and possibly to other central nervous system transient ischemic manifestations. In the cardiovascular system itself, tachyarrhythmias may lead to angina (particularly in patients with coronary artery disease), extension of tissue damage (in patients with myocardial infarction), and cardiac failure.

Cardiac arrhythmias may become an emergency either because of the hemodynamic disturbance associated with very rapid or very slow ventricular rate or because of electrical instability that may lead to ventricular fibrillation. In the following discussion, paroxysmal tachyarrhythmia describes the sudden onset of rapid cardiac (ventricular) rate at 140 or more beats/min. Bradyarrhythmia means a ventricular rate of 50 beats/min or less.

PAROXYSMAL TACHYARRHYTHMIAS

Diagnosis

Paroxysmal tachyarrhythmias include atrial fibrillation with rapid ventricular response, atrial flutter with 1:1 or 2:1 ventricular response, paroxysmal supraventricular tachycardia, and paroxysmal ventricular tachycardia.

The patient may be a previously healthy individual who suddenly experiences palpitations (described as awareness of rapid cardiac activity) or a patient known to be afflicted by disease, cardiac or otherwise. Tachyarrhythmias are often observed in the postoperative period of thoracic and cardiovascular surgery and as complications in noncardiac but critically ill patients. There may be associated symptoms, such as dizziness, lightheadedness, chest pain, or dyspnea. Focal neurologic manifestations are rare, but loss of consciousness may occur in older individuals. In critically ill patients, tachyarrhythmias may induce hypotension, oliguria, or heart failure.

The prominent finding on physical examination is a heart rate of 140 or more per minute. If this is found in a healthy individual, the likelihood of a paroxysmal arrhythmia is very high. But in previously ill patients, sinus

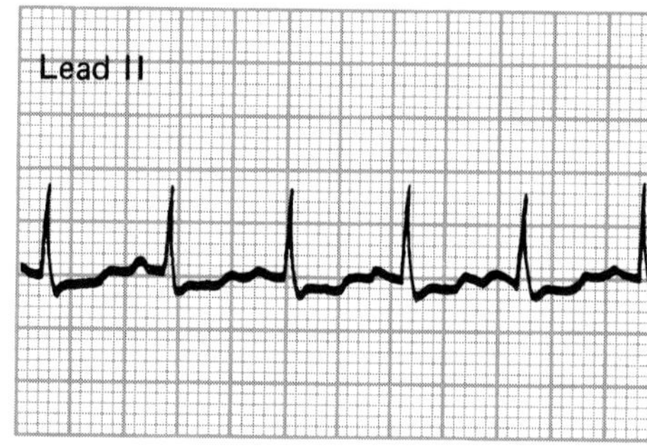

Figure 3.5. Sinus tachycardia.

tachycardia (Fig. 3.5) due to complications (sepsis, pulmonary embolism, fluid-electrolyte imbalance, drug effect) or aggravation of the underlying condition should be considered. Sinus tachycardia should not be interfered with directly because it almost always represents a compensatory mechanism. Such patients may show hypotension and other signs of deterioration if attempts at slowing the heart rate are undertaken without correcting the precipitating cause.

The electrocardiogram shows either narrow (less than 0.10 seconds or 2 mm at standard paper speed) or broad (0.11 or more seconds) QRS complexes. Narrow QRS complex tachycardias are supraventricular in origin, and the differential diagnosis includes sinus tachycardia, atrial fibrillation with rapid ventricular response, atrial flutter with 1:1 or 2:1 response, and paroxysmal supraventricular tachycardia. Broad QRS complex tachycardias are either ventricular tachycardia or supraventricular tachycardia with aberrant ventricular conduction due to rate-related or pre-existing bundle branch block. Reciprocating atrioventricular tachycardia, as seen in the Wolff-Parkinson-White syndrome, is manifested by narrow QRS complexes when the descent of activation from atria to ventricles takes place through the conducting system (antegrade AV junctional conductions) and by wide QRS complexes when the ventricles are activated via the anomalous pathways (with retrograde AV junctional conduction) or when rate-related bundle branch block develops in antegrade AV junctional conduction.

Figures 3.6 and 3.7 summarize the diagnosis of the commonest tachycardia syndromes.

Simultaneous carotid sinus massage and ECG recording is a very useful maneuver for the clarification of rapid supraventricular arrhythmias, and in some cases, it may be both diagnostic and therapeutic. The carotid sinus is identified by gentle palpation just below and behind the right angle of the jaw. Steady pressure is then applied for 3–5 seconds while carefully observing the ECG and glancing at the patient's face to recognize signs of undue distress. If no response is produced, the maneuver may be repeated with both pressure and a rubbing motion of the finger on the carotid sinus. If there is still no response, the left side may then be tried. Simultaneous bilateral carotid sinus stimulation must not be attempted.

In response to carotid sinus massage, atrial fibrillation and flutter will slow the ventricular response so that the irregularity of the rhythm and the characteristic inden-

Narrow (<0.11 sec) QRS complex

	Irregular R-R interval		Regular R-R intervals			
Atrial Activity	F waves or no waves on baseline	Multiform P waves		Abnormal P waves, or long PR interval, or no clear P waves		PR interval shortened in proportion to rate
Likely Diagnosis	Atrial fibrillation	Multifocal atrial tachycardia	Atrial flutter with 1:1 or 2:1 ventricular response	Paroxysmal supra-ventricular tachycardia	Reciprocating A-V tachy-cardia with antegrade A-V junctional conduction	Sinus tachycardia
Carotid Sinus Massage	Rate slows and irregular rhythm becomes more obvious	Usually none	Ventricular rate decreases and flutter waves become obvious	Tachycardia may stop	Tachycardia may stop. Short PR interval and Delta waves may appear	Rate may transiently decrease
Population Bias	Rare in children	Acute on chronic lung disease	Usually patients with cardiac or thoracic disease, or older patients	Usually younger individuals	Any sex, but slightly commoner in younger patients	Shock, infection, heart failure, severe systemic disease

Figure 3.6. Electrocardiographic diagnosis of paroxysmal tachycardias with narrow QRS complex.

tations of the baseline (fine and irregular in fibrillation, coarse but regular in flutter) become apparent. Paroxysmal supraventricular tachycardia may revert to sinus rhythm, but ventricular tachycardia usually remains unaffected or shows only brief interruptions lasting no more than one or two beats. Sinus tachycardia shows a transient slowing of the heart rate.

Patients with atrial fibrillation present with an irregular pulse, both in rhythm and in volume. Rhythm irregularity may be easier to detect at cardiac auscultation. However, atrial fibrillation with very rapid ventricular response may appear deceptively regular until careful measurement of the RR interval is made on the electrocardiogram (Fig. 3.8). In paroxysmal supraventricular tachycardia, the rhythm is regular with a rate of 140–220/min. Carotid sinus massage may be both diagnostic and therapeutic (Fig. 3.9). With rapid rates, aberrant ventricular conduction may occur.

The rhythm strip shown on Figure 3.10 records the onset and termination of a paroxysmal tachycardia. On the top tracing, the fifth complex is a premature supraventricular beat conducted simultaneously to both ventricles (narrow QRS complex). It initiates a run of paroxysmal supraventricular tachycardia in which the subsequent beats show aberrant ventricular conduction. However, the lower strip shows improvement in conduction: the QRS complexes become narrow and remain so until the end of the paroxysm. Note that the first beat after the paroxysm follows a relatively long diastole and is not preceded by a P wave. It is a junctional escape occurring during transient sinoatrial node suppression.

In the majority of cases of atrial flutter, the atrial rate is close to 300/min. With 2:1 conduction, ventricular response is then very close to 150/min (Fig. 3.11). Atrial flutter should, therefore, be suspected whenever the electrocardiogram shows a regular rhythm at a rate of near 150/min. Carotid sinus massage will not affect the atrial flutter itself, but will increase the atrioventricular block, thereby allowing the longer diastoles to show the characteristic indentations of the baseline (Fig. 3.11). Both paroxysmal supraventricular tachycardia and atrial flutter may show the pattern of broad QRS complex tachy-

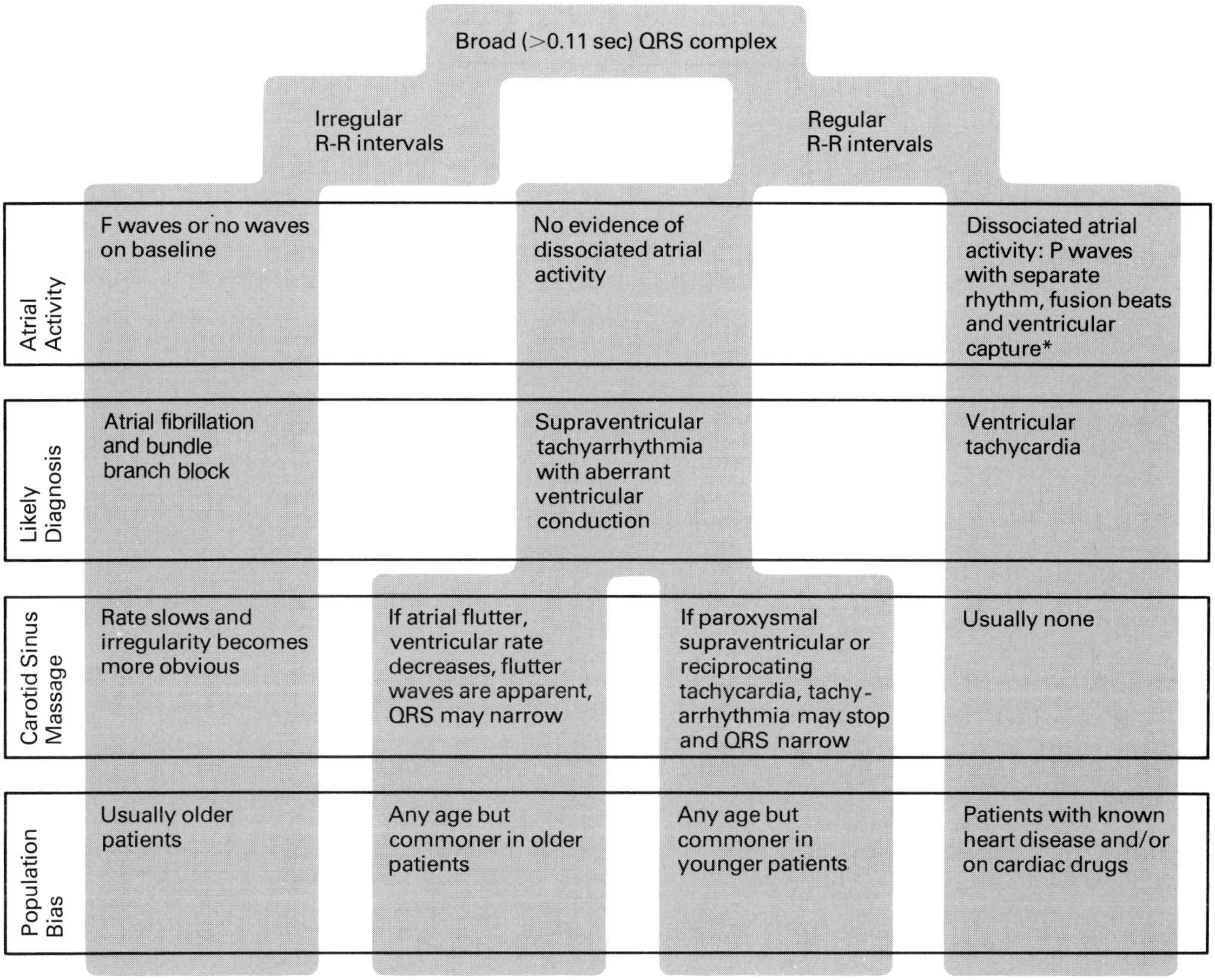

*See text for non-ECG signs of dissociated atrial activity

Figure 3.7. Electrocardiographic diagnosis of paroxysmal tachycardias with broad QRS complex.

cardia on the ECG. Carotid sinus massage may clarify the diagnosis by demonstrating the characteristic flutter waves on the ECG recording. It may also cause transient disappearance of the aberrancy (Fig. 3.12).

A broad QRS complex tachycardia (Figs. 3.12 and 3.13) requires a differential diagnosis between ventricular tachycardia and supraventricular tachycardia with aberrancy. Ventricular tachycardia may be accompanied by subtle signs of dissociated atrial activity, such as intermittent cannon waves on the jugular venous pulse and variation in the systolic blood pressure or in the intensity of the first heart sound. However, in most cases, con-

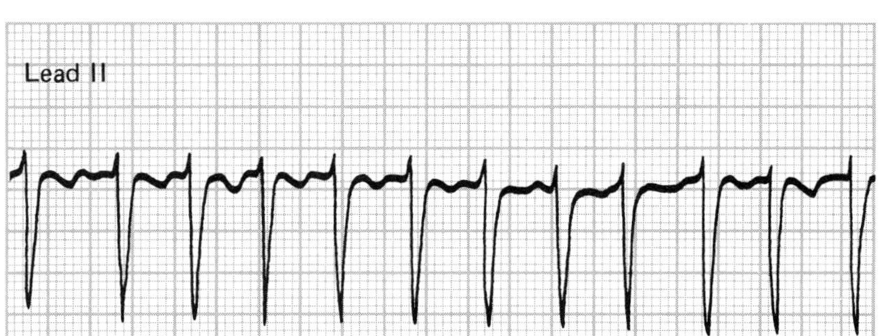

Figure 3.8. Atrial fibrillation with rapid ventricular response. At first sight, rhythm appears to be regular, but closer inspection shows irregularity of RR intervals.

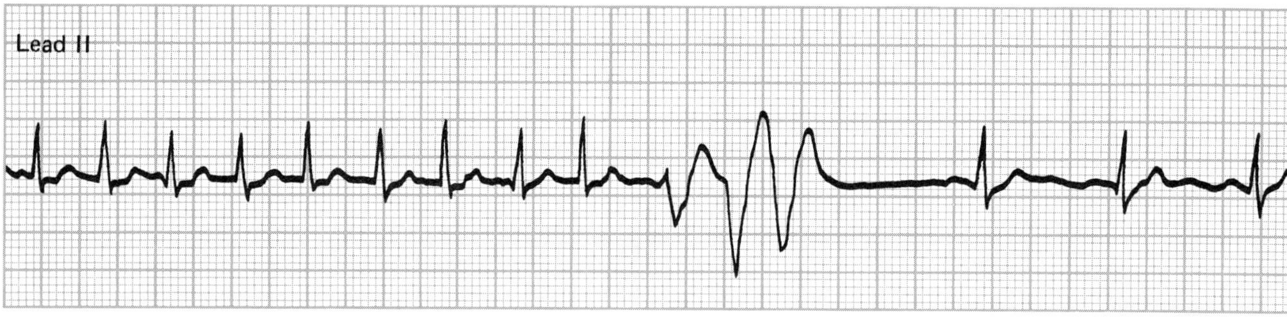

Figure 3.9. Paroxysmal supraventricular tachycardia with narrow QRS complex. Regular rhythm with rate of 175/min. Strip shows conversion to sinus mechanism after 10 mg IV edrophonium. Similar conversion may be achieved with carotid sinus stimulation.

siderable experience is required to rely on these signs for purposes of diagnosis and management. Older patients, particularly with a history of heart disease, are more likely to have ventricular tachycardia, whereas in younger healthy individuals, the chances are that the arrhythmia is supraventricular in origin. The diagnosis may be established by means of carotid sinus massage, which may interrupt paroxysmal supraventricular tachycardia, or by finding definite evidence of dissociated atrial activity. In addition to the clinical signs referred to earlier, dissociated atrial activity may be shown by a dissociated atrial rhythm (P waves) or by the appearance of fusion beats on the electrocardiogram. Fusion beats are atrial impulses that are occasionally conducted to the ventricles (ventricular capture).

Management

Atrial fibrillation with rapid ventricular rate generally responds well to digitalization. This may be accomplished by either the oral or parenteral route; the choice depends on the clinical status of the patient. If atrial fibrillation appears as a complication in an already acutely ill patient, the parenteral route is preferable. A slow intravenous injection of 0.5 mg digoxin is given, followed by 0.25 mg 6 and 12 hours later. Thereafter, the daily maintenance dose is chosen according to the renal function status. The best indicator for this purpose is the blood urea nitrogen (BUN), because renal clearance of digoxin closely parallels that of BUN. With a normal BUN, a daily maintenance dose of digoxin, 0.25 mg, is generally appropriate. If BUN is elevated, a lower maintenance dose, such as 0.125 mg, should be chosen. In either case, it is advisable to determine serum digoxin concentration on the fourth or fifth day after the onset of digitalization for guidance as to the most appropriate maintenance dose.

If an already digitalized patient presents with atrial fibrillation and rapid ventricular response, the adequacy of digitalization should be assessed by determining the serum digoxin level. The result of this test will not be known for several hours; whether any specific action is

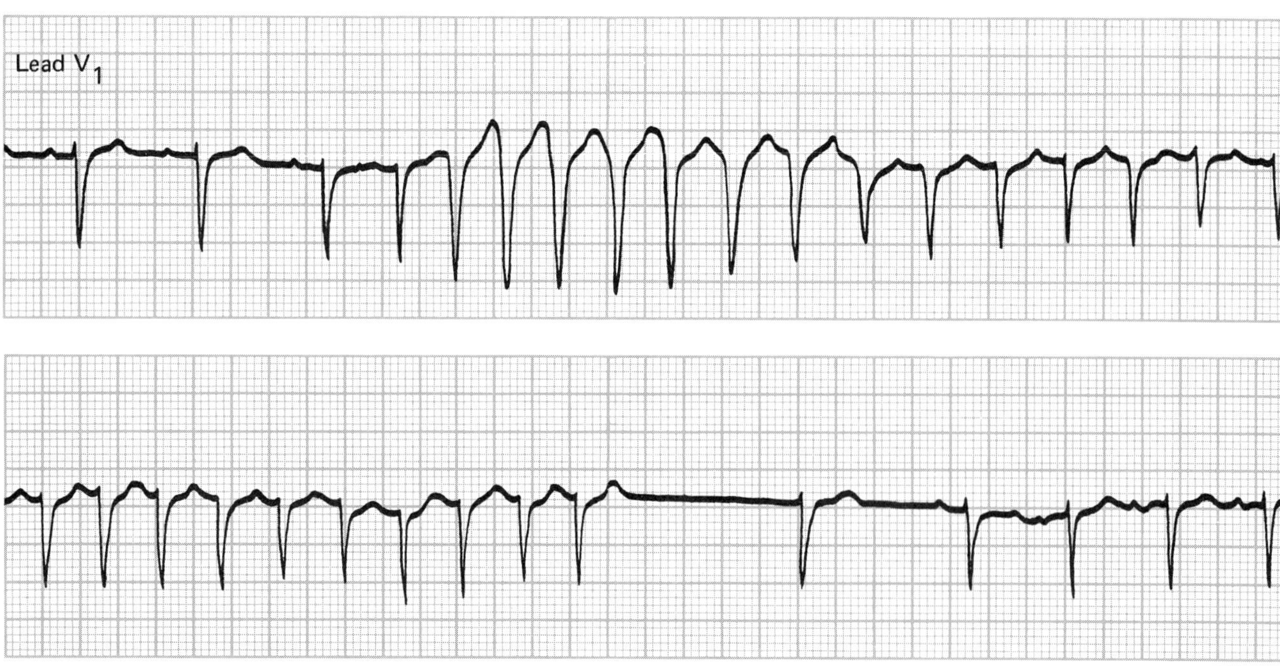

Figure 3.10. Onset and termination of paroxysmal supraventricular tachycardia with aberrant ventricular conduction. The arrhythmia is initiated by a supraventricular extrasystole (*top*); initial aberrant conduction gradually disappears; termination is sudden (*bottom*).

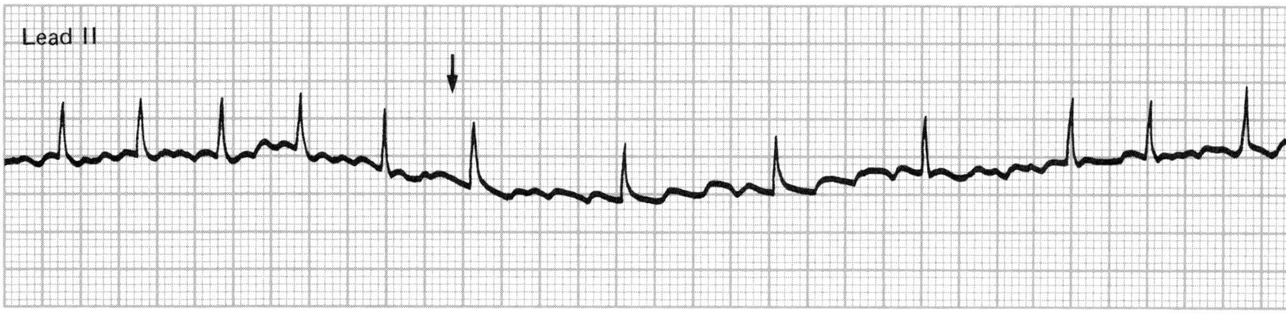

Figure 3.11. Atrial flutter. Narrow QRS complex tachycardia at 150/min. Effect of carotid sinus massage (↓): atrial flutter waves become evident on the baseline as the atrioventricular block changes from 2:1 to 4:1.

required in the interim depends on the clinical and hemodynamic status of the patient. Temporary slowing of the ventricular rate can be accomplished with propranolol, provided the patient is not an asthmatic and gross cardiac failure is not a problem. An initial dose of 1–2 mg may be given intravenously, and if a favorable response (slowing of ventricular rate) becomes evident, oral propranolol therapy may be instituted with an initial dose of 20 mg every 8 hours (q8h).

Quinidine is not recommended for the management of atrial fibrillation with rapid ventricular response. If restoration of sinus mechanism is considered necessary, electric cardioversion is the procedure of choice. However, many patients with recent onset atrial fibrillation will revert to sinus rhythm after the ventricular rate is brought under control with digoxin, propranolol, or both.

Atrial flutter with rapid ventricular response may be treated using the same guidelines given for atrial fibrillation. The combination of digitalization and propranolol is very effective in controlling the rate of ventricular response in atrial flutter by increasing the functional atrioventricular block to 3:1 or 4:1. Reversion to sinus mechanism by pharmacologic means alone is more difficult in the case of atrial flutter. However, atrial flutter easily reverts to sinus rhythm by electric cardioversion in the majority of cases.

Recurrence of atrial fibrillation or atrial flutter may be prevented by maintaining digitalization and using an antiarrhythmic agent. Propranolol 20 mg q8h is recommended. Quinidine may also be effective, but if it is used, the maintenance dose of digoxin must be reduced by half because of the known toxic interaction between digoxin and quinidine. If both these drugs are used together, the status of digitalization should be reassessed by serum digoxin determination.

Paroxysmal supraventricular tachycardia often reverts to sinus mechanism by carotid sinus massage, alone or potentiated by pharmacologic enhancement of vagal tone. Enhancement of vagal tone by itself may revert the rhythm to sinus mechanism. The drug most commonly used for this purpose is edrophonium (Tensilon). A test dose of 1 mg should be given intravenously. If no adverse reactions are noted after 2 minutes, a 10-mg bolus is injected.

Digitalization has been successfully used in the treatment of paroxysmal supraventricular tachycardia. However, a faster response is obtained by the intravenous administration of propranolol—1–2 mg initial dose, repeated after 3 minutes (it is best not to exceed a 6-mg IV dose)—or verapamil 5–10 mg IV. The latter drug is highly effective in reverting paroxysmal supraventricular tachycardia and has become our agent of choice for this syndrome. Because both propranolol and verapamil depress the atrioventricular node by different mechanisms, caution is mandatory when verapamil is given to a patient who has received propranolol, or vice versa.

Cardioversion is effective in paroxysmal supraventricular tachycardia and may be resorted to when other interventions fail.

In ventricular tachycardia, the agent of choice is lidocaine, 1–2 mg/kg body weight given as a rapid intravenous bolus. This is followed by an intravenous infusion at a rate of 2–4 mg/min. A second bolus (50–75% of the initial bolus) may be given after 5 minutes to prevent a therapeutic hiatus in plasma lidocaine concentration. If the patient's hemodynamic status is rapidly deteriorat-

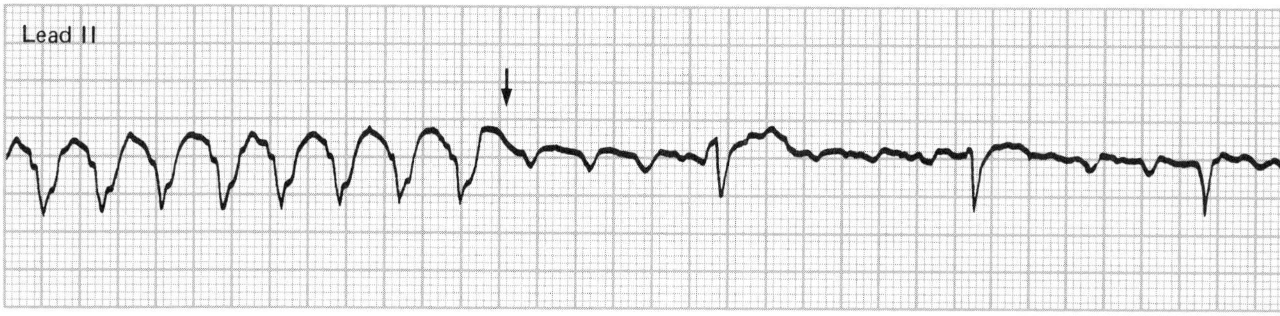

Figure 3.12. Supraventricular tachycardia with aberrancy. Broad QRS complex tachycardia. Slow (200/min) atrial flutter with 1:1 conduction. Aberrant ventricular conduction disappears during carotid sinus pressure (↓), and characteristic flutter waves become apparent.

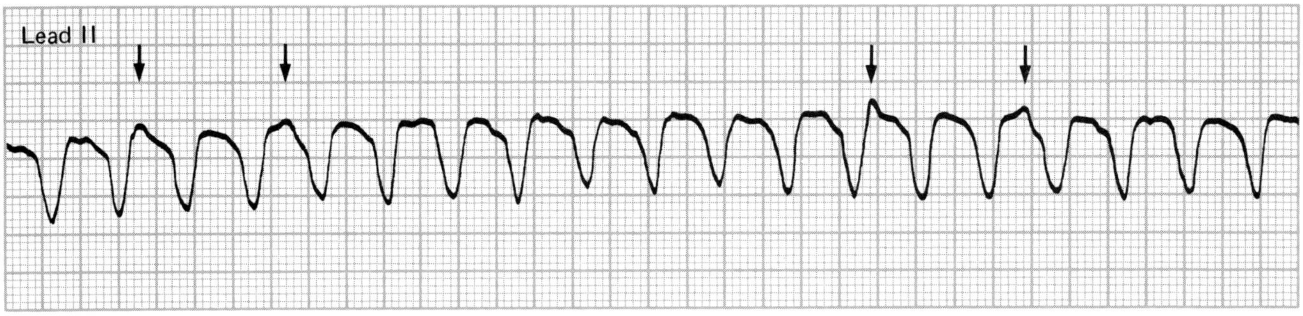

Figure 3.13. Broad QRS complex tachycardia: ventricular tachycardia. Recurrent added irregularities (↓) suggest dissociated atrial activity and therefore the diagnosis of ventricular tachycardia.

ing—manifested by hypotension, mental confusion, or loss of consciousness—electric cardioversion should be done immediately and sedation is often necessary.

Procainamide may be useful when lidocaine fails to revert ventricular tachycardia. Our own choice, however, is to proceed to electric cardioversion, performed under transient sedation with intravenous diazepam (5–10 mg). In elderly or debilitated subjects, care should be taken not to induce respiratory depression with a large dose of diazepam. Dim lights and a quiet room facilitate the action of diazepam. Energy settings for cardioversion of ventricular tachycardia may start at 150 J. If this level is ineffective, subsequent shocks with 250 or 400 J may be attempted. It must be remembered, however, that if digitalis toxicity is suspected or known to be present, initial energy settings of 5–10 J should be utilized. A lidocaine bolus given a few seconds before cardioversion may contribute to the restoration and maintenance of sinus rhythm.

In patients with acute myocardial infarction, ventricular tachycardia may lead to ventricular fibrillation. It can also occur unannounced or be preceded only by ventricular extrasystoles. In any case, ventricular fibrillation must be treated with a 400-J cardioversion without delay. Following cardioversion, an intravenous infusion of lidocaine (2–4 mg/kg body weight) should be maintained to prevent recurrences. Should there be recurrence in spite of adequate lidocaine administration (which may be corroborated in some centers by determining serum lidocaine concentration), subsequent prophylaxis may be attempted with procainamide. An initial loading dose of 300 mg is given over a 5- to 10-minute period, followed by IV infusion of 2–4 mg/min. Procainamide may produce hypotension, both through peripheral vasodilation and myocardial depression. An alternative agent is disopyramide, but unfortunately it is also a powerful myocardial depressant and may induce other side effects, the commonest one being urinary retention. The initial dose of disopyramide is 2 mg/kg over 5 minutes followed, if successful, by a maintenance IV drip infusion of 0.4 mg/kg/hour.

Recurrent ventricular tachycardia or fibrillation, refractory to treatment as described above, may be encountered in the setting of acute myocardial infarction. Advanced left ventricular dysfunction and/or mechanical complications (intraventricular septal rupture, papillary muscle rupture) may be present. Some cases may respond to parenteral bretylium tosylate at a dose of 5 mg/kg, preferably intravenously, followed by 5–10 mg/kg every 6 hours. Adverse effects of bretylium tosylate include hypotension (postural or supine), bradycardia, renal dysfunction, nausea, and mental confusion.

A limited experience with intravenous administration of amiodarone in our institution has shown it to be highly promising in the treatment of refractory, life-threatening ventricular arrhythmias. We have used loading doses between 1 and 2 gm followed by oral or parenteral maintenance dose of 400 mg/day, subsequently reduced to 300 or 200 mg/day under close surveillance. Possible late adverse reactions to amiodarone include abnormalities in thyroid function tests, with or without thyroid dysfunction, and a late, potentially lethal pulmonary interstitial fibrosis syndrome.

BRADYARRHYTHMIAS

Diagnosis

Sinus bradycardia may be the result of sinoatrial node dysfunction in elderly individuals—sick sinus syn-

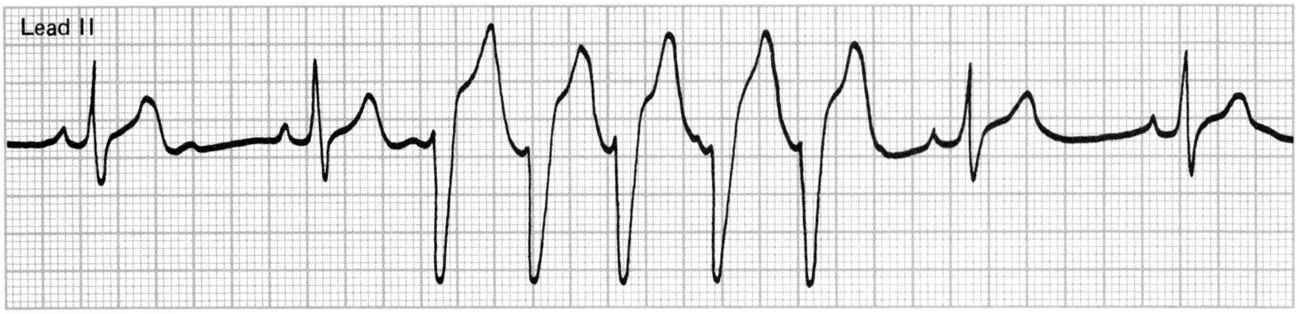

Figure 3.14. Sinus bradycardia with run of ventricular tachycardia.

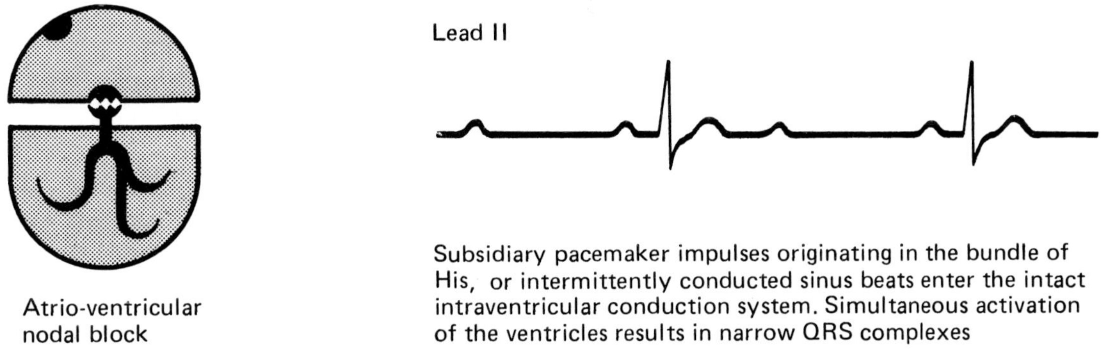

Figure 3.15. Atrioventricular nodal block.

drome—often alternating with rapid supraventricular arrhythmias, or tachycardia-bradycardia syndrome. It may be due to transient enhancement of vagal tone induced by drugs, such as morphine, or by severe pain, as in urinary calculi. It may also be caused by such drugs as digitalis, reserpine or β-adrenergic blocking agents. Sinus bradycardia is common in patients with obstructive jaundice and hypothyroidism and in athletes. Sinus bradycardia in the acutely ill patient, particularly with acute myocardial infarction, may lead to hypotension and facilitate the appearance of arrhythmias (Fig. 3.14).

Second- and third-degree heart block may be the cause of slow ventricular rate. In first-degree heart block, the atrioventricular conduction time (P-R interval on the electrocardiogram) is prolonged, but all sinus impulses are conducted and there is no difference between atrial and ventricular rates. In second-degree heart block, some atrial impulses are not conducted to the ventricles. In third-degree or complete heart block, none of the atrial impulses is conducted to the ventricles, which must be activated by a subsidiary pacemaker situated at or below the AV junction.

The level of the block is suggested by the width of the QRS complex. By narrow QRS complex is meant a QRS duration not exceeding 0.11 seconds. A wide QRS complex is one with a duration of 0.12 or more seconds. In second-degree AV nodal block, also called Mobitz type I, the conducted impulses enter both ventricles simultaneously through an intact intraventricular conduction system (Fig. 3.15). The QRS complex is therefore narrow (Fig. 3.16). In addition, Wenckebach periodicity may be present. In complete AV nodal block, the subsidiary pacemakers are usually located in the bundle of His. From here onward, the conduction system is intact, so the activation wave again enters both ventricles at the same time, producing narrow QRS complexes. The rate of discharge of bundle of His pacemaker sites is usually between 40 and 50 beats/min.

If AV nodal block occurs as a complication of acute myocardial infarction, it is usually found with inferior wall myocardial infarction (Fig. 3.17) due to occlusion of the right coronary artery that supplies the AV nodal artery. In this case the block is usually transient, presumably due to AV nodal improvement as enhanced collateral circulation from the left coronary system develops. Second- and third-degree block distal to the bundle of His must involve all divisions of the interventricular conduction system; that is, the right bundle branch and the two divisions (or the main bundle) of the left branch (Fig. 3.18). In the incomplete or second-degree stage (also called Mobitz type II) the intermittently conducted impulses travel along the least affected branch and spread to the contralateral ventricle through the contractile myocardium, causing a wide QRS complex on the electrocardiogram (Fig. 3.19). If complete block ensues, the subsidiary pacemakers will be located in the specialized myocardium distal to the site of block. The rate of firing of these distal (idioventricular) subsidiary pacemakers is slow, usually 15–30/min (Fig. 3.20). Thus, syncope, Stokes-Adams syndrome, hypotension, or aggravation of heart failure are likely to occur.

If block distal to the bundle of His presents as a complication of acute myocardial infarction, it is usually in anteroseptal infarctions, and its presence implies a large area of necrosis comprising not only the three main divisions of the conducting system but also a substantial

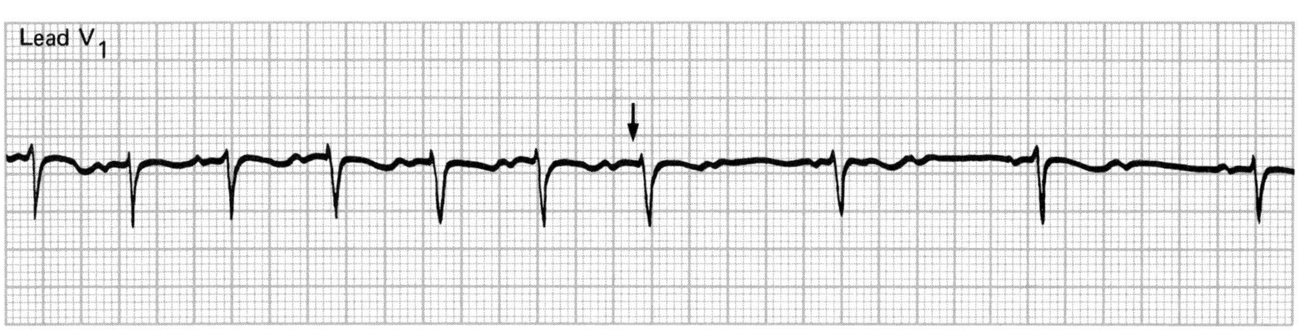

Figure 3.16. Second-degree heart block. Regular rhythm of 90/min. The sudden rate change is due to the development of second-degree heart block. Lengthening of PR interval before rate change (↓) and narrow QRS complexes pinpoint the site of block to the AV junction.

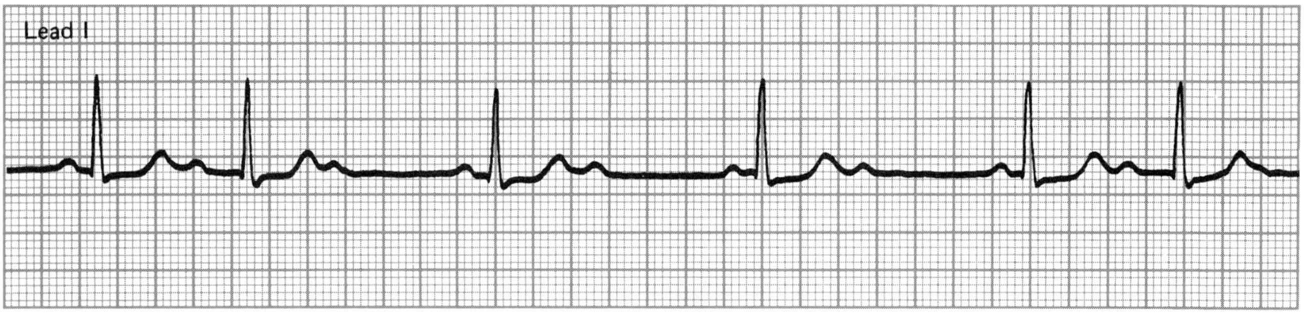

Figure 3.17. Second-degree heart block proximal to the bundle of His. AV junctional block complicating acute inferior wall myocardial infarction. The Wenckebach periodicity (lengthening of the PR interval before the nonconducted P wave) and the narrow QRS complex pinpoint the block at the AV junction level.

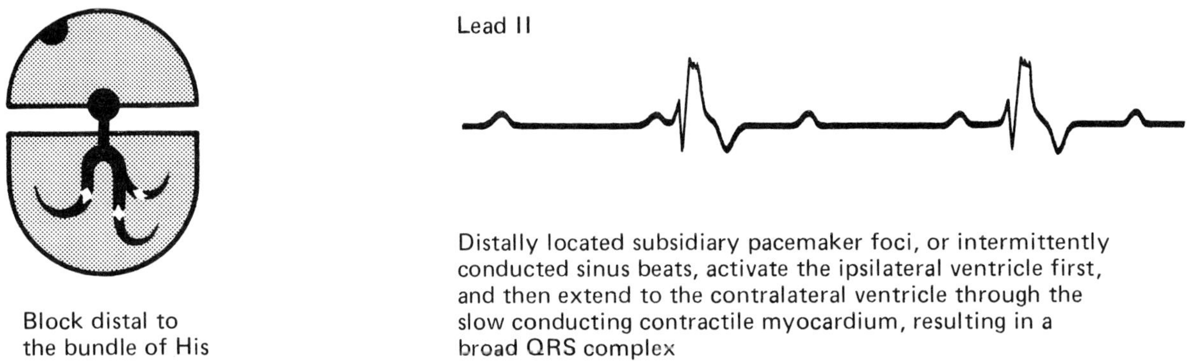

Figure 3.18. Heart block distal to the bundle of His.

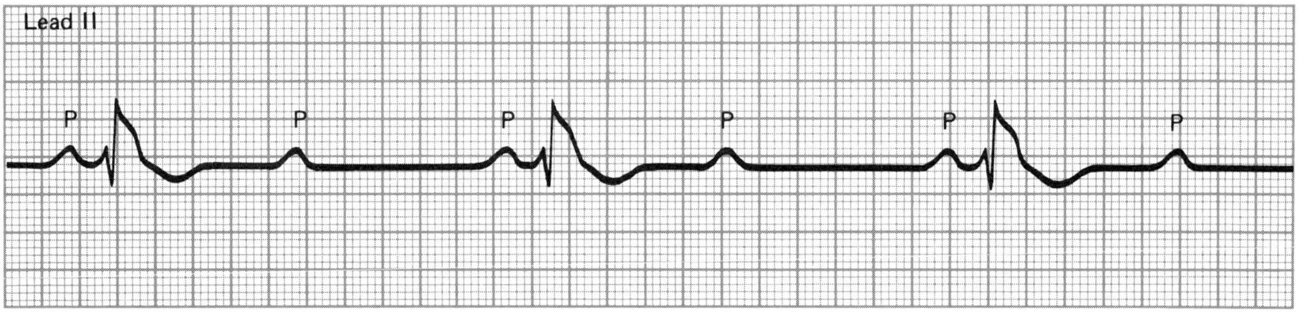

Figure 3.19. Second-degree heart block distal to the bundle of His as suggested by the broad QRS complex (Mobitz type II).

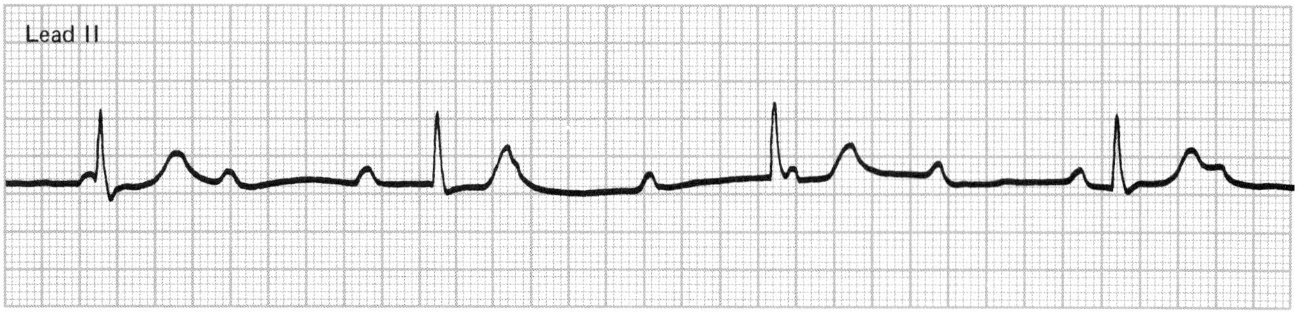

Figure 3.20. Complete heart block distal to the bundle of His. Wide QRS complexes at a slow rate (33/min) identify an idioventricular rhythm and localize the level of the block distal to the bundle of His. Note the dissociated atrial rhythm at 80/min.

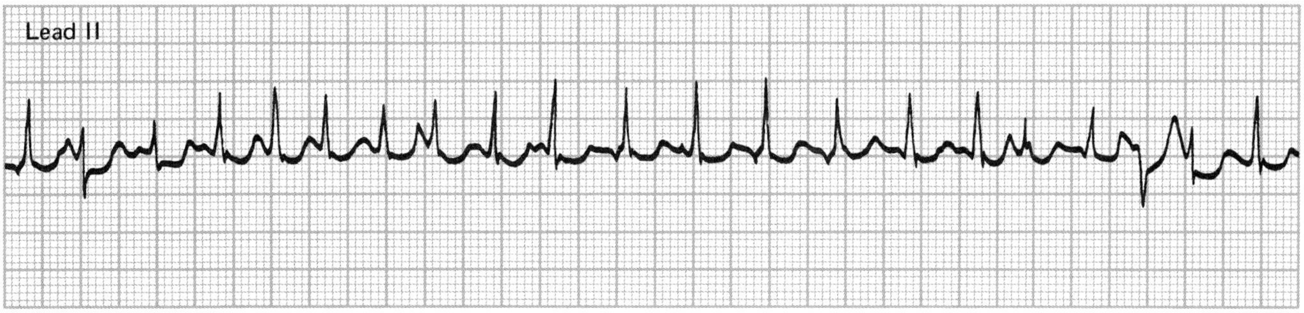

Figure 3.21. Multifocal atrial tachycardia. Rapid irregular tachycardia with a variable rate of 160-240/min. P waves with varying configuration and timing are well shown in this strip.

amount of contractile myocardium; hence, the grave prognosis of these cases.

Treatment

Symptomatic sinus bradycardia should be managed by immediate positioning of the patient in the horizontal or slight Trendelenburg position. Atropine is given subcutaneously (0.6–1.0 mg) or intravenously (0.3 mg). Subcutaneous atropine may then be repeated q3–6h as necessary. Excessive atropine may cause urinary retention or psychotic reactions, particularly in elderly patients. Glaucoma may be aggravated.

AV nodal block, whether incomplete or complete, tends to be benign and transient. Aggravating or precipitating factors, such as digitalis toxicity, should be treated. In some instances, it may persist and produce syncope or other manifestations of circulatory insufficiency, in which case permanent artificial pacing may be necessary. Advanced (second- or third-degree) block distal to the bundle of His generally requires permanent artificial pacing.

In acute anteroseptal infarction, the occurrence of heart block distal to the bundle of His carries a poor prognosis, both due to the block itself and the generally large extent of myocardial necrosis. Temporary artificial pacing must be instituted. If the patient survives the acute phase and block persists, permanent artificial pacing is necessary. It is not yet definitely known whether permanent pacing improves the survival of patients with transient advanced block complicating acute myocardial infarction.

Bundle branch block appearing in the course of an acute myocardial infarction may be the forerunner of advanced block. Insertion of a temporary artificial pacemaker should be seriously considered in these cases.

OTHER ARRHYTHMIAS

Ventricular Extrasystoles

Ventricular extrasystoles are frequently found in critically ill patients. In the setting of acute myocardial ischemia or infarction, they have been related to more serious arrhythmias, particularly if the extrasystoles are frequent, multifocal (different configuration on the same lead), repetitive (two or three consecutive extrasystoles), or occur on the T wave. If acute ischemic disease is suspected, we recommend prophylactic treatment with lidocaine (1–2 mg/kg body weight bolus followed by a 2–4 mg/min infusion and a second smaller bolus 5 minutes later, as previously described). Ventricular extrasystoles in the nonischemic patient do not have the same implications, and attention should be directed toward the possible action of drugs, hypoxia, or electrolyte disturbances.

It must be remembered that ventricular extrasystoles are common in normal individuals without any other evidence of heart disease. In the majority of critically ill patients who have no acute myocardial ischemia or necrosis, ventricular extrasystoles are not the forerunners of more serious arrhythmias and seldom cause any significant hemodynamic derangement. Possible facilitating factors, such as hypoxia, electrolyte imbalance, or drug toxicity, should be corrected, but the use of antiar-

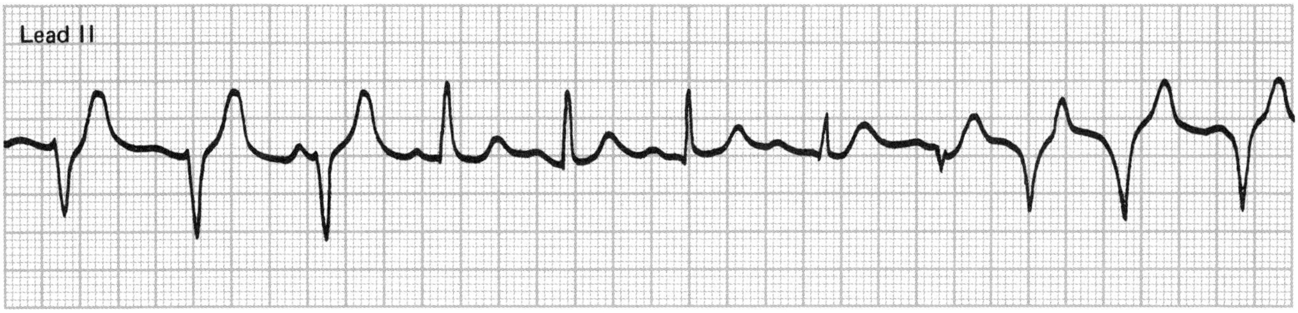

Figure 3.22. Accelerated idioventricular rhythm. Both ends of this strip show an accelerated idioventricular rhythm identified by its regular rhythm at a relatively slow rate (95/min) and broad QRS complexes not preceded by a P wave. Conducted sinus beats show the Wenckebach phenomenon.

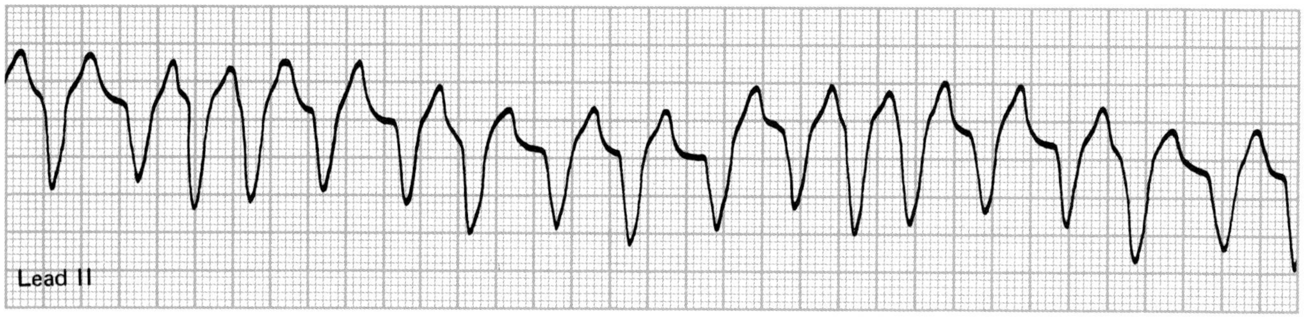

Figure 3.23. Atrial fibrillation with pre-existing intraventricular conduction defect. At first sight this tracing may be mistaken for ventricular tachycardia, but close inspection reveals irregularity of RR intervals, which is the hallmark of atrial fibrillation. The broad QRS complexes are due to a pre-existing intraventricular conduction abnormality.

rhythmic agents should be restricted to those patients in whom a serious arrhythmia (ventricular tachycardia, ventricular fibrillation) does occur.

Multifocal Atrial Tachycardia

Multifocal atrial tachycardia is an arrhythmia characterized by multiple premature atrial beats that probably originate from different foci, as suggested by their variable electrocardiographic configuration and timing (Fig. 3.21). It is almost exclusively found in patients with respiratory insufficiency, usually acute exacerbation of chronic lung disease, and almost invariably in the setting of simultaneous theopylline administration. Multifocal atrial tachycardia is an indication of a high mortality subset and responds poorly to drug treatment or cardioversion. Efforts should be focused on avoiding digitalis toxicity and correcting hypoxia, hypercapnia or hypocapnia, electrolyte abnormalities, and acid-base imbalance. If possible, theopylline should be temporarily discontinued. Some cases may respond to treatment with oral or parenteral verapamil.

Accelerated Idioventricular Rhythm

Accelerated idioventricular rhythm, also known by the misnomer "slow ventricular tachycardia," is a self-limited broad QRS complex rhythm with a rate of 60–110/min, usually in the context of acute myocardial infarction. The majority of cases are benign and require no pharmacologic intervention (Fig. 3.22).

Other Tachycardias

Other tachycardias with a rate of 100–130 beats/min and narrow QRS complexes on the electrocardiogram suggest the possibility of sinus tachycardia or atrial flutter with 3:1 ventricular response if regular, or atrial fibrillation or flutter with variable block, if irregular. Broad QRS complex in this rate range suggests pre-existing bundle branch block (Fig. 3.23) or, if toward the lower end of the above limits, accelerated idioventricular rhythm.

Ventricular Fibrillation

Ventricular fibrillation (Fig. 3.24) is usually the terminal event in death from advanced disease, cardiac or otherwise. It is usually called secondary ventricular fibrillation, and any therapeutic intervention should be viewed in the light of the patient's prospects of surviving the basic illness. Evidently, most cases of secondary ventricular fibrillation do not call for specific action. On the other hand, ventricular fibrillation may occur in an individual whose chances of survival and recovery are excellent, if the arrhythmia can be reverted. This is true in most cases of ventricular fibrillation complicating the early phases of acute myocardial infarction (now largely preventable by the prophylactic use of lidocaine). More rarely, ventricular fibrillation may be the result of accidental electrical shock or the toxic effect of drugs (sympathomimetic agents, tricyclic antidepressants).

The management of primary ventricular fibrillation is

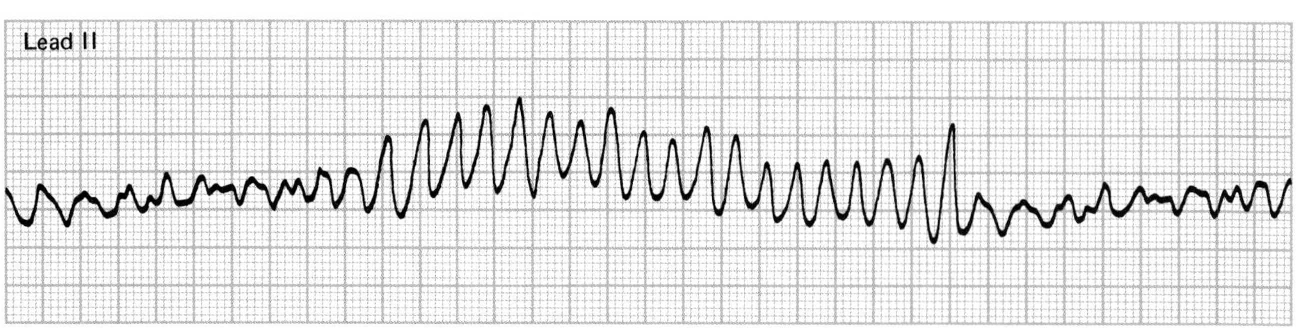

Figure 3.24. Ventricular fibrillation.

direct current cardioversion. For the average size adult it should be performed with a 400-J electroshock, delivered through electrodes applied on the chest wall in the most appropriate position to allow the current flow to go through the ventricular mass. If cardioversion cannot be performed immediately, cardiorespiratory resuscitation should be started without delay.

Ventricular asystole may be due to lack of activation of the ventricles, as in complete heart block, or to absence of mechanical response to electrical stimulation. The latter is often referred to as electromechanical dissociation. It is more often seen following electric cardioversion for ventricular fibrillation and as the terminal event in agonal states. Although evidence of ventricular activation (QRS complexes) is seen on the ECG monitor, no evidence of mechanical contraction is detectable. This is a most serious arrhythmia, but occasionally it may respond to intravenous or intracardiac administration of calcium chloride, 250–500 mg.

Suggested Readings

Braunwald E: *Heart Disease,* ed 2. Philadelphia, WB Saunders, 1987.

Cranfield PF: *The Conduction of the Cardiac Impulse.* Mount Kisco. NY, Futura Publishing, 1975.

Hurst JW (Ed): *The Heart,* ed. 6 Philadelphia, McGraw Hill, 1986.

Marriot HJL: *Practical Electrocardiography,* ed 7. Baltimore, Williams & Wilkins, 1983.

Schamroth L: *The Disorders of Cardiac Rhythm.* Oxford, Blackwell Scientific Publications, 1980.

CHAPTER

4 Hypertensive Crisis

Adam L. Linton, M.D.

A great deal of confusion surrounds the definition of hypertensive crisis, partly because of the use of such inexact terms as severe hypertension, accelerated hypertension, and malignant hypertension. The intention of this chapter is not to discuss the treatment of hypertension in general, but simply to describe the emergency procedure employed to deal with the life-threatening condition known as hypertensive encephalopathy. This condition may be a complication of previously severe hypertension, so-called accelerated hypertension, or it may occur spontaneously in relatively mild hypertension of recent origin. Hypertensive encephalopathy is the only hypertensive syndrome that calls for emergency treatment, usually by the systemic route. It is an acute reversible encephalopathy precipitated by an abrupt sustained rise in blood pressure that exceeds the limits of cerebral autoregulation.

PATHOPHYSIOLOGY

In normotensive individuals, changes in systemic blood pressure are followed by changes in the caliber of cerebral arteries to ensure a constant cerebral blood flow. This phenomenon, termed autoregulation, occurs primarily in the small resistance cerebral arteries: a rise in mean systemic blood pressure results in vasoconstriction, whereas a fall produces vasodilation. The range of blood pressure over which autoregulatory responses can maintain a normal cerebral blood flow is indicated in Figure 4.1. In patients with established hypertension, the range over which autoregulation maintains cerebral blood flow is higher than it is in normotensive individuals, probably because of damage to the small arterial walls.

This adaptation means that chronically hypertensive patients can sustain higher mean pressures without an excessive increase in cerebral blood flow that, in turn, would lead to brain edema and hypertensive encephalopathy. The corollary is also important: it can be seen from Figure 4.1 that chronically hypertensive patients cannot tolerate rapid reductions in mean blood pressure to normal values (around 100 mm Hg) because such a decrease will compromise cerebral blood flow. These observations also make it clear why chronically hypertensive patients are less likely to develop hypertensive encephalopathy than normotensive or recently hypertensive patients.

Hypertensive encephalopathy is the direct result of loss of cerebral autoregulation: the raised hydrostatic pressure causes increased fluid transudation from the capillaries into the brain, producing brain edema. Hypertensive encephalopathy leaves no residual defects if blood pressure is reduced, but in fatal cases pathologic findings usually include brain edema and, occasionally, petechial hemorrhages, minute infarctions, and arteriolar necrosis.

DIAGNOSIS

Hypertensive encephalopathy commonly presents with severe generalized headache, vomiting, and drowsiness or confusion. The full syndrome may require 12–48 hours

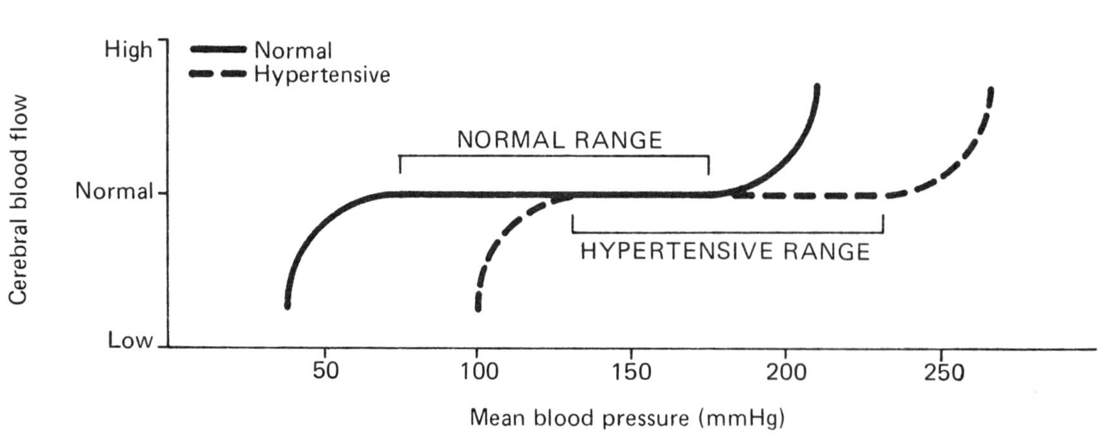

Figure 4.1. Autoregulatory range in normal and hypertensive patients.

to develop, and patients may exhibit generalized seizures, myoclonus, or even focal neurologic deficits, such as hemiparesis or aphasia. It is commonly accompanied by evidence of malignant hypertension with papilledema, retinal hemorrhages, exudates, and constricted arterioles. There is controversy as to whether the syndrome of hypertensive encephalopathy ever occurs without papilledema. In addition to the cerebral symptoms, patients often exhibit cardiac decompensation, rapidly progressing renal failure, and microangiopathic hemolytic anemia. The cerebrospinal fluid is usually clear, but is under increased pressure. The protein content may be normal or slightly increased, and the electroencephalogram shows various nonspecific abnormalities. The brain scan is usually normal. The untreated case will normally progress to coma and death with a few hours.

Table 4.1
Treatment of Hypertensive Encephalopathy

1. Early, uncomplicated: start oral antihypertensive therapy (β-blocker + diuretic)
   a. Nifedipine, 10 to 20 mg, sublingually
   b. IV diazoxide 100 mg: repeat twice if necessary, if unsuccessful, or if
2. Severe, complicated
   a. Establish monitoring
      i. Intra-arterial line central pressure recordings (PCWP; CVP)[a]
      ii. Bladder catheter
   b. Sodium nitroprusside
      i. Continuous IV infusion by pump (0.5–0.8 μg/kg/min)
      ii. Adjust dose as necessary
      iii. Protect solution from light with aluminum foil
   c. Consider IV propranolol and/or α-blockade if all else fails
      i. Start α-blockade first
      ii. Monitor cardiac output for signs of myocardial depression with β-blockade

[a] PCWP, pulmonary capillary wedge pressure; CVP, central venous pressure.

TREATMENT OF HYPERTENSIVE ENCEPHALOPATHY

General

It is obvious from the above description that blood pressure reduction is the immediate objective in the treatment of hypertensive encephalopathy. It must, however, be remembered that, because of the pathophysiology described, no attempt should be made to restore blood pressure to "normal" levels too rapidly, particularly in patients with a history of long-standing hypertension. There is recent evidence to suggest that overenthusiastic blood pressure reduction with intravenous drugs in patients with hypertensive encephalopathy may lead to death or permanent neurologic damage as a result of ischemia. Presumably, in these patients, the mean blood pressure was reduced with aggressive treatment to below the level at which the altered cerebral autoregulation could maintain effective circulation. The objective of treatment, therefore, is a rapid but modest reduction in blood pressure, followed by long-term attempts to control the blood pressure. Careful clinical monitoring and examination are mandatory during acute antihypertensive therapy to ensure that no new neurologic signs appear that could be attributed to a reduction in cerebral perfusing pressure below the critical level necessary for effective brain resuscitation. In the acute phase, if "relative" hypotension is avoided, clinical signs of neurologic dysfunction begin to improve quite quickly.

Drug Therapy

An outline of the treatment of severe hypertension is given in Table 4.1. If the problem is detected early and is not complicated by severe neurologic disturbances, cardiac disease, or pulmonary edema, it is reasonable to start the patient immediately on oral antihypertensive therapy, usually with a β-blocker and a diuretic. Until oral therapy is effective, the blood pressure may be acutely reduced by the administration of nifedipine, 10–20 mg given sublingually. If that fails, intravenous diazoxide can be given in a bolus of 100 mg and repeated twice if necessary. These simple maneuvers may be successful, but if not, there should be no delay in moving to a more aggressive approach.

In the severe or complicated case of hypertensive encephalopathy or if the therapy outlined above is unsuccessful, the patient will undoubtedly require monitoring; at the minimum, it should consist of an intra-arterial line, the establishment of a method for central pressure recording, usually of the pulmonary capillary wedge pressure, and the insertion of a bladder catheter for monitoring of urine output on a continuous basis. If diazoxide has not been successful in lowering the blood pressure, the next drug of choice is sodium nitroprusside. Its advantages are that its effect is immediate and any untoward drop in blood pressure can immediately be reversed by reducing the rate of infusion. This infusion should begin at 0.5–0.8 μg/kg/min with the dose being adjusted as necessary. If the nitroprusside infusion has to be continued for longer than 36 hours, it is important to remember the possibility of cyanide poisoning; thiocyanate levels should be determined in the blood at 36 hours, and the drug should be discontinued if the level is greater than 12 mg/100 ml. The potential for cyanide toxicity is more marked if the patient has renal impairment or if he or she suffers from hypothyroidism. If infusion rates in excess of 0.8 μg/kg/min are required, the possibility of tachyphylaxis or resistance should be considered, and the medication may have to be discontinued. It should also be remembered that, once in solution, nitroprusside tends to deteriorate; it should also be protected from light by wrapping the container of the prepared solution with aluminum foil.

Whichever of the above drugs is required for emergency treatment of hypertensive encephalopathy, its effect may be further potentiated by the administration of furosemide, 80 mg intravenously. This potent diuretic serves to maintain sodium diuresis in the face of falling arterial pressure and counteracts the sodium-retaining effects of diazoxide. Furosemide is of further benefit if the patient concurrently develops cardiac failure. Occasionally, these measures may not be effective, and it is necessary to consider the administration of intravenous propranolol and/or α-blockade. In this situation, phentolamine is begun first at a dose of 0.05–0.10 mg/min and increased in stepwise fashion to the defined blood pressure goal or to a maximum of 2.0 mg/min. Propranolol is never instituted first in combined parenteral α- and β-blockade because, with a pheochromocytoma, a paradoxical increase in blood pressure may be seen. Once α-blockade is established, parenteral β-blockade with propranolol can be cautiously begun at a dose of 0.5 mg/hour and increased slowly until the heart rate falls to less than 60 beats/minute and/or the cardiac index begins to fall. It is imperative to measure sequentially the effect of parenteral β-blockade on cardiac output because of its propensity to depress myocardial contractility. It should be remembered, however, that propranolol is dangerous if the patient is in impending cardiac failure, and its use should be avoided in this situation if possible.

Suggested Readings

Huysmans FT, Thien TA, Koene RA: Combined intravenous administration of diazoxide and beta-blocking agent in acute treatment of severe hypertension or hypertensive crisis. *Am Heart J* 103:395–400, 1982.

Huysmans FT, Sluiter HE, Thein TA, Koene RA: Acute treatment of hypertensive crisis with nifedipine. *Br J Clin Pharmacol* 16:725–727, 1983.

Koch-Weser J: Hypertensive emergencies. *N Engl J Med* 290:211, 1984.

Koch-Weser J: Drug therapy: diazoxide. *N Engl J Med* 294:1271–1274, 1976.

Lebel J, Langlois S, Belleau LJ, Grose JH: Labetalol infusion in hypertensive emergencies. *Clin Pharmacol Ther* 37:615–618, 1985.

Palmer RF, Lassetter KC: Sodium nitroprusside. *N Engl J Med* 929:294, 1975.

CHAPTER

5 Shock

William J. Sibbald, M.D.

Shock is clinically recognized as a decrease in systemic blood pressure, with associated signs and symptoms of perfusion that is inadequate to sustain the essential function of vital organs. Shock may be a consequence of disease resulting in (1) depressed systemic flow and/or (2) a loss of tone within the arterial circulation. Functionally, a depression in systemic flow sufficient to cause shock is associated with a decrease in O_2 transport below critical levels that are required to meet peripheral O_2 demands.

At the cellular level, shock may therefore be regarded as a state of acute nutritional insufficiency for O_2 and other essential substrates. *Cardiogenic, hypovolemic,* and *septic* shock are characterized by a decrease in O_2 availability that, with time, is sufficient to result in cellular anoxia, cellular dysfunction, and, if uncorrected, cell death. Additionally, septic shock may be characterized by a primary defect of O_2 utilization within the cell, again resulting in cellular dysfunction progressing to cell death.

CARDIOVASCULAR PHYSIOLOGY

To appreciate the dynamics of the shock state, as well as to develop a logical plan for treatment, it is important to develop an understanding of the determinants of the blood pressure. Interrelationships of those factors governing blood pressure are expressed schematically and mathematically below (Fig. 5.1).

Level 1 shows that hypotension will result from either a depression in cardiac output or a loss of systemic vascular resistance. With a primary loss of systemic vascular resistance, as seen in septic shock, an increase in cardiac output is one of the compensatory mechanisms available to maintain blood pressure. In cardiogenic and hypovolemic shock, where a primary decrease in cardiac output is characteristic, the compensatory response is an increase in the systemic vascular resistance, mediated by the sympathetic nervous system, endogenously released catecholamines, and other endogenous vasoconstrictors. Therefore, in cardiogenic or hypovolemic shock the periphery is cool and mottled; in septic shock the periphery is usually warm.

Level 2 of Figure 5.1 shows that cardiac output is dependent upon heart rate and stroke volume. Severe brady- or tachyarrhythmias may therefore result in hypotension because of their influence on cardiac output. However, in most forms of cardiogenic and hypovolemic shock, a depression in stroke volume is the primary defect respon-

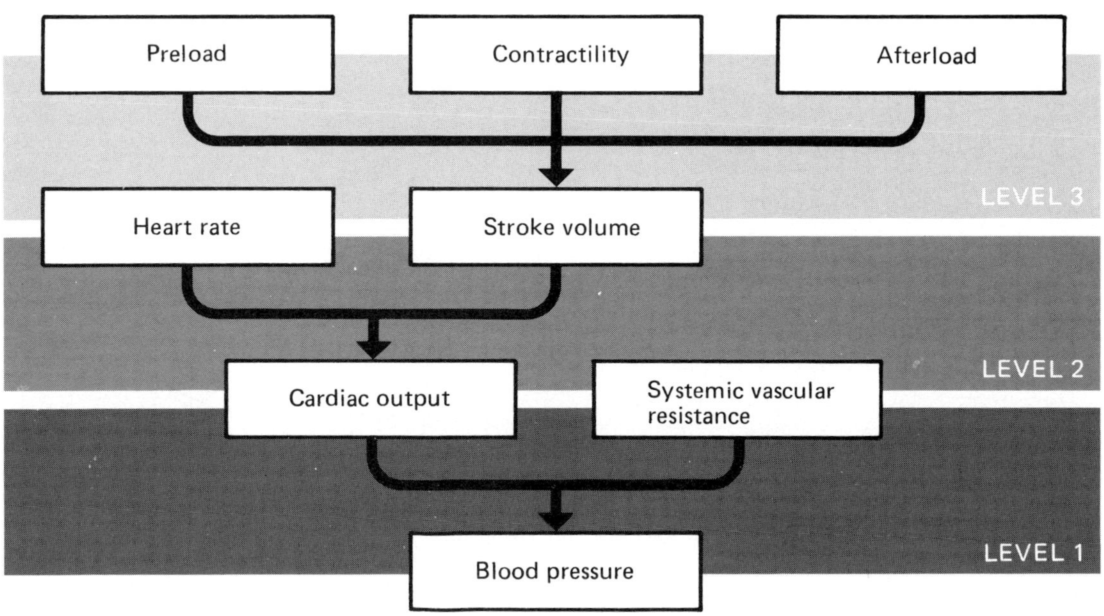

Figure 5.1. Regulation of blood pressure.

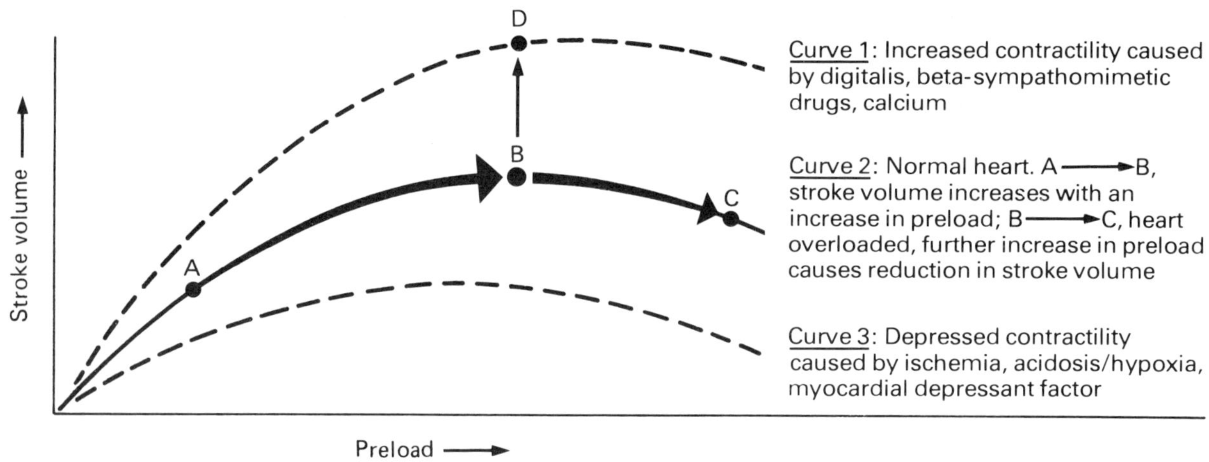

Figure 5.2. The Frank-Starling curve and contractility.

sible for the depressed cardiac output, and any associated tachycardia is simply a compensatory mechanism to attempt defense of the cardiac output.

Stroke volume, the amount of blood ejected with each heart beat *(Level 3)*, is determined by the ventricular preload, the ventricular afterload (or impedance to ejection), and intrinsic myocardial contractility. According to the Frank-Starling principle, which describes heart work as a function of *preload*, a depression in stroke volume (and hence in cardiac output and blood pressure) may occur in situations where the preload is excessively low or high (Fig. 5.2). The greater the degree of stretch between the contractile proteins of the myocardial fibril at end-diastole, the greater will be the subsequent stroke volume—until a point in time when actin and myosin filaments are stretched beyond the point of interdigitation and stroke volume may then actually fall *(Point C)*. At any given preload and afterload, the force developed by a myocardial fibril is dependent upon *contractility*. Although difficult to assess, changes in contractility are assumed when stroke volume changes despite constancy of ventricular preload and afterload, such as when stimulated with a positive inotropic agent *(Points B-D)*. *Afterload* is the tension that must be developed by the ventricle in overcoming the resistance of the arterial tree, and it is elevated with an increased diastolic pressure and/or ventricular cavity size. If both preload and contractility are kept constant, stroke volume is inversely related to afterload; a decrease in an abnormally increased aortic pressure or left ventricular afterload may effect an increase in the stroke volume. Therefore, a depression in stroke volume (and hence cardiac output and blood pressure) may be caused by a reduction in preload by depressed contractility and/or with an excessive increase in the afterload.

It is important to remember that ventricular preload is not measured as an end-diastolic filling pressure (EDP), e.g., pulmonary capillary wedge pressure or central venous pressure. Ventricular preload is most correctly assessed by an end-diastolic volume (EDV) or end-diastolic dimension (EDD). The relationship between EDD and EDV actually describes the stiffness properties of the ventricle; this relationship is not linear and may in fact change to describe a family of stiffness curves (Fig. 5.3). With increasing ventricular volume (Fig. 5.3, points A → B → C), the ventricle becomes stiffer so that a progressively smaller preload is reflected by a progressively higher measured EDP. Similarly, heart disease, such as ischemia, will increase ventricular stiffness properties; following an acute myocardial infarction any given EDV (preload) will be reflected by a greater EDP than would normally be the case in a healthy individual (Fig. 5.3, points A → D).

Because many of the therapeutic agents used in the treatment of shock have the capacity to increase *myocardial oxygen consumption* ($M\dot{V}O_2$), it is important to remember that the $M\dot{V}O_2$ is also dependent upon preload, afterload, contractility, and heart rate. The $M\dot{V}O_2$ will be increased when ventricular end-diastolic tension is increased (increased preload and increased afterload) and when contractility or heart rate is increased. Clinically, the $M\dot{V}O_2$ may be estimated by the product of the systolic blood pressure and heart rate (SBP × HR = "double

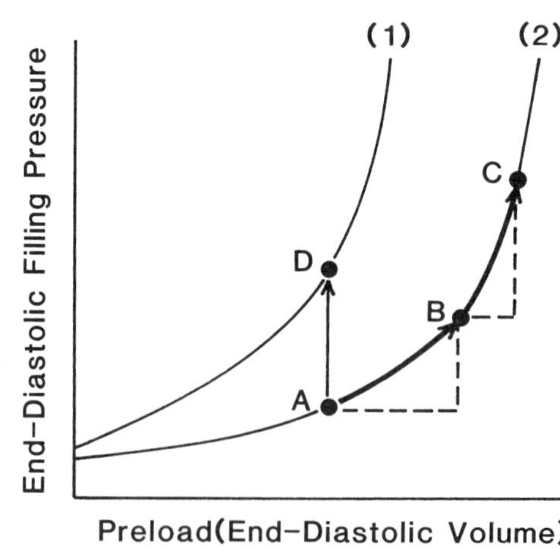

Figure 5.3. Curve 1: Increased stiffness properties (e.g., ischemia) result in increased EDP for any EDV (points *A→D*). Curve 2: Progressive increase in stiffness with increased ventricular filling results in less preload being accommodated for a larger increase in EDP (points *B→C* vs points *A→B*).

product"), an index more useful in determining whether a given change in therapy has been accompanied by a relative increase or fall in $M\dot{V}O_2$, than in determining any absolute degree of $M\dot{V}O_2$.

THE "SHOCK CYCLE" (FIG. 5.4)

Although the effects of the shock state have been defined at a cellular level, it is intuitively clear that the result of protracted hypotension—cellular anoxia—may be the development of multiple organ failure syndrome (MOF) (see Chapter 37) and eventually a perpetuation of the shock state itself.

Cellular anoxia results from reduced O_2 availability, which is characteristic of the hypotensive state. Initial defense includes peripheral vasoconstriction to divert available O_2 transport to teleologically important organs, such as the brain, heart, and liver. Alterations in the Starling forces within the microcirculation initially support the movement of interstitial fluid to the intravascular compartment, as an "autotransfusion" effect attempts to support pressure and flow by augmenting ventricular preload. With ongoing hypotension and reduced O_2 availability, anaerobic metabolism supersedes aerobic cellular activity to maintain ATP production, albeit with the reduced efficiency that is typical of the anaerobic state; considerably less ATP is formed per mole of glucose utilized in the anaerobic than in the aerobic state. Lactic acid is an important by-product of anaerobic metabolism, and the height of arterial lactate correlates with the mortality rate in shock; that is, the more protracted the shock state, the greater the mortality rate.

Lactic acidemia results in increased microvascular permeability. Initial defense of the intravascular volume is lost at this stage as fluid now moves from the intravascular to extracellular compartments; flow is now further depressed as ventricular preload also falls. Cellular swelling in this stage of increased microvascular permeability perpetuates inefficient cellular metabolic activity, and ATP production is further depressed. The metabolic acidosis accompanying excess lactate production may depress myocardial contractility, as may the generation of a myocardial-depressant factor (MDF). Splanchnic ischemia is apparently the cause of MDF production in protracted shock states.

Therefore, protracted hypotension results in a depression of ventricular preload and contractility, both of which contribute to a perpetuation of the shock state.

Although the shock state has been defined at a cellular level, the clinical manifestations of prolonged cellular hypoxia secondary to shock are not only a perpetuation of the shock state itself but also of multiple organ failure—anoxic/ischemic brain injury and ischemic liver failure, renal failure, and acute respiratory failure.

SHOCK: CLINICAL RECOGNITION

Shock is defined quantitatively according to changes in driving pressure. However, determination of the mean

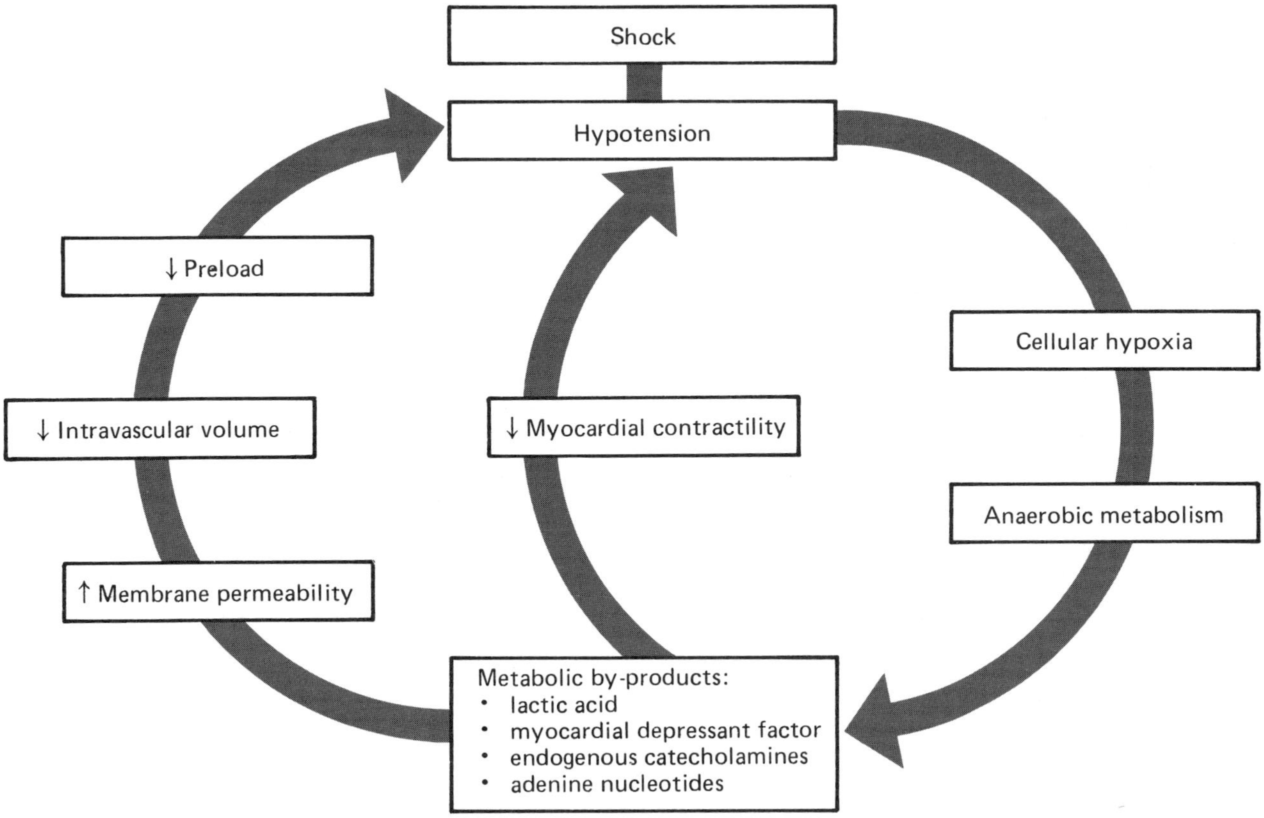

Figure 5.4. The shock cycle.

Table 5.1
Essential Components for the Diagnosis of Shock

Quantitative criteria
↓ BP: <90 mm Hg systolic BP, or a fall of 30–40 mm Hg from previously recorded levels

Evidence of low perfusion
↓ Cerebral blood flow → obtundation/restlessness
↓ Renal blood flow → oliguria
↓ Peripheral blood flow → cool mottled periphery (except in septic shock)

Table 5.2
An Indirect Assessment of Systemic Flow

Measured variable (compared to baseline)	Improved CO	Decreased CO
Blood pressure	Increased	Decreased
Heart rate	Decreased	Increased
(AV) O_2 content	Narrowed	Widened
Arterial lactate	Decreased	Increased
Urine Na^+	Higher	Lower
Urine/serum osmolality ratio	Lower	Higher

blood pressure with a sphygmomanometer may be unreliable in the shock state.

Therefore, to establish that recorded pressures may define shock, confirmation is sought with the clinical correlates of the anticipated response to hypotension. Alterations in the state of consciousness, oliguria, and a cool periphery are all typical of the shock state (Table 5.1). Unlike cardiogenic and hypovolemic shock, it must be remembered that a patient with septic shock may initially present with a warm, vasodilated periphery.

SHOCK: MONITORING AND INITIAL RESUSCITATION

In its early phases, shock dictates urgent treatment, even before the primary cause has been determined or monitoring of the response to therapy has been instituted. Understanding the results of protracted hypotension—the shock cycle—dictates the need to establish a pressure sufficient to restore perfusion to vital organs as expeditiously as possible. If not, the syndrome of "irreversible" shock may become established.

At this early stage, it is useful to attempt clinical assessment of determinants of the blood pressure (BP); that is preload, afterload, contractility, and heart rate. Such an assessment may help delineate the cause of the shock state and establish important guidelines by which to determine and subsequently evaluate the initial therapy. Clinically, heart rate is obtained by simple auscultation of the cardiac apex. Preload is usually high if the jugular venous pulse is elevated, if crackles are obvious on pulmonary auscultation, and if an S3 gallop is heard on cardiac auscultation. Afterload is usually high if the patient is vasoconstricted. Contractility, the most difficult parameter to assess noninvasively, may be crudely appreciated by the thrust of cardiac contraction to palpation of the apical impulse.

All the preceding factors govern the cardiac output (CO) (Fig. 5.1). A low CO is also characterized by a widened arterial-venous oxygen content gradient (>5 vol/%), a high arterial lactate concentration, and a low urine output with associated high osmolality and low sodium content. Sequential monitoring of the above will also enable one to determine whether a therapeutic protocol has resulted in a net improvement in CO or the converse (Table 5.2).

In summary, basic resuscitative measures should be directed at maintaining a mean blood pressure ($\overline{BP}$) over the 70-80 mm Hg necessary for essential core organ perfusion by attention to the ABCs of resuscitation, including:

1. *A*irway: intubation, if not protected
2. *B*reathing: assisted ventilation, to reduce the work of breathing
3. *C*irculation: in cases of obvious volume deficit, rapid infusion of volume replacement (see discussion on hypovolemic shock); with evidence of intravascular excess (e.g., CHF), use Dopamine (800 mg in 500 ml 5% dextrose in water, titrated to desired mean pressure level
4. Other: correction of acidosis, if pH is below 7.20

This stage of shock resuscitation is defined as the "ebb" phase, in which therapy is directed to restoring pressures. Subsequently, once blood pressure is stabilized, concern is directed to management of the "flow" phase, a period where systemic O_2 transport is therapeutically balanced with peripheral O_2 demands.

Emergent management of the ebb phase requires a brief and thorough physical examination and concurrent resuscitation according to the ABCs. The *a*irway is secured by intubation when the patient cannot adequately protect it; *b*reathing is ensured with provision of assisted ventilation, and oxygenation is supported by using 100% inspired O_2 concentration until results of blood gas analysis indicate changes in the need to support oxygenation. Assisted ventilation prevents the emergence of respiratory muscle fatigue, which by itself will cause death in the shock state. By eliminating the O_2 cost of breathing, fully supported mechanical ventilation reduces O_2 transport needs by as much as 20–25% in the shock state; available O_2 is therefore directed to teleologically more important organs. The *c*irculation (pressure) is restored with initial therapy according to the assessment of cause of the shock state. Two large-bore intravenous cannulas (18 gauge) are inserted in the event that rapid fluid replacement is required. Subsequently, the *d*igestive system requires insertion of a nasogastric tube to reduce the likelihood of aspiration, and the *e*xcretory system is evaluated with a catheter to measure urine output.

Once these basic resuscitative measures have been instituted, attention is then given to rapid identification of the primary cause (Table 5.3). The history of the illness is clearly of paramount importance. If a relevant history is not available, a brief but thorough clinical examination assists in initial categorization of the shock state.

Table 5.3
Clinical Signs of the Three Shock States

Type of shock	Septic	Hypovolemic	Cardiogenic
Profile (↓ = predominant feature)			
Blood pressure	↓	↓	↓
Flow (cardiac output)	↑	↓	(↓)
Afterload (SVR)	(↓)	↑	↑
Preload (PCWP)	↓	(↓)	↑ or ↓
Clinical observations			
Peripheral circulation	Warm, vasodilated	Cool, peripherally vasoconstricted	Cool, peripherally vasoconstricted
Peripheral cyanosis	Not usual	Probable	Probable
Pulse	Bounding	Weak, thready	Weak, thready
Central venous pressure	Not raised	Not raised	Usually raised
Cardiac auscultation	None, except from pre-existing cardiac pathology	None, except from pre-existing cardiac pathology	Gallop, murmur, rub
Laboratory investigations			
ECG	Normal	Normal unless traumatic shock is complicated by myocardial injury	Abnormal
Chest x-ray	Edema possible	Clear	Usually edema, ↑ heart size?
Central venous oxygen content	↑	↓	↓
Arterial-venous oxygen content	↓	↑	↑
PCWP	↓	↓	Usually ↑
Cardiac output	↑	↓	↓

Because of the relationship of pressure to cardiac output and systemic vascular resistance, most instances of cardiogenic and hypovolemic shock are the result of a primary decrease in cardiac output and are therefore accompanied by a compensatory increase in the systemic vascular resistance; clinically, one sees a cool mottled periphery. On the other hand, septic shock in the majority of cases is associated with a primary loss of peripheral vascular resistance with a compensatory increase in flow (CO). This hyperdynamic, warm shock state is easily differentiated from the cool vasoconstricted shock state and may give one initial guidance in diagnosis.

Basic laboratory investigations further assist in determining the cause of shock in a majority of cases. Investigations that aid in the initial diagnosis include Hb/Hct, WBC, electrolytes, blood gases, blood sugar, ECG, and chest x-ray. Tests that may serve as a baseline for later management include blood gases, AST, LDH, CPK, creatinine and BUN.

Once the patient's blood pressure has been initially restored with an inotropic agent or volume expansion, and while the search for the underlying cause of the shock state continues, monitoring techniques that are appropriate to the case should be initiated (Table 5.4). It is important to emphasize that therapy based on an isolated measurement of one monitored index may be inappropriate or misleading; a more effective approach to diagnosis and subsequent treatment is based on the understanding that monitored indices give the best information when looked at over a period of time, and especially in response to a therapeutic modality.

HYPOVOLEMIC SHOCK

Hypovolemic shock occurs when left ventricular preload is too low to support an adequate stroke volume; hence, blood pressure falls.

Loss of intravascular volume of up to 1 to 1.5 liters may be adequately compensated for to maintain blood pressure by mechanisms that were previously defined. In volume-depleted states, the intravascular volume is initially defended by autotransfusion of fluid from the interstitial space, decreased urinary free water excretion under the influence of antidiuretic hormone (ADH), and increased sodium reabsorption in the proximal convoluted tubule of the kidney. Only when these mechanisms fail to maintain intravascular volume does hypovolemic shock develop, usually when the circulatory volume is less than 50 to 70% of normal. When the volume falls to lower than that level, intravascular volume loss is too great to maintain the ventricular preload necessary to support an adequate CO; therefore, blood pressure and

Table 5.4
Techniques for Monitoring Shock

Index	Method	Comment
Blood pressure Pulse pressure, postural drop	Sphygmomanometer, Doppler, intra-arterial	Wide pulse pressure in sepsis; orthostatic drop = volume depletion.
Heart rate	Palpation, oscilloscope	Sinus tachycardia usually $<$ 150 beats/min; if $\geq$ 150, consider primary tachyarrythmia.
Filling pressure Preload	CVP, PCWP (Swan-Ganz catheter)	Giant V waves in mitral insufficiency; sequential change is better indication of effect of therapy.
Cardiac output	Fick principle, dye dilution, thermodilution, radionuclide angiography	High CO is typical of sepsis.
Arterial blood gases	Arterial, capillary	Capillary gases may be misleading with vasoconstriction or with ↓ BP.
Central venous gases	Via Swan-Ganz, via CVP	Central venous O_2 saturation varies directly with CO over short periods of observation.
Urine output Urine sodium, urine/serum osmolality	Indwelling catheter	↓ CO = ↓ renal blood flow ↓ UO ($<$30 ml/hr) ↓ urine Na ($<$20 mEq/liter) U/S osmolality ratio $>$2.1)
Arterial lactate	Biochemistry	↑ With poor microcirculatory perfusion = prognostic index.

Derived index	Formula
1. Arterial O_2 content (vol %)	A. % Saturation (Hb $\times$ 1.39) + 0.003 PaO_2
2. Venous O_2 content (vol %)	B. % Saturation (Hb $\times$ 1.39) + 0.003 $P\bar{v}O_2$
3. Arterial-venous O_2 content gradient	Formula A − Formula B above
4. Fick principle	$\text{Flow (CO)} = \dfrac{\text{oxygen consumption}}{\text{arterial-venous } O_2 \text{ content gradient}}$
5. Mean blood pressure	⅓ (pulse pressure) + diastolic (mm Hg)
6. Systemic vascular resistance index	$\dfrac{\overline{BP} - \overline{CVP}}{CI} \times 80\ (\text{dynes}\cdot\text{sec}\cdot\text{cm}^{-5}/\text{m}^2)$
7. Pulmonary vascular resistance index	$\dfrac{\overline{PA} - PCWP}{CI} \times 80\ (\text{dynes}\cdot\text{sec}\cdot\text{cm}^{-5}/\text{m}^2)$
8. Stroke volume index	$\dfrac{CI}{HR} \times 1000\ (\text{ml/beat/m}^2)$

systemic O_2 transport fall to critical levels. A depressed ventricular preload is responsible for the fall in stroke volume along a singular Frank-Starling curve (Fig. 5.2). Without pre-existing disease (e.g., ischemic heart disease), myocardial contractility is not depressed in hypovolemic shock until the duration of the shock state results in lactic acidosis and the release of myocardial-depressant factor from the splanchnic circulation.

When the cause of acute hypovolemia is associated with hemorrhage, the loss of hemoglobin further compounds the decrease in systemic O_2 transport.

Pre-existing disease, such as ischemic heart disease, modifies the compensatory response to hypovolemia, thereby reducing the efficiency of mechanisms meant to defend the blood pressure. For example, augmented contractility to support the CO, under the influence of elevated endogenous catecholamine secretion, is blunted in the patient with heart disease

The primary treatment required is reconstitution of the defect in intravascular volume. Loss of intravascular volume may be primarily due to blood loss (ruptured spleen, upper GI bleed, musculoskeletal trauma), plasma loss (burns, radical surgery involving the retroperitoneum), water loss (Addison's disease, heat stroke), or any combination of the above.

Diagnosis

By definition, hypovolemic shock is associated with a depressed cardiac output secondary to a reduction in effective preload (intravascular volume). Compensatory mechanisms include an increase in the peripheral vascular resistance and heart rate. Therefore, initial diagnosis may be suspected in the presence of:

1. Depressed intravascular volume and ventricular preload: orthostatic hypotension, lack of diaphoresis, depressed CVP and PCWP;
2. Reduced flow (cardiac output): narrowed pulse pressure, reduced central venous O_2 saturation ($<50\%$), widened arterial-venous O_2 gradient (>5 vol %);
3. Increased peripheral resistance: cool, mottled periphery, decreased skin temperature;
4. An obvious source of volume loss.

Monitoring

In the ebb phase of resuscitation from hypovolemic shock, monitoring is directed toward establishing that the blood pressure has been restored to levels compatible with adequate core and peripheral perfusion. This is simply assessed by defining the mean pressure where urine output is $>$ 30 ml/hr, restlessness or obtundation is reversed, and, the periphery is beginning to vasodilate.

In the flow phase of resuscitation, treatment goals are directed toward establishing that systemic O_2 transport now matches peripheral O_2 requirements. With reversal of the O_2 debt of the shock state, arterial lactate falls and central venous O_2 saturation increases.

Treatment

Underlying Disease

Concurrent with resuscitation of the shock state, attention is directed toward controlling the source of volume loss. This is most crucial in hemorrhage, where control of blood loss is mandatory to ensure prompt resuscitation.

Ebb Phase

At least two large-bore IV access sites are established in hypovolemic shock for fluid replacement. As previously discussed, blood is drawn for initial hematologic and biochemical evaluation, as well as for cross-matching.

The pneumatic antishock garment (PASG) may be applied to assist in restoration of the pressure before adequate volume resuscitation is completed. Once applied, the PASG should be removed cautiously and only after pressure is sufficiently restored with volume resuscitation. If hemorrhage occurs, it should not be removed until the patient is in the OR, where definitive control of the site of blood loss is possible.

Intravascular volume replacement is the obvious first-line treatment in hypovolemic shock. Fluid resuscitation restores a constricted ventricular preload and thereby supports an increase in cardiac output and blood pressure. A combination of crystalloid (Ringer's lactate) and colloid (5% albumin) is administered, generally in a ratio of 3:1. Colloid has the advantage of restoring the intravascular volume more rapidly, with effects that are longer-lasting than equivalent amounts of crystalloid.

When inotropic support is needed, Dopamine is our agent of choice for treating hypovolemic shock because it has less of an adverse effect on renal, splanchnic, and hepatic flow than other currently available inotropic agents.

The PaO_2 is maintained above 65 mm Hg with oxygen therapy administered by mask or an endotracheal tube, with mechanical ventilation as necessary (see indications for ventilation). Pulmonary insufficiency (ARDS) may occur with hypovolemic shock and requires early recognition and equally early treatment.

Pharmacologic doses of steroids (e.g., Solu-Medrol 30 mg/kg IV) have been suggested as being of benefit in the treatment of hypovolemic shock. Their efficacy in enhancing myocardial contractility, improving peripheral microcirculatory perfusion, aiding in the delivery of oxygen to the periphery, and "stabilizing" ischemic cells is apparent in some animal models. However, a careful clinical trial in human hypovolemic shock patients is not yet available.

In the hypovolemic patient, it is important to minimize therapeutic interventions that might further decrease the preload. So, if possible, avoid positive end-expiratory pressure, intravenous narcotics, the use of the Trendelenberg position, and excessive rapid warming in the marginally hypothermic patient. If any such therapy is necessary, a further increase in fluid infusion may be required to offset any accompanying decrease in preload.

Flow Phase

Resuscitation of the patient with hypovolemic shock must continue beyond treatment of the ebb phase in which blood pressure is restored to that level commensurate with reversal of the clinical signs of shock (Table 5.5). Major therapeutic goals during the flow phase of this illness include (1) maintenance of the restored perfusion pressure to the core circulation; (2) restoration of a contracted ECF volume, which was initially redistributed to the intravascular compartment during entry into the shock phase to support the blood pressure by augmenting ventricular preload; (3) support of systemic O_2t at the level required to match what is frequently an increased systemic $\dot{V}O_2$ following hypovolemic shock, thereby ensuring adequate cellular O_2 availability; and (4) definitive management of the cause of the hypovolemic state, if not previously accomplished.

Crystalloid is preferentially used to maintain the volume of the intravascular compartment at this time, thereby supporting ECF volume repletion. Lack of an adequately restored intravascular volume to support ECF volume repletion in a patient, who is now presumably normotensive, is determined by these findings on clinical examination: a lack of perspiration, orthostatic hypotension, a cool periphery, and tachycardia. Further, examination of the marginally volume-depleted patient usually demonstrates a low urine output (< 30 ml/hr) characterized by a high urine osmolality and a low urine sodium (< 20 mEq/liter). Management of this portion of the flow phase is usually adequately monitored by such clinical and laboratory examination in the young, previously healthy patient. In elderly patients, however, particularly those with underlying coronary artery disease, a flow-directed right-heart catheter may more safely guide adequate IFV volume and thereby ECF volume restitution.

To improve the systemic O_2t to match systemic $\dot{V}O_2$ (Table 5.5), a sequential approach to management based on the variables defined within the O_2 transport equation is followed. Initially, the arterial O_2 content is maximized by guidelines previously defined, including maintenance of hemoglobin between 11 and 13 gm/dl, a hematocrit between 35 and 45%, and an SaO_2 in excess of 97%. If biochemical evidence for significant, ongoing anaerobic metabolism still exists (e.g., a falling $SmvO_2$ and an increasing aterial lactate), therapy is directed toward improving the cardiac output and therefore, systemic O_2t and using a well-defined algorithm based on monitored hemodynamic parameters. Fluid administration is the initial modality of choice to improve cardiac output when the PCWP is < 15 mm Hg, as stroke volume increases with an augmented LV preload, according to the Frank-Starling principle. The choice of fluid is debatable, assuming that pretreatment goals for the preferred concentration of hemoglobin have been attained. We prefer to use colloid (5% albumin). Fluid is administered in sequential aliquots of 250 to 500 ml boluses over a short time period, and the change in the PCWP with each aliquot of fluid is monitored. When the PCWP approaches 12 to 15 mm Hg, further fluid administration does not usually augment LV preload to enhance the stroke volume significantly because this reflection of the LV end-diastolic pressure usually defies the inflection of the left ventricular end-diastolic pressure, end-diastolic volume (compliance) curve (Fig. 5.3, points B → C). At the inflection of the left ventricular compliance curve, the ability of fluid administration to increase preload marginally, hence to increase stroke volume, is likely offset by the possibility of a sudden rise in the PCWP to levels potentially associated with the development of pulmonary edema. When the PCWP is in excess of 15 mm Hg, either when initially monitored or after one or sequential fluid boluses, and when a defined need exists to augment further cardiac output to support O_2t, therapeutic alternatives include the use of systemic vasodilators or positive inotropic agents.

Table 5.5
Management Protocol for the Flow Phase of Hypovolemic Shock

Treatment goals
Maintain blood pressure and restore systemic O_2 to match systemic VO_2

Investigation
- Hemoglobin/hematocrit
- Arterial blood gases
- Swan-Ganz catheter—measure the cardiac output (calculate the systemic O_2t) and mixed venous gases (evaluate the SvO_2 and the A-VO_2 difference)

Definitive management
O_2 transport = cardiac output × arterial oxygen content
(1) maintain Hb 11 to 13 gm/dl
(2) maintain PaO_2 > 70 mm Hg

(1) Augment LV preload: use IV fluid/RBCs to maintain PCWP 12 to 15 mm Hg.

(2) Consider *cautious* vasodilation if the mean BP is adequate and stable (e.g., nitroglycerine, apresoline, nitroprusside)[a]; with a decline in the PCWP following arterial vasodilation, more fluid must be administered to augment CO by the Frank-Starling mechanism.

(3) Augment LV contractility: HCO_3 if the arterial pH is 7.25 or inotropic support (see Table 5.7)

(4) Augment the chronotropic response if the HR is <70 beats/min: isoproterenol, flow-directed pacemaker.

[a] If the mean BP is less than desired, or unstable, proceed to step 3.

If the mean level of the systemic blood pressure will clinically allow modest arterial vasodilation, vasodilators may be cautiously attempted before inotropic agents are used. Vasodilators usually promote LV relaxation, (Fig. 5.3, points D → A) allowing for the administration of more resuscitative fluid because the LV preload will now be defined by a lower PCWP than previously. With the combination of cautious impedance reduction therapy and concurrent fluid administration, stroke volume—hence systemic O_2t—will be substantially improved as a larger LV preload is now reflected by a lower PCWP. Adminstration of a vasodilator to improve LV compliance, and potentially also to improve microcirculatory O_2 delivery by relaxing precapillary sphincter tone, *must be done cautiously*, with close attention paid to its effects on the mean blood pressure and the PCWP. For an optimal improvement of O_2t, most vasodilators require the concurrent administration of fluid to augment LV preload.

When the mean blood pressure is not adequate to allow the safe use of a vasodilator or when the mean blood pressure falls more than 10 mm Hg with its administration, inotropic agents are employed in the patient with signs of ongoing anaerobic metabolism during the flow phase of resuscitation. We prefer Dopamine in this situation because of its unique spectrum of action. Dobutamine may increase cardiac output while concurrently mediating mild systemic vasodilation. Levophed has been used, particularly in the flow phase of resuscitation of hypovolemic shock, in patients with concurrent acute pulmonary hypertension. Regardless of the positive inotrope chosen, well-defined therapeutic goals should be prospectively established—that is, the level of systemic O_2t desired—and monitoring of appropriate hemodynamic and biochemical indices should then be sequentially performed to ensure when such therapeutic goals are attained.

Once monitored indices define that the systemic O_2t is supporting the $\dot{V}O_2$, all pharmacologic and nonparmacologic interventions that have been used to attain this goal are carefully re-evaluated as to their ongoing need. An orderly approach to withdrawal of supportive therapy with successful resuscitation during the flow phase requires sequential clinical, laboratory, and, when needed, hemodynamic monitoring to ensure that the systemic O_2t continues to match the metabolic needs of the patient during withdrawal. Only one of the previously provided supportive interventions is withdrawn at a time so that, if an untoward change occurs, the clinician is aware which modality of support was responsible for that change.

SEPTIC SHOCK

Septic shock may be due to the sequelae of inflammation on a bacterial, fungal, or viral basis. As a result of the inflammatory process, peripheral vasodilation and an increase in microvascular permeability occur; both events cause a decrease in intravascular volume, which is thereby rendered insufficient to support cardiac output and blood pressure. Additionally, it has been suggested that a circulating myocardial-depressant factor depresses ventricular contractility further in septic shock. Therefore, cardiac output, blood pressure, and O_2 transport fall because of (1) a depressed ventricular preload and (2) depressed ventricular contractility. In contrast, the normotensive septic syndrome is characterized by normal ventricular contractility and profound peripheral vasodilation; an increase in cardiac output is responsible for the hyperdynamic circulatory state most frequently observed in this stage of the host response to severe inflammation.

In the earliest stages of septic shock, peripheral vasodilation is accompanied by an increase in O_2 extraction in the periphery to satisfy cellular O_2 requirements. Later in septic shock, evidence of an inability of cellular utilization of available O_2 predominates, and vasoconstriction may supersede the vasodilated state. Therefore, septic shock is characterized by a hyperdynamic circulation in the presence of peripheral vasodilation (warm periphery), with vasodilation of the resistance (arteriolar) and capacitance (venular) sides of the peripheral circulation, resulting in a functionally volume-depleted state ($\downarrow$ preload) (Table 5.3).

Occasionally septic shock presents primarily as an increase in the peripheral vascular resistance and a normal-to-low flow state. In this situation, the initial phase of vasodilation and relative volume depletion has likely not been clinically recognized or has been of short duration. The vasoconstricted type of septic shock carries a worse prognosis than the vasodilated type, only because it indicates severe sympathoadrenal discharge in response to a prolonged functional volume loss.

The source of the vasoactive mediators responsible for the hyperdynamic state may be the septic focus itself and is not simply the result of endotoxin liberated from Gram negative bacteria. Although the exact mediators remain unknown, it seems that activation of the complement system is necessary for the full clinical picture to emerge. Both Gram negative and Gram positive septicemias present with an initial decrease in resistance, and no clinical feature adequately discriminates between these two types of septic shock.

Diagnosis and Investigation

The hallmark of early septic shock is usually a vasodilated, hyperdynamic circulatory state in the presence of clinical evidence of intravascular volume depletion. The presence of an associated inflammatory focus may or may not be apparent during the initial presentation. The diagnosis may therefore be suspected in the presence of:

1. Increased flow: bounding, full pulses with a narrow arterial-venous O_2 tension gradient (<4 vol %) and a high central venous O_2 saturation (>50%);
2. Decreased resistance: warm, vasodilated periphery with a depressed calculated systemic vascular resistance;
3. Depressed intravascular volume and low preload: orthostatic hypotension and absence of diaphoresis with a low PCWP.

Although oliguria accompanies most types of shock, septic shock may present with a polyuric state. It is not known why a patient with early septic shock is unable to concentrate the urine maximally to defend the intravascular volume, but this inability may be related to abnormalities in intrarenal compartmentalization of blood flow leading to renal sodium loss and a form of "nephrogenic" diabetes insipidus.

Concurrent with resuscitation of the associated hypotension, it is important to initiate investigation of the cause of the septic state. A brief, but thorough history and investigation may raise one's suspicions of an inflammatory focus. Cultures and gram stains of blood, urine, sputum, and, where indicated, of surgical wounds or CSF are obtained before antibiotic administration; three blood cultures should identify a bacteremia, when present, in more than 90% of cases.

Specialized investigative techniques for identification of the inflammatory focus, such as radionuclide scanning, ultrasonography, and computed tomography, should not be conducted until after the patient has been resuscitated in the ebb phase and stabilization of pressures characteristic of the flow phase has been achieved.

Monitoring

Septic shock is frequently associated with multiorgan dysfunction. Appropriate evaluation of the pulmonary (ARDS), renal (acute renal failure), hepatic, hematopoietic (DIC), gastrointestinal (erosive gastritis), CNS (encephalopathy), and cardiovascular (myocardiitis) systems is therefore essential. Monitoring of these organ systems to these identify complications that may accompany septic shock is discussed elsewhere in this text (Chapter 31).

Treatment

As in hypovolemic shock, treatment of septic shock may be discussed under two major headings, the *ebb* and *flow* phases.

Ebb Phase

General resuscitation principles in the ebb phase are the same as those defined in the ABCs of resuscitation. In this state, initial goals are to restore core and then peripheral perfusion and to ensure adequate flow and O_2 transport as rapidly as possible as autoregulation to many organs is lost in the shock state.

If clinical assessment confirms the presence of volume depletion—the usual picture in septic shock—rapid intravenous restoration of the intravascular compartment with Ringer's lactate and colloid (ratio 3:1) is instituted. With concurrent anemia, packed RBCs are used as part of the volume replacement to maintain the hemoglobin between 11 and 13 gm/dl. If, however, clinical assessment suggests the presence of intravascular volume excess, or when there is evidence of underlying heart disease that might progress to dangerous ischemia in the face of ongoing hypotension, an inotrope may be used to gain immediate control of the blood pressure. Depending on pre-existing pressure levels, a reasonable goal is to accept a systolic blood pressure of 90–100 mm Hg; with a history of pre-existing hypertension, evidence of restoration of adequate core perfusion (e.g., increase in urine output) may require a sequential upward titration of inotropic support to establish a level of systolic blood pressure that is considered "acceptable." When an inotrope is required, Dopamine is preferred (Table 5.6). Occasionally, the diastolic pressure remains low even with adequate volume resuscitation and the administration of Dopamine. In that situation, coronary flow may fall, and myocardial ischemia will then complicate the clinical picture; then, Levophed may be cautiously attempted to increase the diastolic pressure.

With the persistence of hypotension following initial fluid resuscitation of a septic patient and the need to consider inotropic support, a right-heart and arterial catheter should be inserted to enable measurement of the filling pressures (can more fluid be safely administered?) and intra-arterial pressure (does the cuff pressure accurately reflect the intra-abdominal pressure?).

After securing appropriate samples for culture, broad spectrum antibiotics are given in the presence of septic shock (see below).

Flow Phase

At this stage in the resuscitation of the patient with septic shock, the primary goals are to (1) match systemic O_2 transport with peripheral O_2 demands and (2) provide other essential cellular nutrients.

The septic patient is hypermetabolic and therefore has greater peripheral O_2 demands than patients with most other causes of shock. Hence, systemic O_2 transport usually needs to be supported at higher levels than, for example, in cardiogenic shock to ensure a normal arterial lactate without undue extraction of O_2 within the periphery (e.g., $S\bar{v}O_2 > 50\%$).

Again, the O_2 transport equation shows that optimization of the CaO_2 is adequately maximized with RBC infusion and support of oxygenation (see Chapter 11); primary resuscitation is now directed at the determinants of CO, in a sequential fashion:

1. If the PCWP is low (< 10 mm Hg), use fluid to expand ventricular preload and thereby increase CO according to the Frank-Starling mechanism.
2. If the PCWP is high (> 15 mm Hg), initially try a vasodilator (e.g., nitroglycerine, see Table 5.6), which may improve CO while the PCWP falls; further augmentation of CO by the Frank-Starling mechanism

Table 5.6
Cardiovascular Medications Commonly Used in Resuscitation of the Patient with Shock[a]

Medications	Primary mechanism of action	Dilution	Average dose (range)
Vasodilators			
Nitroglycerine	+ + + venodilator + arterial dilator	50 mg in 250 ml D5W/NS (max. concentrations- 200 mg/250 ml)	33 μg/min (5–66 μg/min) (no max. dose)
Hydralazine	+ + + arterial dilator	50 mg in 500 ml NS	5 mg/hr (1–25 mg/hr)
Sodium nitroprusside	+ + + arterial dilator + + venodilator	50 mg in 50 ml D5W/NS	2 μg/kg/min (0.5 μg/kg/min)
Phentolamine	+ + + arterial dilator + + venodilator (alpha-adrenergic blocker)	300 mg in 500 ml D5W/NS	1 mg/min (0.1–2 mg/min)
Sympathomimetics/inotropes			
Dopamine	DA: + + +β; + + +	400 mg in 500 ml D5W/NS	0.5–2 μg/kg/min 5–15 μg/kg/min
Dobutamine	+ + + β1 + α	500 mg in 500 ml D5W/NS	5 μg/kg/min (2.5–10 μg/min)
Isoproterenol	+ + + β	2 mg/500 D5W/NS	4 μg/min 1–10 μg/min
Norepinephrine	+ + + β; + + +	4 mg NE (base)/1000 ml NS/D5W	4 μg/min 2–20 μg/min

[a] +—indicates degree of activity.

may now be accomplished with added fluid administration. If a drop in mean blood pressure of > 10 mm Hg occurs with vasodilators infused at minimal concentrations, use inotropic agents to improve the CO and O_2 transport. In septic shock, Dopamine may be preferable to Dobutamine because the vasodilating properties of Dobutamine have been noted to cause a drop in blood pressure in septic patients resuscitated early into the flow phase.

Control of Septic Focus

It is axiomatic that rapid eradication of the septic source is necessary to ensure a favorable outcome. In the absence of cultures, initially use a cephalosporin (e.g., Mandol 1 g q6h IV) and an aminoglycoside (e.g., tobramycin, loading dose 1.5–2.0 mg/kg IV, followed by 1.0 mg/kg IV, q8h). If the clinical examination or history suggests the possibility of an anaerobic organism contributing to the genesis of septic shock (e.g., pelvic abscess, aspiration pneumonitis), clindamycin, 600 mg q6h IV, or chloramphenicol, 500 mg q6h IV, is added to the two previous antibiotics. The dose of the aminoglycoside will have to be altered if renal failure occurs. A useful formula is to give one-half the loading dose every 4 times the serum creatinine, in hours. Blood levels should be closely monitored in this situation to maintain a peak (1 hour postinfusion) of 12–20 μg/ml and a trough (1 hour before next dose) of 1–3 μg/ml. If possible, antibiotic therapy should be guided by available Gram stains of suspected foci. Antibiotics are changed, if necessary, with return of positive cultures and identification of the specific organism's susceptibility. Inaccessible foci (e.g., abscesses) should be surgically drained as soon as the clinical hemodynamic pattern is stabilized.

Nutrition

The septic patient is extremely catabolic. In this state, impaired white blood cell function is often noted. Early attention to nutritional replacement by either the intravenous or enteral route is recommended, providing approximately 30–40 kcal/kg/day.

Corticosteroids

As in the case of hypovolemic shock, the use of high-dose corticosteroids in septic shock remains controversial. Recent work suggests that patients treated with methylprednisolone, 30 mg/kg q8h, do not have a more favorable outcome than those not receiving corticosteroids.

Other Treatment

Maintain the PaO_2 > 65 mm Hg; keep the Hb > 11 g/100 ml; and treat acidosis if pH < 7.3.

The single most important modality in the treatment of septic shock is eradication of the septic focus, by antibiotics or antibiotics plus surgical drainage, once the patient's clinical condition has been stabilized.

CARDIOGENIC SHOCK

A depression in ventricular contractility, which is usually secondary to the effects of ischemia, is the primary cause of a decrease in cardiac output in cardiogenic shock. As a compensatory mechanism, systemic resistance increases to maintain pressure; in cardiogenic shock, however, the increase in resistance is usually not sufficient to offset the effects of a profound decrease in flow and shock thereby results.

In about 10–15% of cases, the systemic resistance does not appropriately increase in cardiogenic shock, perhaps due to the presence of an unrecognized autonomic neuropathy or the effect of drugs that the patient was taking before the acute event. These patients therefore present with a low flow state and, unlike the majority of patients with cardiogenic shock, a warm, vasodilated periphery.

Ventricular preload may be low, normal, or high in cardiogenic shock. In some patients, measured end-diastolic filling pressures (e.g., PCWP) are low as volume and salt restriction before the event leaves the patient functionally volume-depleted, intravascularly. In other patients, the PCWP is 18 mm Hg or greater, which may reflect either a large ventricular preload or the effects of acute ischemia that cause a left-shift of the ventricular stiffness curve. In the latter situation, a low ventricular

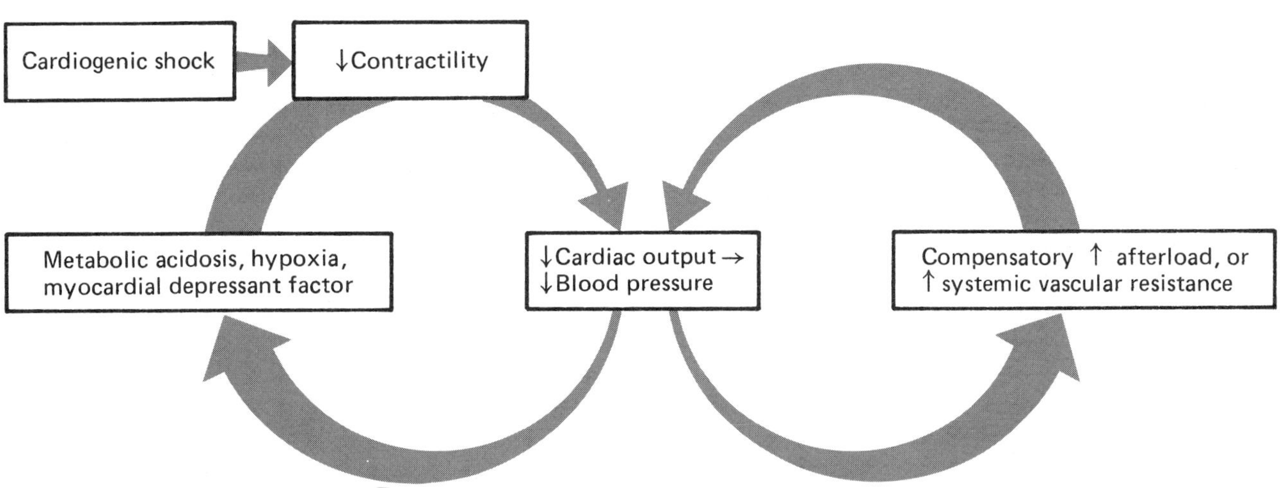

Figure 5.5. Mechanism of cardiogenic shock.

Table 5.7
Causes of Cardiogenic Shock

1. Massive myocardial necrosis following infarction
2. Ventricular septal defect
3. Papillary muscle rupture (mitral insufficiency)
4. Pericardial tamponade
5. Ventricular aneurysm
6. Pulmonary embolism
7. Tachy- or bradyarrhythmias
8. End-stage (severe) congestive/ischemic cardiomyopathy
9. Traumatic myocardiac contusion

preload may very well be reflected by a high measured PCWP (Fig. 5.3).

The outpouring of endogenous catecholamines and other vasoconstrictors (e.g., angiotensin II) in cardiogenic shock supports an increase in the systemic resistance. This increase in left ventricular afterload may further depress cardiac output and, in fact, worsen pre-existing myocardial ischemia. This increase in catecholamines also increases the $M\dot{V}O_2$ and further upsets the balance between coronary blood flow—hence, available O_2—and myocardial O_2 demand. A vicious cycle may therefore be established in cardiogenic shock (Fig. 5.5) because of the effects of further myocardial ischemia; cardiac output may then fall to even greater levels, as will the blood pressure.

Causes of cardiogenic shock other than myocardial ischemia include those conditions listed in Table 5.7. By different means, all these conditions have the same effect: a decrease in cardiac output greater than can be balanced by compensatory factors and a resultant decrease in blood pressure.

Diagnosis

Initially, it is important to establish the myocardium as the underlying cause of the shock state. First, this is accomplished by ruling out hypovolemic and septic shock according to the characteristic historical and physical evidence that distinguishes among the three major types of shock (Table 5.3).

Then, it is necessary to determine that ischemia leading to a critical reduction in ventricular contractile mass is the origin of the cardiogenic shock state and that none of the other clinical conditions listed in Table 5.7 is responsible. History (e.g., pain typical of ischemia) and laboratory examination (e.g., acute ischemia on the ECG, elevated CPK) usually suffice to distinguish ischemia as the cause of the shock state.

A ventricular septal defect (VSD) or papillary muscle rupture leading to acute mitral insufficiency presents with typical murmurs and can be further distinguished by right-heart catheterization; with a VSD, O_2 saturations in the pulmonary artery versus the right atrium show a step-up; with acute mitral insufficiency a characteristic waveform accentuating the V wave is demonstrable with a right-heart catheter in the wedged position. With pericardial tamponade (see Chapter 2) the PCWP and CVP usually increase and show equalization. Ventricular aneurysm, pulmonary embolism, or traumatic ventricular contusion may be suspected from either physical examination or the ECG; contrast ventriculography or scintigraphy is usually required to confirm the diagnosis.

Monitoring

Successful management of cardiogenic shock usually dictates insertion of a right-heart catheter to define the most appropriate method to improve cardiac output, hence blood pressure. Estimating clinically the filling pressures or cardiac output is unreliable in 50% of occasions, which is unacceptable in a disease state that has such a potentially devastating outcome without appropriate therapy.

Monitoring of the patient in cardiogenic shock also involves an ongoing assessment of the work of breathing (respiratory rate) and adequacy of oxygenation (PaO_2), an evaluation of core perfusion (conscious state and urine output), and an assessment, albeit indirect, of the possibility of relief or worsening of myocardial ischemia as indicated by changes in the height of the ST segments (continuous ECG monitoring).

Cardiogenic Shock Secondary to Muscle Necrosis

The remainder of this section discusses cardiogenic shock secondary to massive muscle necrosis. The other causes of cardiogenic shock listed in Table 5.7 are not frequently encountered, yet remain clinically important to identify so that appropriate management can be offered. In order to determine initial therapy and probable prognosis, cardiogenic shock secondary to massive myocardial necrosis may be categorized as follows, using invasive bedside monitoring:

1. Hypoperfusion (cardiac index < 2.2 liter/minute/m^2) *without* pulmonary congestion (PCWP < 18 mm Hg)—mortality rate about 60%.
2. Hypoperfusion (cardiac index < 2.2 liter/minute/m^2) *with* pulmonary congestion (PCWP > 18 mm Hg—mortality rate about 90%.

Following initiation of therapy, it is important to establish that treatment has been appropriate as indicated by an improvement in flow and decrease in systemic vascular resistance (see hypovolemic shock). Similarly, the "double product", the systemic BP multiplied by the heart rate, may be followed as an approximation of whether therapy has been associated with a relative increase or decrease in the $M\dot{V}O_2$.

Treatment

Initial management of cardiogenic shock of any cause involves attention to the general principles of resuscitation prevously discussed and includes the following elements:

1. With obtundation or an increase in the work of breathing, use *intubation* and provision of *assisted ventilation*. Experimentally, the use of assisted ventilation reduces mortality more than 50% when compared to permitting spontaneous ventilation. Such therapy reduces systemic O_2 consumption by omitting

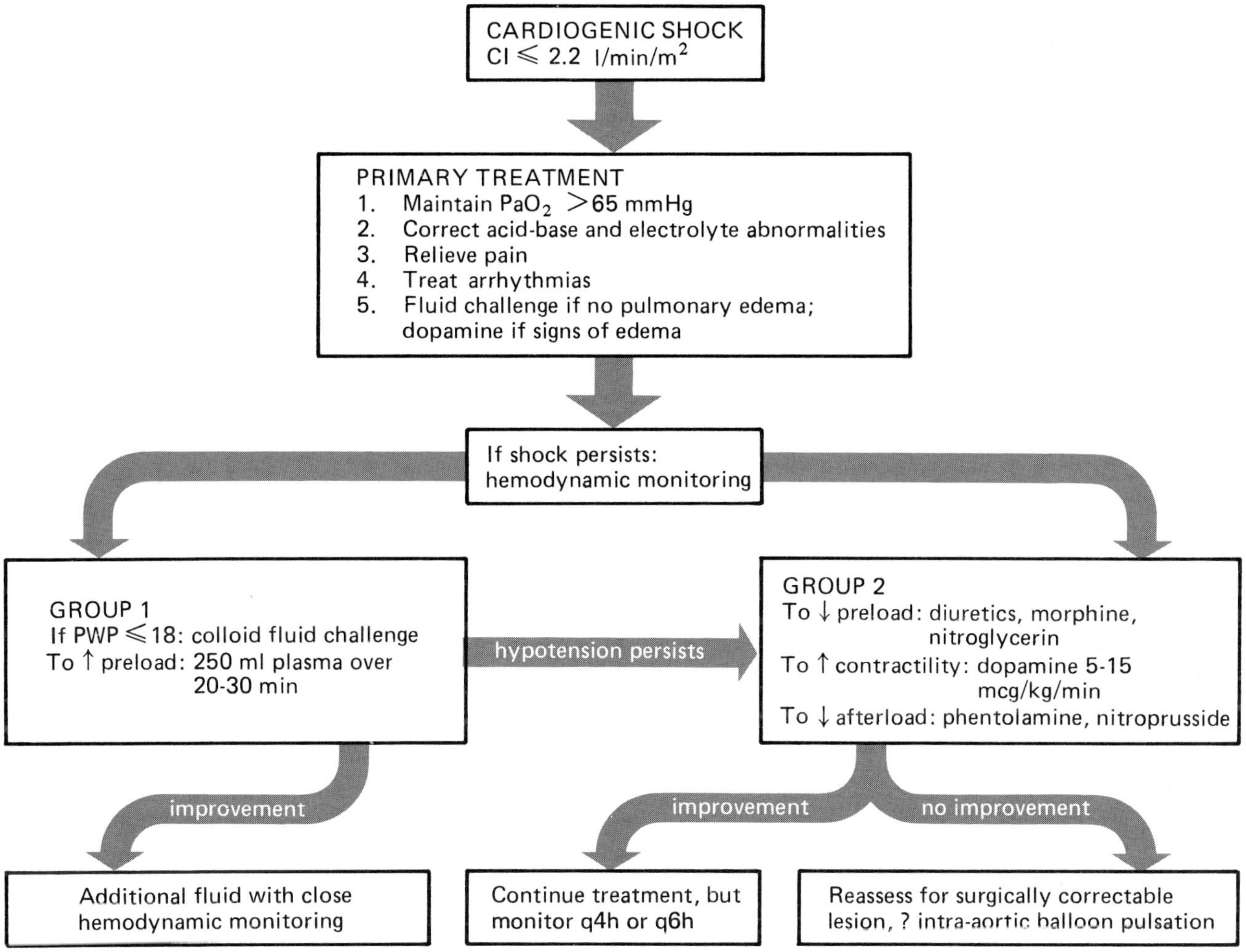

Figure 5.6. Management of cardiogenic shock.

work requirement by respiratory musculature; demands on the myocardium to support O_2 transport are thereby reduced and theoretically, $M\dot{V}O_2$ should fall.

2. *Relief of pain* further reduces $M\dot{V}O_2$ by minimizing peripheral requirements for O_2. *Correction of an acidosis* if the pH is < 7.25 should be accompanied by improved contractility. Management of arrhythmias to ensure, as much as possible, normal sinus rhythm reduces the risk of sudden cardiac death and provides for a better cardiac output by allowing adequate ventricular filling. It remains debatable whether prophylaxis against lethal ventricular arrhythmias can be achieved with the administration of lidocaine (2 mg/min) to reduce the risk of sudden cardiac death in cardiogenic shock; in the light of available evidence and the gravity of the disease state, lethal arrhythmic prophylaxis is probably not unreasonable.
3. If clinical evidence of pulmonary congestion is not initially apparent, one may assume that the patient is functionally volume-depleted and might respond to a fluid challenge with an improvement in cardiac output according to the Frank-Starling mechanism. There are many reasons for volume depletion in patients with cardiogenic shock, including the previous use of diuretics and an inappropriate translocation of intravascular volume from the core circulation to the interstitium. While such a fluid challenge is being administered, the clinician closely monitors the status of the jugular venous pressure, heart rate, pulmonary extravascular lung water (rales, bronchospasm), and heart sounds (gallop). If no response to the fluid challenge is apparent or pulmonary congestion is initially present, Dopamine is infused to keep the mean $\overline{BP}$ over 70–80 mm Hg until further invasive monitoring can be instituted.

   Improvement in cardiac output is accompanied by: ↑ urine output (and ↑ urine sodium, ↓ U/S (urine/serum) osmolality ratio), ↑ PaO_2, ↓ confusion, without evidence of worsening of pulmonary edema. Examination, therefore, often enables the physician to monitor the initial response to primary resuscitative therapy.
4. Hemodynamic monitoring. Persistence of shock, despite a fluid challenge or the requirement for inotropic

support, requires invasive hemodynamic monitoring, with subsequent therapy based on the presence or absence of pulmonary congestion.

Group 1: No Pulmonary Congestion

In this group, a low cardiac output is not accompanied by pulmonary edema. Generally, a PCWP of < 18 mm Hg indicates that cardiac pulmonary edema is unlikely and that the patient's individual Starling curve may initially be manipulated with a fluid challenge in an effort to increase the cardiac output. Although there is still debate about the type of fluid to use, we currently employ Ringer's lactate or plasma at a rate of 250 ml over 30 minutes. At that time, a repeat hemodynamic assessment will delineate if the patient has improved, is still in group 1 and can tolerate another fluid challenge, or has moved into group 2.

If the response to the fluid challenge has been an increase in the PCWP < 5 mm Hg and remains < 18 mm Hg, the patient is on the flat portion of the ventricular stiffness curve and will usually tolerate another fluid challenge to attempt further improvement in the cardiac output. However, if the response to a fluid challenge is an increase in the PCWP > 5 mm Hg (or the PCWP is now > 18 mm Hg), the patient is on the steep, ascending portion of the ventricular stiffness curve (Fig. 5.3) and will not tolerate further fluid without the risk of developing pulmonary edema; this response now dictates management as outlined for Group 2 patients.

It is obvious that a fluid challenge is the least detrimental to the patient because no major increase in $\dot{M}VO_2$ occurs with clinical responsiveness to this type of therapy.

Group 2: Pulmonary Congestion

In this group of patients, a low cardiac output is accompanied by hemodynamic evidence favoring pulmonary edema (e.g., a PCWP > 18 mm Hg). The patient is on the flat portion (plateau) of the Frank-Starling curve and the steep ascending portion of the ventricular stiffness curve; further fluid resuscitation is therefore not indicated.

A high PCWP may indicate a low or a high ventricular preload. Nonetheless, a high PCWP results in an increase in $\dot{M}VO_2$ and promotes the development of pulmonary edema. Intubation and the application of PEEP reduce the effective PCWP by impeding venous return and decreasing ventricular afterload, thereby allowing for improved ventricular ejection. Assisted ventilation also reduces the demands on cardiac performance, as previously discussed. Pharmacologically, the PCWP may also be reduced with diuretics; morphine (5–10 mg IV) and nitrates, including nitropaste (½–1 square inch), sublingual nitroglycerine (0.3 mg), or parenteral nitroglycerine. With shock, however, the use of agents that might reduce the systemic resistance, such as nitrates, nitroprusside, apresoline, or phentolamine, is dangerous because a decrease in resistance can worsen the shock state by further reducing a critical coronary blood flow. Potent vasodilators cannot therefore be recommended in cardiogenic shock until an adequate systemic pressure has been restored with vasopressors/inotropic agents (Table 5.6).

Therefore, concurrent with intubation and application of PEEP with assisted ventilation, restoration of blood pressure in Group 2 cardiogenic shock is accomplished with inotropic agents. Dopamine is used initially and is simply titrated to attain the desired blood pressure. Restoration of the blood pressure to those levels consistent with a normal sensorium, adequate urine output, and reversal of peripheral vasoconstriction is the specific goal of resuscitation in the ebb phase. The level of pressure at which such goals are reached differs among patients; usually, a systemic pressure of 80–100 mm Hg suffices, but in a previously hypertensive patient, this level will likely need to be moved upward. At this time, the effects of Dopamine on the cardiac output, central venous O_2 saturation, and arterial lactate are measured. Dobutamine is felt by some to be superior to Dopamine; however, the ability of Dobutamine to vasodilate at the same time as it increases cardiac output may be of harm if coronary blood flow falls.

Specific Pharmacotherapy in Cardiogenic Shock

Vasodilators

Intravenous vasodilators may be classified into those that exert maximal action on the arterial tree (decrease afterload or resistance), those that exert maximal action on the capacitance or venous system, and those with a combination of arterial and venous effects.

In cardiogenic shock, vasodilators are used only when two conditions are met:

1. Blood pressure adequate to sustain core perfusion has been attained with either fluid or inotropic therapy.
2. The PCWP is elevated (e.g., greater than 16 to 18 mm Hg). In cardiogenic shock, the ability of vasodilators to improve cardiac output further is primarily seen when left ventricular preload is normal to larger than normal.

Generally, the mechanism of action of vasodilators is to facilitate cardiac output by reducing ventricular afterload. If insufficient healthy myocardium has survived the acute ischemic event or if ventricular preload is less than normal, their action may be only one of reducing pressure as an increase in cardiac output is then not sufficient to negate the effect of a depressed systemic resistance.

Use of vasodilators in cardiogenic shock requires clear definition of goals of therapy, such as to decrease the blood pressure by no more than 10% of baseline, followed by an assessment of changes in cardiac output, O_2 transport, and arterial lactate to ensure that any change in flow has been upward *and* is associated with improved O_2 transport, or a tendency for the arterial lactate to fall.

Nitroprusside

Nitroprusside reduces arterial tone and hence BP (afterload), as well as relaxes venous tone. Clinically, it therefore decreases the SVR and PCWP. After pressure has been stabilized at levels to ensure a core perfusion it is an ideal agent for "combination" therapy in cardiogenic shock with an initial dose of 15 μg/minute and increments every 10–15 minutes of 15 μg/minute. The increase in dose is stopped when the BP falls and/or the desired reduction in PCWP is obtained. Nitroprusside can therefore improve CO by improving the patient's position on the Frank-Starling curve, as well as decreasing impedance to ejection and hence shifting the curve up and to the left.

Phentolamine

Phentolamine has its maximum effect on the arterial resistance, with only a minimal effect on the PCWP. When used, it may then improve CO only by impedance reduction and not by lowering the patient's position on the Frank-Starling curve. Intravenous therapy is 0.1 mg/min as a starting dose with careful titration up to a maximum of 2.0 mg/min, according to the reduction in blood pressure that the clinician is prepared to accept.

Nitroglycerin

Intravenously, nitroglycerin has its maximum action on the venous capacitance system and hence reduces PCWP and improves CO by reducing the patient's position on the Frank-Starling curve. Intravenously, we start with 0.5 mg/hour and carefully increase it to a maximum of 2 mg/hour, titrating its effects by the change in PCWP and cardiac output.

Inotropic Agents

Digoxin

Digoxin is not used to increase contractility or decrease preload in cardiogenic shock, even in the presence of a high PCWP, except for treating associated atrial arrhythmias. We prefer instead to use inotropic agents or, when possible, vasodilators (as above) to reduce preload. Further, digoxin may cause splanchnic ischemia, a potentially deleterious complication of any low flow state.

Digoxin is reserved for its effect on AV condition and hence is used with atrial tachyarrhythmias, to slow nodal conduction to the ventricle.

Improved flow with slowing of the ventricular response to PAT, for example, is due to improved ventricular filling during diastole. Conversion of arterial tachyarrhythmias to sinus rhythm with digoxin also supports improved flow because of restoration of the atrial kick.

Sympathomimetic Agents

Dopamine is our agent of choice to increase myocardial contractility in group 2 patients, because it does so while affecting $M\dot{V}O_2$ less than isoproterenol. It is unique in that at low dose ranges (1–6 μg/kg/min) it improves renal, splanchnic, and mesenteric blood flow in addition to improving myocardial contractility. At a dose range of 8–12 μg/kg/min it has effects similar to isoproterenol, and over 15 μg/kg/min, it acts like an α-agonist. Dobutamine is a new agent that is said to have less peripheral vascular effects than Dopamine and is more of a pure inotrope. It is used in dose ranges of 2.5–10 μg/kg min. Isoproterenol is an effective inotrope, but tends to produce its effect with a greater increase in $M\dot{V}O_2$ than the other agents described, because of its relatively greater effect on HR.

Levophed may be required to restore pressure in some patients. The reason why Dopamine or Dobutamine may fail to achieve this clinical goal may be "receptor fatigue." Levophed should only be given to patients who have been adequately volume resuscitated.

Circulatory Assist

The principle of intra-aortic counterpulsation involves the application of electrocardiographically synchronized diastolic balloon pumping so that the aortic diastolic pressures rises, and aortic systolic pressures remain the same or decrease while aortic mean pressures rise. This particular technique of assisted circulation is the only one that has received extensive trial in cardiogenic shock secondary to myocardial infarction. Experimental and clinical studies have shown that counterpulsation systems augment diastolic coronary perfusion and thereby improve nutrition (e.g., O_2 transport) to the myocardium; reduce the aortic systolic and end-diastolic pressures and therefore the workload and oxygen consumption of the heart; and augment the perfusion of peripheral tissues, which reverses somewhat metabolic insufficiency and lactic acidosis. Despite transient reversal of many of the critical hemodynamic and metabolic factors associated with shock, survival during balloon pumping has largely been confined to the period of actual assistance. In-hospital mortality after balloon pumping may differ little from shock therapy where pharmacologic management is the sole approach.

The primary area of application of intra-aortic balloon pumping is in the support of a fragile patient with cardiogenic shock whose candidacy for surgical procedures, such as aortocoronary bypass graft and aneurysmectomy, requires additional studies. Because coronary arteriography and left ventriculography impose additional hazards, circulatory assistance may prevent or offset hemodynamic deterioration before anticipated surgical intervention.

UNRESPONSIVE SHOCK

In a patient who presents with shock unresponsive to one's best diagnostic and therapeutic interventions, it is essential that re-evaluation of diagnosis be considered. Some of the common causes of "unresponsive" shock are outlined in Table 5.8.

Table 5.8
Causes of Unresponsive Shock

Unrecognized pneumothorax
Addison's disease
Unrecognized pericardial effusion
Shock 2° to intestinal ischemia
"Cold" septic shock
Shock 2° to brainstem dysfunction (i.e., neurogenic)

SUMMARY

Response to therapy of shock need not be judged inadequate if previously defined levels of BP are not attained. Many physicians are often not satisfied until the magical "120/80 mm Hg" figure is reached. In reality we should be satisfied with the attainment of any level of blood pressure that is compatible with evidence of improved core perfusion, as monitored by urine output and improved mentation. This level may indeed be below a previously recorded BP for the patient. Any further attempt to elevate the BP is not necessary, and may indeed increase the extent of myocardial damage by increasing oxygen need in ischemic, but not as yet necrotic, tissue.

Suggested Readings

Abraham E, Bland RD, Cobo JC, Shoemaker WC: Sequential cardiorespiratory patterns associated with outcome in septic shock. *Chest* 85:75–79, 1984.

Bregman D, Kaskel P: Advances in percutaneous intra-aortic balloon pumping. *Crit Care Clin* 2:221–236, 1986.

Chatterjee K: Myocardial infarction shock. *Crit Care Clin* 1:563–590, 1985.

Chernow B, Rainey TG, Lake CR: Endogenous and exogenous catecholamines in critical care medicine. *Crit Care Med* 10:409–416, 1982.

Cohn JN: Blood pressure measurements in shock mechanisms of inaccuracy in auscultatory and palpatory methods. *JAMA* 199:972, 1967.

Connors AF, McCaffree DR, Gray BA: Evaluation of right heart catheterization in the critically ill patients without acute myocardial infarction. *N Engl J Med* 308:263–267, 1983.

Forrester JS, Diamond G, Swan HJC: Correlation classification of clinical and hemodynamic function after acute myocardial infarction. *Am J Cardiol* 39:137, 1977.

Goldenheim PD, Kazemi H: Cardiopulmonary monitoring of critically ill patients (Part 1). *Med Intell* 311:717–721, 1984.

Goldenheim PD, Kazemi H: Cardiopulmonary monitoring of critically ill patients (Part 2). *Med Intell* 311:776–780, 1984.

Houston MC, Thompson WL, Robertson D: Shock—diagnostic and management. *Arch Intern Med* 144:1433–1439, 1984.

King EG, Chin WDN: Shock: an overview of pathophysiology and general treatment cells. *Crit Care Clin* 1:547–561, 1985.

Parker MM, Shelhamer JH, Bacharach SL, Green MBV, Natanson C, Frederick TM, Damske BA, Parillo JE: Profound but reversible myocardial depression in patients with septic shock. *Ann Intern Med* 100:483–490, 1984.

Raper R, Sibbald WJ: Misled by the wedge? The Swan-Ganz catheter and left ventricular preload. *Chest* 89:427–434, 1986.

Ross AD, Anaran DM: Colloids vs. crystalloids—a continuing controversy. *Drug Intell Clin Pharm* 18:202–212, 1984.

Sibbald WJ: The influence of cardiopulmonary complications of severe trauma on the systemic response to injury. In Little RA, Frayn KN (eds): *The Scientific Basis for the Care of the Critically Ill.* Manchester, England, 1986, pp 275–292.

Sibbald WJ, Calvin JE, Holliday RL, Driedger AA: Concepts in the pharmacologic and nonpharmacologic support of cardiovascular function in critically ill surgical patients. *Surg Clin North Am* 63:455–482, 1983.

Udhoji VN, Weil MH: Hemodynamic and metabolic studies on shock associated with bacteremia. *Ann Intern Med* 62:966–978, 1965.

Wilmore DW, Aulick LH: Systemic responses to injury and the healing wound. *J Parenteral Enteral Nutr* 4:147–151, 1980.

CHAPTER

6 Cardiopulmonary Resuscitation

H.R. Wexler, M.D. and A.W. Gelb, M.B.Ch.B.

Cardiac arrest is defined as the sudden cessation of the ability of the heart to pump blood. The commonest and most treatable cause is myocardial infarction with ventricular fibrillation. Other common causes are asystole and pulmonary embolus with electromechanical dissociation.

The diagnosis is made clinically. Because the cessation of cerebral blood flow results in the loss of consciousness within 10–15 seconds and, shortly thereafter, respiration stops, the diagnostic features of cardiac arrest are loss of consciousness, absent pulse, and no (or agonal) respiratory efforts.

The aims of cardiopulmonary resuscitation (CPR) are to (1) restore a coordinated, effective heart beat and (2) maintain organ perfusion and oxygenation, especially to the brain, until cardiac output is restored.

Initial resuscitative efforts should focus on the ABCs: the establishment of an airway, breathing, and circulation. External cardiac compressions should be preceded by a "precordial thump," which has been reported to cause defibrillation in some patients.

INITIAL RESUSCITATIVE EFFORTS

Airway

An adequate airway for ventilation should be established first. Early tracheal intubation is optimal because it ensures patency and protection of the airway and reduces the risk of pulmonary aspiration. In the unintubated patient whose airway is being maintained by jaw lift or oropharyngeal airway, the BCLS-recommended pattern of ventilation can result in high peak inflation pressures that may inflate the stomach and lead to the regurgitation of gastric contents. Cricoid pressure by an assistant may reduce the likelihood of this occurrence.

In some patients, especially those with facial trauma, it may not be possible to maintain the airway by jaw lift, oral airway, or endotracheal intubation. Instead, cricothyrotomy or tracheostomy may be required to establish the airway.

Ventilation

The BCLS recommendation for ventilation consists of a tidal volume of 800–1200 ml delivered in 0.5 seconds, 12–20 times per minute. As mentioned, this may result in high peak inflation pressures. This pressure can be reduced by using a smaller tidal volume or by lengthening the inflation time. An inflation time of 1.5 seconds results in "asynchronous" ventilation in that the lungs are still inflated during the cardiac compression. This may augment cardiac output (vide infra).

Cardiac Compression

In adults, external cardiac compression is carried out with the heel of one hand over the lower third of the sternum and the other hand placed on top. Both hands are pushed down to compress the sternum 1½–3 inches (3.8–7.6 cm) 80–100 times/min. This faster rate produces greater blood flow than the previously taught 60 times/min. In infants, two fingers are used over the mid-sternum, often with the other hand under the back, at a rate of 120 times/min.

Contrary to previous belief, the heart is not trapped or compressed between the sternum and vertebral column. Blood flow is caused by the overall rise in intrathoracic pressure associated with the chest wall compression. When intrathoracic pressure is increased, the blood flows out of the heart and thorax along the valveless arterial system while efflux via the venous system is prevented by the venous valves. This mechanism has been demonstrated in animal studies and in patients in whom "cough-CPR" is effective. For this reason, asynchronous ventilation/compression in which the lungs are kept inflated during thoracic compression may be advantageous. An alternative or additional means of raising intrathoracic pressure is abdominal compression or counterpulsation. The effectiveness of these techniques is currently under investigation.

Conventional CPR provides at best marginal organ perfusion: less than 10% of normal cerebral blood flow and less than 5% of normal coronary blood flow. Although the newer techniques, such as asynchronous CPR and abdominal compression, may increase cerebral blood flow to 30% of normal and coronary perfusion to 10% of normal, these marginal flows do not allow survival without significant brain damage beyond 30 minutes of resuscitation. Recent studies have shown that open chest CPR provides blood flow upward of 80% of normal, with good cerebral recovery after 2 hours of resuscitation. Therefore, consideration should be given to this procedure if effective spontaneous cardiac output has not been achieved after 15–20 minutes of closed chest CPR where the etiology is unknown or a reversible cause is suspected.

DRUG THERAPY

Drug therapy during CPR has four goals: (1) stablization of cardiac rhythm, (2) maintenance of organ perfusion, (3) maintenance of a normal electrolyte and acid-base balance, and (4) augmentation of cardiac output. The rapid return of a coordinated, effective myocardial contraction leads to the best recovery after cardiac arrest. All efforts are directed to this end while attempting to maintain organ viability.

Although drugs injected into a fast-running peripheral arm vein do reach the central circulation, peripheral limb flow is greatly decreased during CPR. Therefore, the fastest intravenous route to the coronary circulation is

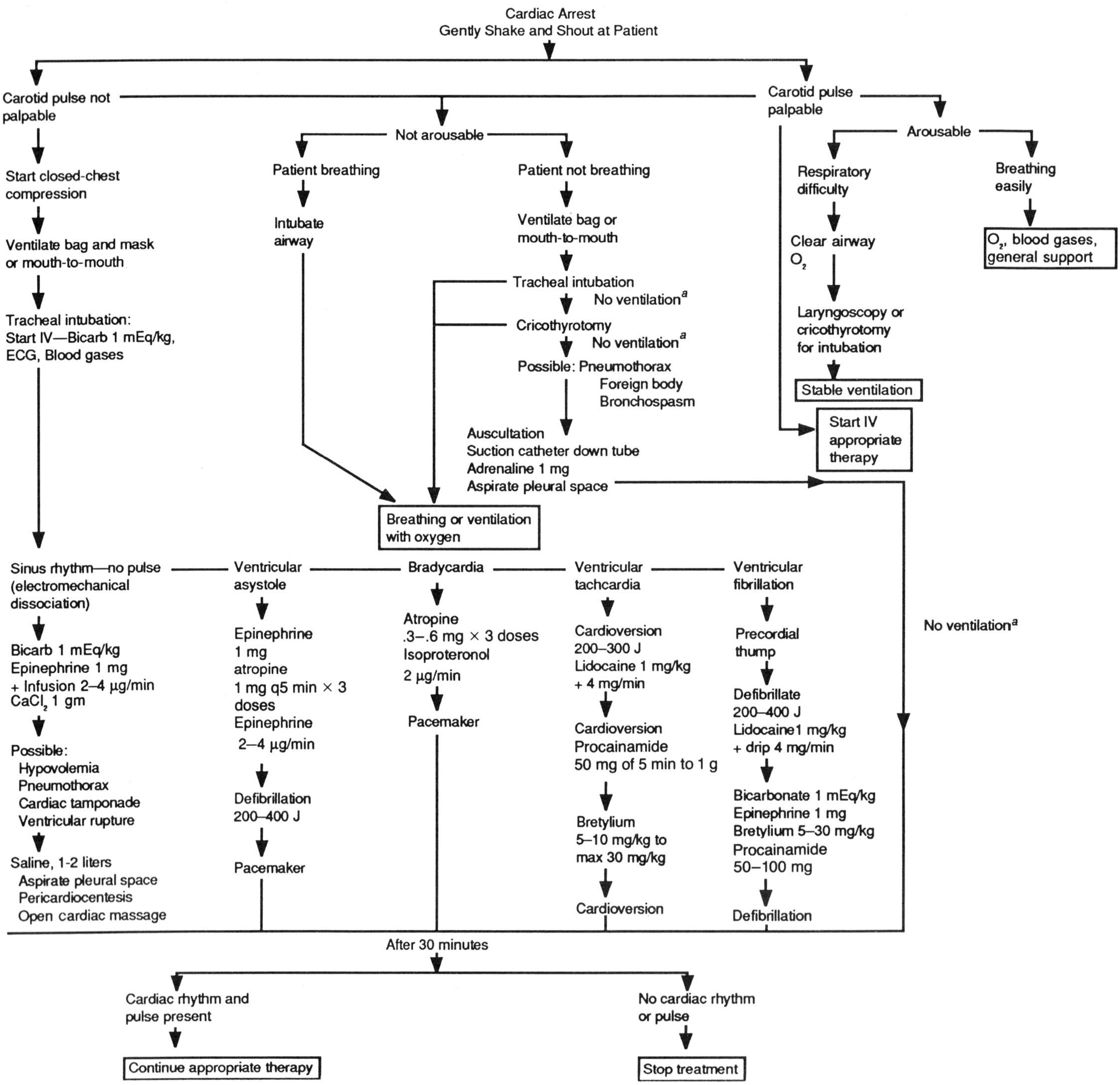

[a] Inability to ventilate mechanically.

Figure 6.1. Flow chart of therapy in cardiac arrest.

via a central venous catheter. Obtaining central venous lines, however, may involve delays and complications, which must be weighed against the usefulness of a *good* peripheral IV.

When a line cannot be secured immediately, endotracheal administration of drugs may be time saving and possibly life saving. Adrenaline, atropine, lidocaine, naloxone, and diazepam have been shown to be absorbed through that route. The optimum dose, pH, and volume of solution to be given by this route have not yet been determined. Venous access, therefore, should still be achieved as soon as possible.

Bicarbonate Therapy

Tissue hypoperfusion leads to metabolic acidosis on the basis of lactate production. Empiric administration of 4 mEq/kg body weight of sodium bicarbonate for each 30 minutes of CPR, usually as 50–100 mEq every 5–10 minutes, maintains an arterial pH of approximately 7.35 if the arterial PCO_2 is normal. Although hypercapnea and hypernatremia are potential hazards of bicarbonate therapy, these are rarely seen with the doses used. (The authors recommend the use of hyperventilation to maintain an adequate pH by decreasing the PCO_2. Only if this is unsuccessful or if blood gases are unavailable should bicarbonate be given.)

Antiarrhythmic Therapy

As noted, the commonest and most treatable cause of cardiac arrest is acute ventricular fibrillation. The first line of therapy for this condition is electrical defibrillation, starting in the adult with an energy output of 200 J and increasing, if required, up to 400 J. Unfortunately, electrical defibrillation may be unsuccessful in restoring or maintaining a coordinated heart rhythm.

Both lidocaine and procainamide elevate the ventricular fibrillation threshold and prolong the refractory period, allowing effective defibrillation. Lidocaine is given initially as an intravenous bolus of 1 mg/kg followed by 0.5 mg/kg every 10 minutes to a maximum of 3 mg/kg. Procainamide is given as an IV bolus of 50 mg every 5 minutes to a maximum of 1 gm *or* until the QRS width increases by 50%. Bretylium tosylate has similar actions to lidocaine and procainamide, but may also induce spontaneous defibrillation, an effect not seen with the other two drugs. Bretylium releases catecholamines that stimulate myocardial contractility and also cause postganglionic blockade and vasodilation. The initial dose is 5 mg/kg. If there is no effect, 10 mg/kg can be given every 15–30 minutes to a maximum of 30 mg/kg. Case reports suggest that more than one drug may be necessary to sustain a normal heart rhythm.

The flow chart (Fig. 6.1) describes the course of therapy in more detail.

Vasopressor Therapy

The main requirement for effective myocardial perfusion during CPR is a diastolic blood pressure of at least 30–40 mm Hg. Alpha-agonist stimulation produces vasoconstriction leading to an adequate diastolic blood pressure. Beta-stimulation, on the other hand, produces vasodilation and a lower diastolic blood pressure, and it increases myocardial oxygen demand. Resuscitative results in experimental and clinical studies are superior with alpha stimulation. Adrenaline, usually given in doses of 1 mg, has more alpha than beta effect. Methoxamine, a pure alpha agonist is reported to be as effective as adrenaline, whereas isoproterenol is less effective.

Atropine

Although atropine increases the heart rate, it is also associated with increased myocardial oxygen consumption and ventricular arrhythmias, including fibrillation. Therefore, the drug should be reserved for patients with bradycardia who have hypotension or inadequate cardiac output. The drug should be titrated in doses of 0.2–0.4 mg IV to increase the heart rate sufficiently to restore blood pressure or cardiac output. A small number of asystolic patients refractory to other drug therapies may respond to atropine, although improved survival has not been shown. In patients with bradycardia or asystole, electrical pacing is the preferred method of support.

Calcium

Calcium does increase myocardial contractility by mediating excitation-contraction coupling. It is useful in treating hypotension after cardiopulmonary bypass, especially in patients on calcium channel blocking therapy or who are hyperkalemic. However, there is no evidence to suggest that calcium converts asystole to ventricular fibrillation or helps in converting fibrillation to a coordinated contraction. In doses of two times the recommended dose, calcium does produce a pulse in about 10% of patients with refractory electromechanical dissociation, but improved survival is questionable. Too, calcium has been implicated in the myocardial and cerebral postischemic reperfusion syndrome, which results in "stone heart" and severe cellular damage to myocardial and brain cells. It should therefore be used judiciously.

Suggested Readings

Standards and Guidelines for Cardiopulmonary Resuscitation (CPR) and Emergency Cardiac Care (ECC). *JAMA* 255:2843–3014, 1986.

Wexler HR, Gelb AW: Controversies in cardiopulmonary resuscitation. In Bregman D (ed): *Critical Care Clinics: New Techniques in Mechanical Cardiac Support.* Philadelphia, WB Saunders, 1986, pp 335–345.

PULMONARY

CHAPTER

7 Respiratory Failure in the Critically Ill

E. Garner King, M.D.

BASIC CONSIDERATIONS

Respiratory Failure—Definitions[a]

Seventy to eighty percent of all patients entering a general systems support intensive care unit (ICU) do so as the result of respiratory failure. *Respiratory failure* has been arbitrarily but usefully defined as a PaO_2 of less than 50 mm Hg and/or a $PaCO_2$ of greater than 50 mm Hg in a patient spontaneously breathing ambient air at sea level. The application of this definition requires, in addition to an understanding of arterial blood gas interpretation, an appreciation of the concept of *incipient* respiratory failure with *relative* hypoxia and/or hypercapnia. This condition is best assessed by (1) measurement of spontaneous ventilatory capability and (2) interpretation of arterial blood gases in the light of V_A. This concept is very important to understand as the successful management of acute respiratory failure depends on its *anticipation* and not on its treatment after the fact. Thus, although established respiratory failure may be defined in terms of arbitrary blood gas values, it can usually be *predicted* on the basis of serial spontaneous ventilatory capability measurements (Table 7.1). These include V_T, f, V_C, and PIP.

On the basis of the above-noted definition, respiratory failure may be roughly categorized into two broad types (Table 7.2): (1) *hypoxemic* (Fig. 7.1), i.e., those patients in whom the PaO_2 is less than 50 mm Hg while the $PaCO_2$ is typically normal or low; and (2) *hypercapneic or hypoventilatory* (Fig. 7.2), i.e., those patients in whom the $PaCO_2$ is elevated. In this latter group, the PaO_2 is also low of course; however, the low value is commensurate with the increase in $PaCO_2$. There may be overlap between these categories.

[a] See the Glossary at the end of the chapter.

Table 7.1
Assessment of Ventilatory Capacity

Subjective	Objective
Is the patient awake, cooperative, alert? Can the patient cough and deep breathe effectively? What are the secretions like, and is there bronchospasm? Can the patient swallow? Is there ventilatory dyscoordination? What is the work of breathing like? Is the patient hemodynamically stable?	**Mechanics** $V_T \gtrsim$ 5–7 ml/kg $V_C \gtrsim$ 12–15 ml/kg PIP $\gtrsim$ 20 cm H_2O f $\lesssim$ 35/minute (in adults) **Oxygenation** A-a$DO_2 \lesssim$ 250–300 Hg **Ventilation** $PaCO_2$ 40 ± 5 mm Hg, with [H+] $\gtrsim$ 40 ± 5 $V_D/V_T \gtrsim$ 0.55

Interpretation of Arterial Blood Gases

PaO_2

In simplistic terms, the arterial PaO_2 is determined by the following relationship:

$$PaO_2; \propto \text{ventilation/“shunt factor”}$$

Table 7.2
Comparison of Hypoventilatory and Hypoxemic Respiratory Failure

	Hypoventilatory	Hypoxemic
Incidence	Relatively uncommon	Common
History	1. Usually longstanding antecedent COPD 2. Evidence of neurologic, muscular bellows, or airways incapacity	Lungs usually normal before acute pulmonary insult
Typical ABGs	↓ PaO_2, ↑ $PaCO_2$	PaO_2 ↓, $PaCO_2$ normal or ↓
Resting lung volumes	High—in the COPD group	Low
Assisted ventilation	1. COPD group: avoid, if titrated O_2 and airways therapy supportive 2. Others: criteria for intubation and assistance noted in Table 7.1	Early
$\dot{V}_A$	↓	↑

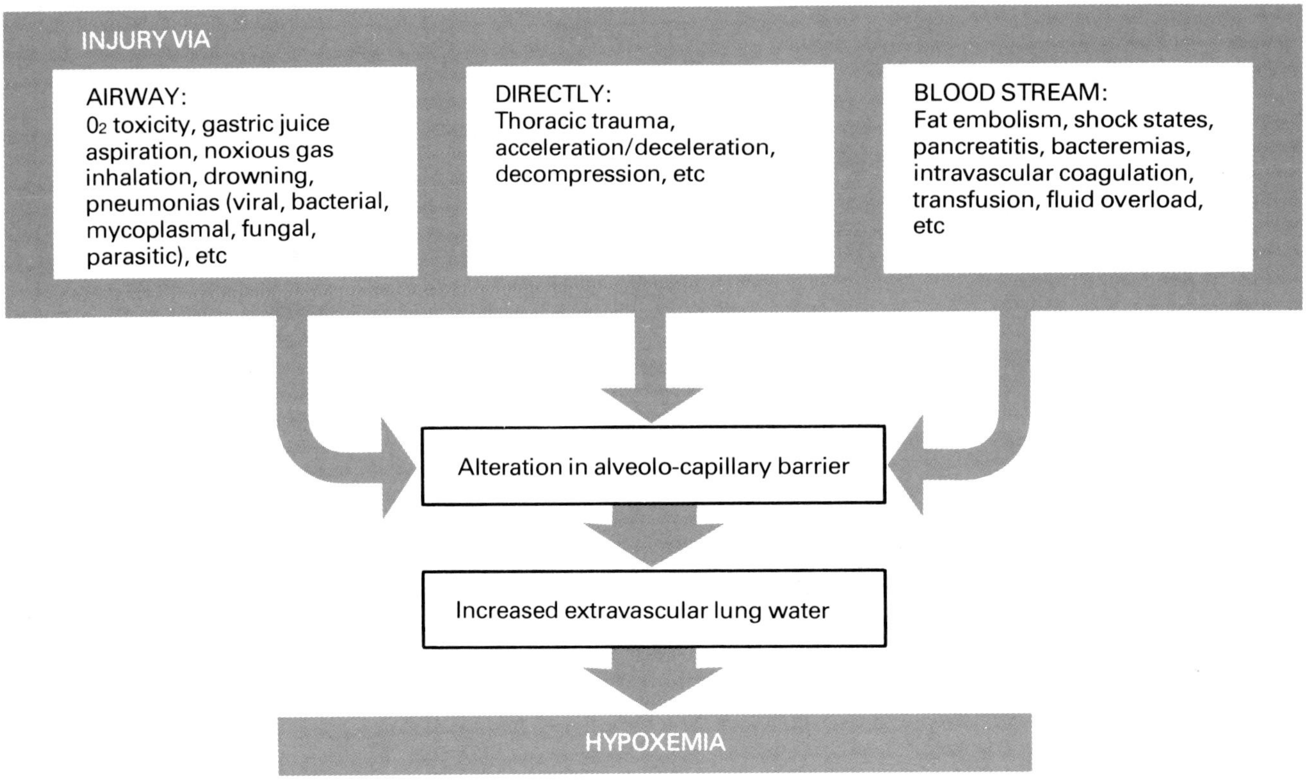

Figure 7.1. Hypoxemic respiratory failure. The final common pathway leading to accumulation of extravascular lung water appears to be alteration in the alveolar capillary membrane.

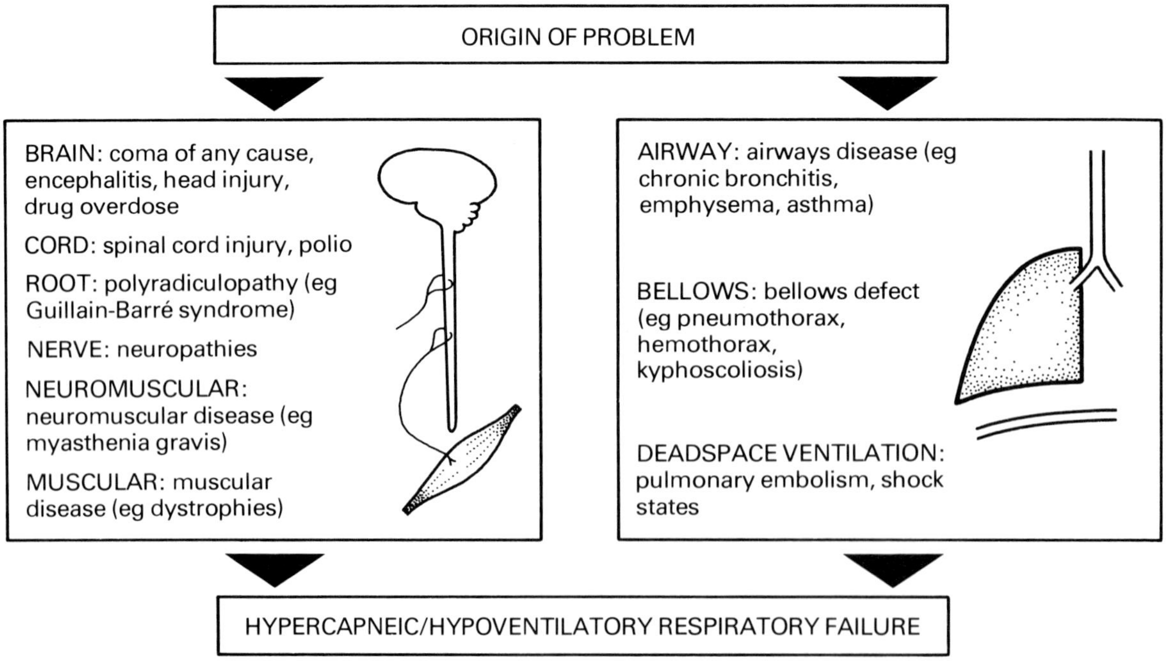

Figure 7.2. Diagrammatic classification of the hypoventilatory or hypercapneic respiratory failure syndromes.

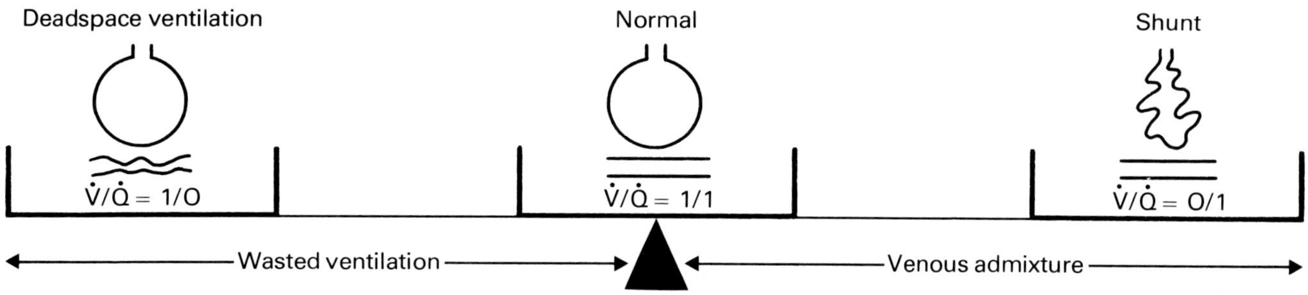

Figure 7.3. Diagram illustrating the continuum of $\dot{V}/\dot{Q}$ relationships from the extremes of dead space and shunt to the situation of perfect matching. Interestingly, each disease state has a distinctive $\dot{V}/\dot{Q}$ pattern. For example, with pulmonary embolism, there is increased dead space ventilation and venous admixture with relatively little shunt, whereas ARDS patients usually manifest predominant shunt.

This gives rise to the conventional *cause of hypoxemia* list:

1. Decreased or inadequate FiO_2;
2. Decreased $\dot{V}_A$;
3. $\dot{V}/\dot{Q}$ mismatch;
4. "Diffusing defect";
5. Absolute shunt.

When reviewing this mental checklist, if the FiO_2 is adequate and the $PaCO_2$ is normal or low, items 1 and 2 can be ruled out. In most hypoxemic patients, the ICU physician is usually faced with the problem of identifying which of the last three mechanisms is operative—they are the "shunt factors" of the denominator in the PaO_2 relationship. Avoiding semantic arguments, diffusing defect is probably best considered to be a mild degree of $\dot{V}/\dot{Q}$ mismatch easily correctable with only a sniff of oxygen and is seldom of concern. $\dot{V}/\dot{Q}$ mismatch and absolute shunt, however, represent degrees of the same basic phenomenon of $\dot{V}/\dot{Q}$ mismatch (Fig. 7.3) and may theoretically be separated by placing the hypoxemic patient on 100% oxygen: the PaO_2 remains unchanged in the patient with shunt, whereas, in the patient with pure $\dot{V}/\dot{Q}$ mismatch, the PaO_2 should rise to approximate that calculated from the alveolar gas equation. In the practical world of the ICU, patients should never be placed on 100% oxygen for purposes of measuring theoretical shunt as this process in itself leads to absorption atelectasis with measurement of a falsely high shunt fraction. In practice, most critically ill patients have a mixture of both $\dot{V}/\dot{Q}$ mismatch and absolute shunt. If there is a preponderance of the latter, as evidenced by an $AaDO_2$ of 300 mm Hg or greater, it becomes necessary to institute a distending airway pressure in order to open up shunting gas exchange units. If the problem is largely that of $\dot{V}/\dot{Q}$ mismatch, PaO_2 can usually be corrected to hemoglobin-saturating levels by the simple expedient of increasing the FiO_2. An illustration of these principles is seen in Figure 7.4.

There is occasionally unnecessary confusion over the terms oxygen tension (PaO_2), oxygen content (CaO_2), and saturation of hemoglobin by oxygen (SaO_2). Tension is measured in mm Hg, Torricelli units (torr), or, most correctly, kilopascals (kpasc)[b]. It is a measurement of the collective forces of bombardment exerted by randomly moving oxygen molecules on the walls of their container, as well as an "escaping tendency," i.e., a force that moves molecules beyond the confines of their container to regions of lesser concentrations (Fig. 7.5). It is not a quantity, but it does indirectly reflect the number of oxygen molecules undergoing active Brownian motion.

CaO_2, in contrast, does represent a quantity (see below) and is a reflection of the volume of oxygen at a defined temperature and pressure being carried by an arbitrarily fixed blood volume (traditionally, 100 ml). The units are therefore ml/100 ml, or ml %, or volumes %. The CaO_2 is largely determined by the amount of O_2 bound to hemoglobin. However, there is a small amount of O_2 physically dissolved in plasma that may be important to

[b]Throughout this chapter, partial pressures of gases are expressed in mm Hg because, despite attempts to establish the terms "torr" (for Torricelli units) and "kilopascals" (in honor of Napoleon, the SI system, and metrification), mm Hg continues to be employed in most North American hospitals. Of the avant garde terms, kilopascals has the most to recommend it scientifically as it truly is an expression of "force per unit area." Should one want to impress one's friends and colleagues, simply divide the mm Hg numeric value by 7.5 to get the approximate partial pressure in kilopascals. In this regard one need remember that 1 kilopascal roughly equals 7.5 mm Hg, which, in turn, is approximately 10 cm H_2O.

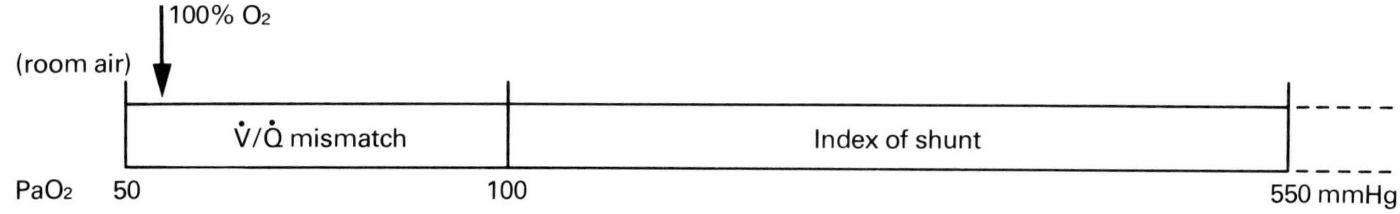

Figure 7.4. Causes of hypoxemia defined by utilizing 100% oxygen. The figure is an example of an ARDS patient placed on 100% oxygen. The minimal improvement in a PaO_2 of 100 mm Hg serves as an index of marked shunt. If the PaO_2 had improved to, for example, 450 mm Hg, the patient would have had more $\dot{V}/\dot{Q}$ mismatch than shunt.

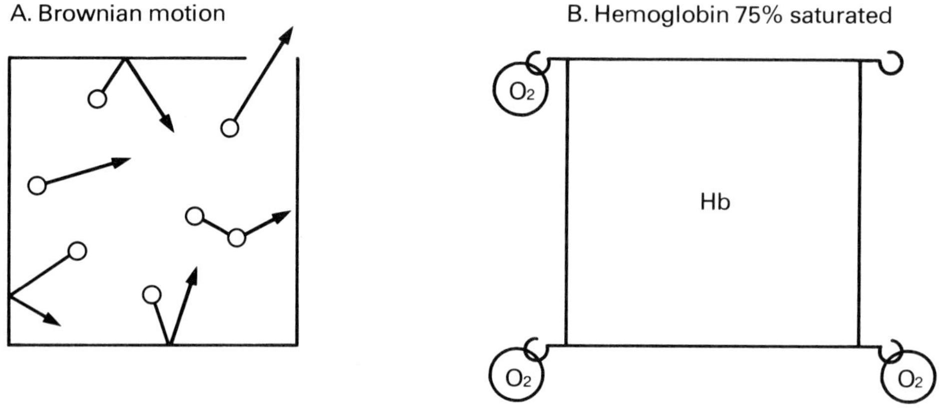

Figure 7.5. Molecular physics of oxygen transport. *A,* Sketch depicting molecules undergoing Brownian activity confined to a box and striking the walls of the container. *B,* A fanciful hemoglobin molecule with three of its four oxygen "hooks" occupied, i.e., the molecule is 75% saturated.

consider in the preservation of "watershed areas" in shock, or in hyperbaric conditions as occur in hyperbaric oxygen therapy or scuba diving.

Finally, SaO_2, does not refer to O_2 directly at all, but refers to the number of hemoglobin-binding sites actually occupied by O_2. The units are percent (%), and the term serves as an index of potential oxygen availability.

$PaCO_2$

The other relationship that most of us intuitively understand is the simplified $PaCO_2$ equation:

$$PaCO_2 \propto CO_2 \text{ production/ventilation}$$

This relationship is often complicated in critically ill patients in whom CO_2 production may be increased due to the increased work of breathing, continued muscle activity, fever, and high glucose total parenteral nutrition regimens, thus taxing the inverse relationship between $PaCO_2$ and ventilation. In addition to overall hypoventilation causing elevations in $PaCO_2$, it must be remembered that decreased perfusion to gas exchange units in the presence of ongoing ventilation ("dead space" ventilation) can also lead to a rise in $PaCO_2$.

How is it that patients in respiratory failure from different causes can present themselves to the puzzled clinician with so many different low PaO_2 and low-normal-high $PaCO_2$ variations? It is estimated that average adult lungs contain some 300 million gas exchange units. At any given time the $\dot{V}/\dot{Q}$ ratios in these gas exchange units vary enormously, giving rise to an almost infinite number of permutations and combinations of $\dot{V}/\dot{Q}$ matching. This is illustrated in Figure 7.3 on $\dot{V}/\dot{Q}$ mismatch, where the theoretical spectrum of $\dot{V}/\dot{Q}$ ratios over the lung is shown as a teeter-totter with perfect matching occurring at the fulcrum and gradations of $\dot{V}/\dot{Q}$ ratios extending toward shunt at one end and dead space ventilation at the other. Even in the normal lung in the upright position, $\dot{V}/\dot{Q}$ ratios range from 3.5 at the apex to 0.63 at the base, and in disease states, this variability of $\dot{V}/\dot{Q}$ matching may be greatly exaggerated.

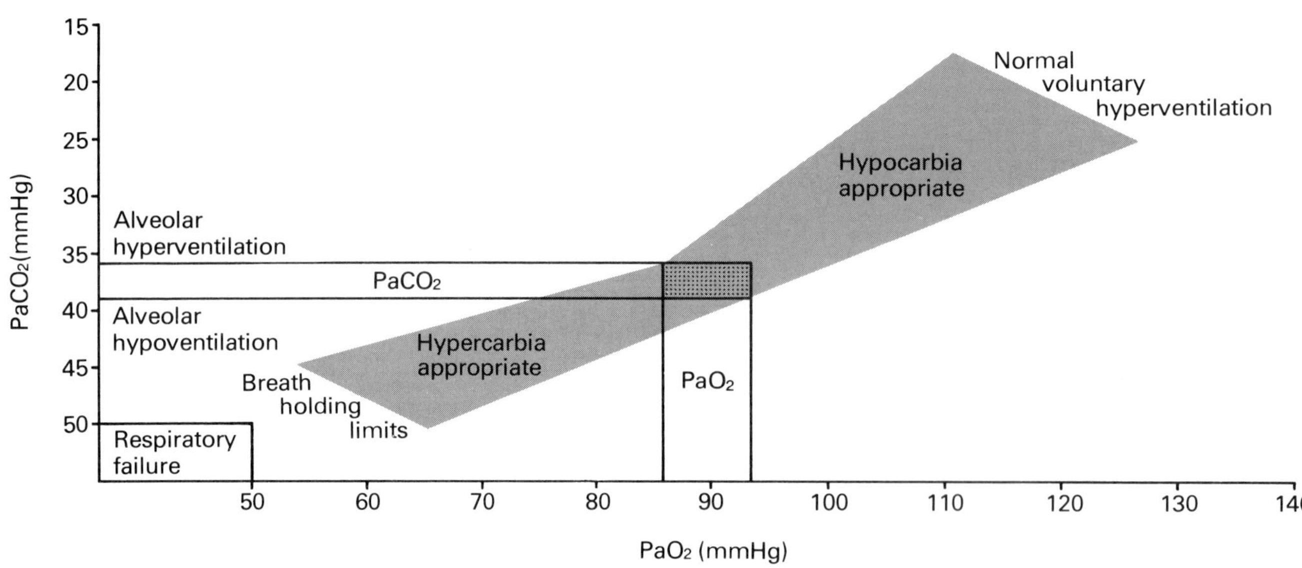

Figure 7.6. Graph depicting the relationship between PaO_2 and $PaCO_2$ over a wide range of $\dot{V}_A$ in normal trained subjects spontaneously breathing at sea level.

It should be evident from this cursory glance at elementary conventional pulmonary physiology that some sort of connection exists in normals between PaO_2 and $PaCO_2$ and that this relationship must be taken into account when interpreting arterial blood gas values. Figure 7.6 pictorially describes this relationship in normal, trained subjects breathing ambient air at sea level. *Note that the PaO_2 must always be interpreted in the light of V_A*. For example, a patient with a PaO_2 of 80 mm Hg and a $PaCO_2$ of 25 mm Hg is *relatively* hypoxemic, although not in respiratory failure by definition. As a second example, note that a patient with a PaO_2 of 55 mm Hg and a $PaCO_2$ of 55 mm Hg is, in all likelihood, hypoxemic simply from hypoventilation and that an element of $\dot{V}/\dot{Q}$ mismatch and/or shunt need not be invoked to account for the hypoxemia in addition to the overall hypoventilation.

Sampling of Arterial Blood Gases (ABGs)

Because of the frequency with which ABGs are sampled in ICU patients it is usually desirable to have an indwelling arterial line. Sites of preference for insertion are (in descending order): radial (nondominant arm with an Allen's test first), femoral (placed by Seldinger technique), dorsalis pedis, and superficial temporal. Blood samples must be drawn in heparinized, air-tight syringes and have their gas tensions measured immediately. The common placement of flow-directed pulmonary arterial catheters within the right-heart circulation makes measurement of mixed venous PO_2 ($P\bar{v}O_2$) and $P\bar{v}CO_2$ levels an easy business. It is often valuable to follow the $P\bar{v}O_2$ when attempting to reduce FiO_2 to a minimum level (see below).

ESSENTIALS OF RESPIRATORY CARE

Criteria for Establishing Airway Access and Assisted Mechanical Ventilation

Many of the subjective and objective criteria for the establishment of airway access and assisted ventilation are arbitrary; however, taken in combination and added to an element of experience they have stood the test of time (Table 7.1). Note that the "greater than" and "less than" signs simply need to be reversed in order to establish criteria for weaning, extubation, and decannulation. The art of medicine must be exercised in making a few fine decisions regarding intubation, but in general the clinician should be able to form reasonably sound judgments on the basis of the material presented in Table 7.1. In the table, the ABGs are the last items to be mentioned. This de-emphasis is deliberate and is because ABGs tend to be defended "to the last ditch" through the autoregulatory $\dot{V}/\dot{Q}$ matching process that occurs in the lungs. Respiratory failure should be anticipated where possible and not simply diagnosed on the basis of abnormal blood gases.

Oxygen Therapy

Oxygen must be regarded as a drug and its dosage titrated to the effects produced. Generally, sufficient oxygen should be administered to produce a hemoglobin-saturating PaO_2, i.e., about 70 mm Hg. There are circumstances, however, in which PaO_2s higher or lower than this level are desirable. For example, in the patient in shock, most physicians feel that a higher than physiologic PaO_2 should be sought in order to protect "watershed areas." Conversely, in patients who are very dependent on their hypoxic ventilatory drive to maintain breathing, such as some COPD patients, great care must be taken when administering oxygen not to exceed a PaO_2 of 55–60 mm Hg and thereby deprive the patient of carotid chemoreceptor stimulation.

Concerns about oxygen toxicity should *never* keep a physician from adequately oxygenating the patient. There is no doubt that the phenomenon of oxygen toxicity is very real and that high FiO_2s also promote atelectasis; however, *hypoxemia kills,* and the capillary-to-mitochondrial gradient for oxygen must be maintained if cells are to survive. PaO_2s of less than 40 mm Hg are a profound stimulus to the development of pulmonary hypertension and right-heart failure. At PaO_2s less than 28–30 mm Hg, widespread death of tissue ensues. Most authorities agree that oxygen toxicity probably does not occur at PIO_2s of less than 250 mm Hg. The duration of exposure to high FiO_2s for the production of toxicity is uncertain, as in experimental circumstances there are large species and individual variations in susceptibility. Furthermore, the additional role, if any, of positive pressure ventilation in the production of lung damage remains controversial. High FiO_2s for short periods of exposure are occasionally necessary and, as such, are probably acceptable; however, every effort must be made to reduce FiO_2s as soon as practical. In this regard, note that patients seemingly requiring very high FiO_2s to maintain hemoglobin-saturating PaO_2s have large shunts, and therefore the FiO_2 can be significantly reduced without interfering to a major degree with the resultant PaO_2. Paradoxically, the addition of the nitrogen "splint" to gas exchange units close to their closing volumes may reduce shunt and enhance oxygenation.

If a hemoglobin-saturating PaO_2 cannot be achieved with a patient spontaneously breathing oxygen by mask, specifically if the $AaDO_2\pm$ exceeds 250–300 mm Hg, consideration must be given to intubation and institution of mechanically assisted ventilation in order to reduce $\dot{V}/\dot{Q}$ mismatch and shunt.[c]

In order to ensure adequate oxygen delivery, the critical care physician must not merely examine the PaO_2 but should assess the whole oxygen transport system as the cells in the periphery are dependent on both respiratory and hemodynamic components. All factors in the O_2 transport (O_2t) relationship must be considered:

$$O_2t = \dot{Q}_T \times CaO_2$$

[c] A useful "guestimate" of the PaO_2 can be obtained from the "rule of 7s" in which the FiO_2 as a percentage is multipled by 7: the measured PaO_2 is then subtracted from the resultant approximated PaO_2. For example, a patient on 40% oxygen with a PaO_2 of 50 mm Hg has an $AaDO_2$ of roughly $280-50=230$ mm Hg. (Another "ballpark" figure worth bearing in mind is that for each 100 mm of $AaDO_2$ gradient, a 5–8% estimate of shunt is usually not far off.)

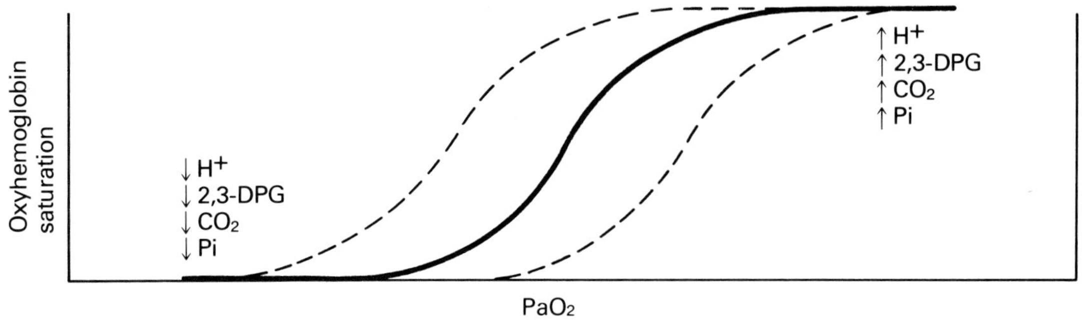

Figure 7.7. The oxyhemoglobin dissociation curve showing the relationship between saturation and PaO_2 and noting some of the factors that move the curve either to the right or the left. (2,3-*DPG* = 2,3-diphosphoglycerate; *Pi* = inorganic phosphates).

where $\dot{Q}_T$ is a function of stroke volume and heart rate and CaO_2 is a function of hemoglobin concentration, chemical character, saturation, and PaO_2. These latter factors are related through the well-known equation:

$$CaO_2 = ([Hb] \times 1.34 \times SaO_2) + (0.0031 \times PaO_2).$$

The relationship between PaO_2 and SaO_2 is depicted by the equally well-known hemoglobin dissociation curve for oxygen (Fig. 7.7), the position of which reflects the tenacity with which oxygen binds to the hemoglobin molecule. Generally, a right shift of the curve produces diminished oxygen-heme binding and is associated with an increased tendency for hemoglobin to give up oxygen at the tissue level: conversely, a left-shifted curve is associated with an increased affinity and binding with an increased ease of oxygen uptake by heme at the lung level. SaO_2 should be both calculated (from PaO_2-SaO_2-[H+] nomograms) and measured in order to detect a "saturation gap," which indicates an abnormal curve position, e.g., in carbon monoxide intoxication.

In order to know how well oxygenated each organ system is, ideally one would be able to measure the venous PO_2 from the tissue in question. To get a general idea, however, about peripheral oxygen uptake, it is often useful to follow $P\bar{v}O_2$s and $S\bar{v}O_2$s as obtained from pulmonary arterial blood. This is particularly true when one is trying to reduce the FiO_2 to a minimum to avoid oxygen toxicity and when $P\bar{v}O_2$s may be kept above the 30–35 mm Hg range. Further, for a relatively fixed oxygen consumption, alterations in SaO_2 and $S\bar{v}O_2$ reflect cardiac output reasonably accurately.

Administration of Oxygen

Table 7.3 outlines the methods by which oxygen may be provided and oxygenation improved: this topic is more completely covered in Chapter 8. Humidification of inspired gases is always required, and in the intubated and mechanically ventilated patient, water balance must be watched very carefully. In these patients, positive free water balance almost always occurs because of (1) reduction of insensible water loss from the airway, (2) addition of large volumes of distilled water to the airway from nebulization systems, (3) positive pressure ventilation that may "turn on" antidiuretic hormone with free water retention, and (4) analgesic, barbiturate, and phenothiazine use—all agents known to stimulate the antidiuretic hormone mechanism. In fact, for most patients in an ICU there is a constant battle to maintain reasonable water balance and a normal serum sodium concentration.

Intubation

Whenever possible, endotracheal intubation should be carried out under topical anesthesia without resorting to the use of muscle relaxants, hypnotics, or profound sedation. This maintains the patient's ability to cough, deep breathe, and look after his or her own airway throughout the procedure and thereafter. Whenever there is a question about cervical bony stability, intubation should be carried out over the fiberoptic bronchoscope or placed "by braille" transnasally *without* manipulating the head and neck. One circumstance in which it is probably preferable to perform endotracheal intubation with the patient

Table 7.3
Means of Improving Oxygenation

- Spontaneous breathing
  - Nasal cannulae
  - Simple mask
  - Mask with reservoir bag
  - Venturi mask with selectable FiO_2
  - Continuous positive airway pressure (CPAP)
- Mechanical ventilation
  - Positive pressure breathing
  - Distending airway pressure application
  - Jet ventilation
  - Oscillatory ventilation
  - Vibratory ventilation

Table 7.4
Comparison of Transnasal and Transoral Intubation

Transoral	Transnasal
Advantages	
Can place a larger tube	Easier to fix in place
Easier to suction	Patient may be able to eat and swallow
Easier to put in	
Disadvantages	
Persistent sialorrhea	Smaller, longer tube
Difficult oral toilet	Harder to suction
Patient must be tube-fed	Blockage of paranasal sinuses
	Nosebleed at insertion

Table 7.5
Indications for Tracheostomy

Upper airway obstruction
Tracheobronchial toilet
Long-term ventilation
Reduction of nonelastic load and dead space facilitation of weaning from mechanical ventilation

paralyzed or under sedation/hypnotic drug influence is that in which a closed head injury with increased intracranial pressure is suspected. Table 7.4 outlines some of the pros and cons of transnasal versus transoral endotracheal tube placement. Intubation should be carried out under full atropinization (0.015 mg/kg IV), especially if the patient is thought to be hypoxemic or has a bradycardia. If it is deemed necessary to paralyze the patient for intubation, succinylcholine may be given IV in a dose of 1 mg/kg. This should be accompanied by cricoid pressure, and suction must be at hand in anticipation of the gastroesophageal reflux that commonly accompanies the use of a depolarizing neuromuscular agent. Ideally, tubes with high compliance, soft cuffs should be used, and the portion passing through the larynx should be made of a soft nonreactive material, such as Silastic. All tubes must be securely fixed in place so that movement in the airway is minimized.

The "safe" duration for maintenance of an endotracheal tube in place can be the source of lively arguments among physicians practicing regularly in ICUs. We commonly leave Silastic high compliance cuff tubes in place for purposes of ventilation and airway access for periods as long as 4–6 weeks. It must be stated, however, that if the ICU physician can clearly "see down the road" and predict a prolonged need for maintenance of airway access, toilet, and ventilation, it is better to establish a tracheostomy early, rather than late. Because of the high incidence of complications from tracheostomy in children and babies, we commonly leave uncuffed endotracheal tubes in place in these patients for the duration of the acute illness. The major current indication for performing a tracheostomy in intubated patients is to maintain tracheobronchial toilet. In addition, many patients with COPD or other mechanical respiratory difficulties may be easier to wean from an established tracheostomy than an endotracheal tube (lower nonelastic load and dead space

Table 7.6
Complications of Tracheostomy

Immediate
Dislodgement
Obstruction
Hemorrhage
Pneumothorax-mediastinum
Delayed
Tracheal stenosis: stomal, cuff, tip
Stomal infection
Erosion into adjacent structures

and better tracheobronchial toilet). In order to minimize the possibility of tube-related upper airway complications, cuffs should be adjusted to a "just leak" position, tube stability should be ensured, and tube size should be selected so as to avoid traumatic intubation and laryngeal distortion. Pressure and mobility related complications of prolonged intubation are noted in Figure 7.8. All patients who have been intubated for longer than 1 week should have follow-up with fiberoptic bronchoscopy, flow volume loops, and, when indicated, tomograms of the upper airway.

Tracheostomy

With the advent of soft, pliable, nonreactive endotracheal tubes with high compliance, low pressure cuffs, the need for tracheotomy has declined markedly over the past few years. Table 7.5 outlines the major indications for establishment of a tracheostomy. The only important principle to be followed in the performance of a tracheotomy is that the airway should be controlled by the presence of an endotracheal tube at all times. Major complications of tracheostomy are noted in Table 7.6

Notes on Airway Care

Suctioning

Clearance of secretions, blood, and pus from the airways should be on a prn basis, rather than by the clock. In addition to the usual signs indicating a need for suctioning, such as obstructive airway noises, patient restlessness, and decreased air entry on one side of the chest, a watchful eye should be kept on ventilatory peak pressures, which may detect secretional trouble in the airway long before it becomes grossly evident. Soft pliable cath-

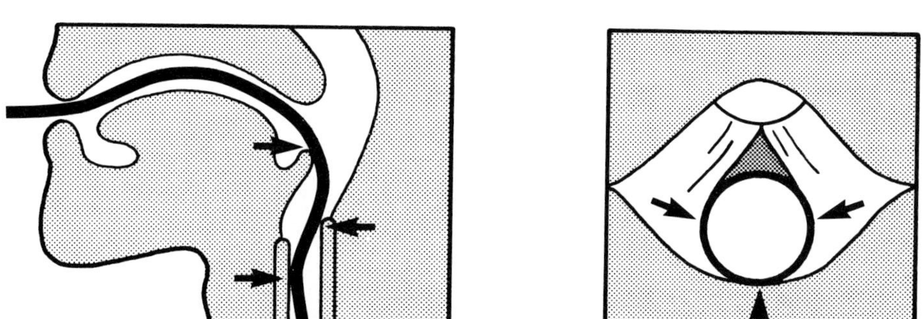

Figure 7.8. Potential pressure points in an intubated patient. Sketches of the upper airway showing pressure effects of an endotracheal tube on the *left,* tip of epiglottis, posterior commissure, anterior cricoid, and *right,* the true vocal cords *(arrows).*

eters should be used that are of a diameter that readily slip down the endotracheal tube, but are large enough to suck up whatever secretions are present. In patients on distending airway pressures (PEEP and/or CPAP) a sealing nipple should be attached to the tube connector so that suctioning minimally disturbs the expiratory plateau. Regrettably, despite all the fancy head-turning maneuvers traditionally practiced by nurses to get catheters to go into the left mainsteam bronchus, most suctioning only clears the right side, and only rarely does the catheter actually enter the left mainsteam bronchus. When effective and specific left-sided toilet is sought, bent-tip catheters or the fiberoptic bronchoscope should be employed. Airway mucosal trauma and bleeding are minimized by using mushroom-tipped catheters.

Bronchoscopy

Directed airway secretion clearance can readily be achieved with the fiberoptic bronchoscope. The combination of fiberoptic bronchoscopic suction and lavage, accompanied by unilateral endotracheal tube placement and/or unilateral IPPB, usually opens up lobes or whole lungs when they have been rendered atelectatic by secretions.

Instillations

The purpose of instillations is to humidify the airways and to liquefy secretions for easier removal: they should not be a part of routine airway care. Although there is some data suggesting that mucolytic agents improve secretion clearance and removal (in comparison to warmed normal saline), these agents must be accompanied by bronchodilators as they are markedly bronchoirritant.

Aseptic Technique

All suctioning, lavage, etc., must be carried out with an aseptic (not just "clean") technique. Most ICU patients are immunologically compromised and have many potentially infected access sites: the most dangerous of these access sites is the airway.

Chest Physiotherapy

The main techniques used are those of *vibration, percussion,* and *postural drainage.* Although the effectiveness of these maneuvers in patient outcome and survival is controversial, there is no question that they play a significant role in maintenance of tracheobronchial toilet. Chest physiotherapy is often more effective and easier to perform in the ICU setting when patients are on circle electric beds.

Weaning from Mechanical Ventilation

Much of the art of weaning falls into the category of dogma, and a good deal of the methodology currently employed has not been subjected to rigorous, critical scientific examination. It has been recognized for years that, when patients have been maintained on mechanical ventilatory devices, a period of gradual separation is necessary before spontaneous unassisted ventilation can take place. This requirement seems to be due to a number of factors, including psychological dependence, respiratory muscle atrophy and weakness, and the phenomenon of ventilatory dyscoordination. The predominance of these various factors varies from patient to patient, but some rules of thumb have evolved over the past 10 years about weaning in general, and these eight basic rules are briefly reviewed below.

1. Never begin weaning unless you think the patient has *some chance of success.* Ideally, the patient should have achieved the reverse of the subjective and objective criteria for intubation and mechanical ventilation noted in Table 7.1, although we often begin weaning with V_Ts of 4–5 ml/kg.

2. *Always quit while you're ahead:* devise a program that allows for watchful expectancy with discontinuance of the weaning routine at the earliest sign of fatigue and discomfort, such as increased respiratory and/or heart rate; diminishing V_T, V_C, or PIP; sweatiness or agitation; and, most importantly, increasing ventilatory dyscoordination.

3. Develop *a program* with appropriate input from all attending staff. There is nothing more discouraging to the patient than to have a new regimen proposed by whoever is "rounding" each day or each week. This is not to say that such a program should not be *flexible,* but that clear-cut objectives and goals should be borne in mind.

4. Keep the patient informed and develop an *incentive* system.

5. The patient must be in an *appropriate nutritional state* and *stable hemodynamically.* This means not only that the patient must be on sufficient nitrogen and calories but that he or she must not have a carbohydrate intake so large that the ventilatory status cannot keep up with the carbon fragment load. The patient must be arrhythmia-free and not in left ventricular failure.

6. *Pain must be controlled,* but the patient cannot require large amounts of narcotics or sedation if weaning is to be a success.

7. Have the patient in a *position* where all respiratory muscles have a fair chance: ideally, spontaneous ventilatory effort should be made with the patient sitting upright in a chair or with the whole bed elevated some 15–20° at the head end to allow the diaphragm to work as well as possible.

8. The final principle is *never to wean at night.* This message is not necessarily to be taken literally, but should be used to remind the medical staff that (1) patients being weaned need their *rest* and (2) weaning is an *active* process demanding the attention of all staff. Unfortunately, IMV in particular has been abused as a weaning technique as patients are often left to be "weaned by the machine." It is a good practice to make all "big moves" (e.g., extubation) about midmorning, i.e. after morning tracheobronchial toilet has been completed and when all nursing, paramedical, and medical staff are in attendance.

A word about *ventilatory dyscoordination* may be necessary. In the normal respiratory cycle, there is a progressive, defined, and orderly sequence of increased tension or contraction of the muscles of inspiration-expiration. The inspiratory muscular action sequence is as follows: (1) accessory muscles, (2) upper intercostals, (3) lower intercostals and lateral diaphragm, and (4) central diaphragm and oropharyngeal (especially genioglossus). In circumstances of weakness and/or fatigue this orderly sequence is disturbed, much as a distance runner becomes incoordinate when exhausted. To the problems of dyscoordination of inspiratory effort are often added the more obvious ones of active expiration with vigorous contraction of abdominal muscles, frequently accompanied by expiratory grunt. In extreme form, there may be pronounced "rocking" respiration between chest and abdomen, but the physician, once aware of the phenomenon, must be on the lookout for subtler degrees of dyscoordination. Sequential coordination of the inspiratory-expiratory sequence virtually always becomes disordered as a prelude to development of frank respiratory failure with arterial blood gas derangement.

The selection of a means of weaning is perhaps less important than attention to the eight basic principles noted above. The two basic weaning routes available are the T-piece or nebulization trial and the IMV method: these are not by any means mutually exclusive, and there is no place for doctrinaire approaches in weaning programs. It is beyond the scope of this chapter to provide an exhaustive critique of each method; suffice it to say that both have merits and deserve application in given clinical circumstances.

Assisted Mechanical Ventilation (AMV)

In implementing the AMV spontaneous ventilation route, the author's practice is to divide the 12-hour day shift into three blocks of 4 hours each. Patients are placed on a cold nebulization, continuous flow, T-piece, CPAP system for progressively longer periods, usually beginning with a "cold neb challenge" during which careful monitoring ends the period at the first sign of respiratory difficulties (falling V_T, rising f, rising HR, sweatiness, agitation, or increased ventilatory dyscoordination). It is important that trends be followed here: there are *no* magic numbers. Note also that arterial blood gases are *not* the major determinant of when to terminate a cold neb challenge. During these spontaneous breathing episodes 3–5 cm H_2O or CPAP is used on the theoretical grounds that it may prevent a decrease in resting lung volumes with the tube-inducing loss of "expiratory retard" that normal upper airways seem to provide. With progress, the 4-hour block becomes 2 hours cold neb: 2 hours AMV and then 2½ hours cold neb: 1½ hours AMV, etc. Once the patient has reached a level of 3½ hours cold neb: ½ hour AMV for the three blocks throughout the day, consideration may be given to extubation or decannulation. We usually leave a "dummy trach" occlusive plug made of dental prosthetic material for a day or so to be sure that decannulation will be successful.

IMV Route

From a theoretical point of view this method offers many potential advantages; however, if improperly applied it may simply prolong the business of weaning. The basic principle is simple: pick an IMV rate that the patient seems comfortable with, gradually reduce it until the rate is 0 or 2, and then extubate or decannulate. The guidelines for easing off of the weaning program as outlined under the cold nebulization system apply equally well to IMV weaning. However, even with IMV, it is still essential to wean intelligently and observe the patient closely. When the patient: IMV rate ratio exceeds three-to-one with patient distress, the patient is probably being weaned on a "trial by ordeal" basis. Great care must be taken to make sure that the patient's spontaneous non-IMV breaths come from a reservoir-continuous flow-past system. Unfortunately, some of the dial-in IMV-CPAP systems on the newer fixed-volume ventilators increase the work of breathing enormously as their demand-CPAP systems provide inadequate peak instantaneous flow delivery.

A word about the "SOS" (sink or swim) approach: there are at least three groups of patients for whom prediction factors about potential success in spontaneous ventilation without endotracheal or tracheostomy tubes and AMV are often wrong or impossible to assess. In these patients it is frequently necessary to perform an "SOS test" in which the endotracheal tube is simply removed and the patient is watched very closely for respiratory distress. These groups are (1) babies and small children, (2) the elderly and those with COPD, and (3) patients with chronic neuromuscular disease.

HYPERCAPNEIC OR HYPOVENTILATORY RESPIRATORY FAILURE

By definition, in this form of respiratory failure, there is either diminished overall alveolar ventilation or increased dead space ventilation (or both), with resultant elevation in $PaCO_2$. This type of respiratory failure is conveniently subclassified as acute or chronic and also on a functional-anatomic basis, starting with the cerebrum, descending on down the brainstem and spinal cord, out through the spinal roots and peripheral nerves, to the neuromuscular junctions and muscles, and finally to the respiratory effector mechanism of the thoracic bellows and airways (Fig. 7.2). Overlap potentially exists between hypoxemic and hypercapneic forms of respiratory failure. For example, asthmatic patients are usually hypoxemic with low $PaCO_2$ levels in the early stages of an acute attack, but with progression and increasing severity they begin to retain CO_2, and in the late stages are both hypoxemic and hypercapneic.

Hypercapneic Respiratory Failure Related to Neuromuscular Disease

Table 7.7 outlines the major conditions in this category that are likely to be found in an ICU. It is essential to *anticipate* the development of respiratory failure in this group of conditions. The objective and subjective assessments noted in Table 7.1 should be serially followed, and whenever spontaneous ventilatory capability is either impaired or there is a clearly deteriorating trend, intervention should be considered. Again, one must remember that arterial blood gases are well defended and that active treatment should begin *before* the $PaCO_2$ rockets up with a decompensating $[H+]$. Occasionally, patients in respiratory failure related to neuromuscular disease re-

Table 7.7
Hypercapneic Respiratory Failure Related to Neuromuscular Disease

Condition	Disease state	Management concerns
The unconscious patient	Closed head injury	Maintenance of clear airway
	CNS infections	Avoidance of increases in intracranial pressure with suctioning, etc. (IV or intratracheal xylocaine). Nursing: head up, optimizing PEEP levels. Use of mannitol and ?barbiturates.
	Drug overdose	Removal, lavage, saline purgation, charcoal, *N*-acetyl-cysteine (IV or po) for acetaminophen, hemoperfusion, hemodialysis. Protection of airway, especially during gastric lavage.
Guillian-Barré syndrome		Anticipation of impending bulbar problems and/or respiratory failure. Nutrition. Physiotherapy. Anticipation of autonomic problems (hyper-, hypotension, gut distension, arrhythmias). Prevention of GI hemorrhage.
Myasthenia gravis		Anticipation of respiratory failure, aspiration. Coordination of treatment with other consultants. High dose steroids, immunosuppressives, anticholinesterases, thymectomy, plasmaphoresis.
Cervical fracture-dislocation	Trauma	*Early* stabilization of neck. C1–C4: ongoing respiratory support. C6–C7: anticipate impending respiratory problems. Early and aggressive physiotherapy.

quire prolonged or ongoing ventilatory support, and efforts must be directed toward offering them a variety of supportive systems in order to ensure their future mobility and participation to the fullest extent possible in life. These other ventilatory devices include portable positive pressure ventilators, negative-phase ventilators, cuirass-type respirators, rocking beds, pneumobelts, etc.

Hypercapneic Respiratory Failure Related to Airways Disease

Table 7.8 outlines the major management concerns related to asthma (more completely covered in Chapter 13) and chronic obstructive pulmonary disease (COPD). When patients with COPD go into respiratory failure it is often useful to categorize them, when possible, into those with panlobular emphysema and those with predominantly chronic bronchitis as the latter condition tends to be more readily treatable. COPD patients are usually pushed into respiratory failure by *intercurrent infection,* and every effort must be directed toward establishing a specific bacteriologic diagnosis so that appropriate antibiotic therapy can be begun early. In contrast to most other circumstances in which respiratory failure occurs, as a general rule mechanical ventilatory assistance should be employed only as a last resort in patients with chronic lung disease because of the danger of producing muscle

Table 7.8
Hypercapneic Respiratory Failure Related to Airways/Bellows Disease

Condition	Aggravating factors	Management concerns
Asthma	Allergy, infection	Danger signals: unresponsiveness to usual inhaled β-mimetics, silent chest, pulsus paradoxus > 20 mm Hg systolic, FVC < 10 ml/kg, FEV_1 < 6 ml/kg, normal or ↑ ġ $PaCO_2$, PaO_2 < 50 poorly responsive to ↑ FiO_2. Treatment[a]: β-mimetics—aerosolized *and* IV, IV methylxanthines, IV steroids, intubation and mechanical ventilation, lobar lavage, paralysis, appropriate antibiotics.
COPD	Infection, allergy, heart failure	Attempt to avoid mechanical ventilatory support. Treatment[a]: use of antibiotics for *infection,* digoxin and diuretics for heart failure (but with great care in cor pulmonale), methylxanthines IV, β-mimetics by aerosolization and IV, steroids, intubation and mechanical ventilation, tracheobronchial toilet, tracheostomy to facilitate tracheobronchial toilet for weaning.

[a] Drugs for management of airways disease

Aminophylline	Maintenance of therapeutic range of 10–20 μg/ml. Check blood levels! Load: 5–6 mg/kg, IV Maintenance: 0.7–0.9 mg/kg/hour, IV
Salbutamol	Aerosol: 1:4 dilution, nebulized over 10-minute intervals q1–6h. Load 10 μg/kg, IV Maintenance 0.2 μg/kg/min. Titrate to relief of bronchospasm or appearance of cardiovascular side effects.
Isoproterenol	1–2 mg in 200–500 ml D5W and titrate to HR 140–160 and/or relief of bronchospasm
Methylprednisolone	10 mg/kg IV q8h until objective improvement, then progressively one-half dose to 10–15 mg prednisone/day equivalent. In extrinsic asthma, follow eosinophil count as index of steroid effectiveness.

atrophy and ventilatory dyscoordination. The mainstay of therapy in this group is carefully controlled titrated oxygen, delivered to provide a PaO_2 of 55–60 mm Hg without withdrawing hypoxemic ventilatory drive. Oxygen may be provided via nasal cannula, calibrated Venturi mask, or face hood; but the O_2 must be treated like a drug, with the FiO_2 being titrated to effect. In patients who are oxygen-unresponsive and in those with a rising $PaCO_2$ and decompensating [H+], intubation and mechanical ventilation may have to be instituted. When this has occurred, every effort must be made to get the "chronic lunger" off the ventilator and breathing on his or her own as soon as possible so as to prevent the development of serious ventilatory dyscoordination and respiratory muscle atrophy. IMV may be useful in this situation, but its effect should be assessed carefully. In order to promote early weaning, sedation and analgesics should be used sparingly, if at all. Occasionally the added nonelastic load of an endotracheal tube makes weaning by cold nebulization or T-piece trial impossible, and, in this situation, one must resort to the SOS approach. Similarly, it may be necessary to perform a tracheotomy in the COPD patient on the ventilator in order to improve tracheobronchial toilet and facilitate weaning (diminished nonelastic load and anatomic deadspace).

Table 7.8 describes some of the specific management concerns for COPD patients in respiratory failure, which are similar to those described for asthmatics, although the role of steroids in managing the COPD patient is controversial. Salbutamol may be employed as an aerosolized medication in a 1:4 dilution administered either at intervals or continuously. Methylxanthines in the form of aminophylline are conventionally given in a loading dose of 5–6 mg/kg followed by 0.7–0.9 mm/kg/hour, although care must be taken to follow aminophylline blood levels, rather than relying on a "cookbook" approach. Ideally, one should strive to attain a blood level of 10–20 μg/ml and be aware of problems of drug metabolism when other drugs are used or when there is liver disease. Emphasis must be placed on combating infection, and Gram smears of sputum, as well as appropriate cultures, should be examined to determine which antibiotic is most appropriate.

Some of these patients present as cor pulmonale with marked peripheral edema and pulmonary hypertension. The inclination to treat these individuals with large doses of diuretics must be resisted as they require their preload in order to maintain an adequate cardiac output. Because cardiac output is the major determinant of arterial oxygenation in the presence of a fixed pulmonary shunt, any maneuver resulting in a potential decline in cardiac output, such as using furosemide to get rid of the edema, should be pursued with caution. The drug of choice for control of the pulmonary hypertension or cor pulmonale is oxygen. In panlobular emphysema patients, the abrupt institution of intermittent positive pressure breathing via endotracheal tube may precipitate a sudden fall in cardiac output and demise. This fall can be avoided by full atropinization of the patient along with augmentation of preload through volume infusion.

Table 7.9
Functional Changes in Hypoxemic Respiratory Failure

$\downarrow$ PaO_2
$\downarrow$ Or normal $PaCO_2$
$\uparrow$ $\dot{V}_A$
$\uparrow$ Work of breathing
$\uparrow$ V_D
$\uparrow$ f
$\downarrow$ RV and FRC

HYPOXEMIC RESPIRATORY FAILURE (HRF)

Many of the conditions associated with HRF can be conveniently lumped together under the heading of the adult respiratory distress syndrome—ARDS. This condition is covered in some detail in Chapter 11, and only a few of the most important points are emphasized here.

Although the term ARDS is and has been valuable, it is important always to seek a more specific cause of the hypoxemia, particularly of specifically treatable conditions, such as the bacterial pneumonias. It seems that a final common pattern of lung injury can occur regardless of how the lung is assaulted. Injury to the blood-gas interface may occur via the airway, the bloodstream, or directly (Fig. 7.1). The lung seems to have a stereotyped way of responding to these diverse insults—with an alteration in the alveolocapillary membrane that permits net egress of fluid from the vascular compartment into the interstitium and alveolar space of the lung. Table 7.9 summarizes the major functional abnormalities seen in ARDS.

Although there is considerable controversy over the precise pathogenetic mechanisms involved in the production of this syndrome, our supportive management of the condition is relatively straightforward. The major supportive techniques available are noted in Table 7.10. Again, it is to be emphasized that continued attempts must be made to secure a primary diagnosis (this may

Table 7.10
Support Principles for Patients with Hypoxemic Respiratory Failure

A. Oxygenation: titrated O_2
1. Nasal cannulae
2. Mask
3. Mask and reservoir

B. Alteration of lung volumes
1. CPAP
2. High V_T
3. Sighs
4. PEEP

C. Careful fluid balance: $\dot{Q}_T$ optimized for O_2 transport
1. Attention to crystalloid overload
2. Negative fluid balance
3. Diuretics
4. Diuretics and ECFV maintenance with oncotic load
5. Dialysis: ultrafiltration
6. Pharmacologic manipulation of $\dot{Q}_T$, "afterload," "preload"

D. Changes in posture: side-to-side, prone/supine

E. Membrane oxygenation

Table 7.11
Indications for Initiation of PEEP

$PaO_2 < 75$ mm Hg with $FiO_2 > 0.5$
Requirement for $FiO_2 > 0.45$ for > 12 hours to produce Hb-saturating PaO_2
Diffuse relatively homogeneous lung disease
"Prophylactic PEEP"—high risk ARDS patient
Relative contraindications to PEEP application
↓ ECFV
Patchy, necrotizing, nonhomogeneous pulmonary process
Unilateral lung disease
Panlobular emphysema

involve lung sticks with fine needles or transbronchial or open lung biopsy), particularly when specifically treatable infective agents may be involved in the septic or febrile patient. Seeking out a treatable cause is perhaps most important in those immunologically impaired individuals who develop "whited out lungs" with HRF.

The mainstay of support, however, remains *oxygenation*. Some of the milder forms of ARDS may be successfully managed by simply elevating the inspired oxygen fraction. This action is usually unsuccessful, however, due to the large shunt component that most of these patients manifest. Generally the application of some form of distending airway pressure becomes desirable or mandatory. The author has not found the mask application of CPAP in spontaneously breathing adult patients to be very successful. The added work of breathing, the unpleasantly tight-fitting, claustrophobia-producing mask, and the inevitable distention of the gut are more than most patients can tolerate. Generally, intubation with mechanical ventilation is required, with the subsequent application of PEEP. The indications for the initiation of PEEP are outlined in Table 7.11. Some physicians also use PEEP prophylactically in those patients considered to be at great risk of developing hypoxemic respiratory failure. Anecdotal evidence would support this view, but should be weighed against the attendant and perhaps unnecessary barotrauma imposed. In this regard, there is some evidence that PEEP is associated with an increase in extravascular lung water and may, in itself, be damaging to alveolocapillary partition in the long run.

A PEEP level is sought by progressive increments that allow maintenance of a hemoglobin-saturating PaO_2 without significant compromise of cardiac output and oxygen transport. This is often difficult to determine without serial measurements of cardiac output, and of CaO_2 and $P\bar{v}O_2$. The author has found the concept of "best PEEP" to be unhelpful as most of these patients are on the top flat part of their compliance curve. Cardiac output can, of course, be maintained by augmentation of preload through fluid administration, as well as by pharmacologic manipulation; however, here the physician must be careful, as "pushing the cardiac output" with fluids may produce a larger shunt fraction. Conversely, as noted previously, in the presence of a fixed pulmonary shunt, the $P\bar{v}O_2$ and hence PaO_2 may be dependent upon cardiac output level, with low cardiac outputs producing low PaO_2 levels. As a general rule, it is sensible to keep ARDS patients a bit "on the dry side" and to de-emphasize crystalloid fluid replacement.

Position is extremely important in the support of ARDS patients. We use the circle electric bed in order to find positions that optimize VQ relationships. Figure 7.9 demonstrates the improvement in oxygenation that may be seen in an ARDS patient when moved to a prone position. It should be stressed, however, that it is the *change* in position that is important, rather than the position itself, and that side-to-side changes can also result in significant improvements in PaO_2—thus allowing a reduction in damagingly high FiO_2 levels.

From a prognostic point of view, despite fancy ventilators, positive end expiratory pressures, careful fluid therapy, antibiotics, titrated oxygen, etc., the overall mortality for the ARDS remains around 30–50% in the best institutions. This high mortality rate obviously reflects to some degree the underlying conditions, e.g., the ARDS associated with abdominal sepsis and other organ system failure, such as acute tubular necrosis, has a particularly bleak outlook. Aside from the prognostic implications of attendant illness, other prognostic indices include PEEP and dehydration responsiveness, and the

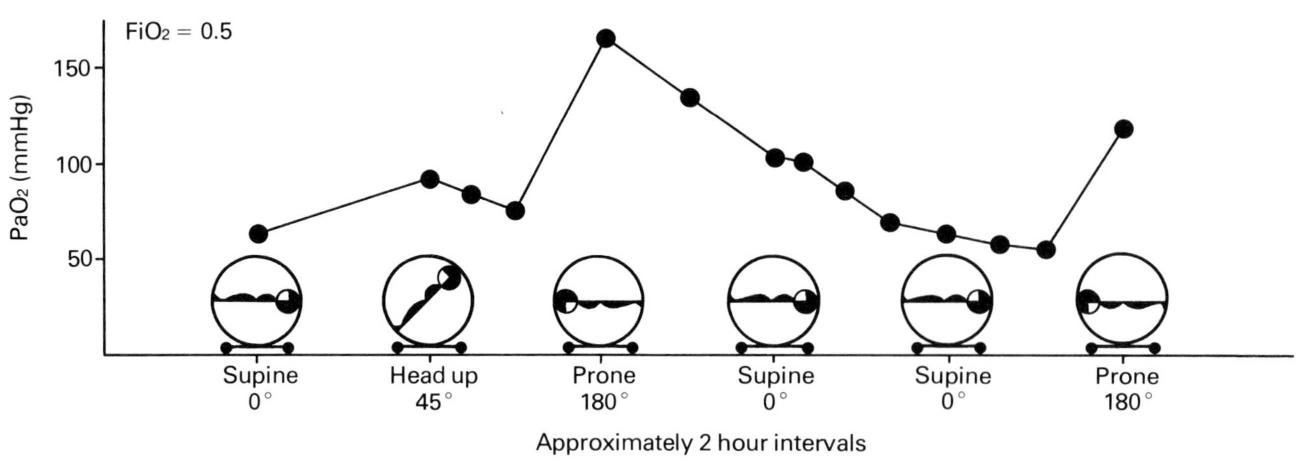

Figure 7.9. Diagram illustrating the effects on PaO_2 of alterations in body position in a patient on a fixed FiO_2 and $\dot{V}_A$.

findings on lung biopsy. It is not uncommon for long-term ARDS patients to demonstrate an improvement in their $AaDO_2$. Despite this improved matching of ventilation with perfusion in the few remaining normal lung regions, diminishing effective compliance, progressive pulmonary hypertension, and a lung biopsy that shows alveolar, ductal, and interstitial fibrosis are harbingers of ultimate demise.

Glossary of Abbreviations

$AaDO_2$	Alveolar to arterial difference (gradient) for oxygen (mm Hg)
ABGs	Arterial blood gases
ARDS	Adult respiratory distress syndrome—virtually synonymous with hypoxemic respiratory failure
CaO_2	Content of oxygen carried in arterial blood (ml/100 ml, ml%, vol%)
COPD	Chronic obstructive pulmonary disease
CPAP	Continuous positive airway pressure (distending-airway pressure in a spontaneously breathing patient)
D5W	5% dextrose in water
ECFV	Extracellular fluid volume
f	Respiratory frequency or rate
FEV	Forced expiratory volume
FiO_2	Fraction of inspired oxygen (a decimal, e.g., 0.4, or %)
FRC	Functional residual capacity
FVC	Forced vital capacity
$[H^+]$	Hydrogen ion concentration (mEq/liter)
[Hb]	Hemoglobin concentration (g/100 ml, g%)
HR	Heart rate
HRF	Hypoxemic respiratory failure
IMV	Intermittent mandatory ventilation (regularly applied mechanical breaths superimposed on a spontaneous breathing pattern)
IPPB	Intermittent positive pressure breathing
O_2t	Oxygen transport
PaO_2	Partial pressure of oxygen in arterial blood (mm Hg)
$PaCO_2$	Partial pressure of carbon dioxide in arterial blood (mm Hg)
PEEP	Positive end expiratory pressure (distending airway pressure in a mechanically ventilated patient)
PiO_2	Partial pressure of inspired oxygen (mm Hg)
PIP	The maximum subatmospheric pressure that a patient can exert against a closed system from functional residual capacity (FRC) (mm Hg or cm H_2o)
po	by mouth
prn	Pro re nata; as required
q6h	Once every 6 hours
$\dot{Q}$	Perfusion (ml/unit time)
$\dot{Q}_T$	Cardiac output (ml/min)
SaO_2	Saturation of hemoglobin by oxygen (%)
$\bar{v}$	Venous
$\dot{V}$	Ventilation (ml/unit time)
$\dot{V}_A$	Alveolar minute volume (ml/min)
V_C	Vital capacity (ml)—the volume of air moved when breathing out from total lung capacity (TLC) down to residual volume (RV)
V_D	Dead space volume
V_T	Tidal volume (ml)—the volume of an average tidal breath

Suggested Readings

Bendixen HH, Egbert LD, Hedley-White J, et al: *Respiratory Care*. St. Louis, CV Mosby, 1965.

Brandstetter RD: The adult respiratory distress syndrome. *Heart Lung* 15: 155–164, 1986.

Dantzker DR (ed): *Cardiopulmonary Critical Care*. Orlando, FL, Grune & Stratton, 1986.

Kirby RR, Sun RA, Desantels DA: *Mechanical Ventilation*. New York, Churchill-Livingstone, 1985.

Sykes MK, McNicol MK, Campbell EJM: *Respiratory Failure*. Oxford, Blackwell Scientific, 1976.

CHAPTER

8 Mechanical Support of Respiration

John H. Gallant, R.R.T.

The importance of proper and effective application of respiratory and ventilatory support cannot be overemphasized. To provide incorrect support is, at least, ineffective and, at its worst, dangerous. Patients cared for in an intensive care unit require a wide range of respiratory support, from humidification of their inspired air to total ventilatory control. The purpose of this chapter is to describe on a basic level the various types of respiratory and ventilatory equipment in use, their function, and application.

OXYGEN THERAPY AND ANCILLARY EQUIPMENT

Oxygen therapy takes place when an FiO_2 (fractional concentration of inspired oxygen, expressed as a decimal) delivered to a patient's airway is higher than that provided by room air ($FiO_2 = 0.21$). There are a number of methods available for providing oxygen therapy. Outlined below are the devices* most often used in the intensive care setting.

Simple Oxygen Mask (Fig. 8.1)

The simple oxygen mask is a clear green vinyl mask with perforations on each side and a small-bore green oxygen supply tubing attached. It must be remembered that therapeutic oxygen is totally dry due to the process of its production. Inspired gas must be 100% humidified at body temperature before it reaches the alveoli because dry gas can result in reduced mucociliary clearance and airway epithelial damage. With the use of this mask oxygen is humidified by passing through a bubble-through type humidifier mounted under the flowmeter. The mask's FiO_2 delivery is fit and flow dependent. That is, the FiO_2 delivered to the patient is a product of how well the mask fits the patient's face and whether the flow of oxygen through the humidifier and to the mask is sufficient to meet a predicted percentage of the patient's inspiratory demand. If it is not, the patient will supplement this delivery with ambient air through the side vents in the mask, thereby reducing the predicted FiO_2. This device should not be one's first choice for long-term therapy.

Venturi Oxygen Mask (Fig. 8.1)

To some extent this is a misnomer but because the name "Venturi Oxygen Mask" is in popular use to describe this device, it will be referred to as such in our text.

This mask is available in several forms, but all will have a Venturi somewhere near the patient. A Venturi is a device constructed so as to utilize a principle first expressed by Daniel Bernoulli in the mid-1700s. Essentially what Bernoulli described was that the lateral pressure of a gas flowing through a tube varies inversely with the velocity of that gas. In other words, as a gas is accelerated through a restriction, lateral pressure drops. Giovanni Venturi then applied this principle to construct a device that would entrain fluids from a secondary source.

In the Venturi mask the oxygen is accelerated through a restriction or jet, and the secondary source entrained is room air. The dilution is controlled by a calibrated jet or the size of the entrainment holes, so that a controlled fixed oxygen concentration is delivered. Some varieties have color-coded and changeable Venturis. These are calibrated to deliver a specific FiO_2, e.g., 0.24, 0.28, 0.31, 0.35, 0.40. Another type can be adjusted manually to deliver an FiO_2 of 0.24, 0.26, 0.28, 0.31, 0.35, 0.40, or 0.50. Still others have adjustable dials on the Venturi that alter the size of the entrainment ports.

Flow of oxygen through the bubble-through type humidifier must be set according to the instructions on the Venturi in each of the above examples. The ability of this type of mask to deliver a controlled, low FiO_2 makes it especially useful for patients who, because of long-standing airflow limitation, have become CO_2 retainers and could become apneic if the PaO_2 (partial pressure of oxygen in arterial blood) were allowed to increase too much. These patients risk CO_2 narcosis and death if the hypoxic stimulus to breathe is removed.

High Concentration Mask (Fig. 8.1)

These masks are basically of two types: the partial rebreather and the nonrebreather. The essential difference between the two is the presence of a valve between the reservoir and the patient. The approximate expected FiO_2 is 0.60 with the partial rebreather and greater than 0.80 with the nonrebreather mask. Safe management of these masks includes assuring sufficient oxygen flow to retain some volume in the reservoir bag during all phases of the patient's breathing cycle. It should be noted that the degree of fresh gas in-flow with the partial rebreather mask will change the amount of carbon dioxide in the reservoir. However, because the first gas to enter the reservoir on patient exhalation is upper airway gas, which is low in carbon dioxide, the resultant pCO_2 of the inhaled gas mixture is not high.

*Becton, Dickinson Canada, 2464 South Sheridan Way, Mississauga, Ontario L5J 2M8, Canada.

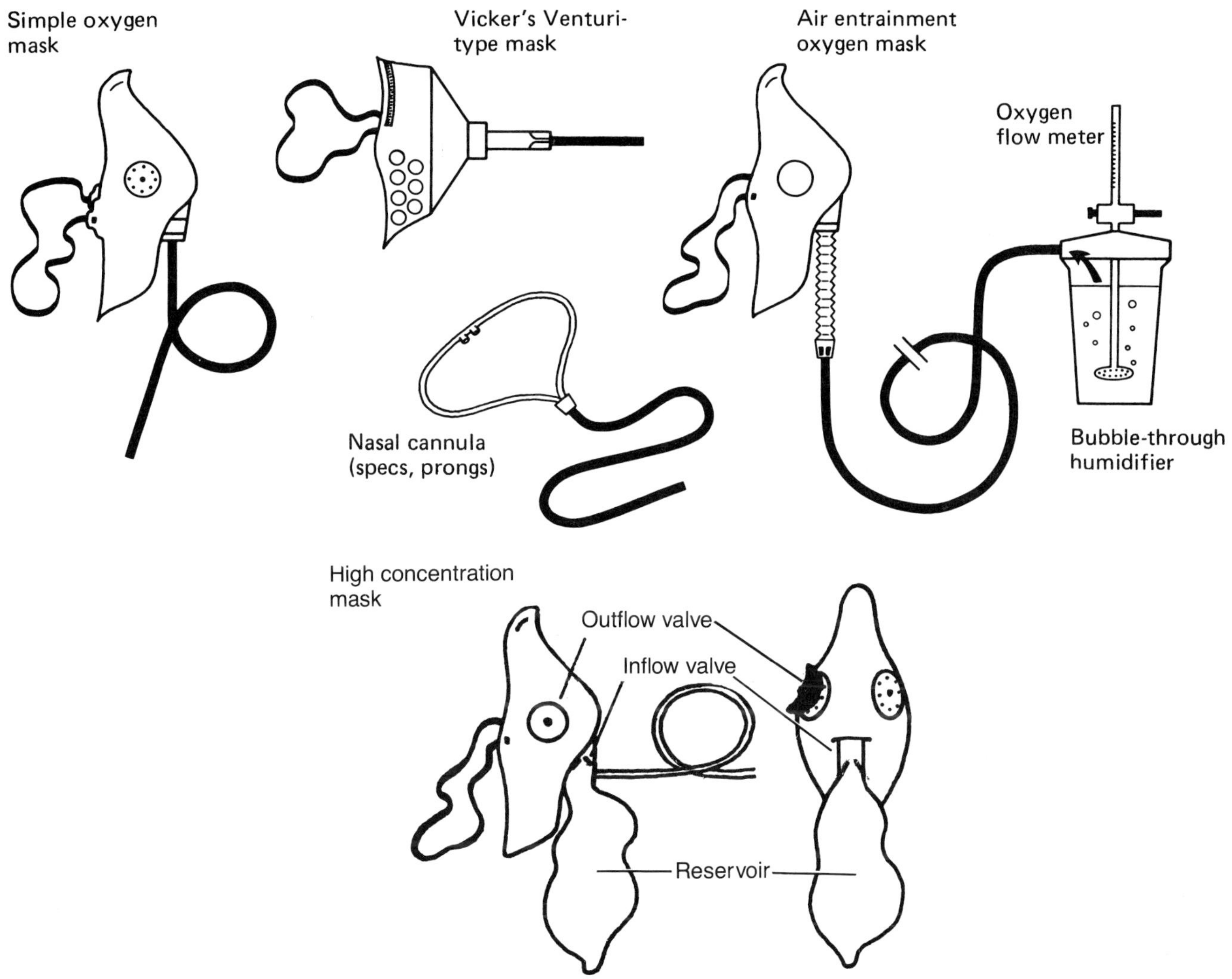

Figure 8.1. Simple oxygen mask, Venturi-type masks, nasal cannula, and bubble-through humidifier.

Nasal Cannula (Specs, Prongs) (Fig. 8.1)

This device is also fit and flow dependent. If properly fitted to the patient, the FiO_2 will vary more or less in proportion to changes in flow. A third factor that will affect an expected FiO_2 from this or any of the above-mentioned devices is the patient's respiratory pattern. A large tidal volume (V_T) inhaled quickly will result in a lower FiO_2 than a small V_T inhaled slowly. The patient's pharynx and tracheobronchial tree act as a mixing chamber. With the oxygen flow constant, concentrations will vary with any change in the amount of room air inhaled. The FiO_2 does not vary appreciably between mouth and nose breathing patients receiving oxygen therapy by a nasal cannula provided the nasal passages are patent.

Bubble-Through Humidification (Fig. 8.1)

This device is so named because the gas delivered flows from a flowmeter at the wall, or cylinder and regulator, through a water reservoir via a tube that terminates in a porous disperser several inches into the water. The gas is passed through the disperser to minimize the bubble size, which increases the gas/water interface and allows for better humidity. Now partially humidified, the gas passes up and out into a small diameter tube and on to any one of the above-mentioned oxygen therapy devices.

This device is less than ideal for increasing the relative humidity of the totally dry oxygen. The many different types of bubble-through humidifiers that have been tested yield a relative humidity range of 30–38%. For long-term oxygen therapy, a better system is required because of the workload that inadequate humidification places upon the mucous membranes to complete the job of totally humidifying the inspired gas.

Nebulizer Humidification (Fig. 8.2)

This device is a better humidifier of inspired air/oxygen than a bubble-through device. It draws water up from its reservoir, and a jet of gas (either oxygen or air) atomizes the water into tiny particles. These particles are further baffled and end up very small (0.5–5.0 μm). By greatly increasing the gas/water interface, relative humidity is increased to at least double that of the bubble-through

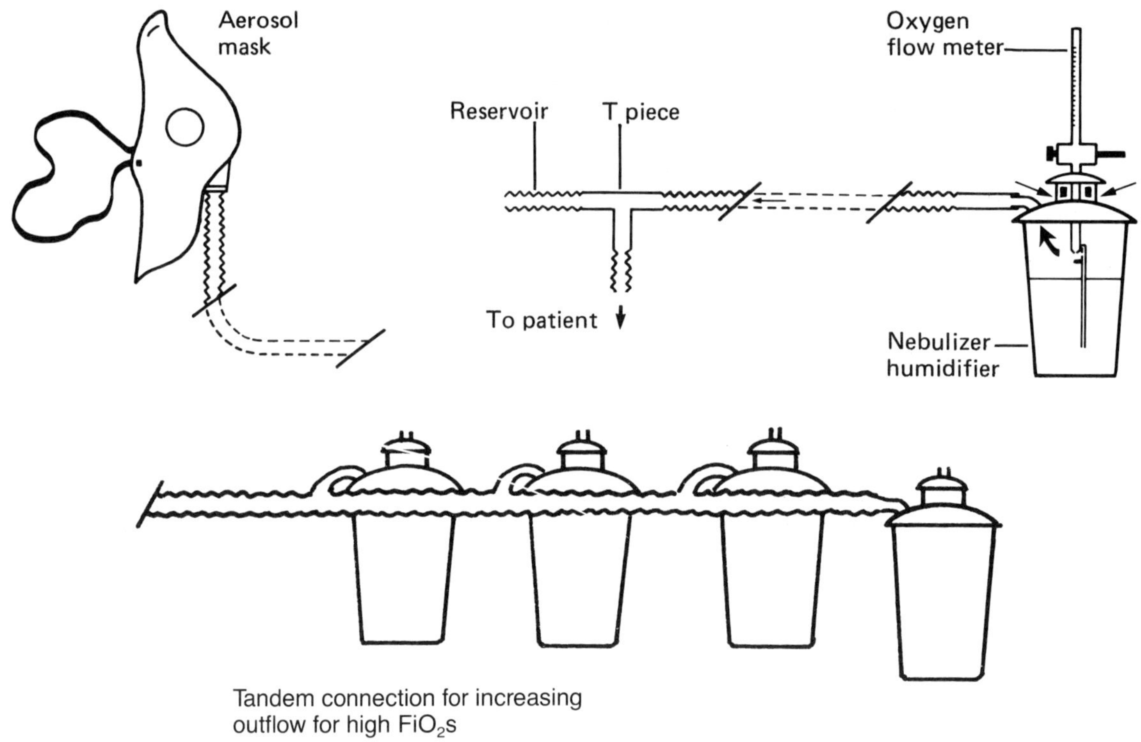

Figure 8.2. Aerosol mask and nebulizer humidification.

humidifier. This can be further increased by heating the water because this heat transfers to the gas passing through it and thus increases its ability to hold water vapor.

It must be noted that gas and water leaving the nebulizer are conveyed by a large diameter tube (22 mm), which is made of corrugated opaque plastic and is light weight. The large volume of this tubing allows vaporization of the water to continue as it travels to the patient's mask or other device.

Aerosol Mask (Fig. 8.2)

In appearance this mask is much like the simple oxygen mask except it has a 22-mm connector for aerosol tubing attachment and has large round holes on each side. An important point is that the nebulizer used with the aerosol mask should also be an oxygen-diluter nebulizer. That is, it should function much like the Venturi mask—dilution by entrainment. Adjusting the diluter for a specific FiO_2 would allow it to deliver a very close approximation of the FiO_2 indicated on the dial. It does this by changing the size of the entrainment holes. The thing to remember about this device is that it is not flow dependent and will retain the selected FiO_2 through a wide range of flowmeter settings.

When setting up an aerosol mask, the clinician should adjust the diluter on the nebulizer to the desired FiO_2 and then open the flowmeter to at least 5–6 liters/min. Before placing the mask on the patient, check that an aerosol can be seen at the mask. After fitting the mask to the patient, adjust the flowmeter either up or down until, during the patient's peak inspiration, aerosol spill from the large round holes in the sides of the mask all but stops. With this procedure, the clinician can be sure the correct flow is being used to provide the patient with the desired oxygen therapy. Failure to do this results in substantial changes in delivered FiO_2 and makes control of therapy difficult.

It must be noted here that all nebulizer jets will have a maximum flow capacity, which is usually between 10–15 liters/min. If one assumes a patient's normal peak inspiratory flow to be 30 liters/min it can be readily seen that it is not going to be possible to deliver an FiO_2 of 1.00 to the patient. It is also common for a patient with hypoxia to increase his or her inspiratory flow significantly, perhaps to three times the normal flow or higher.

One method of overcoming this problem is to arrange several of these nebulizers in tandem. The use of quick-connect plumbed Y-adapters makes this possible. Inserting one Y into the wall outlet and one in each of these limbs provides mounting for four nebulizers and a total outflow of up to 60 liters/min at an FiO_2 of 1.00.

Intubated or Tracheostomized Patients (Fig. 8.2)

A large percentage of patients treated in the ICU are intubated or tracheostomized and, as such, are denied much of the natural means of humidifying their inspired air. Humidification must therefore be supplemented. Where no further therapy or ventilatory assistance is needed, humidification is accomplished by a nebulizer powered by compressed air and the conveying of aerosol to the patient by means of a T-piece. This is a simple device that gives the end of the patient's tube access to the flow of nebulized water and oxygen through the aerosol tube.

On the distal end of the T-piece is attached a short length of aerosol tubing (6–12 inches) that acts as a reservoir.

The flowmeter is set the same way as indicated for the aerosol mask (spill of aerosol all but stops on peak inspiration). Often V_T is not constant. However, the reservoir provides for the occasional small increase in V_T, thereby maintaining consistency of the FiO_2. It is advisable not to use too long a reservoir, because the aerosol supply tubing may become disconnected from the nebulizer or gas flow to the nebulizer may somehow be interrupted. Either of these situations would dramatically increase the patient's dead space if a long, large volume reservoir were used. Dead space (mechanical) is the volume of gas that must be rebreathed before fresh gas can reach the patient.

VENTILATORS

Intubated patients will, for one reason for another, often require ventilatory support. This section reviews ventilating equipment currently available and indicates the preferred choice to suit individual patient requirements. Ventilators are classified by how they cycle from the inspiratory phase to the expiratory phase or how inspiration is terminated.

Pressure-Cycled Ventilators (Fig. 8.3)

The Bird MK VII and MK VIII* are examples of pressure-cycled ventilators that deliver gas (inhalation) until a preset pressure limit is reached in the circuit. At that point the exhalation valve opens, and the patient exhales. This limitation makes it difficult to deliver consistently a specific volume of gas to the patient. However, by assessing airway resistance encountered and the dynamic compliance of the patient's lungs, flow rates and pressure limits can be adjusted to alter the volumes delivered. One can monitor this performance with a respirometer, a device that measures gas volumes.

*Bird Corporation, Palm Springs, CA 92262; telephone (714) 327-1571.

As a general rule, if the patient has higher than normal airway resistance and the V_T needs to be increased while using the Bird, then the flow should be decreased. This produces more laminar flow, which decreases the back pressure generated by the high flow through a resistance and prolongs inspiration, thereby increasing V_T. It may also be necessary to increase the pressure limit. Tidal volume management on a pressure-cycled ventilator therefore is a function of both flow and pressure limit, which are determined by the clinician.

The types of patients suitable for the pressure-cycled ventilator are (1) patients who do not have a high degree of pulmonary pathology; (2) postoperative patients admitted to an ICU for monitoring and ventilation to lessen the work of breathing; and (3) patients in emergency situations, because pressure-cycled machines are simple to operate and quickly set up.

Time-Cycled Ventilators

The Bourns BP-200† is an example of a time-cycled ventilator, which is frequently employed in the ventilation of pediatric patients. It is called a time-cycled ventilator because the length of the inspiratory phase is controlled by a timer. The machine has a master timer and integrates several timed functions:

1. The respiratory rate—the length of time between the closings of the exhalation valve.
2. The inspiratory/expiratory (I:E) ratio, which is determined by the portion of the respiratory cycle time devoted to inspiration. Inspiratory time is the length of time the exhalation valve remains closed. The remainder of the respiratory cycle is expiratory time.
3. The inspiratory time limiter serves as a safety control and limits the constant flow to a maximum time while adjusting the respiratory rate and I:E ratio controls to a new setting.

†Bourns Life Systems Division, 9335 Douglas Drive, Riverside, CA 92503. It is recognized that there are a number of excellent time-cycled ventilators available for use, e.g.: Healthdyne, Marietta, Georgia, Sechrist, Anaheim, California.

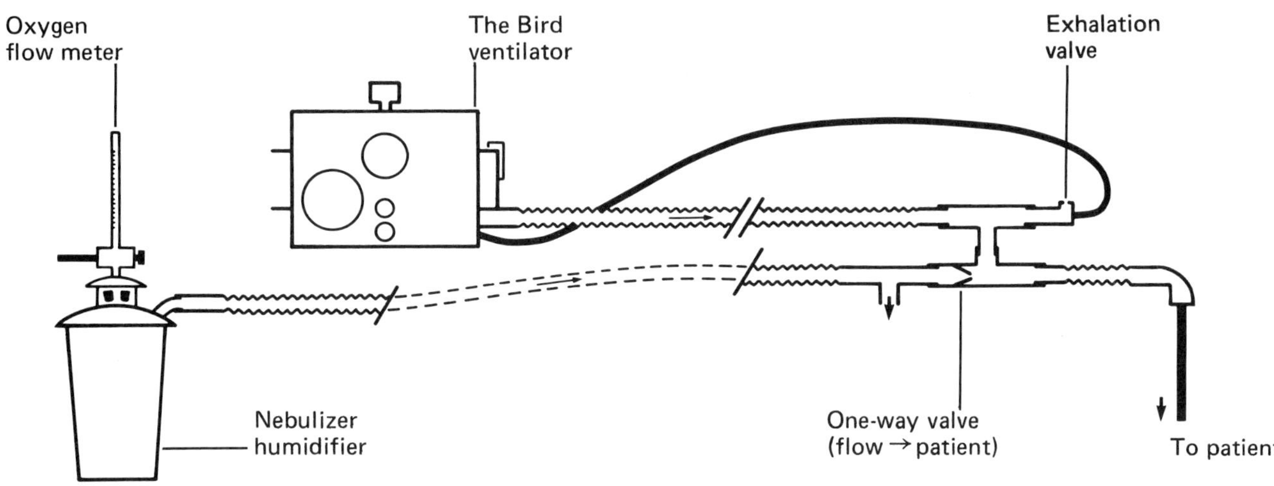

Figure 8.3. Circuit for the Bird intermittent mandatory ventilator.

It is important to mention that the gas flow through the BP-200 is controlled by a flowmeter built into the face of the unit. Once turned on, the gas flow is constant through the circuit and would simply spill into the air if the exhalation valve did not close. Because the timer, once set, closes and opens the exhalation valve intermittently and because the patient is connected to the circuit between the flowmeter and exhalation valve, the continuous flow shunts to the patient's lungs while the valve is closed. When the exhalation valve opens, the flow (together with the patient's exhalation) follows the path of least resistance and passes through the valve.

Because of the way the machine works, the BP-200 is an intermittent mandatory ventilator. Flow is continuous across the patient's airway and, as the mandatory ventilations from the ventilator are reduced in weaning, the patient simply supplements by breathing spontaneously from the passing fresh gas flow.

Other modalities available to the patient on the BP-200 are positive end-expiratory pressure (PEEP) and continuous positive airway pressure (CPAP). A high pressure jet of gas against the exhaled gas flow, which is controlled on the face of the machine, gives the clinician access to these two additional modes. The opposing gas flow results in increased pressure throughout the circuit, as well as the patient's lungs. This increase in pressure in the lung results in prolonged patency of soft terminal airways. Without this positive pressure, airways might close early and thus trap gas in the alveoli high in carbon dioxide ($PaCO_2$). More importantly this early closure will result in increased physiologic shunt by reducing the oxygen gradient in these areas.

This maneuver is particularly useful in increasing the PaO_2 in patients with ventilation/perfusion ($\dot{V}/\dot{Q}$) deficiencies. Essentially it is a matter of assisting the alveolar-capillary membrane to function more efficiently. This is done in two ways: (1) by airway splinting as mentioned above and (2) by increasing the functional residual capacity (FRC) of the lung. This increase in FRC simply supplies more O_2 molecules to the functional membranes for diffusion into the blood by prolonging the gradient. The application of these techniques usually results in an increase in oxygen tension in the blood.

The only difference between PEEP and CPAP is that PEEP is interrupted periodically by a controlled ventilation from a ventilator. To use CPAP on the BP-200, the mode selector on the face of the machine so marked is turned; the previously set respiratory rate and I:E ratio are suspended. The main gas flow and opposing gas flow will continue as before. The result is the patient will exhale against a controlled resistance and small airways are kept open.

Spontaneous CPAP (Fig. 8.4)

Spontaneous CPAP provides continuous airway pressure to a patient breathing spontaneously. Although it is possible, with difficulty, to provide CPAP to patients without an endotracheal tube or tracheostomy tube in place, this discussion will deal only with the intubated patient.

Several studies have shown that intubated patients on T-piece therapy for extended periods of time may have increased alveolar closure. It is felt that loss of lung volume is due in part to the removal of normal glottic airway resistance to exhalation resulting from emplacement of the tube.

With the use of the opposing gas flow principle and various properly placed pieces of tubing it is relatively simple to construct a spontaneous CPAP device (Fig. 8.4). The first requirement is a nebulizer and aerosol tubing. Attach a Bird #999-1757 Venturi T. Another T installed between the Venturi T and the patient provides access to the system to monitor the pressure. Then a short flextube and swivel connector of the type normally used on ventilators are added for patient connection.

The second requirement is a gas source for the opposing flow to the Venturi T. One can use either an oxygen blender with a needle valve to control the flow, or two flowmeters (air and oxygen) with the two supply tubings connected together before connection to the Venturi T. The mix must then be analyzed and the air and oxygen flows adjusted to yield both the desired CPAP (5, 10, or 15 cm H_2O) and the same FiO_2 as being supplied from the nebulizer. The patient's V_T is monitored by inserting a respirometer between the manometer T and the patient in such a way as to collect exhaled volumes.

Another method, a little more difficult to assemble but superior in several ways, provides blended gas, high humidity, ample patient flow, and safety systems (Fig. 8.4A).

Assembly requirements include a wheeled stand on which is mounted an oxygen blender fitted with two flowmeters as per the figure, an exhalation valve from a disposable volume ventilator circuit and a variable popoff of the spring/disk type, a manometer, and a disconnect alarm. Mount a heated nebulizer or heated pass-over humidifier to one of the flowmeters and a T-connector to the outlet. On one end attach a 3-liter anesthetic reservoir bag and, on the other, a length of ⅜-inch tubing. For the patient circuit use a Bain breathing circuit.®* Assemble the exhalation end to the pressure-monitoring T-connector and then to the pressure popoff and exhalation valve assembly.

The continuous positive airway pressure is provided by attaching a length of ¼-inch tubing to the second flowmeter and connecting it to the exhalation valve. This tubing has a T'd in restricted bleed. One that functions well is a Bird® inspiratory power-drive line center body brass fitting. Over this fitting is attached a short length of ¼-inch tubing with several linear cuts to prevent occlusion. CPAP is managed by manipulation of this gas flow. Patient gas, sufficient to distend the reservoir, is provided by the other flowmeter.

Occlude the patient end, fitted with a two-way swivel connector, before attachment to set the level of positive pressure. Set the popoff by opening it until it begins reducing level of CPAP and then closing it slightly. If an increase in positive pressure is required, remember to close the popoff before adjusting the CPAP flowmeter. Then re-

*Bain Breathing Circuit, Kendall Company, Hospital Products, Boston, MA 02101.

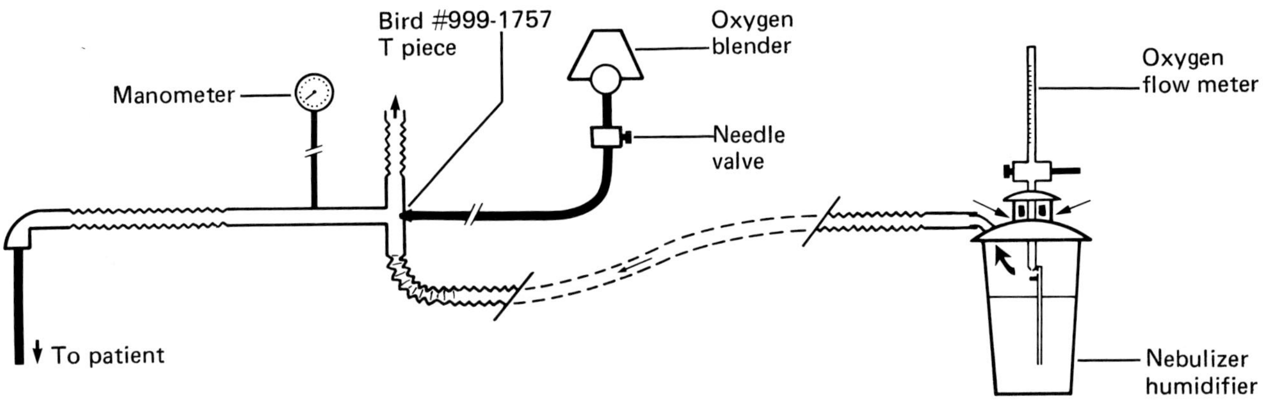

Figure 8.4. Apparatus for spontaneous CPAP.

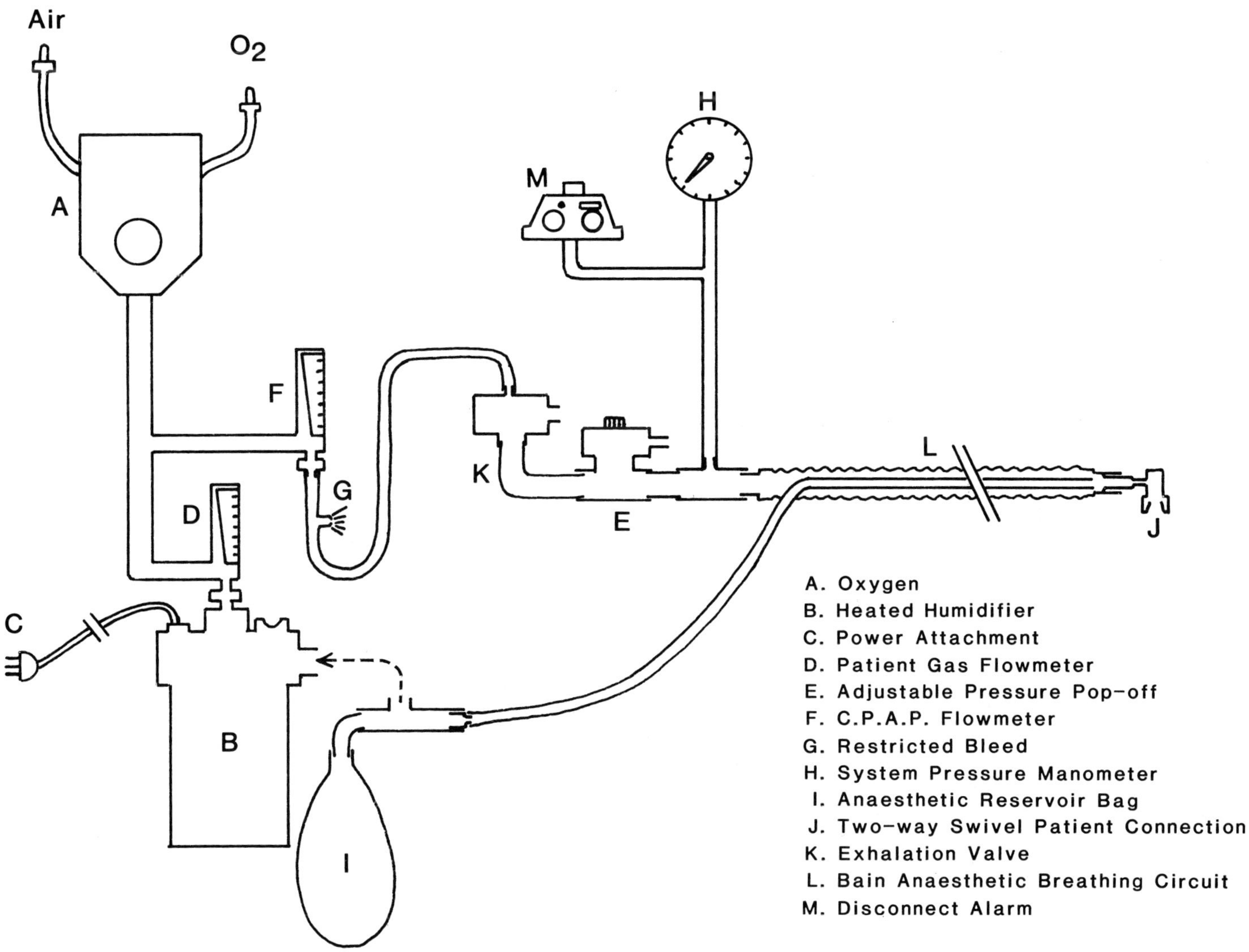

Figure 8.4A. Blended gas, high humidity CPAP apparatus.

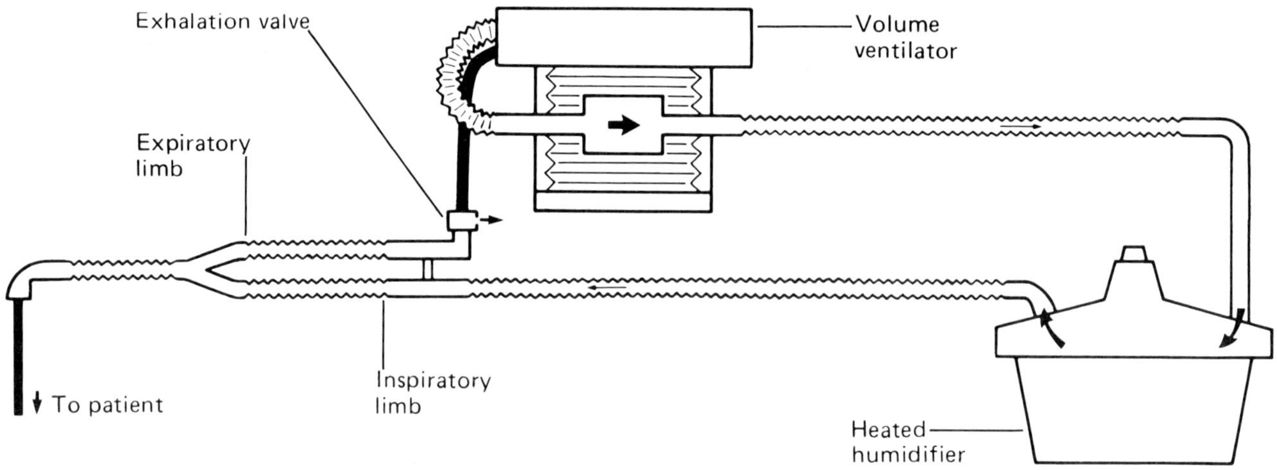

Figure 8.5. Volume-cycled ventilator circuit.

set the popoff as described above. This device provides excellent CPAP therapy for short-term or continuous therapy.

Volume-Cycled Ventilators (Fig. 8.5)

The Bennett MA1* and the Monaghan 225† are just two examples of the many different models of volume-cycled ventilators available. Each of these machines has a different internal circuitry that controls its functions, but as far as the patient is concerned they are the same. Each can be set to deliver a specific volume of gas, and each has FiO_2 control devices, variable flow controls, pneumatic exhalation valve control, adjustable pressure limit control, medication nebulizer control, and PEEP control. Essentially a ventilator is a volume ventilator when inspiration is terminated by delivery of a preset volume. There can be little argument with the statement that alveolar ventilation can best be controlled when an appropriate volume of fresh gas is tidally moved into and out of the lungs an appropriate number of times each minute.

For a variety of pathologic reasons, pumping a specific volume of gas into a patient's lungs can produce a variety of reactions. The compliance of the patient's lungs and thorax and obstructions in the airways causing resistance to gas flow are conditions that must be considered when setting up a ventilator. The volume ventilator is far more suitable for ventilation of patients with low compliance ("stiff" lungs) and high resistance because it will deliver a preset volume regardless of the pressure these conditions reflect. It must be restated here that these ventilators do have pressure limit controls that are usually adjusted to a level slightly higher than the peak airway pressure generated by the delivery of the preset volume.

An important consideration in volume ventilation is the flow rate of the preset volume. Flow rate should be adjusted either up or down after the patient is connected and ventilating, with attention paid to both the lowest possible peak airway pressure and the patient's I:E ratio. As a general rule, the presence of pathology, such as obstructive lung disease, for example, will require a lower flow rate in order to lower resistance. This prolongs inspiration and shortens expiratory time. Some volume machines have warning devices to indicate when the I:E ratio falls below 1:1. In this situation the clinician may encounter problems setting the ventilator to optimize ventilation and oxygenation. This type of patient should have a longer time for exhalation than patients without obstructive disease. In some cases an I:E ratio of 1:3 or 1:4 may be desirable for complete passive exhalation, especially in the patient with emphysema or chronic bronchitis. The consequence of these ventilator settings is reduced cycle rates with resulting hypoventilation and possible hypoxemia. One of the ways we deal with this problem is by adding PEEP. Its splinting effect on the airways facilitates the exit of expiratory gas and allows for a reduction in arterial carbon dioxide, an improvement in arterial oxygen, and a shorter expiratory time. This reduced exhalation time allows us to use lower flows for delivery of the V_T and a higher rate if required.

Unlike the time-cycled ventilator mentioned earlier, these volume-cycled machines (Fig. 8.5) are not inherently intermittent mandatory ventilators (IMV), although some machines can be modified to provide this modality. They do not supply a continuous flow of gas during the expiratory phase of ventilation. As a result, to use IMV a supplementary circuit must be attached to the ventilator. In our critical care/trauma units we do this by attaching a reservoir bag that is supplied with a mix of both air and oxygen to the same proportions as used in the ventilator (Fig. 8.6). This circuit is fitted to the inlet port of the heated humidifier by way of a one-way valve. This valve is necessary to close the circuit against volume loss into the supplementary circuit when the ventilator delivers a mandatory breath. Most of the state-of-the-art ventilators provide synchronized IMV

*Puritan-Bennett Corporation, Oak at 13th, Kansas City, MI 64106.
†Monaghan Corporation, 40 East Dry Creek Road, Littleton, CO 80122; telephone (303) 770-2700.

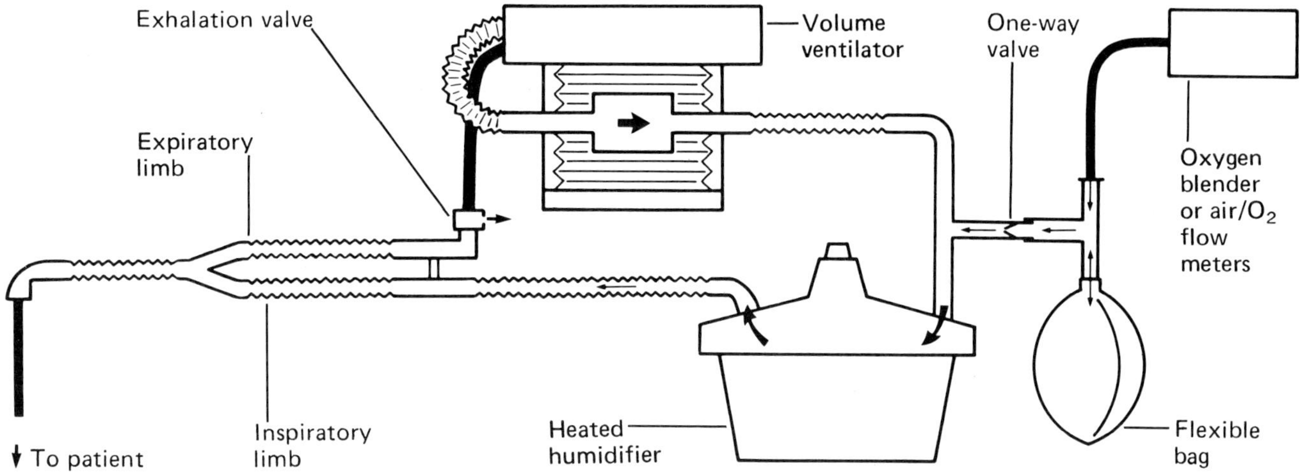

Figure 8.6. Supplementary circuit to volume ventilator for IMV.

mode with ample gas flow potential to meet the patient's peak inspiratory flow demand and would not require the addition of this supplementary gas circuit. However, they are rather costly.

MONITORING VENTILATOR PERFORMANCE

Although the volume ventilators are calibrated so that the clinician can dial the required volume, this does not mean the patient will necessarily receive that volume. Several factors will reduce the generated volume to the delivered volume: poor patient compliance, flow rate too high, small undetected circuit leaks, and, to a lesser degree, the temperature of the water in the humidifier.

Compliance and resistance are the two adversaries of volume delivery in mechanical ventilation. In simple terms, compliance is a measure of the chest's "willingness" to be inflated by the delivery of a volume of gas by a ventilator. Compliance is reduced by a stiff chest wall, an edematous lung, or pneumothorax. Resistance is primarily concerned with the tubes of the respiratory organ—the airways. If the airways are restricted by secretions, neoplasm, or bronchospasm then serious decreases in gas volume delivered to the respiratory unit for a given driving pressure result. Volume ventilators will, however, deliver volume in spite of this increase in resistance, but only at the cost of increased peak and mean airway pressures unless the preset peak pressure limit is reached. Reaching this pressure causes the machine to terminate respiration and would result in reduced volume delivery.

Monitoring for an accurate delivered V_T is done by inserting a respirometer, a hand-held device that meters flow and indicates volume, in the circuit to measure the volumes of gas exhaled by the patient. Adjustments are made to the ventilator with respect to this volume and not the volume indicated on the ventilator. This method of volume adjustment automatically allows for compliance losses and assures the clinician of desired volume delivery to the patient.

A close approximation of the volume lost to circuit compliance can be calculated by multiplying the peak airway pressure noted on the ventilator by a volume appropriate for the circuit and ventilator in use. For example, the circuit that we use on our volume ventilators has a compliance loss of 3 ml for every cm H_2O pressure resulting from volume delivery. Therefore if a patient's ventilator indicates a volume of 800 ml and this volume delivery results in a peak airway pressure of 30 cm H_2O, the volume loss to circuit compliance would be $3 \times 30 = 90$ ml. The volume actually received by the patient, provided no other leaks were present would then be $800 - 90 = 710$ ml.

Other parameters that require frequent monitoring are respiratory rate, ventilating pressures (both mean airway and peak airway), PEEP when used, FiO_2, heat level of the humidifier, and minute ventilation.

Disconnect alarm devices, if not inherent in your ventilator, are a required accessory. By tapping into the breathing circuit at a convenient location and properly setting the pressure sensor control one gains assurance of audible notification of a patient/circuit disconnection. This device may require frequent checks for safe function.

In our unit, the policy is to monitor patients and their ventilatory equipment q2h or according to their needs. This routine includes auscultation of the chest for bilateral air entry and location of loose bronchial secretions: if secretions are present they are removed by tracheobronchial suction. The oral cavity and pharynx are also suctioned. The integrity of the cuff around the endotracheal or tracheostomy tube is assessed by placing the diaphragm of the stethoscope on the trachea and listening for air leaking between the tracheal membrane and the cuff on peak inspiratory pressure from the ventilator. Only a minimum occluding volume should be used in the cuff. Attention to this volume assures that the lowest possible cuff to mucosal membrane pressure is used, thereby minimizing mucosal ischemia and necrosis. This pressure should be monitored at least twice a day. One method of monitoring this pressure is as follows: A manometer is connected to the cuff pilot line by means of a

T-connector with a syringe attached that is preloaded with 2–3 cc of air for additional volume if required. Add 1 cc of air to the system to compensate for cuff volume shift to the added manometer and tubing. While monitoring for leaks with the stethoscope, remove all gas from the cuff with the syringe. Note the position of the piston in the syringe and quickly replace most of the gas. Add gas in small amounts from the remaining volume in the syringe until the leak just stops. Note the position of the piston and calculate the volume used. Note the pressure on the manometer and record both numbers. This method assures that a minimum occluding volume of gas is used to seal the cuff.

At this point we turn our attention to the ventilator circuit (Fig. 8.5). If water condensation is evident in all limbs except the expiratory limb (the tubing from the patient Y to the exhalation valve), the heat level on the ventilator humidifier should be increased. This increase will further heat the water, and the gas passing through it will have a higher level of humidity. Continue to increase the heat until condensation in this limb of the circuit begins to appear. The use of thermometers that are commercially available and designed for the job make control of humidification much easier. Simply install one in the circuit near the patient connection and adjust the heat level of the humidifier to maintain temperature at, or just below, normal body temperature. Should you find that condensate levels are high in the circuit, even to the point of pooling in the dips in the circuit tubing, this water should be removed. Quickly disconnect, empty, and reconnect each limb of the circuit. Ideally the inspired gas should be close to normal body temperature.

Note the water level in the humidifier, and if necessary add sterile water by bypassing the humidifier temporarily with the circuit. This bypass can easily be done by connecting the tubing from the inlet port on the humidifier to the tubing from the outlet port. Remove the top of the humidifier and fill. Replace the top and reverse the bypass procedure, checking that all connections are secure.

The FiO_2 is monitored even though volume ventilators tend to have a sophisticated oxygen blender built in. This monitoring is done with an oxygen analyzer. There are several types available.* The type used in our unit at present is fuel-cell powered and indicates the concentration of O_2 in proportion to the molecules passing through the cell membrane. It comes with a T-piece that exposes the membrane to the ventilator gas while not causing volume loss. If a supplementary gas circuit is used in conjunction with the volume ventilator, remember to analyze both the ventilator gas and the supplementary gas. The ventilator gas should be measured at the main gas outlet before the humidifier and the supplementary gas proximal to the one-way valve (Fig. 8.6).

Tidal volume, minute volume, and respiratory rate are monitored by insertion of a respirometer in the circuit, as previously explained in the CPAP section. The respirometer is turned on for 1 minute and allowed to collect a total volume exhaled, and the number of exhalations are counted. This information is recorded on the patient's chart, as well as the average V_T obtained by dividing the minute volume by the rate. When using IMV the mandatory ventilation and the patient's spontaneous ventilation must be averaged separately. This separation is easily done by deducting the product of the known mandatory volume and rate from the total minute volume collected for 1 minute and dividing the remaining volume by the spontaneous rate. The peak airway pressure indicated on the ventilator manometer at peak inspiration is also recorded. This pressure determination is very important in monitoring volume ventilation because a change in this pressure, either up or down, can tell us a great deal about the patient's changing airway resistance.

Some examples of the reason for a rapid increase in airway pressure may be mucus plug, endotracheal tube slipping into the right mainstem bronchus, or pneumothorax. A slow increase in pressure might indicate developing pulmonary edema or other interstitial disease, perhaps adult respiratory distress syndrome (ARDS). A rapid decrease in pressure usually indicates a ventilator, circuit, or endotracheal cuff problem. A gradual decrease in pressure may indicate improvement in patient lung compliance and/or decrease in airway resistance.

An essential noninvasive monitoring technique used during mechanical ventilation is the daily chest x-ray. In addition to allowing the clinician to assess the resolution or progression of the primary disorder of the lung, it also provides for the monitoring of proper placement of the endotracheal tube, the degree of cuff inflation, and the presence of barotrauma. Action can then be initiated to treat or correct the problem.

As a means of reducing the routine use of blood gases, an invasive procedure, several other methods of patient monitoring have gained favor in recent years.

Transcutaneous, $TcpO_2/TcpCO_2$, monitors measure blood gases from heated skin sites that "arterialize" the capillary bed in the skin. It has been found that Tc gases correlate well with arterial blood gases in a high percentage of patients.

Capnometers are used to monitor alveolar CO_2 (end-tidal) by attaching a sensor or sensor sampling line to the patient's airway. A high degree of accuracy when compared to arterial pCO_2 has been shown.

Pulse/oximetery, a technology gaining popularity, is able to assess hemoglobin saturation noninvasively by passing appropriate light frequencies through a digit, the nose, or the ear. These devices also boast a pulse-counting sensor. They have been shown to be extremely sensitive and accurate.

The metabolic analyser is another tool that has found increasing favor in the management of the critically ill. The preprogramming, the entry of certain data, and the monitoring of the patient's expired gas yield a wealth of information, not the least of which is oxygen consumption versus CO_2 production and patient dead space. This

*Beckman Instruments, Irvine, CA; and Hudson Oxygen Therapy Sales Company, 27711 Diaz Street, PO Box 66, Temecula, CA 92390; telephone (714) 676-5611.

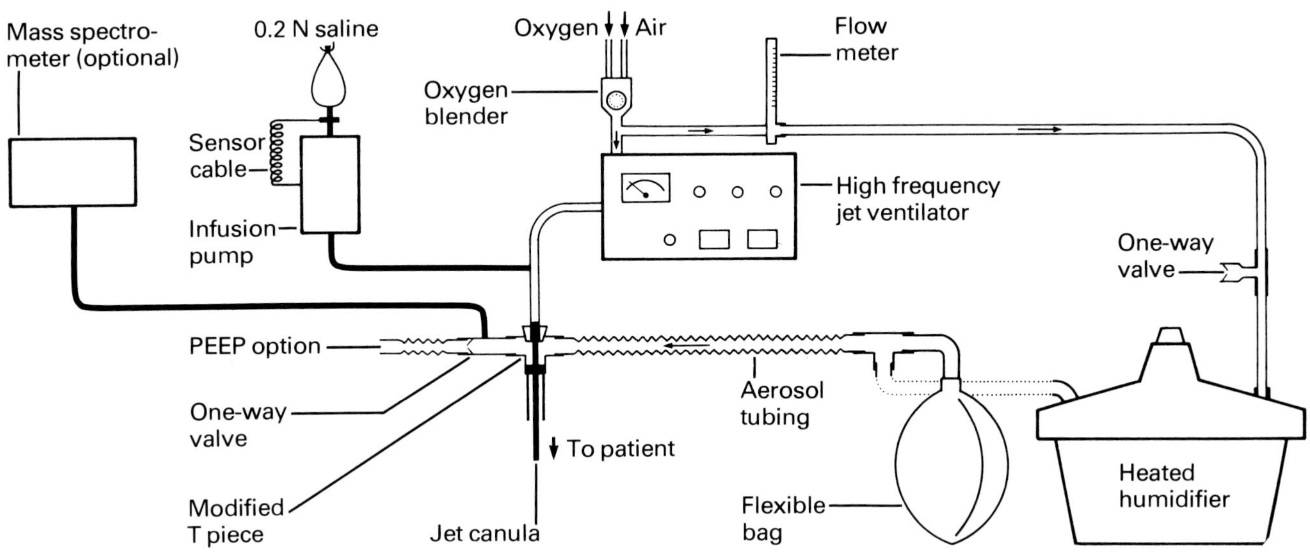

Figure 8.7A High frequency jet ventilation apparatus.

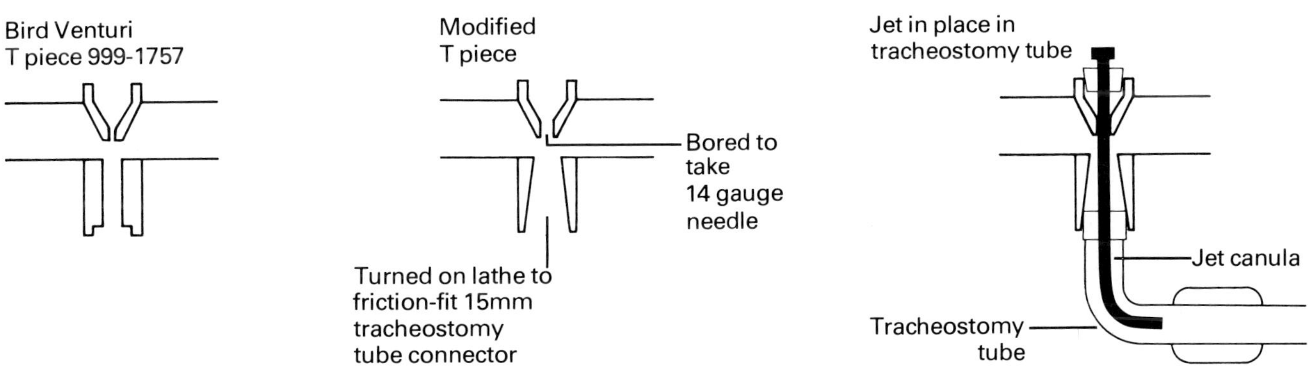

Figure 8.7B Modification of Bird Venturi T for use in jet ventilation apparatus.

machine has proven to be very helpful in the management of patient weaning in the presence of respiratory muscle fatigue.

Careful monitoring of certain lab results are essential for effective ventilatory control. Particular notice must be taken of hemoglobin levels to assure that satisfactory oxygen content in arterial blood can be maintained. Arterial lactate should also be noted as an indicator of sufficient oxygen delivery to the tissue. It is also important to note arterial pH to help assess the degree of right or left shift of the oxygen dissociation curve. These measures are essential for accurate assessment of oxygen delivery.

Problems may arise when the patient has received large amounts of acid citrate dextrose (ACD) stored blood in which the 2,3-DPG level has fallen. Ventilated patients being transfused with several units of blood stored with this preservative should be ventilated with a higher FiO_2 than would seem indicated to assure total saturation of the hemoglobin. Patient temperature also needs consideration as to its effect on the oxygen dissociation curve and allowances made in setting the FiO_2.

Tidal volume requirements based on 10–12 ml/kg of ideal body weight can be calculated, and a cycle rate of 10–14 breaths per minute used, but the real test of what minute alveolar ventilation to use is done by monitoring the $PaCO_2$. Normal range in controlled ventilation is 35–40 mm Hg and if the results indicate hypoventilation (not applicable in treating cerebral edema with hyperventilation), one has two options: reduce V_T or reduce respiratory rate. If the results indicate hypoventilation ($PaCO_2$ higher than normal) then consider increasing V_T or the respiratory rate. In both of these examples it would be usual to adjust the rate first.

High Frequency Jet Ventilation (HFJV) (Fig. 8.7A)

HFJV is a relatively new and dramatically different type of ventilation. Its development during the 1960s through the late 1970s in Europe and elsewhere probably resulted from the need to provide ventilation during bronchoscopy. It consisted of jetting gas through a needle placed into the trachea by either a transverse insertion or placed directly into the trachea by the mouth. At this time, more or less traditional rates were used. Acceptable ventilation and oxygenation resulted. Later experimentation during the late 1970s in North America revealed that a shorter insufflation time together with a more rapid rate also resulted in good gas exchange and, most importantly, at a very low peak intrabronchial pressure. This feature is important from the standpoint of barotrauma to the chest resulting from conventional positive pressure ventilation. Another application of this ventilatory mode is in patients with a patent bronchopleural fistula. Conventional positive pressure ventilation may keep the pulmonary tear open, and a large portion of the tidal volume delivered by the ventilator would then be lost through the chest tube. Because the peak intrapulmonary pressures, when using HFJV, do not generally reach more than a quarter to a third that of conventional ventilators, the "opening pressure" of the tear is not reached.

Why does it ventilate so successfully with an inspiratory time perhaps as short as 0.12 seconds and a cycle rate of 150/min? There are several postulated and, to some degree, documented reasons: first, because the system is not unlike a T-piece with the jet inserted through the middle, it is an open system. It depends on the very high flow of gas through the jet, together with the volume entrained from the T-piece and the resistance to exhalation gas escaping upward through the endotracheal lumen that partially limits the outflow rate, to build up a moderate pressure in the lung. In other words, some "exhalation" takes place during the latter part of insufflation, as well as between insufflations. Second, this activity so agitates the gas throughout the entire airway network that airways, which might otherwise close during the conventional ventilation expiratory phase, tend to remain open. This prolonged opening of the airway, in part, contributes to the enhanced diffusion reported in the literature. Kinetic activity of the gas in the airways is very much higher than with conventional ventilation due to the very high driving pressure of the jet gas. This activity too appears to be a factor in diffusion enhancement. Lastly, by increasing the driving pressure of the gas through the jet and thereby increasing the flow, one can increase the expansion volume of the lung in the face of unchanged pulmonary resistance. It should be evident that if the expiratory route (the remainder of the endotracheal tube lumen) remains constant and the jet flow is increased due to increasing the driving pressure, the result will be an increase in expansion volume.

Much remains to be learned concerning HFJV, but in certain clinical situations it has already shown great promise. The literature reports its use in neonatal respiratory distress syndrome (RDS), ventilation during CPR, bronchoscopy, general anesthesia, ARDS, postpneumonectomy, bronchopleural fistula, and others. Although these reports are quite positive, HFJV applicability for routine use in ventilating critically ill patients is not yet completely defined.

One of the systems we use is built on a VS-600* and comprises a circuit constructed in this hospital (Figs. 8.7A and B). Another (not pictured here) is the Healthdyne Impulse Ventilator.†

The future use of HFJV remains to be more completely elucidated. Further research and development may reveal new applications of this means of mechanical ventilation.

CONCLUSION

Mechanical support of respiration and ventilation has demonstrated undeniable therapeutic benefit in the management of the critically ill. Oxygen therapy in all its forms—artificial airway management, mechanical ventilation to control gas exchange in patients unable to breathe, the use of adjunct therapy such as PEEP to improve arterial oxygenation at lower FiO_2s, special circuitry such as the CPAP apparatus mentioned in this chapter, the monitoring techniques employed, and the use of HFJV—are examples of the contribution made to patient care by mechanical support of respiration.

Suggested Readings

Cherniack RM: *Current Therapy of Respiratory Disease.* St. Louis, CV Mosby, 1986.

Comroe JH: *Physiology of Respiration,* ed 2. Chicago, Year Book Medical Publishers, 1974.

Dorsch JA, Dorsch SE: *Understanding Anaesthesia Equipment.* Baltimore, Williams & Wilkins, 1984.

Dupuis YG: *Ventilators, Theory and Clinical Application.* St. Louis, CV Mosby, 1986.

Egan DF: *Fundamentals of Respiratory Therapy.* ed 3. St Louis, CV Mosby, 1977.

McPherson SP: *Respiratory Therapy Equipment,* ed 3. St. Louis, CV Mosby, 1985.

Slonim NB: *Respiratory Physiology.* St. Louis, CV Mosby, 1986.

West JB: *Pulmonary Pathophysiology—The Essentials.* Baltimore, Williams & Wilkins, 1982.

*I.D.C. Pittsburgh, PA

†Healthdyne, Marietta, Georgia

CHAPTER

9 Basic Principles of Chest X-Ray Interpretation in a Critical Care Unit

Michael S. Lefcoe, M.D.

The anteroposterior supine chest radiograph is the mainstay of radiology of the chest in a critical care environment. The examination is easy to perform and only minimally disturbs the patient. It offers an easily reproducible picture from day to day and allows good visualization of the lungs. Its drawbacks are that it does not allow diagnosis of small amounts of air and fluid in the pleural space. If one does anteroposterior supine chest films as the routine radiographs, then one must be prepared to do lateral decubitus films on the slightest suspicion of abnormalities in the pleural space. An upright anteroposterior film has the advantage of detecting small amounts of air and fluid in the pleural space and air fluid levels in the lung and, therefore, is the film of choice if technically possible. However, upright radiographs are not easily reproduced because the angle to which the trunk is elevated varies from day to day. It is mainly for these reasons that, in our institution, we employ the anteroposterior supine radiograph in most instances and use lateral decubitus films frequently to supplement this radiograph. In a few patients who are able to be put upright, an upright film is made.

In chest radiology, one cannot overemphasize the importance of having previous films available to compare on a day-to-day basis. Older films, if available, are very valuable because chronic processes in the lungs may be mistaken for acute life-threatening situations.

For optimal comparison and assessment of the lungs, especially in assessing pulmonary edema, the film must be made with the lungs well inflated to about the same degree with each radiograph. If patients are not on a respirator, this may be difficult. If the patient is on a respirator, the radiology technologists are instructed to expose the film when the lungs are maximally inflated. A technique useful for accomplishing this is to watch the respirator bellows. When patients are not on respirators but are unable to take an adequate inspiration, the respiratory technologist "bags" the patient in order to obtain films with an adequate volume of air in the lungs. If the patient is on intermittent mandatory ventilation (IMV) then the lungs will be variably inflated. In this case, the technologist must watch a few cycles of breathing before deciding on the most optimal cycle in which to make the exposure.

COMMON TECHNICAL PROBLEMS

When the radiologist or physician views the radiographs, certain technical abnormalities may be present that could lead to misinterpretation. Common abnormalities are listed below. If it is possible to repeat the film and eliminate these technical problems, this should be done. If this is not possible, then the interpretor must take into account these technical abnormalities and not mistake them for pathology.

Exposure

The chest radiograph is properly exposed when one can identify the disk space behind the heart, and the vessels behind the heart in the left lower lobe and still see vascular markings in the outer portion of the lung within 1 cm of the pleural surface without using a bright light.

If one cannot see the disk space behind the heart or vessels behind the heart, then the film is underpenetrated. If the film is too dark, then the vessels and markings in the outer portion of the lung cannot be visualized. A too-dark film can be assessed using a bright light, which is essential if one is not to interpret overexposed films as pneumothoraces, etc.

Motion Unsharpness

If the patient moves, if respiratory motion occurs during the exposure, or if exposure times are long, unsharpness of the radiograph is seen.

Rotation

Rotation can be assessed by marking the inner ends of the clavicles as an anterior structure and the spinous process of the thoracic vertebrae at the same level as the posterior structure. The distance between the inner end of each clavicle and the spinous process should be the same on both sides. In general, when the patient is rotated, the lung that is more dependent is poorly inflated and smaller and that side of the chest is whiter than the opposite side. An exception to this occurs with large breasts or soft tissue masses anteriorly that, when the patient is turned with that side down, may move out of the field and make the more dependent lung less white. In addition, when the patient is rotated, the trachea and other midline structures are displaced toward the dependent side in the supine position. The mediastinum appears abnormal. These findings can be mistaken for collapse of the lung or overinflation of the opposite lung by the unwary observer.

Degree of Expansion of the Lungs

Figure 9.1 demonstrates an inspiratory and expiratory film of the same patient. Notice the marked difference in

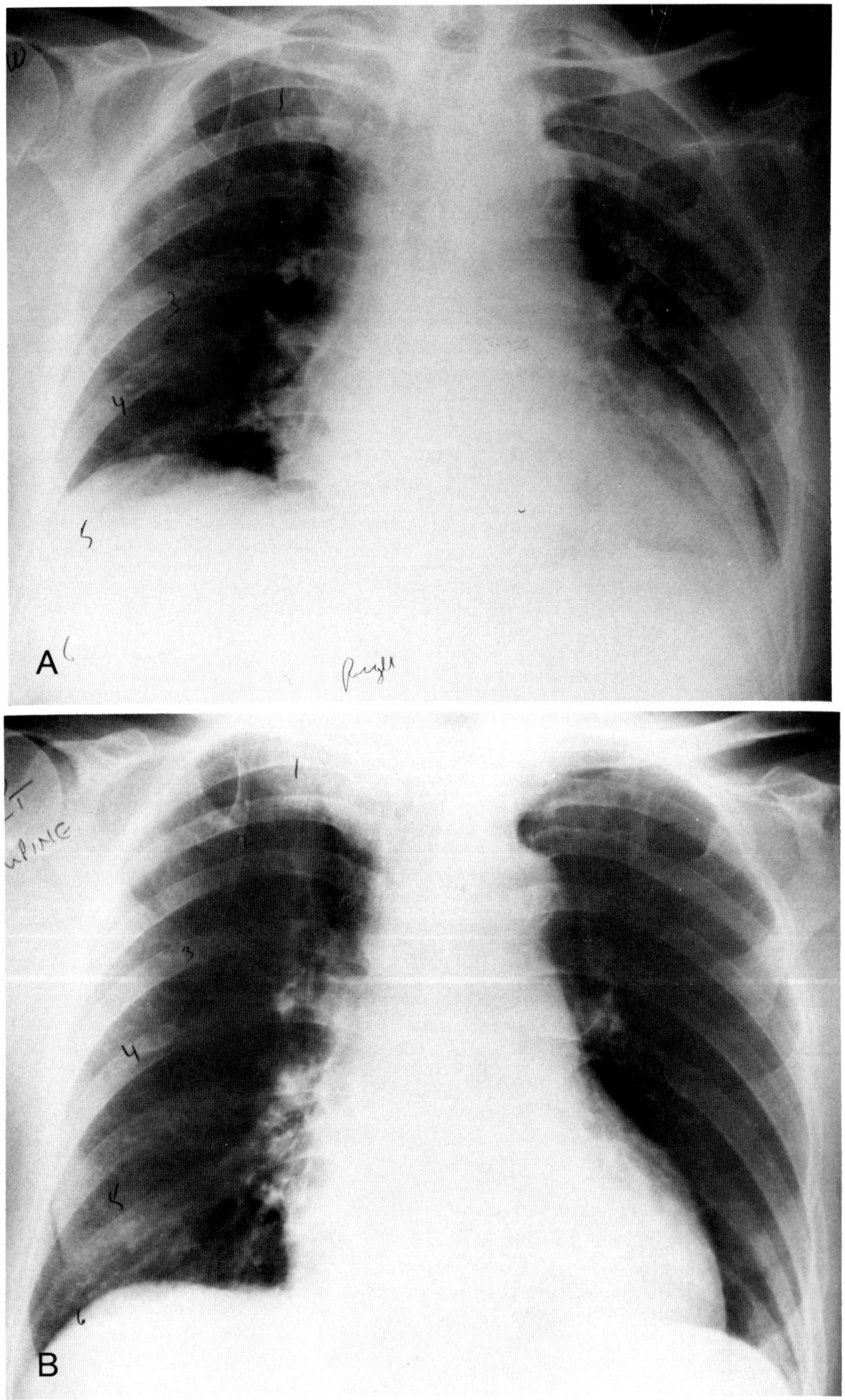

Figure 9.1. Degree of expansion of the lungs. *A*, Expiratory. *B*, Inspiratory.

the appearance of the heart and mediastinum and the whiteness of the lungs. It is for this reason that the size of the lungs must be assessed on every film and compared with previous radiographs to be sure that one is assessing lungs that are the same volume. If this is not done, then it is easy to see how a slightly underexposed poorly inflated lung can mimic pulmonary edema. In general, a rough estimation can be made by counting the ribs down to the level of the apex of the hemidiaphragm. In a proper inspiratory film, the apex of the hemidiaphragm should be at the fifth anterior interspace or at least the fifth anterior rib. Posteriorly, the eighth posterior rib at the apex of the hemidiaphragm is a similar measurement. However, this varies from patient to patient, and the best practice is to compare with previous films if they are available.

SPECIAL CHEST VIEWS

Following the anteroposterior supine or upright portable chest radiograph, the next most useful film and the one most often obtained in the critical care unit is the lateral decubitus view. This film is essential in assessing the amount of pleural fluid or the presence of a pneumothorax. Air fluid levels are also detected on these horizontal beam films. To detect a pneumothorax, the suspected side is elevated, and air can be seen separating the lung from the ribs. The lateral decubitus film, when pleural fluid is present, will demonstrate an opacity separating the ribs from the lung when the side suspected of having the pleural fluid is placed dependent (Fig. 9.2).

It must be remembered that, on the supine chest film, just a slight increase in density on one side of the chest may be the only abnormality seen in the presence of considerable amounts of pleural fluid (up to 700–1000 ml).

INTERPRETATION OF THE CHEST RADIOGRAPH

If available, any previous film should always be obtained for comparison. The chest radiograph is then assessed with respect to the technical factors mentioned above, i.e., motion unsharpness, degree of inspiration, rotation, and exposure factors. In intensive care work, it is very important to know the location and appearance of all tubes and catheters. The most important of these is the endotracheal tube.

Following this initial examination, a systematic search of the films should be made as is done in the routine radiograph. One should assess the bones, soft tissues, trachea, mediastinal outlines, outline of both hemidiaphragms, pulmonary hila, and, finally, the lungs, comparing the two sides of the way down. It is very important to remember that the loss of any normal interface between two immediately adjacent different radiographic densities (i.e., lung and upper portion of the hemidiaphragm) indicates that these two contrasting ra-

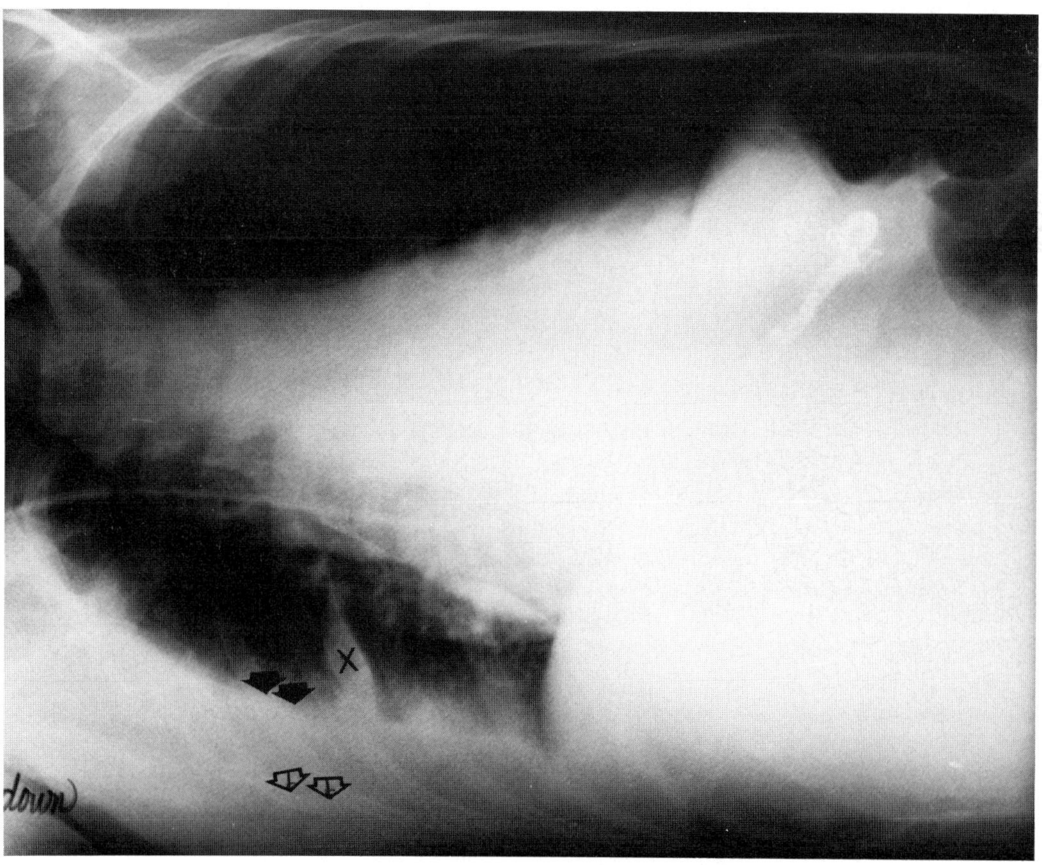

Figure 9.2. Lateral decubitus film. Right side down demonstrating right pleural effusion showing an opacity separating the ribs *(open arrows)* from the lung margin *(closed arrows)*. Note also the fluid tracking up into the minor fissure (X).

diodensities are no longer in contact or that one of these structures has changed its radiographic density to be the same as the adjacent structure. No structure is seen radiographically, unless it is in immediate contact with a structure of different radiographic density. For example, if the normal air present in the left lower lobe is replaced with fluid in the alveoli secondary to secretional retention in the smaller airways, then one loses the normal line indicating the upper margin of the left hemidiaphragm on the film. In addition, if the normal contrast between the pulmonary vessels that are of unit density, contrasted with the immediate adjacent air-containing lung, is lost, then these vessels become indistinct. This indicates that the adjacent air-containing parenchyma in the lung is no longer of 0 density, but now is of unit density, the same as the pulmonary vessels, such as might occur in pulmonary edema. As a further illustration, one does not see a line or margin between the right atrium and right ventricle because both these structures contain blood and are of unit density, as is the muscle of their wall. However, one does see a margin corresponding to the lateral wall of the right atrium as this is touching the right lung, which is air containing and therefore of contrasting radiographic density.

In the supine portable film, because of physiologic changes in the patient and shortening of the tube to the film distance, one must be aware of changes in the appearance of the mediastinum. It appears wider than on an upright 6-foot posteroanterior chest film. There may be a change of up to 2 cm in the transverse diameter of the cardiac silhouette with varying degrees of inspiration and expiration, systole and diastole, making assessment of daily change in cardiac silhouette fraught with problems. Changes in appearances in air and fluid collections in the lungs and pleural spaces must also be adjusted for on the supine films, as compared to the upright 6-foot posteroanterior film.

In general, although the chest radiograph in the critical care unit is comparable to the chest radiograph made on any patient in the x-ray department, there are certain very important differences. The detection of smaller abnormalities is difficult because often there is some motion unsharpness on the film and the resolving power of the supine system is not as good as the posteroanterior chest film made in the x-ray department. It is important in working with such cases not to “miss the forest for the trees.” Fundamental observations, such as the presence of pneumothorax, shift of the trachea, opaque hemithorax, localized opacities, and diffuse edema, are all significant, whereas the finding of a small pulmonary nodule is not of the same importance in the acutely ill patient.

TUBES AND CATHETERS

When interpreting a chest radiograph in the critical care unit, following assessment of the technical factors, the

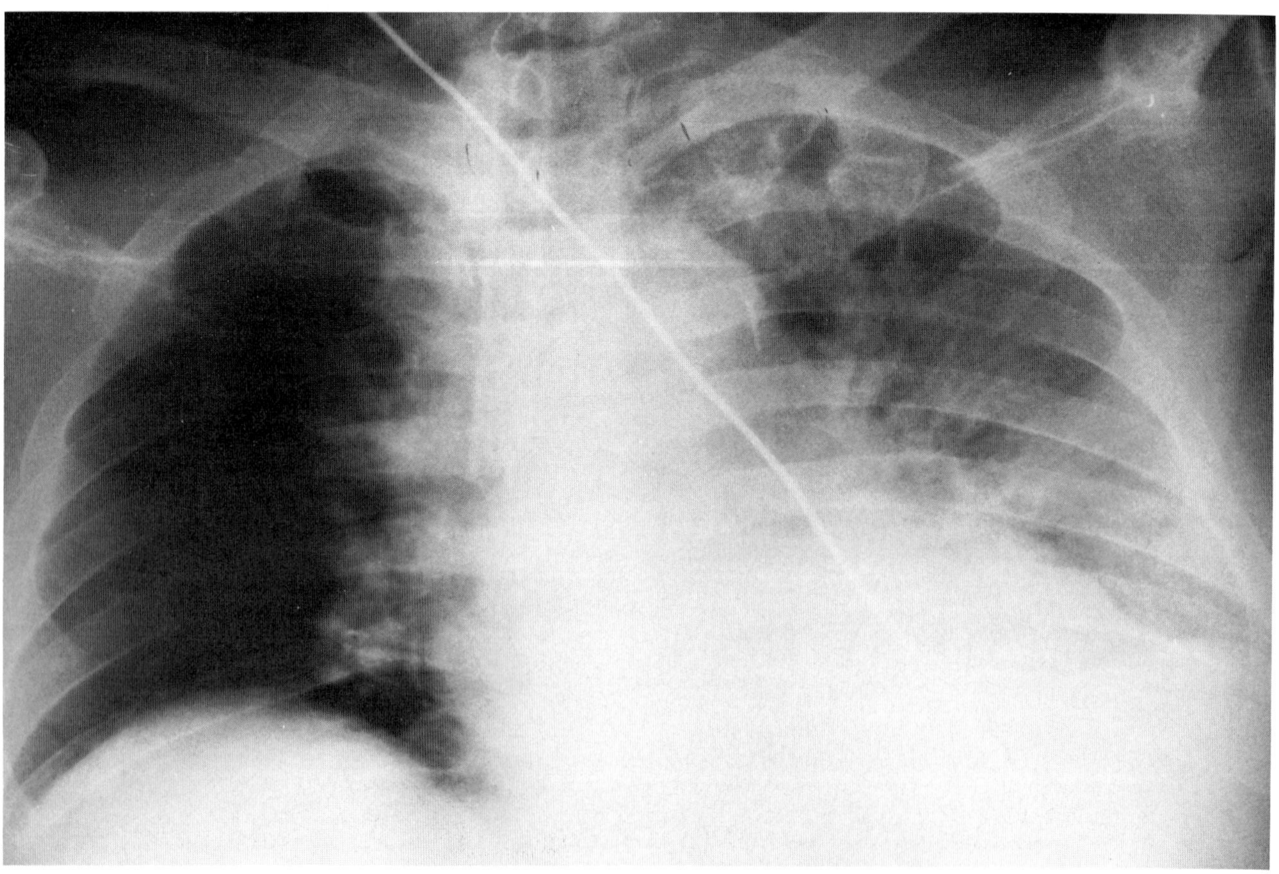

Figure 9.3. Endotracheal tube in right mainstem bronchus with partial collapse of the left lung.

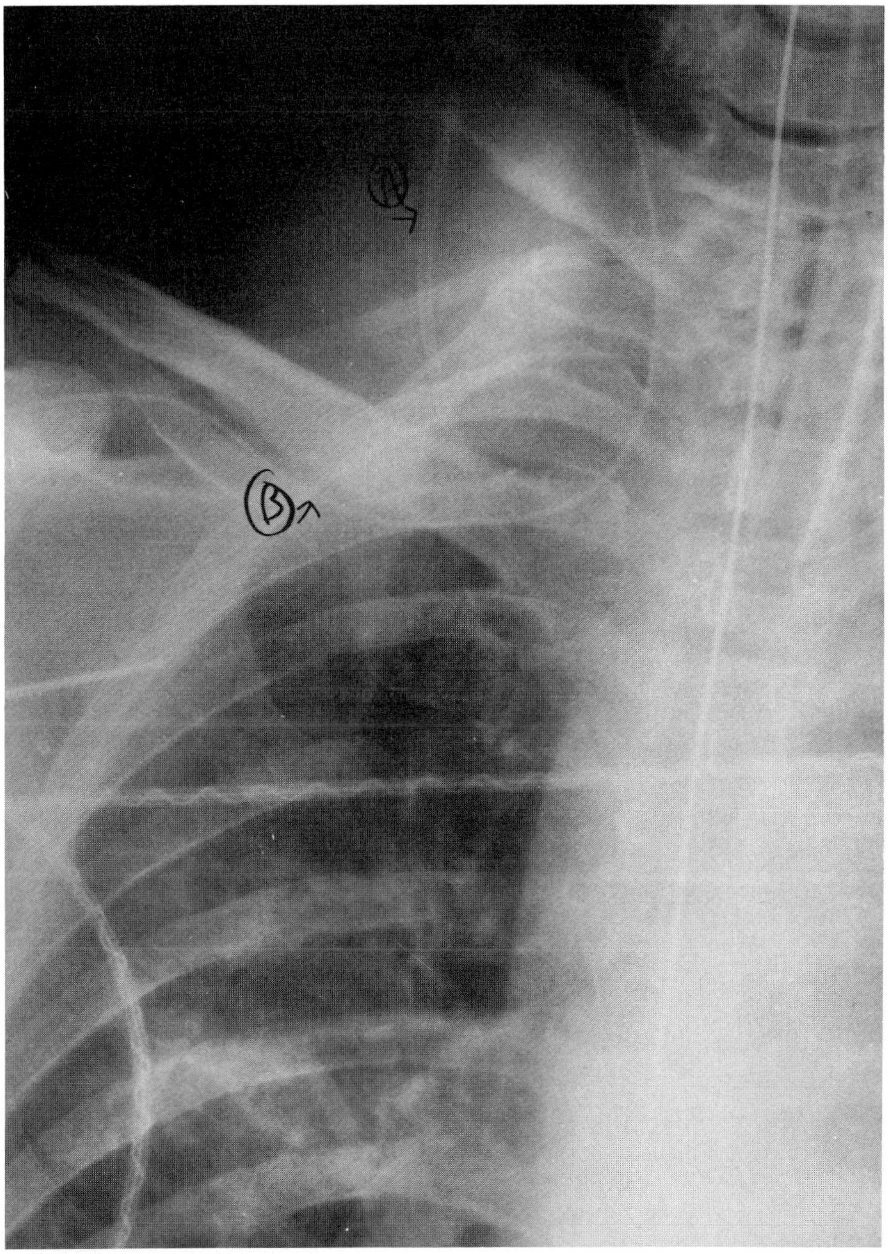

Figure 9.4. Location of internal and external jugular veins. *Catheter A* is in the external jugular vein. *Catheter B* has been placed into the right subclavian and has gone up the internal jugular vein, showing the relative locations of these veins on the radiograph.

next area to examine systematically is the location and types of tubes, wires, and lines that are present on the film.

Endotracheal Tube

The endotracheal tube is extremely important, and its position should always be noted on each film. The ideal location is at the level of the medial ends of the clavicles. Tubes above this level must be lowered because the cuff will damage the trachea. Tubes lower down produce difficulties in suctioning the left lung and, if low enough, are in the right mainstem bronchus, thereby occluding the left mainstem bronchus and producing collapse of the left lung to varying degrees (Fig. 9.3). In addition, if the tube is in one or the other mainstem bronchi and the total tidal volume is delivered to one lung, barotrauma is a common complication.

One must also assess the tube cuff. Overinflated cuffs, even of the more modern low pressure type, still may produce damage. It is also possible for the cuff to be progressively overinflated over a period of weeks and then to produce a rather large degree of local tracheal dilation.

The angle of the tracheostomy tube is important to assess. Traction by the plastic conductance tubing or pressure by these external tubes may result in the tracheostomy tube being tilted and a tip erosion occurring where the tip of the tube impinges on the thin wall of the trachea with the overlying pulsating innominate artery. Disastrous ruptures of the innominate artery into the airway have occurred secondary to these complications.

Nasogastric Tube

Opaque nasogastric tubes should be used in the critical care unit so that their location can be assessed. Often the tube, although clinically felt to be in the stomach, is either in the lung or is not fully down in the stomach. Regurgitation of tube feeds produces areas of aspiration pneumonia in these situations. In some cases, esophageal lines are placed in the esophagus to monitor pressures, especially if the patient is on high levels of positive end-expiratory pressure (PEEP). These tubes are best located at the level of the left atrium.

Intravascular Catheters

One should always note the location of intravascular catheters on the radiograph. Figure 9.4 shows the appearance of an external jugular catheter as compared to an internal jugular catheter. In our experience, external jugular catheters are most prone to complications. They often do not pass into the superior vena cava and instead remain in veins outside the chest cavity. Extravasation of fluid from badly placed catheters or catheters that have eroded through the veins are not rare complications. Widening of the mediastinum in a patient with any type of intravascular catheter, subclavian or jugular, should raise the possibility of a vascular leak induced by this catheter. Subclavian catheters may be put in either above or below the clavicle, and their ideal location depends on their purpose. Generally, they should be in the superior vena cava near the superior vena cava/right atrial junction. Bleeding from puncturing of the subclavian artery produces a characteristic opacity over the apex of the lung, pushing the lung down as blood accumulates in the extrapleural space. Leaks may occur extrapleurally or into the pleural space. Pneumothorax is a recognized complication of these catheters and should always be looked for with a radiograph immediately after insertion.

Wedge Balloon Catheters (Swan-Ganz Catheters)

The position of these catheters should always be noted. Ideally, they are placed at the level of the interlobar artery on the right side or in the left upper or lower lobe arteries.

If they are far out in the lung, the possibility that they are permanently wedged should be considered. It is often possible to see the balloon inflated if it is inflated with air, as the air contrasts with blood in the pulmonary vessel. Complications are rare, but do occur. Figure 9.5 illustrates an infarct in the distribution of the Swan-Ganz

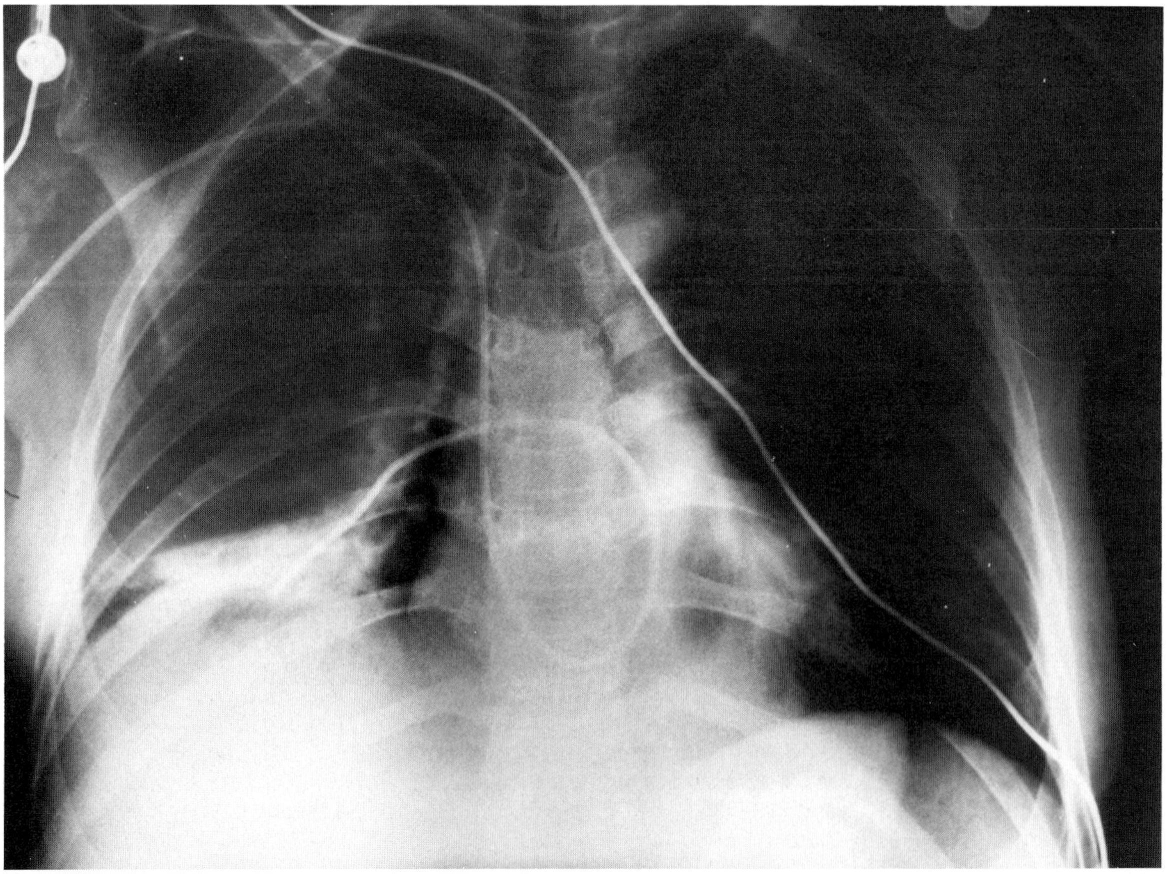

Figure 9.5. A complication of the Swan-Ganz catheter in which it has been wedged in the right lung base for 24 hours. Note the wedge-shaped opacity at the right base representing an area of infarction.

catheter that had remained wedged for over 24 hours in this position. In addition, the balloon may occasionally be overinflated in a very small vessel, and an area of pulmonary hemorrhage may occur at this site. Extra loops in the ventricle may also be seen. Knotting may occur, and in this case, percutaneous retrieval is possible via the femoral vein using fluoroscopy and a wire retrieval system. This type of retrieval is also possible for broken-off fragments of other intravascular catheters.

Intra-Aortic Balloon Pump Catheter

The normal appearance and location of this catheter are illustrated in Figure 9.6. The balloon can be seen also when it is inflated. If the balloon catheter is too low, it may obstruct the renal mesenteric artery supply and, if too high, the brachiocephalic vessels.

Pleural and Mediastinal Drains

The location of pleural and mediastinal drains is also important. When improperly inserted, the side holes may be in the soft tissues of the chest, resulting in significant subcutaneous emphysema. Other complications of pleural drains include drains that are located too close to major vascular bundles at the apex or in the mediastinum. Localized injuries to the lung producing small hematomas can also be seen when the drains are removed.

DIFFUSE OPACITIES THROUGHOUT BOTH LUNGS: PULMONARY EDEMA

It is probably a bit of a gross generalization, but nonetheless a useful one, that any patient who develops any bilateral opacity in the chest radiograph should be considered to have pulmonary edema as the most likely diagnosis. In the very earliest cases, the picture of pulmonary edema can be simulated by slight motion unsharpness, a slightly underexposed film, or a partial expiration film. In the earliest changes, the chest x-ray reveals slight blurring of the vascular markings and an increase in interstitial linear markings in the lung. *It is of utmost importance to remember that the assessment of pulmonary edema is very dependent on the volume of air in the lungs.* In this regard, Figure 9.7 illustrates the complete radiographic clearing of pulmonary edema in a patient with cardiac failure and a high pulmonary capillary wedge pressure when the lungs were inflated with 15 cm of PEEP. Figure 9.8 shows that the edema is still there, but is now spread out, lining overinflated alveoli. Therefore, in order to assess the degree of pulmonary edema in the lungs, one must compare films made with the same degree of expansion and with the same amount of PEEP. It is therefore possible that, if the patient is on PEEP, the radiograph may appear normal despite the presence of significant pulmonary edema.

Pulmonary edema, as seen on an anteroposterior chest radiograph in a critical care unit, is not a diagnosis in itself, but rather is consistent with a number of different etiologic agents. Table 9.1 lists the common causes of pulmonary edema seen in the author's critical care unit.

Table 9.1
Radiographic Pulmonary Edema Pattern in Critically Ill Patients

A. High pulmonary capillary wedge pressure
   1. Left-sided cardiac failure and fluid overload[a]
   2. Neurogenic edema[a]
   3. Near drowning
B. Usually low pulmonary capillary wedge pressure
   1. ARDS[a]—capillary leak syndrome secondary to
      a. Sepsis
      b. Hypovolemic shock
   2. Liquid gastric aspiration[a] (Mendelson's syndrome)
   3. Other capillary leak syndromes
      a. Fat embolism
      b. "Pump lung"
      c. Transfusion reaction lung
      d. Heroin overdose
      e. Near drowning
   4. Bilateral pneumonia—viral, Legionnaire's, *Pneumocystis carinii*
   5. Pulmonary hemorrhage
   6. Other
      a. Pulmonary arteritis
      b. Loeffler's syndrome
      c. Alveolar proteinosis
      d. Bronchiolo-alveolar carcinoma
      e. Acute alveolitis
         (1) Diffuse fibrosing alveolitis desquamative phase
         (2) Extrinsic allergic alveolitis (farmer's lung, etc.)

[a] Denotes most common.

It is extremely important to realize that, on a single radiograph at a single point in time, it is not possible to distinguish one of these types of pulmonary edema from another. Having accepted this fact, it is nonetheless true that certain generalizations can be made about the capillary leak pulmonary edemas (or ARDS, adult respiratory distress syndrome) and their radiographic pattern as compared to cardiac pulmonary edemas. In general, it is true that, for the same severity of radiographic picture, the PaO_2 tends to be worse in low pressure edema than in high pressure edema. The response to diuretics is much less in low pressure edema, which also maintains a remarkable persistence in severity from day to day. PEEP is more effective in clearing cardiac or high pressure edema than in clearing edema secondary to capillary leakage syndromes. In both types of pulmonary edema (low and high pressure), pleural effusions, especially right sided, may be associated. In practice, definition of cardiac size may be of little value in distinguishing the causes of pulmonary edema; many cases of cardiac edema have normal cardiac silhouettes, and many cases of capillary leakage syndromes have dilated ventricles and large cardiac silhouettes.

Clinical Correlation

From the clinical point of view, probably the most sensitive indication of the presence of pulmonary edema is a drop in the PaO_2. If a radiograph is done at this time, it may be normal. This is fairly well documented in cases of ARDS where the first radiographic changes may only become apparent 24 hours after the initial drop in the PaO_2. However, radiographic findings may often be present in the absence of any physical findings in the chest, such as rales. This is especially true with early changes, such as interstitial edema.

Provided there are no great differences in the state of

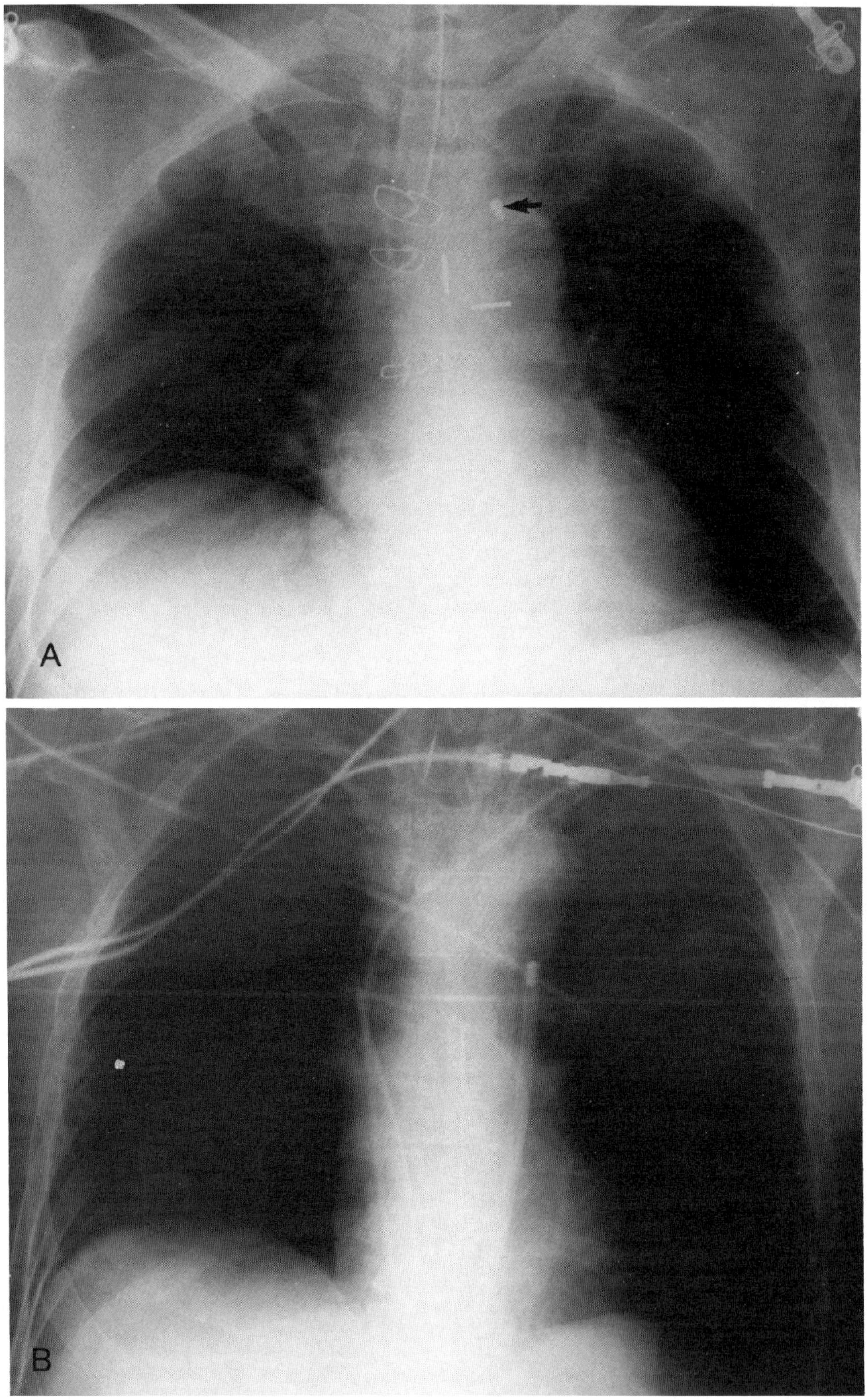

Figure 9.6. Intra-aortic balloon pump catheter. *A,* High position with tip of catheter near the origin of the great vessel *(arrow)*. *B,* In good position just at or below the transverse arch in the descending aorta.

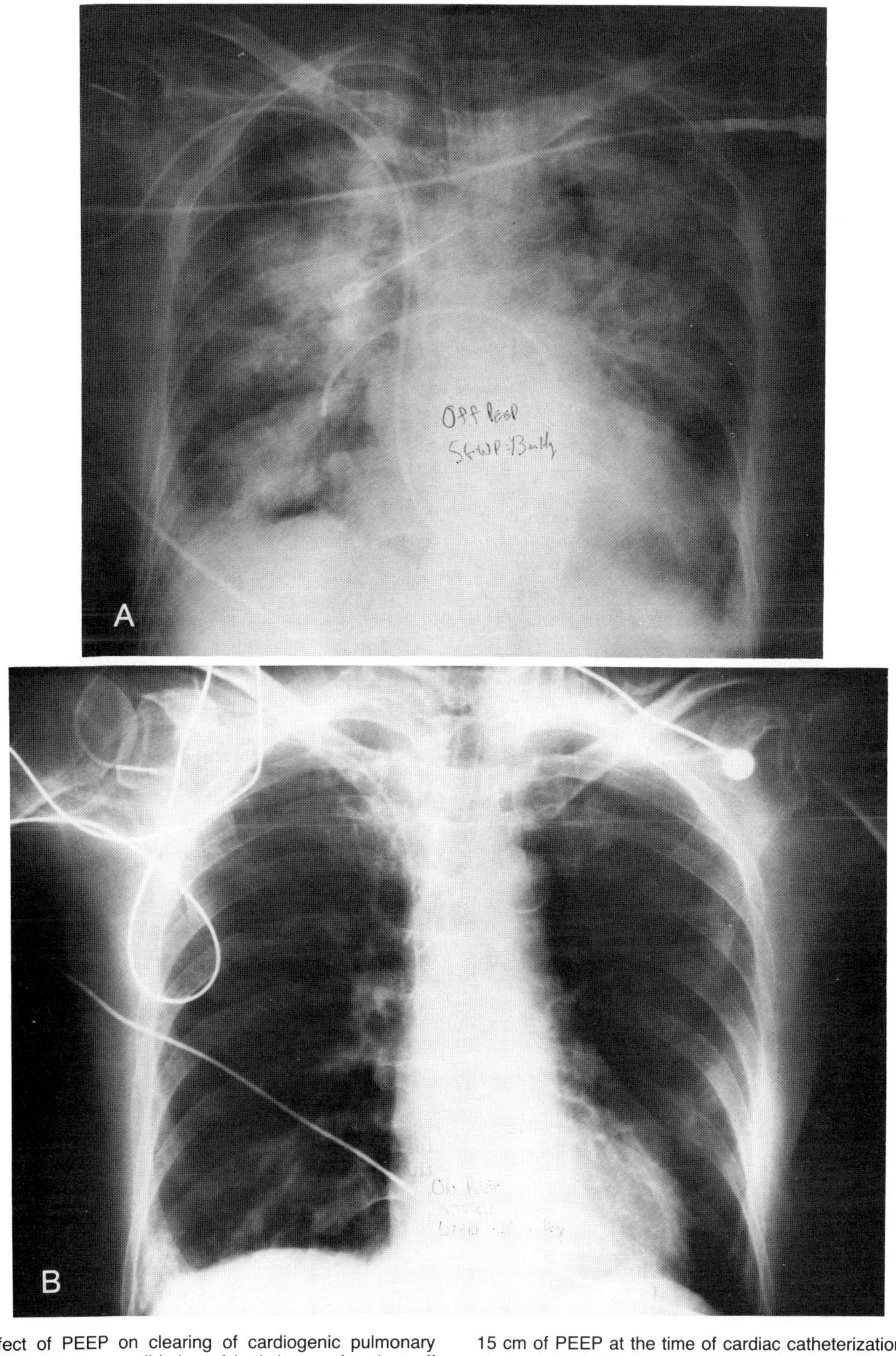

Figure 9.7. Effect of PEEP on clearing of cardiogenic pulmonary edema. *A,* Fluffy air space consolidation of both lungs of patient off PEEP. Swan-Ganz wedge pressure is 43 mm Hg. *B,* Same patient on 15 cm of PEEP at the time of cardiac catheterization, with left ventricular end-diastolic pressure of 38 mm Hg.

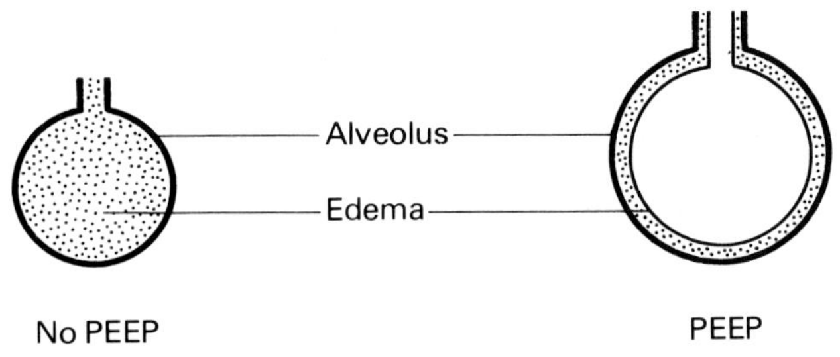

Figure 9.8. Effect of PEEP on edema in alveolus.

inflation of the lungs, sequential chest radiographs are of value in assessing changes in pulmonary edema from day to day, and they correlate well with the pulmonary capillary wedge pressure (PCWP) in cases of cardiogenic pulmonary edema (Figure 9.9 *A-E*).

LOCALIZED OPACITIES ON THE CHEST RADIOGRAPH

It is an oversimplification, but perhaps a useful generalization, that a localized opacity in the lung represents either secretional retention, pneumonia, or infarction in the vast majority of critically ill patients. By far, the commonest localized opacities are those produced by various forms of secretion retention.

Secretion Retention

Opacities produced on the chest radiograph secondary to various forms of secretion retention or atelectasis vary greatly in appearance. This variation is likely due to different etiologies of the shadows and location of the problem. If a major mucous plug is obstructing a major bronchus and there is no collateral air drift, a wedge-shaped collapse of a lobe is produced and there is no air bronchogram or air in the bronchi, because the mucous plug is obstructing the major airway (Fig. 9.10). The two lobes that commonly collapse are the left lower lobe and the right upper lobe. In children, the right upper lobe is very prone to collapse, especially in the immediate postoperative period.

Secretion retention in smaller airways, such as subsegmental or segmental bronchi, produce various types of shadowing. Small triangular shadows may be produced by segmental collapse, and occasionally, line shadows are produced by subsegmental collapse secondary to mucous plugging in smaller airways. Following re-expansion of a collapsed lobe, line shadows often remain at the site of residual segmental collapses that are not totally resolved. Secretion retention and mucous plugging in the bronchioles may also produce relatively homogeneous opacification of a lobe or an area of lung with an air bronchogram and without a great deal of loss of volume. This type of secretion retention is indistinguishable from so-called post-bypass adhesive atelectasis produced by surfactant deficiency and local mechanical factors in the left lower lobe following cardiopulmonary bypass surgery. In addition, minor degrees of loss of volume may be noted by crowding of the basilar lung markings, indistinctness or loss of the outline of the hemidiaphragm, or elevation of a hemidiaphragm. Left lower lobe secretion problems are often indicated by loss of the hemidiaphragm as the aerated lung in the periphery of the lower lobe is replaced by edema fluid in alveoli secondary to secretion retention either in smaller or larger airways. Secondary signs of loss of volume in secretion problems are evident to varying degrees. These include displacement of the fissures, displacement of the trachea toward the side of loss of volume, displacement of the heart and mediastinum toward the side of loss of volume, and elevation of the hemidiaphragm. In addition, in the case of fairly high degrees of loss of volume in the upper or lower lobes, the remaining normal lobes are often overinflated and show increased radiolucency and spreading vascular markings.

In general, the chest radiograph is a valuable tool in assessing problems with retained secretions in these patients. It is also of value in following the effects of treatment, such as posturing, physiotherapy, and, in the more resistant cases, bronchoscopy. Persistent signs of secretion retention in one or both lung bases, especially associated with small or moderate amounts of pleural fluid, must always raise the question of problems underneath the hemidiaphragm that may be causing secondary poor expansion of the lung bases. Examples of abnormalities producing these basal lung changes are pancreatitis, subphrenic abscess, or cholecystitis.

Pneumonia

Localized areas of pneumonia in the chest radiograph may have exactly the same appearance as those described above secondary to secretion retention, with the exception of classic lobar collapses without air bronchograms. However, in many cases pneumonic consolidations are not segmental or wedge shaped, and fluffy alveolar opacities are seen, rather than the more segmental wedge-shaped or linear shadows produced by secretion retention. In the final analysis, the clinical picture must be correlated with the localized opacity on the radiograph.

Pulmonary Infarction

The third and perhaps least common localized opacity in the critically ill patient is a pulmonary infarction. These opacities are almost always basal and may again mimic the minimal crowding of markings or localized segmental opacities seen in secretion retention. For this reason, the diagnosis of pulmonary infarction based on the chest radiograph alone is really quite difficult. In this regard, lung scans are of value, and perfusion and ventilation scans are discussed elsewhere (see Chapter 11). In difficult cases, pulmonary angiography may be required to establish a diagnosis. Classical infarcts occur in a small number of patients with pulmonary emboli. These shadows are wedge-shaped and homogeneous and often are seen in the costrophrenic angles (Fig. 9.11). Some cases have the so-called Hampton's hump, which has an inverted cone appearance with the margin of the consolidation toward the hilum having a convex contour.

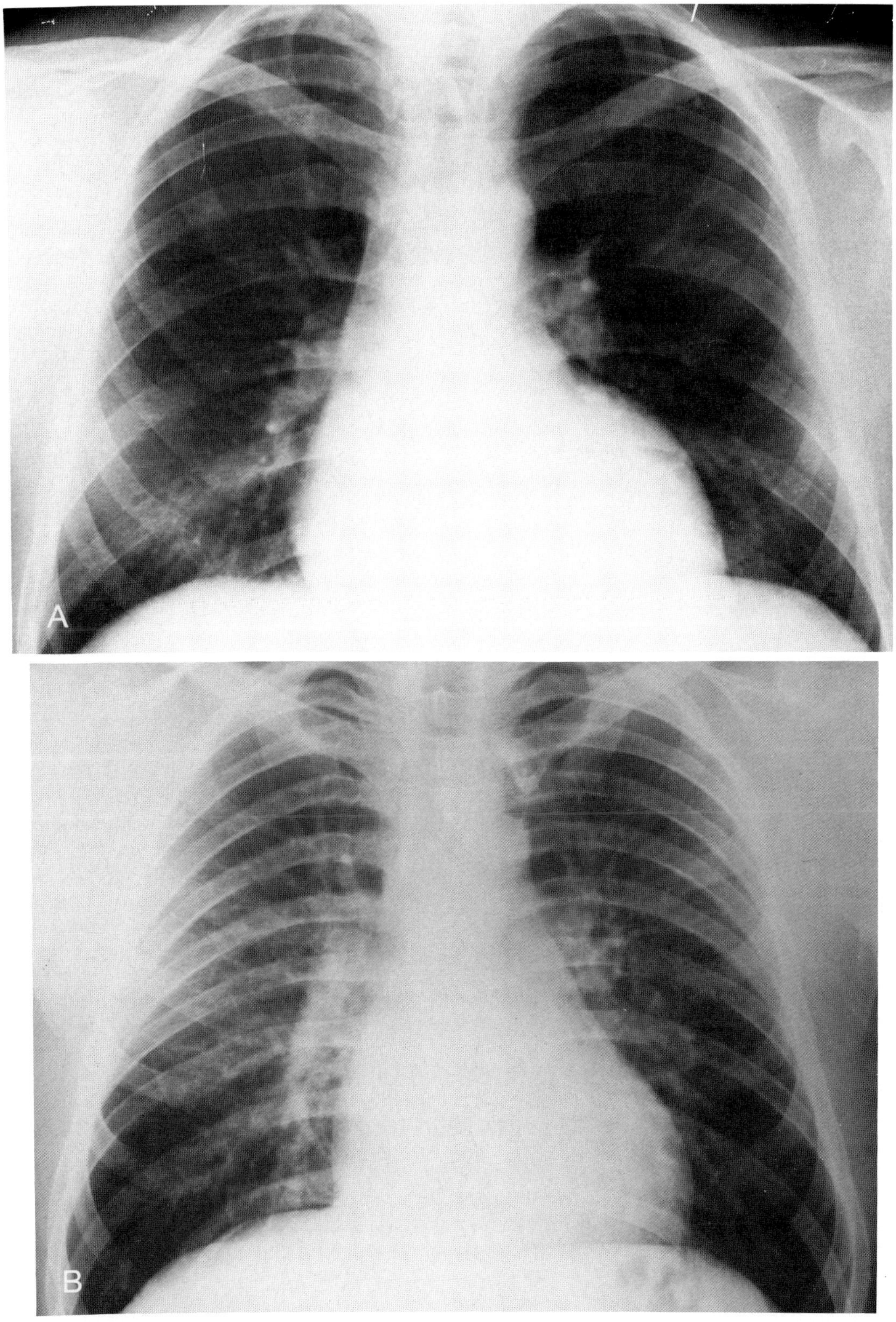

Figure 9.9*A, B*. Pulmonary edema—progressive severity. *A,* Normal. *B,* Probably early interstitial edema and redistribution of blood flow to the upper lobes. Note slight increase in markings and mild venous engorgement.

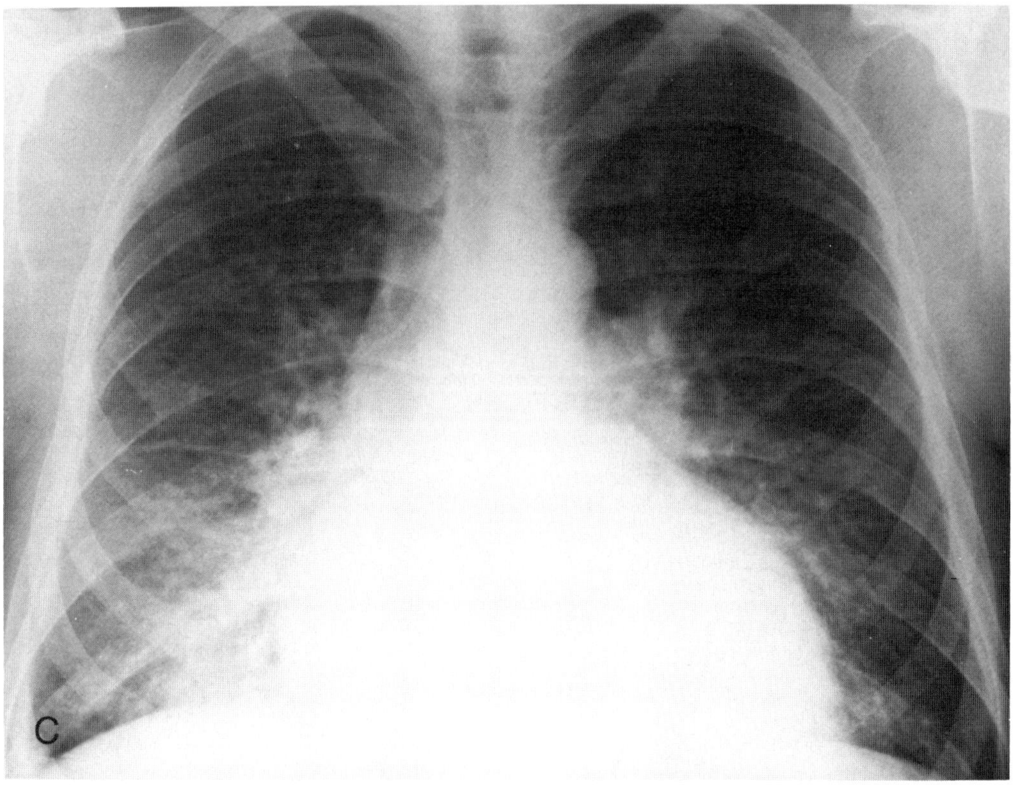

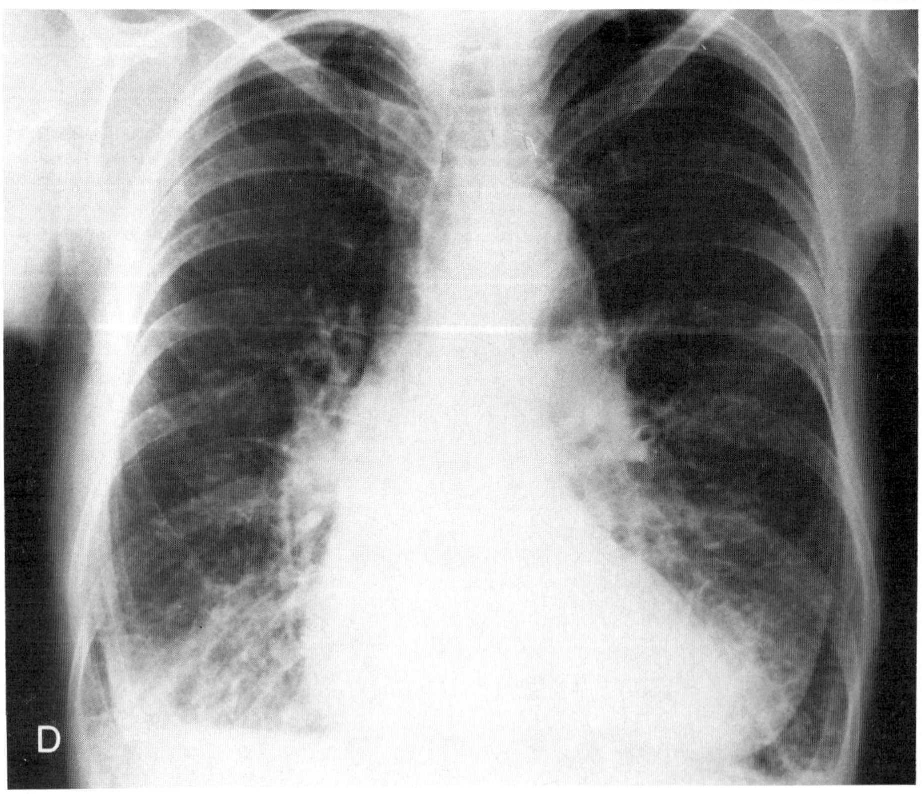

Figure 9.9 ***C, D.*** *C,* Definite interstitial edema with blurred vessels, increased interstitial markings, a small amount of fluid in the right pleural space, and thickening of the right minor fissure due to fluid. *D,* Interstitial edema with Kerley B lines.

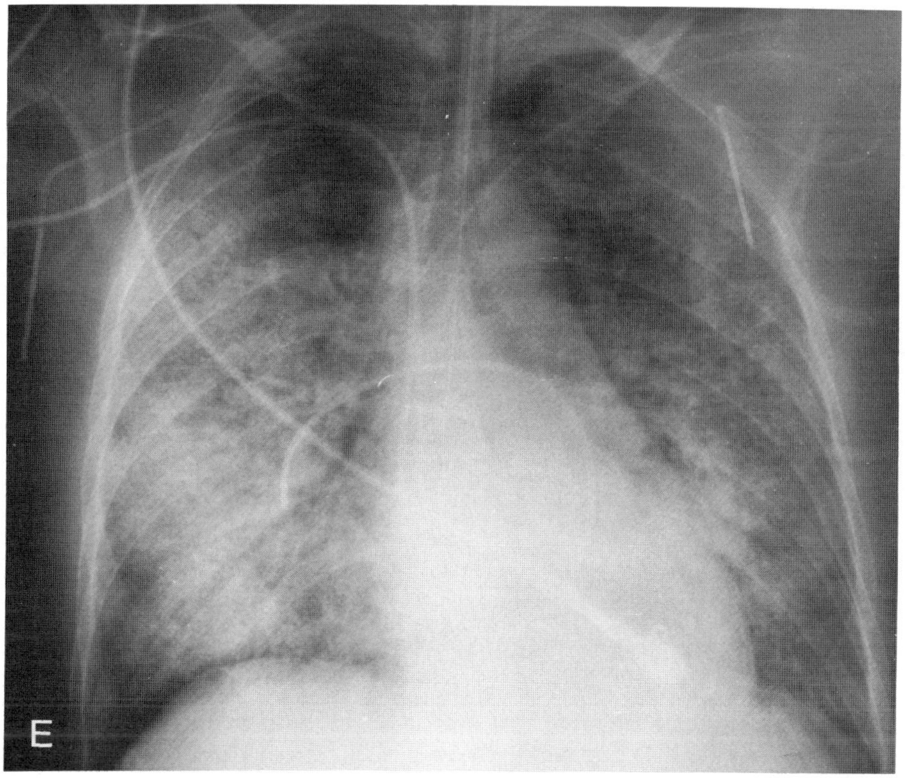

Figure 9.9. *E,* Bilaterial air space edema.

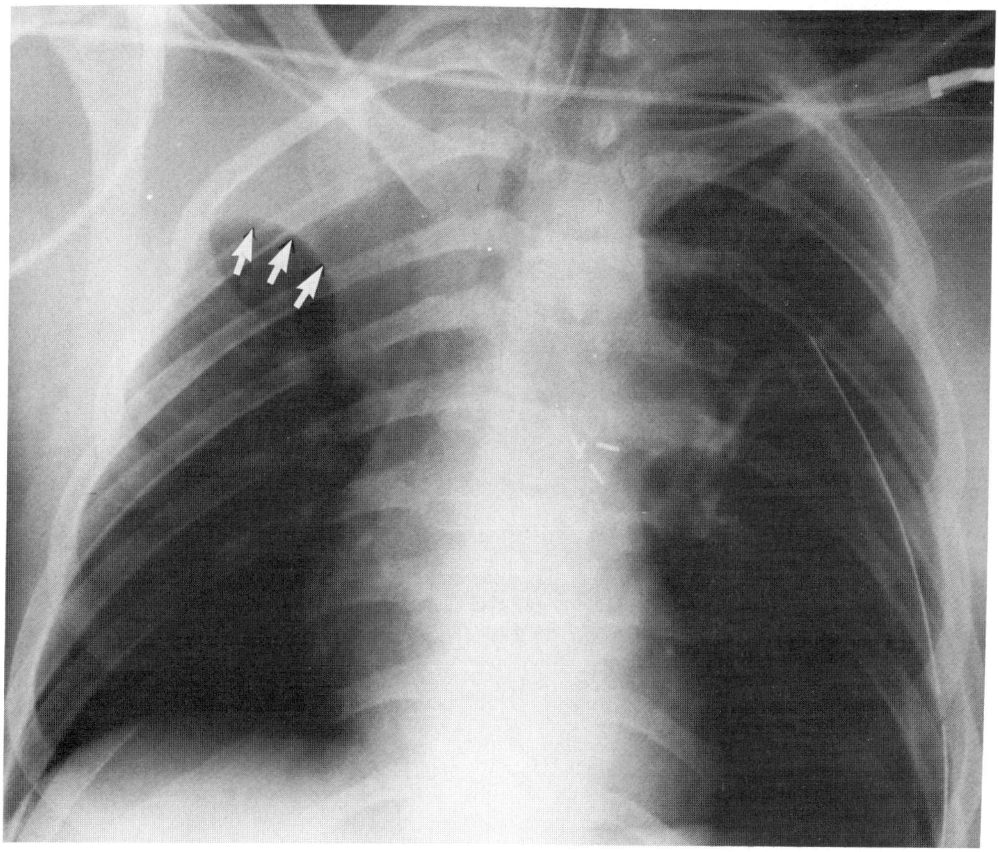

Figure 9.10. Right upper lobe collapse—mucous plug. Homogeneous wedge-shaped opacity without an air bronchogram. The trachea is displaced toward the right side. Note the bowed upward displacement of the minor fissure *(arrows)*.

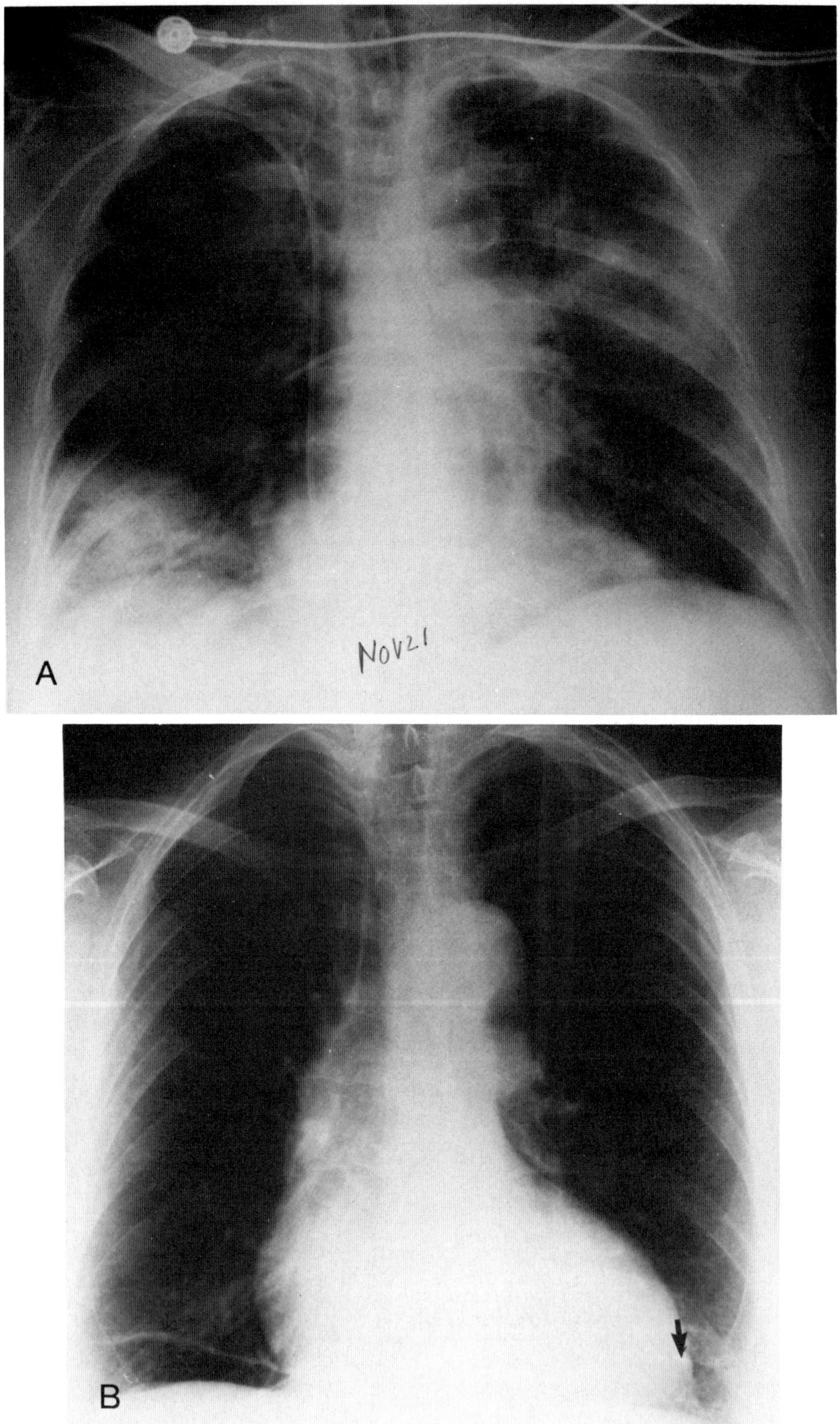

Figure 9.11. Bilateral lower lobe pulmonary infarcts. *A,* On the left side, a rather nondescript ill-defined area of increase in density. In the right base, a more defined opacity is seen with a sharp medial margin in the costrophrenic angle. This opacity is more suggestive of an infarct. *B,* Basal line shadows secondary to pulmonary thromboembolism *(arrow).*

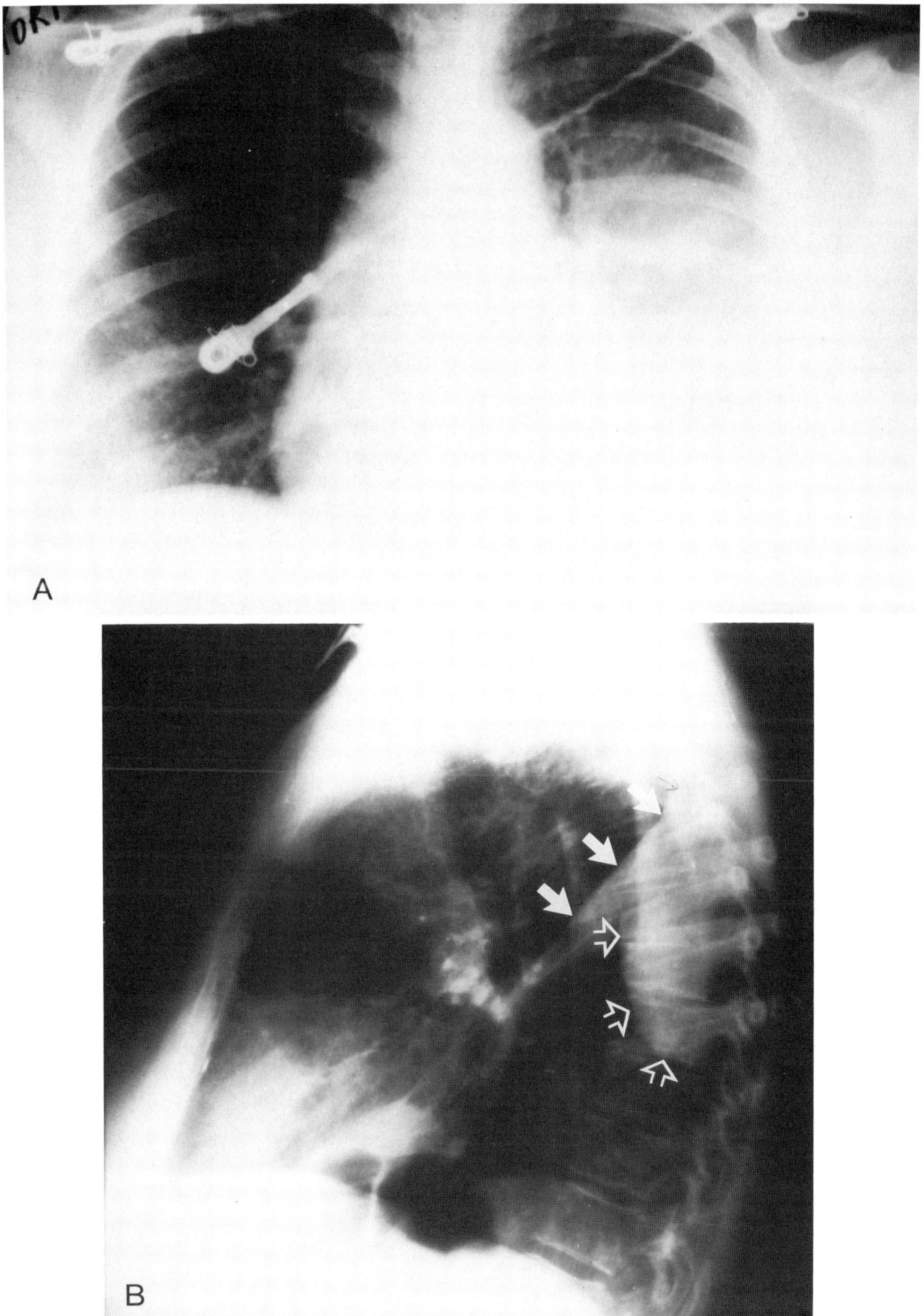

Figure 9.12 ***A, B.*** *A,* The supine film reveals an opacity over the lower left hemithorax in a febrile patient with a history of pneumonia. *B,* A lentiform opacity is seen posteriorly on the lateral film *(open arrows)*. Some fluid is also tracking down the chief fissures *(closed arrows)*.

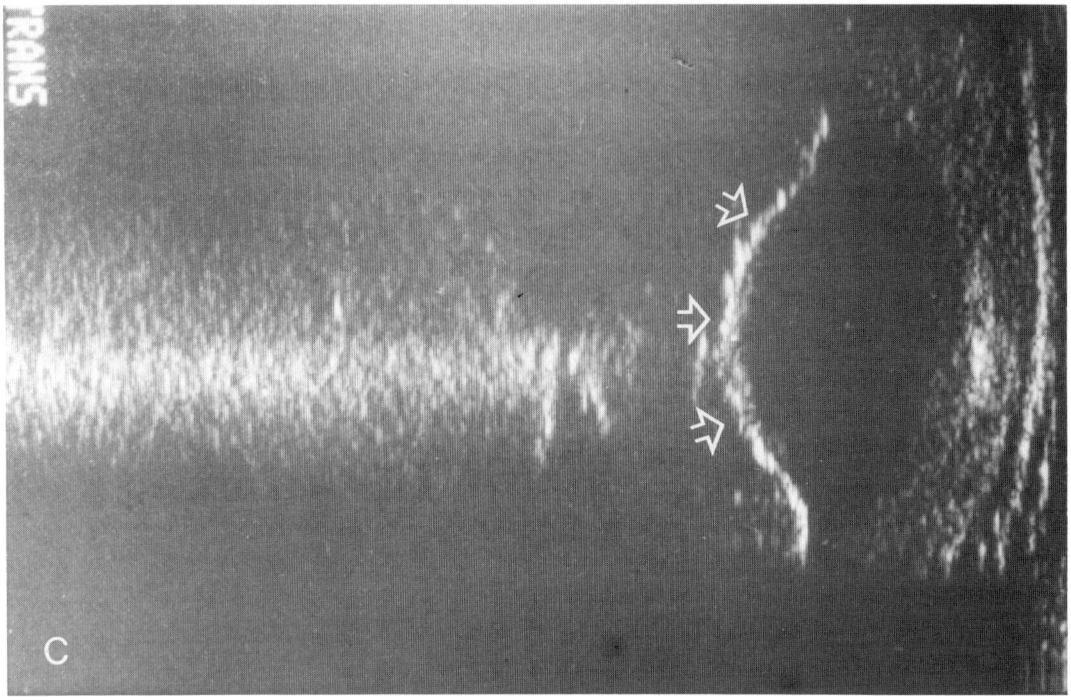

Figure 9.12 *C*. Bedside real-time ultrasound examination reveals lentiform collection of fluid, confirming loculation of loculated posterior empyema before needle aspiration.

PLEURAL DISEASE

It is in the assessment of abnormalities in the pleural space that the lateral decubitus chest film, or upright film, finds its greatest value in the critically ill patient. However, as most films are made supine, one must become familiar with the distribution of air and fluid in the pleural space in the supine position.

Free pleural fluid lies behind the lung in the supine position and produces a slightly increased opacity of that hemithorax as compared to the other side. From 700-1000 ml of fluid may accumulate and lie behind the lung before it begins to creep up the lateral aspect of the lung and separates the aerated lung from the ribs on the frontal film, making its presence obvious. (Fig. 9.2).

The slight opacity produced over the hemithorax by pleural fluid creates a general haze over the hemithorax. It may, at times, be difficult to distinguish it from parenchymal lung disease. The most helpful finding is that, in parenchymal lung disease, the vascular markings are obscured in the area of involvement, whereas in pleural effusion, there is an overlying haze and the vascular markings remain intact. In addition, the presence of an air bronchogram is helpful in indicating a pulmonary parenchymal abnormality as opposed to isolated pleural fluid.

If the pleural fluid is free, a lateral decubitus film allows it to move between the lung and the chest wall, showing an area of opacity separating the lung from the ribs.

Diagnostic ultrasound and computed tomography (CT) examination of the chest are of considerable value in helping sort out problems of pleural fluid and empyema in critically ill patients. A portable ultrasound machine may be brought to the bedside and can be used to detect localized or loculated pleural fluid collections before needle aspiration or placement of chest tubes (Fig. 9.12). In addition, CT of the chest can be done in the supine position without disturbing the patient and gives excellent visualization of the pleural space and mediastinum (Figs. 9.13 and 9.14).

PNEUMOTHORAX

In the supine posture, air tends to rise to the highest portion of the thorax, which is in the anterior costophrenic angles and, on the left side, the cardiophrenic angle anteriorly. Figure 9.15 demonstrates a collection of air in the pleural space in the supine film. Notice the blackening of one hemidiaphragm as compared to the other side. If enough air is present, it will separate the lung from the chest wall further up and permit visualization of the visceral pleural line.

In all cases, a lateral decubitus film with the suspected side elevated is of value in confirming the presence of free air in the pleural space.

WIDENING OF THE MEDIASTINUM

Mediastinal widening is an important observation on the chest film in critically ill patients. Following severe chest trauma, it should always raise the possibility of rupture

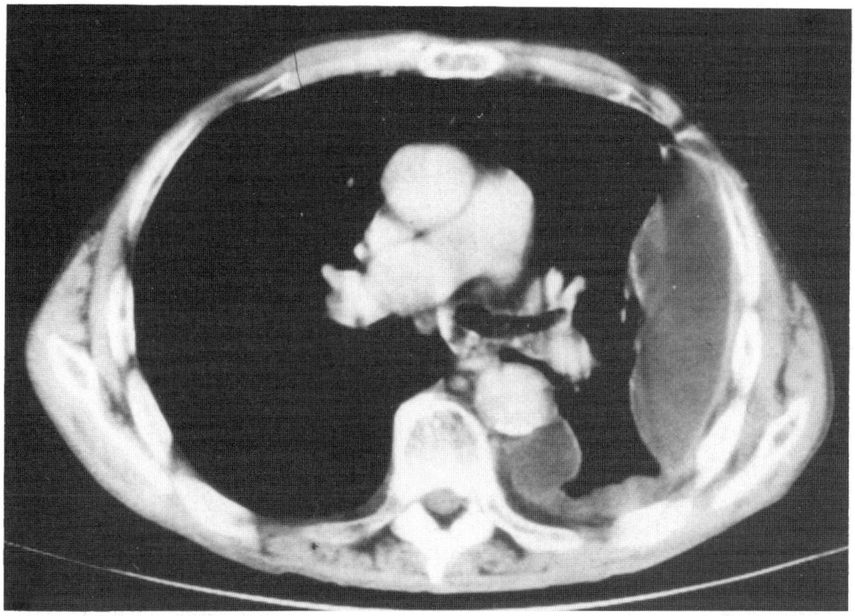

Figure 9.13. Loculated empyema in the left pleural space as it appears on CT of the chest.

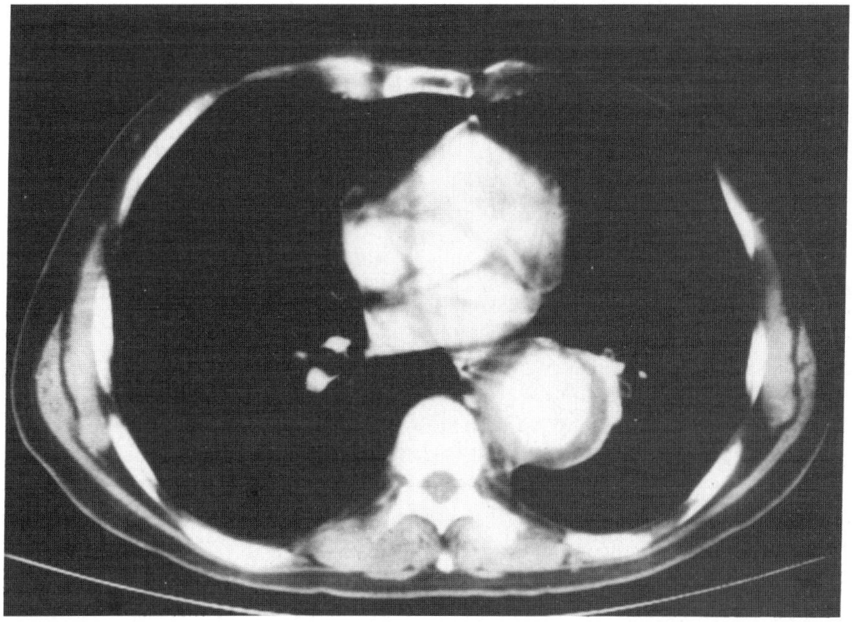

Figure 9.14. The value of CT in the mediastinum. CT examination of the chest following injection of contrast medium reveals atherosclerotic aneurysm of the descending aorta with clot surrounding the opacified lumen.

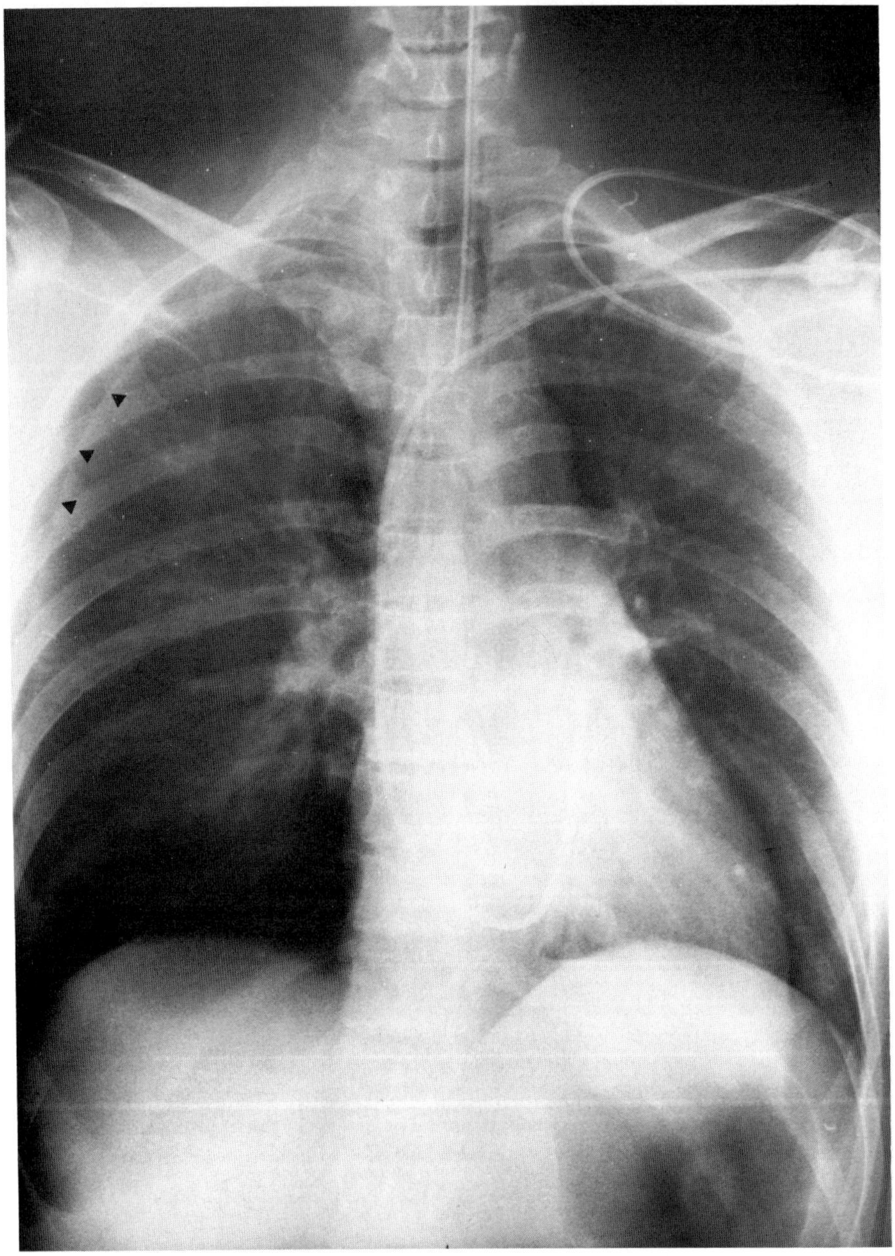

Figure 9.15. Right-sided pneumothorax on supine film. Note the radiolucency overlying the right hemidiaphragm, which represents air in the right anterior costophrenic angle. Enough air is present also to separate the lung from the chest wall, revealing the visceral pleural line *(arrows)*.

of the thoracic aorta, and an aortogram should then be done. Other local causes of increase in mediastinal width are postoperative cardiac surgery with bleeding and leakage of extravasated fluid from badly placed intravascular catheters. Lesser degrees of mediastinal widening may be seen in systemic situations of increased capillary permeability, such as burns and widening of the vascular pedicle of the superior mediastinum as seen in generalized hypervolemic states and right-sided cardiac failure. Early mediastinal widening and edema with or without gas shadows may be seen in mediastinitis. CT of the chest provides the best imaging of the mediastinum (Fig. 9.14).

Suggested Readings

Fraser RG, Paré PJA: *Diagnosis of Diseases of the Chest,* vol 3. Philadelphia, WB Saunders, 1979.

Goodman LR, Putman CE: *Intensive Care Radiology: Imaging of the Critically Ill.* St. Louis, CV Mosby, 1978).

CHAPTER

10 Airway Emergencies in Children

Trevor R. Lobb, M.D.

Croup, epiglottitis, and airway obstruction are all potentially life threatening in the young child (2-6 years of age), with epiglottitis being the most malignant. Because the laryngotracheal airway is small in comparison to the volume of air that must pass through it, even marginal compromises of its cross-sectional area can quickly lead to distress. These conditions therefore are absolute medical emergencies demanding rapid diagnosis and treatment.

CROUP

Croup (laryngotracheitis) is an insidious viral inflammation developing over several days with mild-to-moderate cold symptoms preceding its development. The disease is progressive as it descends into the lungs, and other people in the household may also be affected. The brassy cough and stridor vary with excitement and are frequently nocturnal. Treatment consists of humidification, hydration, and possibly steroids.

EPIGLOTTITIS

Within hours, epiglottitis progresses in some children to complete airway obstruction. A sore throat, including an inability to swallow, often leads to drooling as the child sits bolt upright with neck extended forward in an obvious effort to breathe. Laryngoscopy shows a characteristically red inflamed epiglottis. The offending microbe is usually *Haemophilus influenzae* type B (blood and throat cultures) associated with a definite leukocytosis. Management consists of oxygenation followed quickly by establishment of a tracheal airway and antibiotics. The present trend is toward combined therapy with ampicillin (100–200 mg/kg/24 hours) and chloramphenicol (50–100 mg/kg/24 hours) given intravenously in divided doses every 4 hours until cultures have established sensitivity to one or the other. The one to which sensitivity has been established is then continued in reduced dosages for 7–10 days. The need for the tracheal airway diminishes after the first day.

AIRWAY OBSTRUCTION

The manifestations of an aspirated foreign body are usually sudden in onset and are associated with choking, rather than coughing. Treatment obviously consists of bronchoscopy and removal.

DIAGNOSIS AND TREATMENT

Although the diagnosis may be aided by a good history (Fig. 10.1 and Table 10.1) and lateral soft tissue radiographs of the neck can often demonstrate characteristic deformities, inspection of the larynx and trachea is the only sure way of defining the problem. However, direct examination is not without risk of reflex laryngospasm

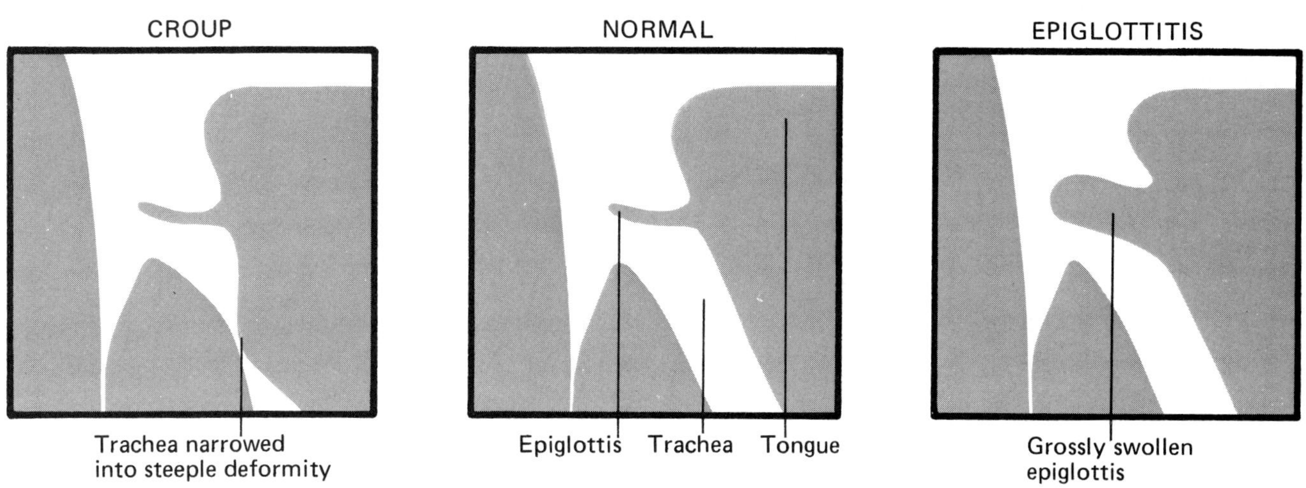

Figure 10.1. Soft tissue changes in croup and epiglottitis.

Table 10.1
Diagnosis of Airway Emergencies in Children

	Foreign body	Croup	Epiglottitis
Onset	Sudden	Days	Hours
Position	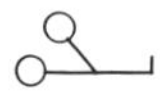	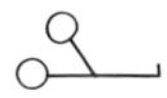	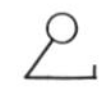
Temperature	Normal	Possible	Very high
Leukocytosis	Normal	Possible	High
Stridor	Inspiratory/expiratory	Inspiratory	Inspiratory
Cough	Present	Barking	Possible
Endoscopy	Foreign body	Edematous trachea	Red epiglottis
Treatment	Removal	Croupette/steroids (± airway)	Airway/ antibiotics

and complete obstruction and therefore must never be attempted casually. It requires the coordinated skills of an otolaryngologist and an anesthetist in an operating room equipped for endoscopy and with provisions for emergency tracheostomy and cardiopulmonary resuscitation.

Preparation is essential. The patient should have an indwelling venous catheter and administration of supplemental oxygen by mask. The actual technique depends on experience: some physicians insist on awake laryngoscopy with anesthetic standby, whereas others prefer examination after a smooth induction of anesthesia by mask inhalation. Although general anesthesia is probably more pleasant for the patient, it involves additional risks depending on the physician's experience and skills. Muscle relaxants are extremely dangerous because airway patency may depend solely on the patient's intense muscular effort. Once the bronchoscope is through the larynx or an endotracheal tube passed on laryngoscopy, the patient can be quickly and safely anesthetized by conventional methods (intravenous or inhalational), making subsequent examination more controlled. The key is to secure the airway as soon as is safely possible. The diagnosis is then easily established by examination.

At present tracheostomy is considered radical because of its possible complications—tracheal stenosis and pneumomediastinum. Although an oral endotracheal tube is just as adequate, nasal intubation is preferred with children because of better fixation, freedom from chewing, and easier subsequent review by laryngoscopy. Substitution of an endotracheal tube through a bronchoscope after anesthesia is relatively simple as long as the scope is not removed until the anesthetist can see the larynx with his or her own laryngoscope. These patients must be kept sedated to minimize accidental extubation and then nursed in a unit familiar with endotracheal tubes and their problems. In the case of epiglottitis, the endotracheal tube is usually safely removed after 1–2 days of antibiotic treatment, but a bronchoscope or laryngoscope should be available. Should the diagnosis be severe croup and require tracheostomy, generalizations about convalescence are less defined because this condition frequently requires special tracheal care.

CHAPTER

11 Pulmonary Edema

William J. Sibbald, M.D.

Pulmonary edema may be defined as an abnormal increase in water outside the vascular compartment in the lung. An understanding of how pulmonary edema may occur in many varied clinical circumstances begins with an understanding of the Starling equation. This formula describes forces responsible for movement of fluid and solutes from the pulmonary intravascular compartment to the interstitium and, eventually, to the alveoli. The Starling equation states that:

$$\text{Filtration} = \text{conductance} \times \text{driving pressure.} \qquad (1)$$

The *driving pressure* is the difference between the hydrostatic pressure and the colloid osmotic pressure (COP) within (intravascular) and outside (interstitial) the pulmonary microvasculature. The intravascular colloid osmotic pressure is determined by the plasma proteins and can be measured with an oncometer or calculated according to the equation described by Landis and Pappenheimer: COP (mm Hg) $= 2.1 + 0.16\ c^2 + 0.009\ c^3$, where c = total serum protein in grams per 100 ml. The intravascular hydrostatic pressure is clinically measured as the left ventricular end-diastolic pressure (LVEDP), or the pulmonary capillary wedge pressure (PCWP). *Conductance* describes the unique permeability of the pulmonary microvascular membrane to fluid and solutes. The Starling equation may thus be written:

$$\dot{Q}f = K[(Pmv - Ppmv) - \sigma(\pi mv - \pi pmv)] \qquad (2)$$

where $\dot{Q}f$ = net transvascular flow of fluid; K = endothelial fluid conductance, which is determined by the permeability of the lung's exchanging membrane together with the surface area of the microvasculature across which fluid exchange might occur; Pmv = microvascular hydrostatic pressure; Ppmv = interstitial hydrostatic pressure; σ = protein reflection co-efficient; πmv = plasma protein osmotic pressure; and πpmv = interstitial protein osmotic pressure.

PATHOPHYSIOLOGY

Increased Fluid Flux

The *normal* values for the pressures affecting fluid filtration across the lung's microvascular membrane are shown in Figure 11.1. When summed, it can be seen that, even in health, there normally exists a pressure gradient that allows the flux of a protein-poor filtrate from the intravascular compartment to the interstitial compartment. To retard the development of edema, defense factors normally become operative when the filtration of water across the lung's exchanging membrane increases and include (1) a decrease in the πmv, (2) an increase in the Ppmv, and (3) an increase in pulmonary lymphatic flow. Therefore, with any increase in filtration across the microvascular membrane, lymphatic flow increases to drain excess fluid from the interstitium. At the same time, a decrease in the πpmv augments the osmotic pressure differences across the membrane and thereby operates to maintain fluid within the intravascular space. And, an increase in the Ppmv also reduces the tendency for fluid filtration by negating, in part, the effect of any increase in the Pmv. Eventually, however, these defense factors will be overwhelmed by the forces favoring egress of fluid from the intravascular compartment; a net increase in extravascular water thereby occurs, resulting in interstitial pulmonary edema. The alveolar flooding stage of pulmonary edema is the most severe form and occurs as interstitial fluid migrates down to the terminal airways and overflows into the alveoli. Therefore, pulmonary edema results when filtration across the pulmonary endothelial membrane exceeds the lymphatics' capacity to maintain the "dryness" of the interstitium and is seen with (1) increased driving pressures, (2) increased conductance or permeability of the membrane, and (3) lymphatic dysfunction. Table 11.1 lists causes of pulmonary edema according to this classification.

The most common cause of pulmonary edema is congestive heart failure, referred to as "hydrostatic" or "cardiac" pulmonary edema (CPE). Edema occurring with increased permeability of the pulmonary microvessels is referred to as "permeability" or "noncardiac" pulmonary edema (NCPE) and is most commonly seen in association with systemic sepsis, as in the adult respiratory distress syndrome (ARDS) (see Chapter 8).

Sequelae of Increased Lung Water

Regardless of the underlying cause, pulmonary edema is characterized by hypoxemia, a depression in the arterial oxygen tension ($\downarrow$ PaO_2). The hypoxemia is a result of changes in the normal ventilation:perfusion ($\dot{V}/\dot{Q}$) relationships within the lung. Narrowing or closure of small airways and the filling of alveoli with edema fluid lead to nonventilation of well-perfused alveoli; intrapulmonary shunting ($\uparrow$ $\dot{Q}s/\dot{Q}t$) of blood thereby occurs (Fig. 11.2).

Shunting occurs when venous blood entering the pul-

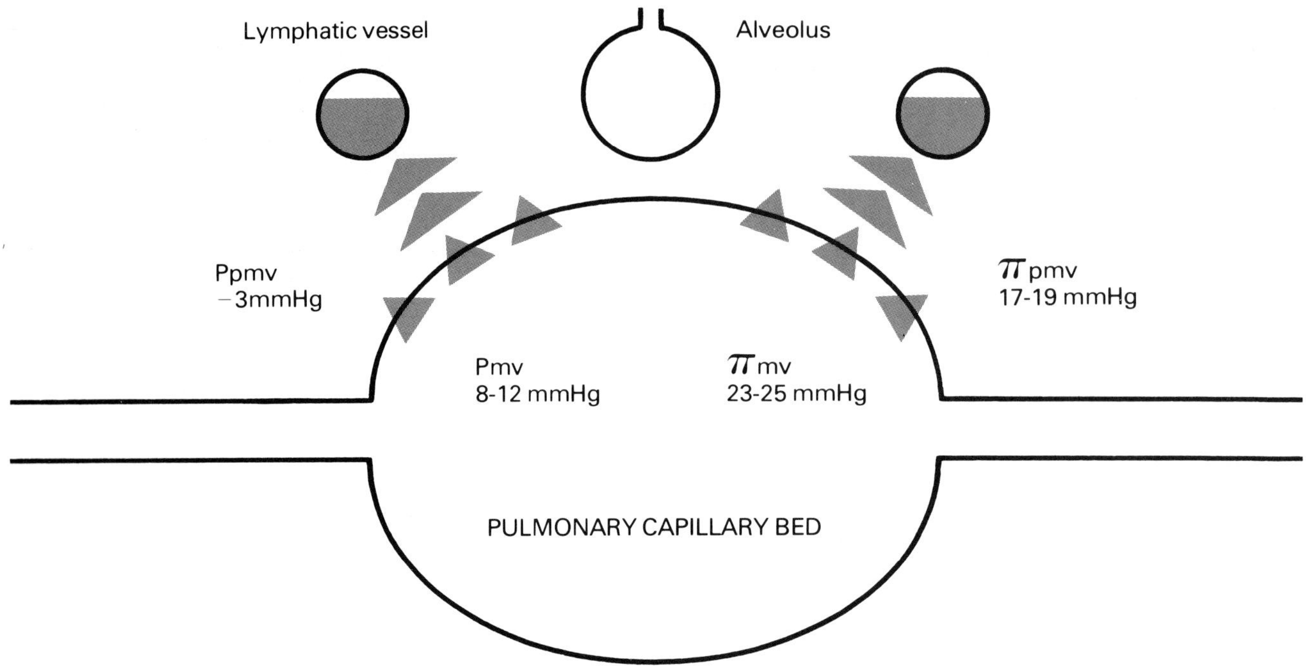

Figure 11.1. Normal pulmonary water flux. In health, the balance of the Starling forces favors a net movement of fluid out of the vessel. The pulmonary interstitium/alveoli are kept dry by the drainage effect of the pulmonary lymphatics, as well as by changes in interstitial hydrostatic and osmotic pressures.

monary microcirculation is not adequately oxygenated because fluid-filled or collapsed (atelectatic) alveoli prevent the delivery of oxygen from the environment to the deoxygenated blood entering the lungs from the right heart.

Hypocarbia (↓ $PaCO_2$) usually accompanies acute hypoxemic respiratory failure due to pulmonary edema. With pulmonary edema, the respiratory rate is elevated (tachypnea) due to stimulation of stretch receptors in the pulmonary interstitium by edema and stimulation of aortic and central chemoreceptors by the low arterial oxygen tension. An increased minute ventilation (respiratory rate × tidal volume) results in CO_2 excretion in excess of production and low arterial CO_2 tensions (hypocarbia) follow.

Increased extravascular fluid within the lungs also causes increased stiffness of the lungs, clinically referred to as decreased compliance. Noncompliant or "stiff" lungs

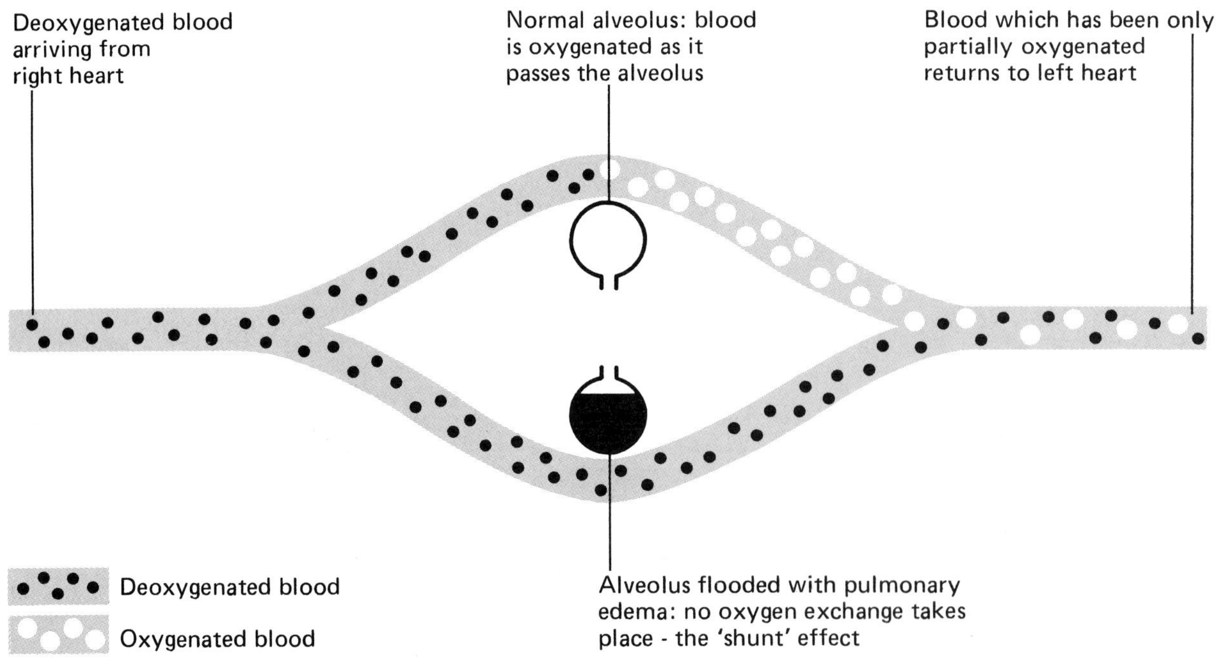

Figure 11.2. Effect of pulmonary edema on oxygenation.

Table 11.1
Common Causes of Pulmonary Edema[a]

Increase in driving pressures
↑ Pmv: congestive heart failure; mitral stenosis
↓ Ppmv: re-expansion of collapsed lung
Increase in permeability (ARDS)(↑ K)
Systemic sepsis
Pancreatitis
Shock
Head injury (neurogenic)
Fat embolism syndrome
Aspiration of liquid gastric juices
Pulmonary embolus
Multiple transfusions
Amniotic fluid embolism
Lymphatic dysfunction
Lymphangiocarcinomatosis
Postirradiation lymph fibrosis

[a] This table defines some of the common causes of pulmonary edema according to the pathologic alterations found within the Starling equation.

require a greater inspiratory pressure to produce a constant tidal volume than do healthy lungs.

When the patient is mechanically ventilated, changes in pulmonary compliance may be approximated by this equation: tidal volume/peak inspiratory pressure. This equation, in fact, reflects the stiffness properties of the chest wall, as well as the stiffness or noncompliance of the lungs themselves; normal values are usually in excess of 30 ml/cm H_2O.

In summary, pulmonary edema, an abnormal increase in extravascular lung water, results in arterial hypoxemia, hypocarbia, and stiff lungs.

HYDROSTATIC (CARDIAC) EDEMA

The most common cause of hydrostatic or cardiac pulmonary edema (CPE) is reduced left ventricular compliance (increased stiffness) due to ischemia, constrictive pericarditis, or valvular heart disease. With changes in left ventricular compliance, the end-diastolic filling pressure increases and is reflected back to the fluid-exchanging surface of the pulmonary microcirculation. This effect may be approximated by measuring the PCWP, which is usually in excess of 20 mm Hg in the presence of florid edema documented by chest radiography. It must, however, be remembered that a lowered plasma COP effectively allows for the development of pulmonary edema at a PCWP less than 20 mm Hg because the COP gradient across the lung's exchanging membrane acts to negate the effect of increasing hydrostatic pressures within the lung's microcirculation. Thus, if the plasma COP is less than normal, as in malnutrition or albumin depletion from whatever cause, the P_{CRIT}—the critical hydrostatic pressure (i.e., PCWP) at which pulmonary edema becomes radiographically apparent and clinically significant—is correspondingly reduced (Fig. 11.3).

As an increase in the PCWP promotes further transvascular flux of a protein-poor fluid, defense mechanisms that normally maintain the alveoli in a dry state, as previously discussed, are overcome and first interstitial and finally alveolar edema result (Fig. 11.4).

Diagnosis (Fig. 11.5)

Clinically, pulmonary edema is recognized in a patient usually complaining of the relatively sudden onset of dyspnea. Wheezes and crackles are found with auscultation, an S_3 gallop may be heard, the JVP may be elevated, and the chest radiograph provides confirmatory evidence. The chest radiograph initially demonstrates interstitial edema and, finally, diffuse air space disease.

Arterial blood gases confirm the presence of arterial hypoxemia and hypocarbia; a metabolic acidosis may be noted if systemic O_2 transport (O_2t) is significantly depressed below tissue O_2 needs.

Once the diagnosis of type 1 (hypoxemic) failure due to pulmonary edema is confirmed, differentiation must then be made between edema on a cardiac and that on a non-

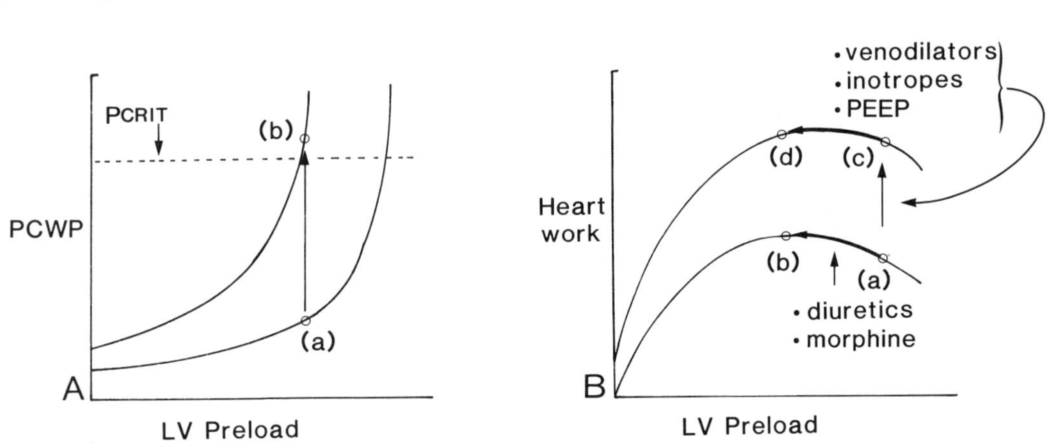

Figure 11.3. *A,* LV pressure-volume curves. With acute edema, increased stiffness of the LV results in a higher PCWP for unchanged preloads (point a-b), thereby exceeding the PCRIT, the hydrostatic pressure beyond which pulmonary edema rapidly accumulates. Some drugs reverse this process (i.e., point b-a), thereby allowing constancy of LV preload, yet at a lower PCWP. *B,* Frank-Starling Relationships. With acute edema, diuretics and morphine reduce LV preload on a constant Frank-Starling curve (point a-b). Venodilators, inotropic agents, and PEEP commonly shift the patient to a high Frank-Starling curve (points a-c) in addition to their preload-reducing actions (points c-d); hence, heart work is more substantially improved while the PCWP falls with the better management protocols.

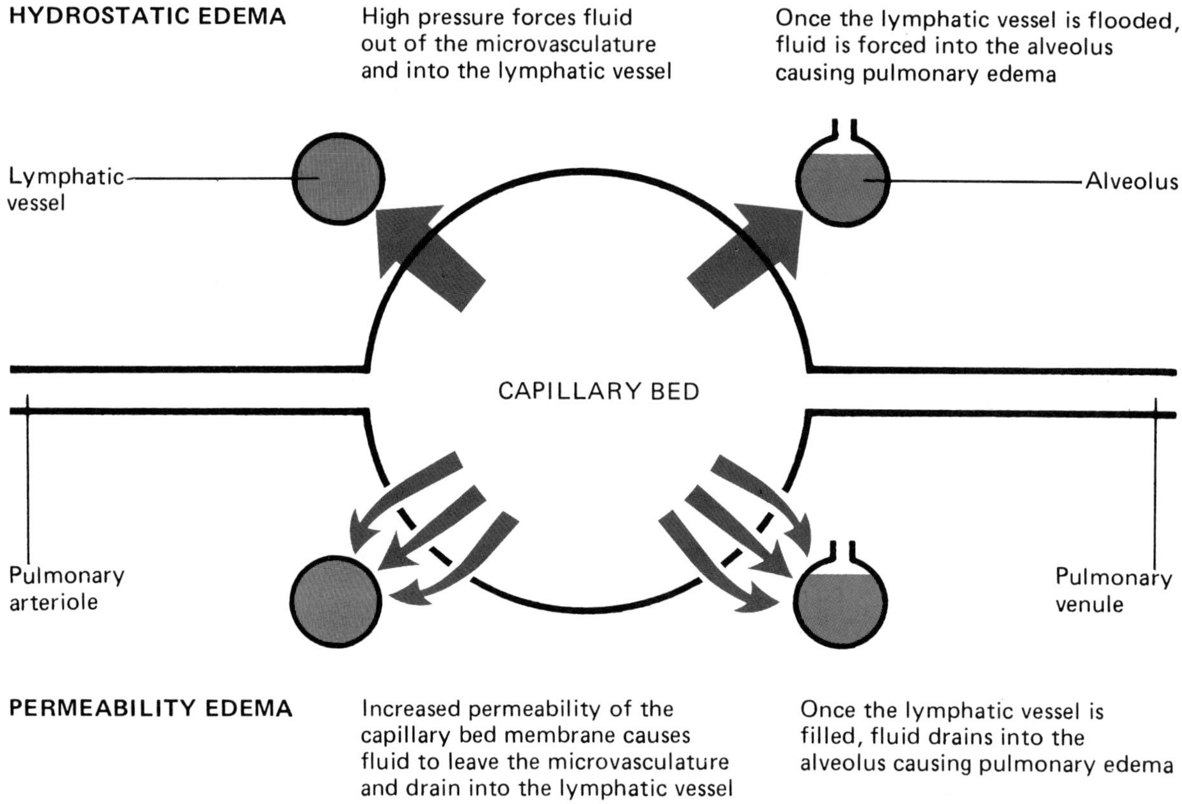

Figure 11.4. Mechanism of hydrostatic and permeability edema.

cardiac basis. Often, the initial differentiation between CPE and NCPE (ARDS) is suspected on the basis of the associated underlying disease, remembering the clinical conditions that are associated with either type of edema (Table 11.1).

In CPE, a history of chronic congestive heart disease or an acute event preceding the edema, such as myocardial infarction or pulmonary embolus, may assist in making an accurate diagnosis. Because edema complicating heart disease is due to an increase in hydrostatic pressures and often is accompanied by a low cardiac output, a number of physical findings may also be of help in supporting the differential diagnosis: a cool mottled periphery, a rapid weak pulse, or a narrow pulse pressure are more frequently found in CPE than in NCPE. Physical findings are supplemented by laboratory investigation to identify the myocardium as a primary cause of disease, including an ECG (acute infarct? left ventricular hypertrophy?); a chest roentgenogram (heart size increased?, Kerley B lines?); and cardiac enzymes (acute infarct?).

Invasive right-heart catheterization may occasionally be necessary to differentiate between the two types of pulmonary edema. In CPE, the PCWP is usually greater than 20 mm Hg, and normalization of the PCWP is accompanied by clearing of the chest roentgenogram within 24 to 36 hours; in NCPE, a normal PCWP is not usually associated with any substantial clearing of change in the chest roentgenogram over a 24- to 36-hour period, unless the underlying disease with which NCPE is associated has been effectively managed.

In the intubated patient with pulmonary edema, analysis of edema fluid may also assist in diagnosis; with a primary permeability defect, such as ARDS, more protein gains access to the alveoli than in hydrostatic edema. Therefore, in cardiac edema, the lung protein:serum protein ratio is <0.6, and in permeability or noncardiac edema the ratio is >0.7.

In summary, differentiation of CPE from NCPE may be difficult because the clinical presentation of acute respiratory failure is similar in both. However, relating the presence of edema to an underlying primary disease, with appropriate use of clinical signs and laboratory investigation, may be adequate for diagnosis in the majority of cases. In those cases where diagnosis is still in doubt, central monitoring of intravascular pressures (Swan-Ganz catheterization) is invaluable by providing a direct measurement of the PCWP.

Treatment (Table 11.2)

Treatment of the patient with acute pulmonary edema may be divided into two phases: (1) acute resuscitation and (2) specific management.

Acute Resuscitation

The treatment goals of this phase are to ensure that the airway is secure, that the patient is ventilating ade-

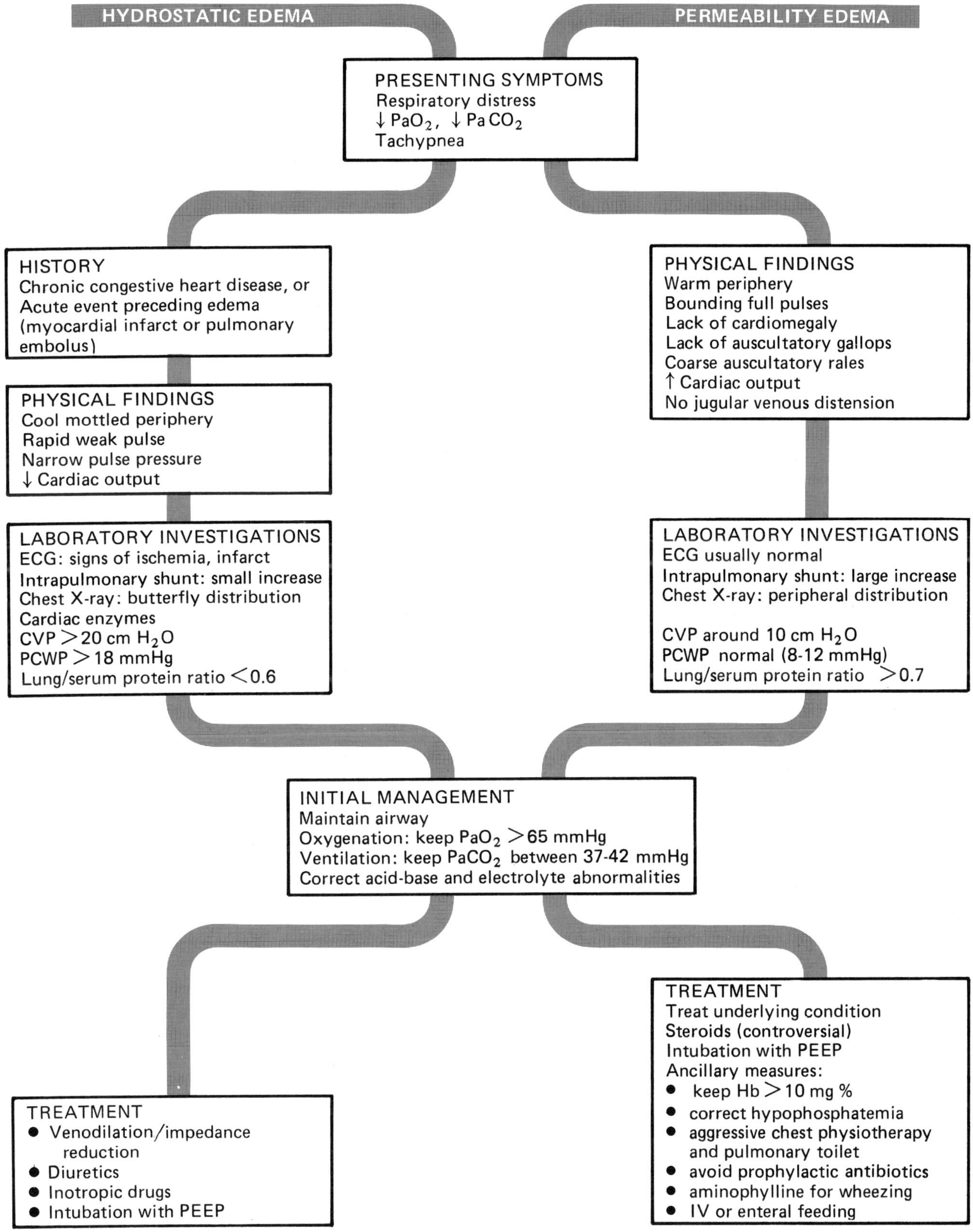

Figure 11.5. Diagnosis and management of hydrostatic and permeability edema.

Table 11.2
Acute Management of Cardiac Pulmonary Edema[a]

Intubation with PEEP, 5–10 cm H_2O
Morphine—5–15 mg, IV push over 3–15 minutes
Lasix—40–80 mg, IV push
Aminophyline—5–6 mg/kg, IV over 15–30 minutes
Nitroglycerine
1. 0.3–0.6 mg SL
2. 1/2–1 square inch topically
3. Continuous infusion

Sodium nitroprusside—continuous infusion

Other
Ethacrynic acid—25–50 mg IV
Inotropic agents
1. Digitalization
2. Dopamine
3. Dobutamine

[a] The options chosen depend upon the severity of the disease presentation.

quately, and that cardiopulmonary function is sufficient to meet the O_2 needs of the periphery.

When there is evidence of respiratory fatigue or in the presence of obtundation, elective intubation is performed and volume-cycled ventilation provided. Assisted ventilation reduces the O_2 cost of breathing and thereby enables available O_2 transport to be distributed to organs that may be teleologically more important than the respiratory muscles.

Oxygenation is supported by increasing the amount of inspired O_2 delivered to the patient via a face mask, or with intubation. If the use of supplemental O_2 by mask does not restore the PaO_2 to levels greater than 70 mm Hg on 50% inspired O_2, or less, or if signs of respiratory fatigue are not alleviated with supplemental O_2, intubation is performed and PEEP is applied. PEEP improves the PaO_2, and hence systemic O_2 transport, in patients with CPE by several mechanisms, including (1) the reduction of an abnormally elevated left ventricular preload, (2) the opening of alveoli to participate in gas exchange, and (3) an "unloading" of the left ventricle, which thereby improves cardiac output, hence O_2 transport at the same time as the PCWP falls.

Specific Management

Subsequently, therapy is directed at measures that will reduce the PCWP, thereby decreasing the major hydrostatic force responsible for pulmonary edema. Concurrently, the effect of all acute and specific management goals is assessed to ensure that systemic O_2 transport has not been adversely affected by the therapy chosen. For example, PEEP may improve the PaO_2 by opening previously closed alveoli. But, if PEEP induces a depression in the cardiac output, net O_2 transport may fall (Fig. 11.6).

Reducing Blood Volume and Venodilation

Increasing the size of the venous capacitance system redistributes volume from the central to the peripheral circulation.

In the acute situation, intubation with the use of PEEP is effective in impeding venous return, thereby reducing left venticular preload and the PCWP. Morphine, 5-15 mg IV, given slowly (over 3-5 min) effects sufficient venodilation to decrease the PCWP modestly; it also reduces anxiety and the work of breathing. Lasix (40–80 mg IV) establishes a diuresis, assuming there is adequate renal blood flow (i.e., absence of shock) and concurrently increases the size of the venous capacitance system, thereby reducing central blood volume. The addition of a loading dose of aminophylline (5–6 mg/kg) with Lasix may result in a diuresis greater than that achieved with the diuretic alone because aminophylline augments cardiac output and renal blood flow; it also improves the $\dot{V}a/\dot{Q}$ mismatch, hence the PaO_2, because of its bronchodilating properties.

Other Vasoactive Agents

Other vasoactive agents useful in reducing the PCWP are nitroglycerine and sodium nitroprusside. In acute pulmonary edema, the stiffness properties of the left ventricle may be increased, especially if the cause of the increased PCWP is myocardial ischemia. With an increase in stiffness properties, any volume in the left ventricle will be reflected by a higher PCWP. Parenteral drugs, such as nitroglycerine and nitroprusside, cause a redistribution of central volume to the periphery by their venodilating properties. Additionally, they may improve the stiffness properties of the left ventricle, thereby allowing left ventricular volumes to be reflected by a lower PCWP (Fig. 11.4). Commitment to a continuous infusion of venodilators is most safely done with hemodynamic monitoring to monitor their effects on the PCWP, as well

EFFECT OF PEEP ON O_2 TRANSPORT

	O_2 TRANSPORT	=	Cardiac Index	x	Arterial O_2 Content
PRE-PEEP	392 ml/min/M²	=	2.84 Liters/min/M²	x	13.79 vol%
POST-PEEP	303 ml/min/M²	=	2.08 Liters/min/M²	x	14.57 vol%
NET EFFECT	-89 ml/min/M²		-0.76 Liters/min/M²		+0.78 vol%

Figure 11.6. Effect of PEEP on O_2 transport.

as on cardiac output, mean blood pressure, and systemic O_2 transport.

Diuretics

Diuretics, by reducing the intravascular volume, reduce the PCWP. They may be ineffective, however, in situations in which reduced renal blood flow complicates a shock state with a significant depression in cardiac output. With good renal function, in nonemergent situations, it is probably safer to reduce LV preload, and the PCWP, with diuretics, before using parenteral vasoactive agents.

Diuretics are given parenterally in acute illness because erratic absorption often follows oral administration.

For reasons not completely appreciated, ethacrynic acid 25–50 mg IV may initiate a diuresis where Lasix has failed, especially in the presence of mild renal insufficiency.

Inotropic Agents

If both the clinical picture and monitored indices suggest a reduced cardiac output, inotropic agents are of benefit in that they improve heart work (hence cardiac output) for any given left ventricular preload. This often results in improved perfusion of the core circulation, with subsequent improvement in both myocardial and renal function. Inotropic agents, by increasing myocardial contractility, also reduce the left ventricular preload, which translates into a reduced PCWP.

It is emphasized, however, that all inotropic agents increase myocardial oxygen consumption and may increase infarct size. Digoxin does not have an immediate effect, but will improve contractility within 2 hours. Digoxin is given as 0.5 mg immediately, infused over 10–15 minutes, and repeated in 4–6 hours. Maintenance dosage depends on renal function (see Chapter 15). Dopamine (5–10 μg/kg/min), may be preferable to digitialization in patients with a normal heart size because digoxin may have adverse effects on myocardial oxygen consumption in this group of patients. Dopamine may also selectively increase renal blood flow and thereby promote a substantial diuresis. Dobutamine (5–10 μg/kg/min) also increases cardiac output and may reduce the PCWP more than comparable doses of dopamine.

NONCARDIAC PULMONARY EDEMA (ARDS)

There are many risk factors for the development of ARDS, with the chance of developing this syndrome increasing according to the number of risk factors present (Table 11.1). Pulmonary edema characterizes ARDS and may lead to acute hypoxemic respiratory failure, because of the development of a permeability lesion within the pulmonary microvasculature. This permeability defect allows the egress of protein-rich fluid from the intravascular compartment to the pulmonary interstitium and alveoli *at normal hydrostatic* (i.e., PCWP) *pressures*. The Starling forces, however, remain operative; in the presence of a permeability lesion within the lung's microvasculature, an increase in the PCWP increases fluid flux across the lung's exchanging membrane at a greater rate than would be noted with a similar increase of the PCWP in CPE.

ARDS also has well-defined systemic effects, although the majority of patients present clinically with signs and symptoms relating to its effects on the gas exchange function of the lungs, such as acute respiratory insufficiency. With ARDS, a permeability defect also occurs in the systemic microvasculature; nondependent peripheral edema results. The extraction of O_2 at the cellular level is also deranged in ARDS as the extraction ratio, or efficiency of O_2 utilization, is reduced. This is particularly of concern because ARDS is characterized by a heightened systemic O_2 consumption. ARDS may lead to the syndrome of multiple organ failure (see Chapter 37), particularly if O_2 delivery is less than peripheral O_2 requirements over a sustained period.

The cause of this multiplicity of derangements in the lung and periphery in ARDS is not well understood. However, animal models of this syndrome have found an important role played by neutrophils. Diseases with which ARDS is associated result in activation of the complement system. A by-product of C activation, C5a, activates neutrophils, which subsequently become entrapped in the pulmonary microvasculature. The interaction between the activated neutrophil and the endothelial cell then results in increased permeability of the lung's exchanging membrane, possibly due to the release of toxic O_2 radicals from the neutrophil. The same sequence of events may result in the increase in systemic permeability seen with ARDS. Only correction of the underlying process (e.g., pancreatitis, sepsis) will result in ultimate resolution of the permeability defect.

Diagnosis (Fig. 11.5)

Noncardiac edema must be recognized as only a symptom of another disease process. Once diagnosed, concurrent and parallel investigation must proceed toward identification of the underlying associated disease.

Differentiation between edema due to a permeability defect and that due to an increase in hydrostatic pressures can be difficult, as earlier discussed. In general, however, permeability edema or ARDS should be suspected when acute hypoxemic respiratory failure secondary to pulmonary edema occurs in association with the diseases listed in Table 11.1. Other features characteristic of ARDS may include a warm periphery with bounding, full pulses (ARDS is usually a hyperdynamic, high cardiac output state); lack of cardiomegaly and lack of auscultatory gallops; no jugular venous distension; coarse, auscultatory rales in contradistinction to the fine, moist rales of CHF; normal central filling pressures (normal CVP/PCWP); and an edema fluid/serum protein ratio >0.7.

The diagnosis of ARDS is usually, therefore, one of suspicion when associated disease processes and concurrent physical examination make it difficult to invoke a cardiac cause. It may take time to confirm the diagnosis. As previously mentioned, CPE will show roentgenologic clearing during the 24–36 hours after normalization of the PCWP, i.e., PCWP <18 mm Hg. In contrast, NCPE, if initially associated with a high PCWP, will not show roentgenologic clearing in the same time period with normalization of the PCWP because the permeability defect remains; that is, the egress of protein-rich fluid across the alveolocapillary membrane continues.

Specialized investigative techniques may differentiate CPE from NCPE edema, although their investigative nature prohibits their routine use. Scintigraphy of the lung following an injection of I^{131}-HSA shows increased extravascular accumulation in ARDS compared to CHF. Extravascular lung water (EVLW), measured by the thermal-green dye technique, demonstrates a greater quantity of EVLW in ARDS compared to CHF.

Treatment

Treatment of noncardiac pulmonary edema (ARDS) is based primarily on adequate and expeditious therapy of the underlying precipitating condition (Table 11.1). Because there is still little known about the exact cause of the increase in permeability of the pulmonary microvasculature seen in ARDS, no specific pharmacologic approach either to restoring normal permeability or preventing the progression of the injury can be recommended. However, it is well recognized that with resolution of the underlying process (e.g., sepsis, pancreatitis) the primary pulmonary lesion will resolve. With this consideration then, initial therapy is directed at the primary disease process while at the same time supportive therapy is provided to correct the hypoxemia accompanying ARDS.

Treat the Underlying Condition

The underlying disease process with which ARDS is associated, such as sepsis or pancreatitis, must be aggressively sought out and corrected as quickly as possible. The following principles of care are described briefly because management of acute respiratory failure is detailed in Chapter 7.

General Resuscitation

Because no specific therapy is effective in restoring to normalcy the lung's microvascular defect in ARDS and its sequelae, and because this disease is characterized by a hypermetabolic state and increased systemic consumption, general resuscitation is aimed at maintaining systemic O_2 transport at levels commensurate with peripheral O_2 requirements. The O_2 transport equation demonstrates those factors that may be supported to accomplish previously defined goals of resuscitation:

$$O_2 \text{ transport} = \text{arterial } O_2 \text{ content} \times \text{cardiac output}$$

Optimize Cardiac Output

Evidence of inadequate tissue O_2 availability, such as a low mixed venous O_2 content or elevated lactate, necessitates the institution of measures to augment cardiac output. Cardiac output can be increased by increasing preload or contractility and decreasing afterload.

Optimize Arterial O_2 Content

The hemoglobin should be maintained between 11 and 13 gm/dl and hypophosphotemia prevented to reduce its impact on the position of the oxyhemoglobin dissociation curve.

Attempt to keep the PaO_2 above 65 mm Hg with supplemental humidified oxygen by mask or, if necessary, with intubation and assisted ventilation. Indications for intubation and assisted ventilation are given in Chapter 8. If intubation is necessary, positive end-expiratory pressure (PEEP) is added in increments of 3–5 cm H_2O until lung compliance changes with therapy indicate that further addition of PEEP may only expand already maximally expanded alveoli. This principle is easily judged at the bedside by calculating "effective compliance," which is tidal volume (V_T) divided by peak inspiratory pressure (PIP). With initial institution of PEEP the lungs should become less stiff (i.e., more distensible), which is indicated by an increase in V_T/PIP ratio. When the inherent stiffness of the lungs prevents further expansion of atelectatic and edematous alveoli, further addition of PEEP will then actually cause reduced compliance. The level of PEEP at the last increment is referred to as "best PEEP," a level where the maximal beneficial effect of PEEP is realized. The inspired oxygen concentration is then adjusted to keep the PaO_2 over 65–70 mm Hg.

Both PEEP and ARDS adversely affect cardiac output (CO), and hence blood pressure. Generally, ARDS is a hyperdynamic state, and the presence of a low cardiac output in ARDS is a poor prognostic sign. When a low flow state is associated with PEEP or ARDS, a fluid challenge with a colloid solution or inotropic support with dopamine should be attempted to maximize the CO, and maintain peripheral oxygen delivery. Clinically the sum effect of PEEP on oxygenation and cardiac function is monitored by changes in oxygen delivery, the cardiac output × the arterial oxygen content (Fig. 11.6).

High microvascular hydrostatic pressures measured as the PCWP and/or low colloid osmotic pressures encourage water movement out of vessels into the pulmonary interstitium, over and above the increased egress of a protein-rich fluid caused by the permeability defect itself. Therefore, diuretics and/or venodilators may be used to keep the PCWP in "normal" ranges, i.e., 8–14 mm Hg. Because the PCWP also reflects left ventricular preload, if it is reduced too low, cardiac output will fall, core organ perfusion will suffer, and multiple organ failure might result. We therefore accept the fact that pulmonary edema formation is an ongoing process in these patients and try to reduce its effects on oxygenation with PEEP. We maintain the PCWP in the normal range (8–12 mm Hg) and do not believe that the "dehydration" therapy suggested by some authors reduces morbidity or mortality. Indeed it may increase both because of the danger of multiple organ failure from an established low flow state.

Recent studies have shown that high-dose corticosteroids do not enhance recovery from ARDS, and their use is no longer recommended. However, other drugs are currently undergoing clinical trial in ARDS; in experimental models of ARDS, both nonsteroidal anti-inflammatory agents and prostaglandin E reduce the progression in the permeability defect of the lung's microvasculature. Until the results of clinical trials are available, pharmacologic approaches to reducing the permeability lesion of ARDS must be considered experimental.

Optimize Ventilation

CO_2 production is usually increased in ARDS. Therefore, minute ventilation requirements are increased. In addition, dead space, the presence of ventilated but nonperfused alveoli, is increased. In severe ARDS it may therefore be necessary to treat a high $PaCO_2$. This is done with adjustments of the respiratory rate or tidal volume on the ventilator. We generally prefer the use of high tidal volumes (10–15 ml/kg) to reduce a tendency to atelectasis and then further adjust the minute ventilation (and hence $PaCO_2$) as necessary by primary changes in the respiratory rate. The $PaCO_2$ is maintained at 37–42 mm Hg.

Other

Crystalloid and colloid are used to maintain the PCWP between 8–12 mm Hg. Fluid infusion greater than this pressure guideline is unlikely to be associated with any significant increase in cardiac output according to the Frank-Starling principle because the stiffness properties of the left ventricle will define an increase in end-diastolic pressure with little increase in end-diastolic volume or preload when the PCWP is between 10 and 16 mm Hg.

If a further increase in cardiac output is required with optimization of preload, inotropic agents are used. Dopamine may be more effective than Dobutamine because of the systemic vasodilating properties of the latter, which can result in hypotension.

Suggested Readings

Andreadis N, Petty TL: Adult respiratory distress syndrome: problems and progress. *Am Rev Respir Dis* 132:1344–1346, 1985.

Berkowitz D, Cross MN: Malabsorption as a complication of congestive heart failure. *Am J Cardiol* 2:43, 1964.

Brigham KL: Mechanisms of lung injury. *Clin Chest Med* 3:9–24, 1982.

Colice GL: Neurogenic pulmonary edema. *Clin Chest Med* 6:473, 1985.

Danek SJ, Lynch JP, Weg JRD, et al: The dependence of oxygen uptake on oxygen delivery in the adult respiratory distress syndrome. *Am Rev Respir Dis* 122:387–395, 1980.

Fowler AA, Hamman RF, Good JT, et al: Adult respiratory distress syndrome: risk with common predispositions. *Ann Intern Med* 98:593–597, 1983.

McHugh TJ, Forrester JS, Adler L, Zion D, Swan HJC: Pulmonary vascular congestion in acute myocardial infarction: hemodynamics and radiologic correlations. *Ann Intern Med* 76:29–33, 1982.

Pistolesi M, Miniati M, Milne ENC, Guintini C: The chest roentgenogram in pulmonary edema. *Clin Chest Med* 6:315, 1985.

Rackow E, Fein A, Siegel J: The relationship of the colloid osmotic pulmonary artery wedge pressure gradient to pulmonary edema and mortality in critically ill patients. *Chest* 82:433, 1982.

Sibbald WJ, Cunningham DR, Chin DN: Non-cardiac or cardiac pulmonary edema? A practical approach to clinical differential in critically ill patients. *Chest* 84:453–461, 1983.

Sibbald WJ, Short A, Warshawski F, Harris J, Lefcoe M, Holliday R: Clinical studies of measuring extravascular lung water by the thermal dye technique in critically ill patients. *Chest* 87:582–595, 1985.

CHAPTER

12 Acute Pulmonary Embolism

Albert A. Driedger, M.D., Adel G. Matter, M.D., and William J. Sibbald, M.D.

Pulmonary embolism may be a cause of death in previously well people: an incidence of 2.7/year per million people has been noted for adults, excluding pregnant women in whom the incidence is about 50% greater. Among hospitalized patients, pulmonary embolism is the cause of death in 4–7% of autopsied cases, a contributing factor in another 7–8%, and an associated finding in as many as 60% of cases.

By extrapolation from both prospective studies and autopsies pulmonary embolism is estimated to occur in about 2% of hospitalized patients. The majority of episodes are asymptomatic or present with nonspecific symptoms, with an antemortem diagnosis being established in only 10–30% of fatal cases. Prompt diagnosis and treatment reduce the mortality of thromboembolism from as high as 38% to less than 8%. It is therefore necessary for physicians to think of the possibility early and to have formulated an effective approach to the diagnosis and management of pulmonary embolism.

PATHOPHYSIOLOGY

Venous thrombosis is a necessary precedent of pulmonary thromboembolism. The factors that predispose to venous thrombosis, collectively known as Virchow's triad, are (1) stasis, (2) venous injury, and (3) a hypercoagulable state. Extensive deep venous thrombosis of lower extremities and pelvic veins may be clinically undetectable, and only about 50% of all patients with deep venous thrombosis manifest typical clinical signs. Only 20–25% of patients with pulmonary embolism have clinical evidence of venous thrombosis, even if it is carefully sought for, possibly because the offending vein (e.g., the internal iliac system) is inaccessible for investigation or the thrombus has been cleared by the embolic event.

In the majority of cases of pulmonary embolism, a predisposing cause of deep venous thrombosis relating to one or more of the elements of Virchow's triad will be found. The reduced activity and associated venous stasis associated with cardiovascular disease, chronic obstructive lung disease, bed rest for any reason, or obesity are common precursors of embolism. Lower limb trauma, orthopedic surgery (especially hip surgery), and peripheral vascular surgery all have a recognized incidence of venous thrombosis and embolism. The hypercoagulable state as a precursor of embolism is best exemplified by oral contraceptive use and malignant disease.

If death does not occur from the acute event, then the natural history of the single episode is one of progressive resolution, with partial or complete restoration of lung perfusion over several weeks in most cases. The factors operating to reopen the arterial channels are both fibrinolysis and organization of the embolus. However, untreated pulmonary embolism is prone to potentially fatal recurrence for as long as there is a continuing opportunity for thrombus formation.

Pulmonary infarction occurs in only about 10% of cases of pulmonary embolism. The viability of the embolized lung is maintained in most cases by a combination of blood flow from the bronchial circulation and continued alveolar ventilation.

The manifestations of embolism are largely determined by two factors: (1) the extent to which the pulmonary vascular bed is obstructed by the embolus and (2) the pre-existing functional status of the cardiopulmonary system. Patients with a previously normal cardiopulmonary system can tolerate obstruction of approximately 50% of the pulmonary vasculature without any sustained rise in pulmonary artery pressure. With massive embolization the dominant mechanical effects are exemplified by acute cor pulmonale. When emboli are superimposed on an already diseased heart or lungs, the effects are more variable; smaller emboli may produce symptoms that are no more than an unexplained exacerbation of the patient's recognized illness. In order even to suspect pulmonary embolism in this situation, it is necessary to pay attention to subtle clinical details.

The clinical manifestations of an embolic event are best considered in relation to the effects on pulmonary and cardiac function. Pulmonary embolism alters the regional relationship of alveolar ventilation to perfusion in the lung so that dead space ventilation is increased. Immediately following the embolic event, mediator release from the embolus causes bronchospasm, thereby increasing intrapulmonary shunting and lowering the arterial oxygenation (PaO_2). The increased pulmonary artery pressure will result in increased extravascular water by operation of the Starling forces and in reduced lung compliance.

With massive embolism, in response to the acute pulmonary artery hypertension, the right ventricle will dilate, causing the septum to shift toward the left ventricle. The net effect of septal shift is reduced compliance of the left ventricle, which occurs along with a reduction in

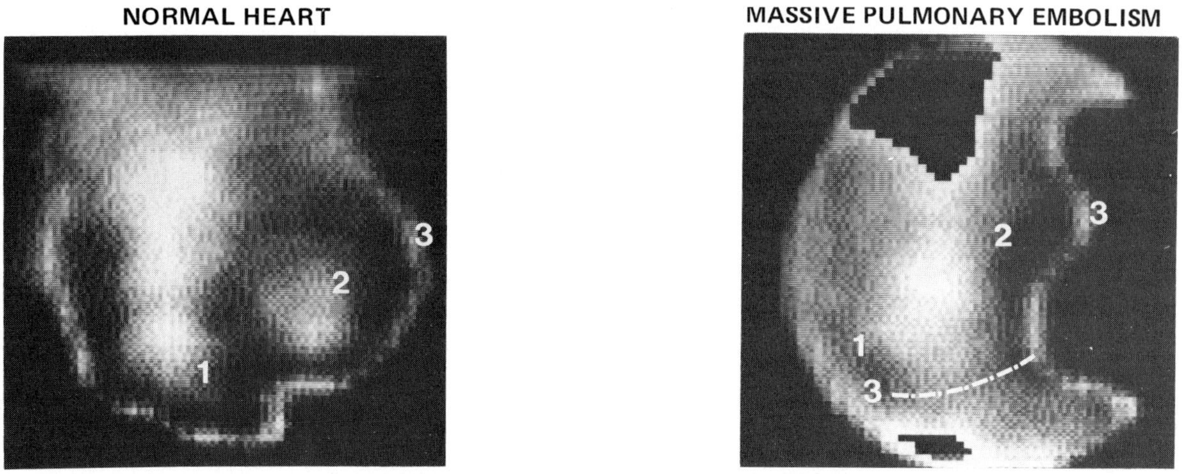

Figure 12.1. Blood pool radionuclide ventriculogram. Left anterior oblique projections of gated equilibrium blood pool images in the normal state and immediately after massive pulmonary embolism. *1,* Right ventricular (RV) blood pool in systole. *2,* Left ventricular (LV) blood pool in systole. *3,* Blood pool perimeter in diastole. The space between the diastolic perimeter and the systolic blood pool represents contraction. In massive embolism, note the large RV, but small LV, which is responsible in part for the low cardiac output in this disease.

the diastolic filling of that ventricle because of right ventricular dysfunction. In comparison to the normal state it can be shown by radionuclide ventriculography that the left ventricular end-diastolic volume decreases significantly after a large embolism (Fig. 12.1). This acute reduction in preload therefore results in diminished cardiac output, according to the Frank-Starling mechanism. The generation of other abnormal reflexes by the interaction of the embolus and the pulmonary vascular bed may also depress cardiac contractility to produce hypotension.

Therefore, the first therapeutic priority is prevention of deep venous thrombosis. The second priority is the prevention of recurrent embolism. The third, although often the most immediate consideration, is treatment of the hemodynamic and respiratory complications of pulmonary embolism.

CLINICAL PRESENTATION

Only infrequently do patients present with the complete picture of a well-identified predisposing factor, clinically apparent deep venous thrombosis, dyspnea, pleuritic chest pain, and hemoptysis. This presentation is typical of embolism, with infarction of the lung causing the hemoptysis. Another presenting pattern is dyspnea, cyanosis, right heart failure, and hypotension reflecting acute cor pulmonale with massive embolism. The third and perhaps most common presentation is that of otherwise unexplained dyspnea. Any one of these symptom complexes may be incomplete and may vary in severity.

The physician who entertains the possibility of pulmonary embolism is obliged to verify these suspicions promptly. Tests performed after several days are likely to be inconclusive or falsely normal. Clearly, if the patient is in shock, the first efforts are directed toward resuscitation and stabilization of hemodynamic and respiratory dysfunction (see Chapter 6). Definitive investigation should begin as soon as the patient's condition permits.

LABORATORY CONFIRMATION

Which biochemical, imaging, or functional tests should be performed? The testing procedures selected should not only be able to verify or exclude pulmonary embolism but also should assist in the recognition of other possible causes of overlapping symptomatology, such as pulmonary infection, myocardial infarction, congestive heart failure, and an exacerbation of chronic obstructive pulmonary disease. The sequence of the tests may have to be varied in accordance with locally available facilities. Figure 12.2 suggests an "optimal" and orderly sequence of investigation.

The hematologic and biochemical tests are entirely nonspecific with respect to pulmonary embolism, and the results are chiefly of value only if they suggest another diagnosis. With embolism, the white cell count is typically less than 10,000 and seldom greater than 15,000.

Serum enzyme values are no longer considered to be helpful in the diagnosis of embolism, but the serial elevation of serum CK-fraction, SGOT, and LDH enzymes may assist in recognition of myocardial infarction. The ECG is chiefly of value in excluding myocardial infarction. Apart from right-axis shift, which is seen with massive embolism and acute right-heart strain, ECG changes are nonspecific and may include tachycardia, T-wave abnormalities, arrhythmias, and ST segment changes.

Hypoxemia ($PaO_2 < 80$ mm Hg on room air) is a frequent finding in embolism. Because it is a nonspecific finding, hypoxemia cannot be used in isolation to make the diagnosis. The PaO_2 is valuable in excluding pulmonary embolism in younger patients with previously normal respiratory function. In older individuals and those with pre-existing pulmonary disease, a low PaO_2 is frequently not of diagnostic value unless a preceding baseline value is known.

The chest x-ray is rarely diagnostic and most often shows nonspecific findings or is normal in pulmonary embolism. The radiographic findings include a raised

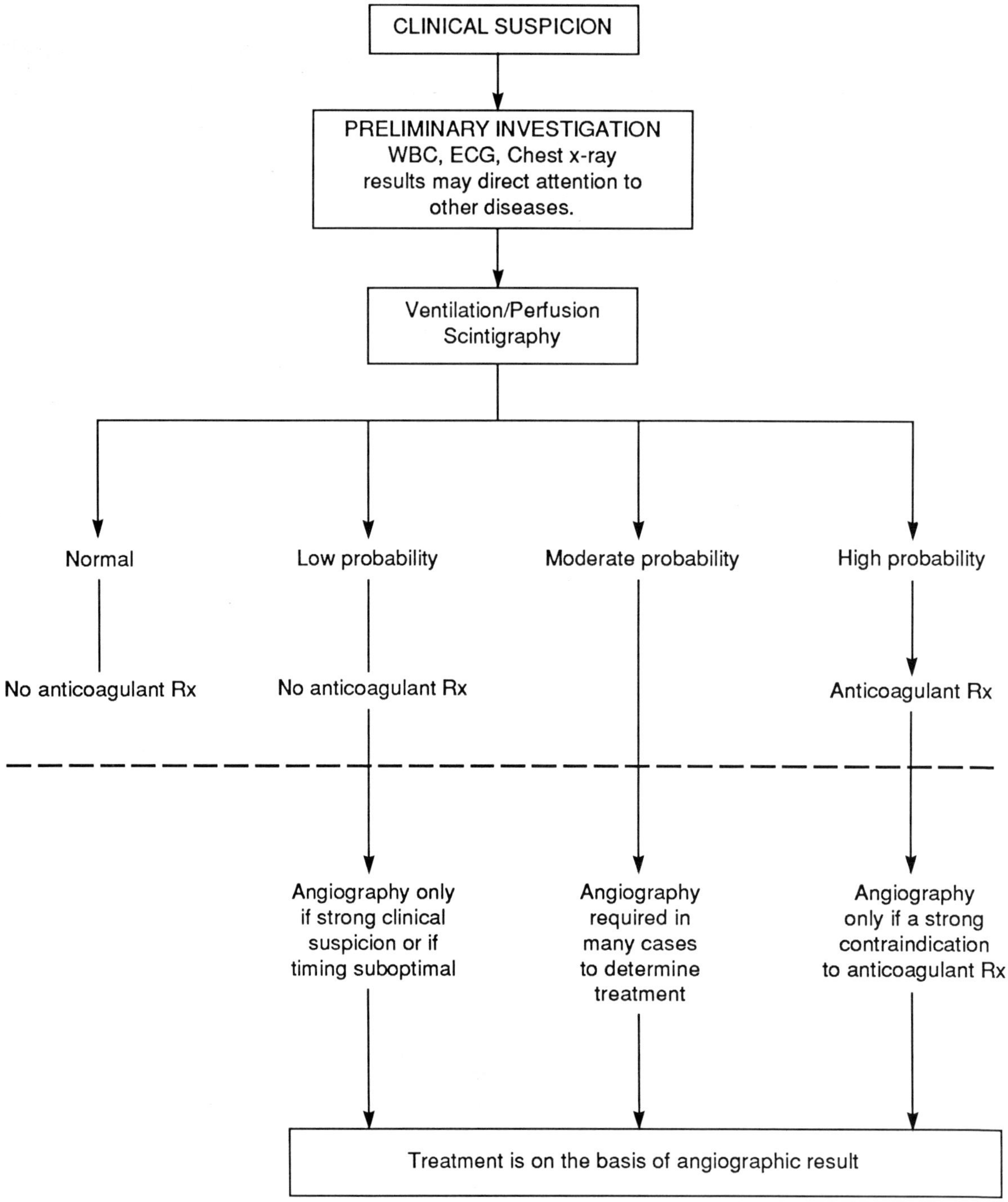

Figure 12.2. Investigation of suspected pulmonary embolism.

hemidiaphragm, cut off or a prominence of a pulmonary artery, linear atelectasis, pleural effusion (usually small), an avascular-appearing region of the lung (oligemia), or an area of consolidation or Hampton's hump. On the other hand, the x-ray may conclusively demonstrate other causes of acute respiratory distress that may be initially confused with embolism, such as pulmonary edema, pneumothorax, pneumonia, and interstitial lung disease.

Combined ventilation/perfusion imaging of the lungs with a combination of inhaled and intravenously injected radiopharmaceuticals should be performed promptly when pulmonary embolism is suspected. It is not appropriate to delay the examination through a weekend or holiday because perfusion may be extensively restored within a 24-hour interval and the diagnosis thereby obscured. A completely normal study obtained in proper temporal relation to the onset of symptoms virtually excludes pulmonary embolism.

Abnormal studies should be categorized according to a low (<10%), moderate (20–35%), or high (>90%) probability of embolism. In a population of patients who were not clinically ill before the onset of suspected embolism, none was subsequently shown to have that diagnosis or to have further episodes if the scan was interpreted as low probability. High-probability interpretation signifies a ventilated perfusion defect(s) of at least one segment, the majority of one segment, or of two medium-sized subsegments; the chest x-ray should have no corresponding abnormality or the abnormality should be substantially smaller in size than that of the perfusion abnormality. Moderate-probability interpretations may be due to inappropriate timing of the examination, concurrent radiographic abnormalities, diffuse chronic obstructive airways disease, or the presence of one medium-sized perfusion defect. The low-probability scan is indicated by matching ventilation and perfusion abnormalities with no corresponding radiographic abnormalities or by small perfusion defects even without matching ventilation abnormalities. When radiographic abnormalities are much larger in size than the corresponding perfusion abnormalities, the probability of pulmonary embolism is also low; in this situation the underlying cause is likely to be parenchymal in origin. In many critically ill patients the interpretation is complex because of the coexistence of pre-existing lung disease.

In some instances the scintigraphic interpretation is at variance with a strong clinical impression. In some patients with both clinical and scintigraphic diagnoses of embolism there may be reluctance to use anticoagulants because of known contraindications unless the diagnosis of pulmonary embolism is established beyond any doubt. In still other situations, insertion of an umbrella into or ligation of the inferior vena cava, thrombolytic treatment, or embolectomy may be contemplated. In all of these instances, pulmonary angiography must be done with reasonable promptness. Although angiography carries a small risk and can detect only clots greater than 2 mm in diameter, it is nonetheless the standard technique against which all other tests are evaluated. Selective angiography directed to the zones of lung that were abnormal on the scintigraph is the most sensitive and preferred technique. Relative contraindications to angiography include allergy to contrast media, recent myocardial infarction, and ventricular irritability.

Digital subtraction angiography is a relatively new technique that has not yet been fully evaluated, but appears to be promising. Its demonstration of small pulmonary emboli is less sensitive than the standard pulmonary angiogram. However, it has the advantage of requiring less contrast injection, which could be given in a peripheral vein or via a pulmonary artery catheter.

At the same time as the investigation for embolism is being conducted, the possibility of venous thrombosis should also be evaluated. The radiographic contrast lower limb venogram is the most widely available test for this purpose and is also the reference against which other tests are assessed. However, the test has limitations. It is invasive, requiring the injection of a large volume of contrast medium. Because it is uncomfortable for the patient, it is unsuitable for screening or for repeated patient monitoring. In addition to the usual general side effects of radiographic contrast, thrombophlebitis could result from the test itself in a minority of patients. The test is useless in evaluating the internal iliac venous system and other deep veins in the pelvis.

Radionuclide venography may be performed with the same tracer material as pulmonary perfusion images, if the injections are made into the veins on the feet. The radionuclide venogram is highly effective for the detection of occlusive venous disease proximal to the knee. By contrast, the leg I-125 fibrinogen uptake test (FUT) is sensitive for the detection of clots in the calves. The FUT has been used widely to study the epidemiology of deep venous disease, but is of limited value as a clinical test. For technical reasons the test is insensitive in the upper thighs and is useless in the pelvis. Therefore, in the context of pulmonary embolism, it is of value only in the region between the knee and lower thigh. Moreover, because the thrombotic process must still be going on while the test is being conducted, the FUT may be rendered negative by early introduction of effective therapy, i.e., anticoagulation. The need for accurate confirmation of acute venous thrombosis has similar implications for anticoagulation as the diagnosis of pulmonary embolism. Doppler ultrasonography and electrical impedance plethysmography can provide useful information, but the results are not consistently reliable.

MANAGEMENT

Prophylaxis

The importance of prophylaxis in the susceptible population cannot be overemphasized. In practical terms prophylaxis consists largely of measures that combat venous stasis in bedridden patients with early ambulation wherever possible. "Prophylactic" low-dose (mini) heparin (3000–5000 units every 8–12 hours) seems to reduce the risk of deep venous thrombosis in patients for whom a prolonged period of immobilization is projected, particularly those with major surgical procedures.

Definitive Therapy

When pulmonary embolism is known or suspected to have occurred, two concurrent therapeutic objectives emerge: (1) maintenance of cardiopulmonary function until resolution of the embolus occurs and (2) prevention of recurrent embolization. The degree of supportive management required depends on the severity of the associated cardiopulmonary effects of embolization. There are three interrelated considerations in cardiopulmonary support: (1) maintenance of circulation, (2) maintenance of oxygenation, and (3) maintenance of ventilation. The main objectives are shown in Figure 12.3.

Maintenance of Circulation

A small group of patients present with hypotension following pulmonary embolism. The hypotension associated with pulmonary embolism is a form of hypovolemic shock, i.e., "pseudohypovolemia." The acute effect of an embolus is to obstruct the pulmonary vasculature, reduce the flow of blood to the left heart, decrease the preload of the left

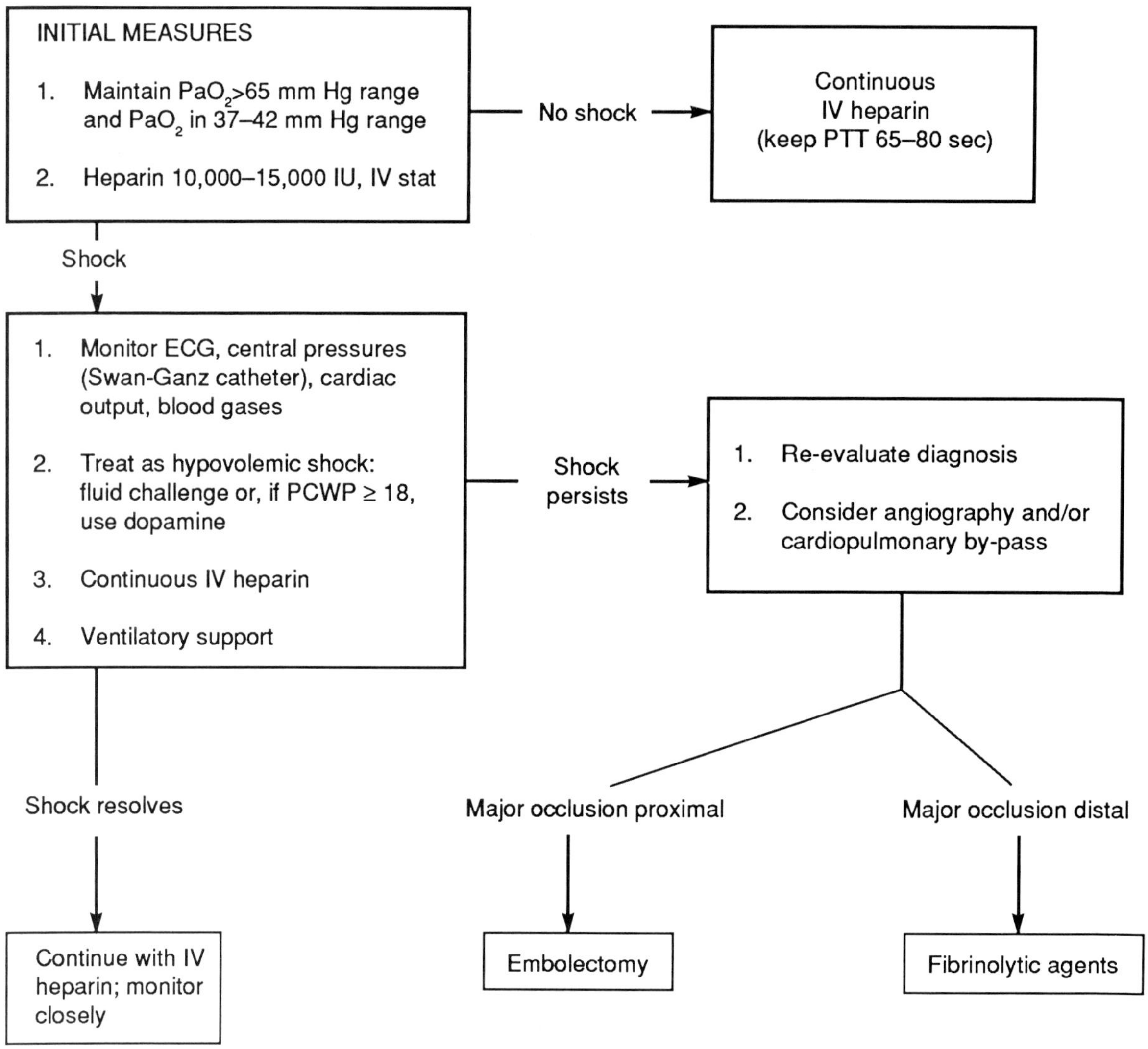

Figure 12.3. Management of pulmonary embolism.

heart, and thereby reduce cardiac output and blood pressure by the Frank-Starling mechanism. Concurrently, the embolic episode may elicit certain reflexes within the pulmonary vasculature that result in systemic peripheral arteriolar vasodilation. This results in relative volume depletion. Hence, a patient in shock following pulmonary embolism should be treated as any other patient in shock (see Chapter 5). Management should include invasive monitoring and, provided that pulmonary edema is not present, consideration of intravascular volume expansion to raise blood pressure. If there is concern about the status of the intravascular volume before the initiation of monitoring, then the blood pressure may be adequately and temporarily supported by means of an inotropic agent, such as dopamine (Fig. 12.3). Because these patients are relatively volume depleted, the use of inotropic agents as definitive therapy for shock may in itself be harmful, in that these agents can increase pulmonary vascular resistance and further augment the cor pulmonale that has been induced by the embolism. The radionuclide ventriculogram (Fig. 12.1) shows the acute hemodynamic imbalance produced by massive pulmonary embolism in causing reduced left ventricular cavity size consequent upon pulmonary hypertension and septal shift. With reduced cavity size a smaller preload is accommodated with high end-diastolic filling pressures. The reduced preload causes hypotension according to the Frank-Starling mechanism.

Maintenance of Oxygenation

The basic principles pertaining to the management of hypoxemia from whatever cause should be followed. If obtundation is associated with either severe hypoxemia or shock, the airway should be protected with intubation to prevent aspiration. Oxygen should be administered either by face mask or by mechanical ventilation if intubation has been necessary. The PaO_2 should be maintained over 65 mm Hg with whatever inspired oxygen concentration is necessary to achieve this level. Positive end-expiratory pressure ventilation usually provides no major benefit in the management of hypoxemia due to pulmonary embolism, unless associated pulmonary edema exists.

Maintenance of Ventilation

The excretion of carbon dioxide is not usually a problem for patients with pulmonary embolism unless the embolus is massive and is associated with severe obtundation. The problem is easily managed by intubation and mechanical ventilation, with appropriate adjustment of the tidal volume and respiratory rate to maintain the $PaCO_2$ between 37 and 42 mm Hg (see Chapter 6).

Prevention of Recurrent Embolization

Anticoagulant Therapy

The major goal of anticoagulant therapy is to prevent further formation of intravascular clots with embolic potential. Heparin has the advantages of having an immediate action and blocking platelet/thrombin interactions on the embolus that may lead to serotonin release with associated bronchospasm and enhancement of hypotension. There is no need to withhold the initiation of heparin infusion pending the completion of diagnostic testing if there are strong clinical grounds to suspect embolism. An initial large intravenous dose of 15,000 units should be followed by a maintenance dosage that will keep the partial thromboplastin time (PTT) to 2–3 times above the baseline level. Two additional advantages of heparin are that it enhances fibrinolytic activity on fresh thrombi and that its anticoagulant effects are promptly reversible if bleeding occurs. The preferred and acceptable modes of heparin administration are summarized in Table 12.1. This therapy should be maintained for a minimum of 8–10 days. After the first week, any pre-existing venous thrombi will be firmly adherent to the vein, and the patient may be allowed to ambulate.

Long-term anticoagulant therapy is indicated in all circumstances where a continuing predisposition to venous thrombosis exists. For this purpose, the coumarin drugs are preferable. Because their action is mediated through altered production of vitamin K-dependent coagulation factors in the liver, the onset of action is not immediate. Therefore, in 2 or 3 days, the patient should receive both coumarin therapy and heparin therapy at a slightly reduced dosage. The prothrombin time is monitored to assess effectiveness of coumarin therapy. When on coumarin therapy, attention must be paid to the interaction of other drugs that alter its effectiveness.

Table 12.1
Heparin Therapy for Pulmonary Embolism

Optimal Treatment
Continuous IV, bolus 10,000–15,000 IU, followed by 1000–1200 IU every hour, as determined by PTT/clotting time
Acceptable Treatment
Intermittent IV, bolus 10,000–15,000 IU, followed by 5,000–6,000 IU q4h, as determined by PTT/clotting time
Not Recommended
Intermittent subcutaneous
Indices to Monitor
Lee-White clotting time and partial thromboplastin time (PIT)
Goal: Two to three times the control level

Table 12.2
Streptokinase Therapy for Pulmonary Embolism

Dosage
250,000 units over 30 minutes followed by 100,000 u/h × 24 hours[a]
Discontinue heparin; normalize PTT before therapy
Monitoring
Initiation of therapy
Platelet count
PT, PTT, thrombin time, fibrinogen level
Four hours after streptokinase is begun: Lytic state achieved if
Thrombin time is increased
PTT is 2 × the control
Fibrinogen is decreased
Fibrinogen degradation products are increased

[a] If lytic state is not achieved, give a second dose of 250,000 units or consider another thrombolytic agent.

Fibrinolytic Therapy

Fibrinolytic therapy may be used to accelerate clot lysis in patients who have had a massive event and when pulmonary hypertension must be relieved promptly. In clinical practice, however, fibrinolytic therapy is currently reserved for patients who have experienced massive pulmonary embolism resulting in systemic hypotension that is not quickly responsive to volume resuscitation or sympathomimetics.

Thrombolysis has been associated with earlier clot resolution, a greater reduction in pulmonary artery pressure, and more improvement in cardiac output than is observed with heparin. There is also evidence that thrombolytic therapy may reduce subsequent alterations in pulmonary diffusing capacity that may be seen after acute embolic episodes. However, there remains a reluctance to administer thrombolytic agents due to the real risk of hemorrhagic complications, which is approximately three times that of heparin therapy.

Streptokinase is an effective fibrinolytic agent that, when used for pulmonary embolus, is given in doses of 250,000 units followed by an infusion of 100,000 u/hr for 24 hours. Therapy should be monitored as outlined in Table 12.2. If heparin has been administered to the patient before the initiation of streptokinase, it must be discontinued and the PTT allowed to normalize before thrombolytic therapy is begun. Likewise, anticoagulants should be withheld for 2–4 hours after streptokinase has been discontinued to minimize the risk of bleeding.

Surgical Therapy

The indications for surgical intervention in pulmonary embolism fall into two categories: procedures for preventing recurrent embolization and surgical embolectomy.

Operations to interrupt the inferior vena cava may be life saving (1) if pulmonary re-embolization continues, despite adequate anticoagulation; (2) if because of previous bleeding problems, anticoagulation is contraindicated; (3) as prophylaxis for a free-floating thombus; and (4) in the presence of septic embolization. Caval interruption carries a substantial morbidity and may not in the long term continue to protect against re-embolization. Interrupting the vena cava with a transvenously inserted umbrella positioned just below the renal veins has been associated with less morbidity than operative intervention.

Pulmonary embolectomy is a salvage procedure that may occasionally be life saving when massive embolization into large vessels has occurred. Because the procedure is associated with at least a 50% mortality, its use is limited to circumstances where severe hemodynamic decompensation has not responded to medical measures and to medical centers where facilities for prompt embolectomy are available. Transvenous catheter embolectomy is a recent innovation that may be useful in selected cases.

Suggested Readings

Biello DR, Matter AG, McKnight RC, Siegel BA: Ventilation-perfusion studies in suspected pulmonary embolism. *AJR* 133:1033–1037, 1979.

Heim CR, Des Prez RM: Pulmonary embolism: a review. *Adv Intern Med* 31:187–212, 1986.

Hyers TM (ed): Symposium on pulmonary embolism and hypertension. *Clin Chest Med* 5:383–554, 1984.

McIntyre KM, Sasahara AA, Sharma GVRK: Pulmonary thromboembolism: current concepts. *Adv Intern Med* 18:199–218, 1972.

Moser KM: Pulmonary thromboembolism. In Petersdorf RG, et al (eds): *Harrison's Principles of Internal Medicine,* ed 10. New York, McGraw-Hill, 1983, pp 1561–1567.

Rubenstein R: Thromboembolism. *Sci Am Med* 18:1–14, 1986.

Sabiston DC: Pathophysiology, diagnosis and management of pulmonary embolism. *Am J Surg* 138:384–391, 1979.

Sharma GVRK, Sasahara AA: Diagnosis and treatment of pulmonary embolism. *Med Clin North Am* 63:239–250, 1979.

Sharma GVRK, Tow DE, Parisi AF, et al: Diagnosis of pulmonary embolism. *Annu Rev Med* 159–166, 1977.

CHAPTER

13 Status Asthmaticus

Nigel A. M.. Paterson, M.B.

Asthma is a common problem, afflicting 4% of the adult population. Each year many asthmatics suffer an acute, severe attack requiring hospital admission, and a few die. Death from asthma in hospital thus reflects therapeutic failure at two levels: failure of prophylactic treatment and failure to treat the acute attack. Clearly an efficient prophylactic program is the ideal goal, not only because it prevents the morbidity and the mortality from acute attacks but also because many fatal attacks of asthma occur suddenly, thereby precluding successful secondary intervention. Nevertheless, even with the most skilled prophylaxis, some patients still develop severe acute attacks. With ideal management, however, the morbidity of such episodes should be minimized, and mortality should approach zero.

PATHOPHYSIOLOGY

Asthma is probably a syndrome, rather than a single disease. The commonly used subdivision of asthmatic patients into extrinsic asthmatics (in whom allergic mechanisms can be identified) and intrinsic asthmatics (in whom such mechanisms are not apparent) is an acknowledgment of the different mechanisms involved in asthma. A majority of patients present with clinical features of both types of asthma. Furthermore, the precipitant(s) of the acute attack often do not conform to the categorization of the patient's type of asthma; a common example is the young atopic asthmatic whose acute attack is precipitated by a viral respiratory infection. Nevertheless, several pathogenetic effector mechanisms have been identified, and an understanding of these mechanisms permits more astute management of the attack (Table 13.1).

Because these mechanisms make variable contributions to the acute attack, the pathologic consequences are also varied. Widespread narrowing of airways is a prerequisite finding, but there is wide variation in its predominant site (central versus peripheral) and the cause of the narrowing. In very severe asthma, several processes may evolve simultaneously so that the most florid pathologic findings are more predictable. There are two general findings. First, the lungs are massively overinflated and at autopsy may remain distended for several hours after their removal from the thoracic cavity. Second, the cause of the narrowing of both central and peripheral airways is not only smooth muscle constriction with or without hypertrophy but also mucosal swelling (basement membrane thickening, neutrophilic and eosinophilic infiltrate, and edema) and intraluminal debris (cells, inspissated mucus, exuded serum proteins). The intraluminal plugs may totally occlude the airway and are often extremely tenacious, resisting removal even with forceps at autopsy.

Table 13.1
Pathogenesis of Asthma

Mechanism	Effects	Therapeutic intervention
Mediator release	1. Bronchospasm: histamine, leukotrienes, prostaglandins 2. Airway inflammation: ECF-A, NCF-A, PAF 3. Mucociliary stasis: leukotrienes, eosinophil major basic protein, oxygen species 4. Airway edema and erythema: histamine, prostaglandins, leukotrienes, PAF	1. Inhibit mediator release: DSCG, β-agonists, theophylline (steroids) 2. Antagonize end-organ responses: antihistamines (not clinically useful), leukotriene, and PAF antagonists (experimental) 3. Treat inflammation: steroids
Bronchomotor reflexes	Increased cholinergic efferent traffic: bronchospasm, mucus hypersecretion	1. Reduce afferent traffic: eliminate pollutants, irritants, infectious agents, etc. 2. Efferent (muscarinic) blockage: ipraptropium bromide
β-Blockade	Decreased effect of endogenous and exogenous β-agonists: bronchospasm	1. Avoid β-blockers 2. Restore β-responsiveness with steroids
Smooth muscle hypertrophy	Increased response to a given stimulus	Bronchodilators

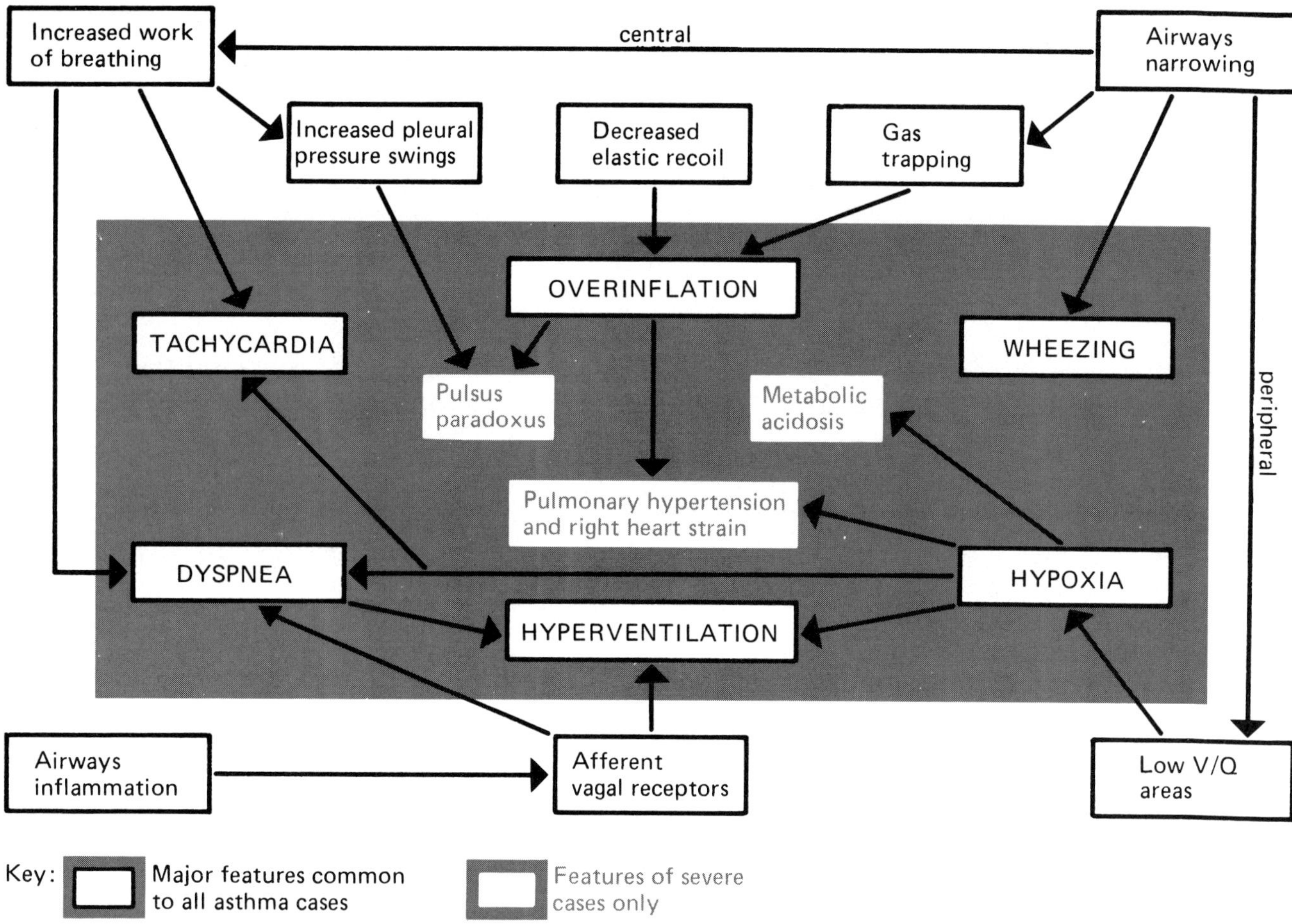

Figure 13.1. Pathophysiology of asthma.

The pathophysiologic consequences of these pathologic events are summarized in Figure 13.1. The principal features are (1) hypoxemia (↓ PaO_2—arterial oxygen tension) due to areas with low ventilation/perfusion ratios; (2) hyperventilation (↓ $PaCo_2$—arterial carbon dioxide tension, ↑ pH) due to peripheral stimuli (airway irritant receptors, increased work of breathing) with or without hypoxia; (3) increased airways resistance, indicated by decreased expiratory flows, e.g., forced expiratory volume in 1 second ($FEV_{1.0}$) or peak expiratory flow rate (PEFR); (4) overinflation—increased total lung capacity and functional residual capacity; and (5) gas trapping—increased residual volume, reduced vital capacity. Most of these features can readily be assessed by the history, physical examination, and simple laboratory tests, and thus it is possible to construct a reasonably accurate picture of what is occurring in the lungs.

ASSESSMENT

The assessment of the patient with an acute attack of wheezing is directed toward three questions:

1. *Is this an attack of asthma?* The diagnosis of acute asthma is usually clear-cut. In the patient who has a personal and/or family history of allergies, a history of recurrent wheezing, previous relief with bronchodilators, and a plausible precipitating cause for the current episode, and who exhibits the physical findings outlined below, there is little doubt that asthma is the cause. Sometimes, however, the diagnosis is less clear-cut, and the clinician must always be conscious of the venerable dictum: all that wheezes is not asthma. Table 13.2 outlines some other conditions that can present with wheezy dyspnea.

Of these diagnoses, perhaps the most difficult to rule out is a greater or lesser component of chronic airflow limitation. The presence of chronic airflow limitation should be suspected in an older smoker who has had a long-standing productive cough and exertional dyspnea and whose dyspnea is not conspicuously wheezy. On auscultation of such a patient, the dominant finding is usually a generalized reduction in the intensity of breath sounds with or without wheezes. Clinical or laboratory evidence of pre-existing right-heart dysfunction or specific radiologic evidence of emphysema (vascular attenuation, bullae) should strengthen one's suspicion of airflow limitation. At first glance, the value of establishing a greater or lesser component of irreversible obstructive disease may not be apparent, because bronchodilators and steroids may be administered in any event. However, recognition of chronic airflow limitation should modify one's therapeutic expectations. More importantly, sev-

Table 13.2
Differential Diagnosis of Asthma

Condition	Diagnostic clues: Symptoms	Diagnostic clues: Signs	Diagnostic clues: Lab data	Further evaluation
Pulmonary embolus	Predisposing cause, pleuritic pain, hemoptysis, precipitous onset	Leg swelling, pleural rub, consolidation, right-heart strain, hypotension	X-ray: oligemia, infiltrate, Hampton's hump ECG: right-heart strain	Lung scan and/or pulmonary angiogram
Acute left ventricular failure	Orthopnea, edema, PND, angina, frothy expectoration	Gallop rhythm, basal crackles, dependent edema	X-ray: cardiomegaly, pulmonary edema ECG: ± ischemia	Response to diuretics, hemodynamic monitoring
Acute exacerbation of chronic obstructive pulmonary disease	Older, smoker, chronic cough, less variation in dyspnea, recent sputum purulence, no well-defined trigger	↓ Breath sounds without much wheezing, signs of chronic cor pulmonale	X-ray: signs of bronchitis and/or emphysema Gases: acute-on-chronic hypoventilation ECG: chronic right-sided strain with hypertrophy Blood: polycythemia	Nil definitive
Upper airway obstruction (e.g., epiglottitis, angioedema, laryngeal edema, tracheal stenosis, tumor, tracheomalacia, goiter)	Inspiratory dyspnea ± whoop, history suggests anaphylaxis, previous intubation, symptoms of thyroid dysfunction, etc.	Inspiratory prolongation and/or stridor	X-ray: central airway lesion Gases: usually normal	CT of upper airway, flow volume loops, including inspiration, direct inspection (laryngoscopy and/or bronchoscopy)
Localized obstruction (e.g., tumor, broncholith, foreign body, etc.)	Postural variation in wheeze	Localized wheeze and/or postural change	X-ray: localized volume loss	CT Bronchoscopy
Pulmonary aspiration	Rapid dyspnea, predisposing cause	± Consolidation: as well as wheeze	X-ray: infiltrates Gases: profound hypoxemia	Acute: aspiration of swallowed marker Recurrent: esophageal motility, etc.

eral aspects of the management of acute asthma—notably, oxygen supplementation, fluid balance, and the use of assisted ventilation—should be reconsidered if there is a major irreversible component.

For the other conditions, presentation as acute asthma is atypical, but it is important to rule out these conditions by the further tests outlined in Table 13.2.

2. *What precipitated the attack?* Although the trigger(s) of the acute attack may often be difficult to identify, there are two reasons for asking this question. First, a knowledge of the trigger and the duration of exposure allows an educated guess about the subsequent course of the attack, e.g., exposure to an acute trigger, such as cold air, may be rapidly reversible, whereas a prompt response is less likely if the trigger is a persistent respiratory infection of 2 weeks' duration. Second, the trigger may not have been removed—this applies particularly to drug-induced and infectious asthma. The mechanism of drug-induced asthma is not necessarily allergic: for example, a nonallergic mechanism accounts for aspirin-induced asthma, which is being increasingly recognized in adult nonatopic asthmatics, and exclusion of nonsteroidal analgesic intake requires a careful documentation of both prescription and proprietary medications.

3. *How severe is the the attack?* In general, most of the clinical assessment of the acute asthmatic should be directed toward answering this question. Table 13.3 outlines the parameters that are useful in assessing the severity of asthma.

History

Often an indication of the likely severity of the attack can be gleaned from the patient's track record. Features that warn of a possible severe attack include previous severe attacks, a requirement for steroids, or failure of previously adequate therapy.

Physical Examination

As indicated in Table 13.3, a careful physical examination can provide an accurate indication of the severity of asthma, provided that valid parameters are used. As a rough guide, if the patient can respond in sentences, the attack is mild; if dyspnea has reduced the patient to monosyllables, the attack is moderate; and if the patient is too breathless to talk, the attack is severe. Patients with severe asthma are often sweaty and unable to lie flat. Some signs may be misleading: extreme dyspnea and anxiety may be present in an otherwise mild attack, and the loudness and pitch of wheezing, although roughly correlated with the level of obstruction, may also create

Table 13.3
Assessment of Acute Asthma

Examination/test	Severity of asthma			
	Mild	Moderate	Severe	Very severe
Clinical				
Speech	Sentences	Words	Nil	—
Heart rate (/min)	<100	90–130	>110	>130
Pulsus paradoxus (mm Hg)	0–10	5–20	10–40	>20
Accessory muscles	±	+	+ +	+ + + +
Breath sounds	N	N	N or ↓	↓ ↓
Wheezes	+/+ +	+ +/+ + +	+ + +/+	+/0
Blood pressure	N	N or ↑	N or ↑	↑, N or ↓
Cyanosis	—	—	—	+
Respiratory muscle fatigue	—	—	—	+
Impaired consciousness	—	—	—	+
Laboratory				
Blood gases				
PaO_2 (mm Hg)	>70	55–70	45–55	<45
$PaCO_2$ (mm Hg)	35–45	30–35	25–55	>55
HCO_3 (mEq/liter)	24	22–24	20–24	<20
pH	7.35–7.45	7.45–7.55	7.30–7.55	<7.30
Forced expiration				
FEV_1 (l)	1.5–3.5	0.8–2.0	<1.0	<0.5
FVC (l)	3.0–5.0	2.0–4.0	0.8–2.0	<1.0
PEFR (l/min)	>200	100–200	50–100	<50
Chest x-ray				
Overinflation	+	+ +	+ + +	+ + + +
Extrapulmonary air	−	−	±	±
ECG: Right-sided strain	−	−	±	+

an erroneous impression if viewed in isolation, as can be seen from Table 13.3.

On the other hand, bona fide use of accessory muscles, as assessed by inspiratory fixation of the sternocleidomastoid muscle with lifting of the clavicle (usually accompanied by supraclavicular indrawing) suggests a severe attack, provided that a clear distinction is drawn between it and simple hyperventilation without excessive work of breathing. A second valuable sign is the sphygmomanometric detection of pulsus paradoxus, i.e., accentuation of the normal inspiratory fall in systolic pressure. A drop of greater than 10 mm Hg is abnormal and usually indicates an attack of at least moderate severity. Third, although there are clearly a multitude of reasons for tachycardia (anxiety, sympathetic activity, medications, infection), a pronounced tachycardia (e.g., >130 beats/min) usually denotes a severe attack and correlates inversely with SaO_2 (arterial oxygen saturation).

Finally there are some signs that indicate impending disaster and demand immediate intervention. Obvious exhaustion, clinical evidence of respiratory muscle fatigue (abdominal paradox, respiratory alternans), hypoxia (altered level of consciousness usually with restlessness, sweating, pallor), hypotension, and cyanosis usually denote very severe asthma that may soon, if not immediately, require assisted ventilation. Similarly, the ominous "silent chest" or clinically apparent extrapulmonary air indicates that the situation is precarious.

Laboratory Evaluation

A typical routine for the laboratory evaluation of asthma is listed in Table 13.4. Of these tests, only the arterial blood gases and chest x-ray are essential although expiratory flows should be obtained whenever possible.

In mild asthma, the arterial blood gases are often within the normal range or simply indicate acute (± on-chronic) hyperventilation (↑ $PaCO_2$, ↑ pH). With increasing severity, hypoxemia becomes increasingly prominent (Table 13.3). With very severe attacks, the $PaCO_2$ may paradoxically revert to normal levels; however, this reversion should not be construed as a favorable finding because the normal $PaCO_2$, in fact, is an inappropriate response to the ongoing respiratory stimuli (airway irritation, increased work of breathing, hypoxemia). Finally, in very severe asthma, hypercapnia may supervene—an ominous sign—and acidosis with both respiratory (hypercap-

Table 13.4
Laboratory Evaluation of Acute Asthma

Blood gases
Chest x-ray
Expiratory flows (spirometry, peak flow meter, etc.)
ECG
Hemoglobin, hematocrit, white cell count and differential, eosinophil count
Electrolytes, blood sugar level, BUN, creatine
Serum theophylline level
Sputum smear for Gram stain and culture

nia) and metabolic (lactate, etc.) components may be seen. Often the chest x-ray is not useful, although overinflation is usually present in severe cases and such complications as pneumothorax, pneumomediastinum, mucoid impaction with atelectasis, and pneumonia may occasionally be confirmed by the x-ray. A simple measurement of expiratory air flow (spirometry or peak flows) is very useful (representative interpretations are listed in Table 13.3) in mild-moderate asthma, but impractical if the asthma is severe because the patient will be too breathless to perform a forced expiratory maneuver.

The other tests are useful but not essential. The ECG may show right-sided strain; the hemoglobin, hematocrit, BUN (blood urea nitrogen), creatinine, and electrolytes are used to manage hydration; the sputum examination and white cell count are used to evaluate infection; and the blood sugar level forms a baseline for monitoring drug side effects (see discussion of β-adrenergic agonists).

If there is any suggestion of abnormal liver function it should be evaluated because abnormalities critically influence theophylline clearance (see section on theophylline derivatives). A baseline serum theophylline level should be obtained if the patient has recently received a theophylline compound.

Overall Evaluation

Finally, the clinician arrives at an overall assessment of the severity of the attack based on the criteria outlined in Table 13.3 and decides on an appropriate intensity of management. If the attack is mild, the patient can be treated in the office or emergency department and, if a suitable response is obtained and there is no recurrence, sent home. A moderate attack (by the criteria in Table 13.3) requires hospital admission, and a severe attack is best handled by monitoring in an intensive care setting, with or without assisted ventilation. If the attack is very severe, the patient must be treated urgently and intensively, and ventilatory assistance will almost certainly be required (see discussion of assisted ventilation).

TREATMENT

The basic components of the therapy of acute asthma are oxygenation, hydration, bronchodilators, steroids, and (if necessary) ventilatory support.

Oxygenation

It is important to correct hypoxemia in the acute asthmatic patient, with the therapeutic aim being a $PaO_2 > 65$ mm Hg. This can usually be achieved with a Ventimask that delivers an inspired oxygen fraction (FiO_2) of 0.24, 0.28, or 0.35, but occasionally a higher FiO_2 is required. There are two reasons for correcting even mild hypoxemia.

In the acute asthmatic, a $PaO_2 < 60$ mm Hg may be associated with clinical hypoxia (i.e., impaired function of a vital organ, such as the brain) because of insufficient oxygen delivery. There are three possible reasons for this association. First, the asthmatic often has a respiratory alkalosis (↓ $PaCO_2$, ↑ pH) that, by shifting the oxygen-hemoglobin dissociation curve to the left, decreases the unloading of oxygen in the tissue. Second, hypocapnia causes cerebral vasoconstriction, thereby decreasing the oxygen delivery to the brain. Third, in contrast to the patient with chronic airflow limitation, the asthmatic has not usually been chronically exposed to hypoxemia and therefore is not protected by adaptive mechanisms, such as raised 2,3-diphosphoglycerate levels, polycythemia, etc. Hence, the asthmatic may develop symptoms of cerebral hypoxia even with a PaO_2 of 45–55 mm Hg, which is often seen in ambulatory outpatients with chronic obstructive pulmonary disease.

The second reason is that hypoxia probably predisposes the patient to dangerous cardiac arrhythmias, and such a mechanism may be operative in asthmatics who die suddenly before reaching hospital. Furthermore, it is likely that any arrhythmogenic potential of the bronchodilators (β-agonists and theophylline derivatives) is enhanced in the presence of hypoxia. Some bronchodilators—notably nonselective β-agonists, such as isoprenaline—cause a fall in PaO_2, probably by abolishing compensatory vasoconstriction in areas with hypoventilation, thereby increasing the $\dot{V}/\dot{Q}$ mismatch in these areas. Thus in the severe asthmatic, adequate supplemental oxygen should be started immediately, without waiting for the results of arterial blood gases, both to treat symptomatic hypoxia and to minimize the risk of side effects from bronchodilator administration. Clearly this treatment presupposes an accurate diagnosis, because liberal administration of oxygen to the patient with chronic airflow limitation carries the risk of profound hypoventilation by removal of hypoxic drive.

Method

1. Draw blood gases.
2. Begin oxygen at FiO_2 of 0.28 or higher, depending on clinical severity.
3. Repeat blood gases in 15 minutes.

Hydration and Tracheobronchial Toilet

The patient with acute asthma has often been too breathless to eat or drink for many hours, and water losses have been increased by hyperventilation. Furthermore, as discussed in the pathophysiology section, the basic pathologic process leads to the accumulation of inspissated tenacious plugs of intraluminal debris. Hence, it is of paramount importance to ensure adequate hydration and to prevent further airway drying by humidifying the inspired air. On the other hand, hypotonic mists should not be used because they induce bronchospasm in asthmatics. Mucolytics and expectorants are generally considered of little use in acute asthma, and some, notably acetylcysteine, may actually aggravate the brochospasm. In some centers, bronchoscopy and airway lavage have been performed in an attempt to remove the luminal plugs—this therapy is sometimes effective, but carries the risk of provoking additional bronchospasm or further compromising gas exchange. Hence, most centers have concluded that, in general, the risks of lavage outweigh the possible benefits.

Method

1. Replenish fluids, orally if tolerated, or by IV, e.g., 4.3% dextrose/0.3 normal saline plus 20 mEq/liter KCl, 1–2 liters over 2 hours then 150 ml/hr.
2. Humidify inspired gas.
3. Do not use mucolytics, expectorants, or antitussives.
4. Bronchoscopic lavage is generally not indicated.

Bronchodilators

Bronchodilators are the mainstay of treatment of acute asthma. Although anticholinergic agents, such as ipratropium bromide, are beginning to be evaluated, the bronchodilators currently in general clinical use fall into one of two categories: β-adrenergic agonists or theophylline derivatives. For mild asthma, a single agent may be employed, e.g., a β-agonist if the patient has been taking an oral theophylline preparation, or vice versa. In moderate or severe asthma a representative drug from each class should be used in combination (Table 13.5) because the two types of drugs act on different receptors, leading to additional bronchodilation when they are used together.

β-Adrenergic Agonists

A bewildering variety of β-adrenergic agonists are commercially available. Those commonly used include ephedrine (contained in Tedral, etc.), isoprenaline (Isuprel), adrenaline, orciprenaline (Alupent), terbutaline (Bricanyl), fenoterol (Berotec), and salbutamol (Ventolin). These drugs are formulated as pills, metered dose inhalers, solutions for nebulization, and solutions for parenteral administration. The choice of a particular agent and the route of its administration is thus somewhat arbitrary. Several of the newer agents, such as fenoterol, terbutaline, and salbutamol, offer the dual advantage of a selective β-2 effect (which means less cardiac stimulation and probably less predisposition to arrhythmia) and a more prolonged duration of action (due to resistance to catechol-*o*-methyltransferase).

The route of administration is subject to debate. Most agree that metered dose inhalers should be confined to mild attacks and that the delivery of an aerosol by an IPPB apparatus offers no advantage over a simple nebulizer circuit. However, for severe cases it is not clear whether a nebulized aerosol or parenteral administration is preferable. On the one hand, nebulized aerosol maximizes local drug concentrations while minimizing the dose to the rest of the body (although some of the aerosol is deposited in the mouth and absorbed). On the other hand, the airways may be almost totally occluded in very severe cases, and aerosol delivery via a ventilator circuit is uncertain, thereby warranting parenteral administration despite the systemic side effects. The following method takes into account these considerations.

Method

1. Do not use metered dose inhalers, except in mild cases.
2. Correct hypoxemia before using β-agonists.
3. In moderate asthma, use nebulized salbutamol (0.5% solution), 0.5 ml (2.5 mg) in 2 ml saline and repeat in 1 hour as required, then once every 4 hours (q4h).
4. In severe asthma, use nebulized salbutamol (0.5%), 1 ml/2 ml saline, and repeat in 1 hour as required. After initial use of salbutamol, continue with nebulized salbutamol q3h–q4h. In severe cases, particularly those in which assisted ventilation is necessary, a reasonable alternative is to use intravenous salbutamol (5 to 15 μg/min as a continuous infusion).
5. Particularly if using IV salbutamol, watch for, and correct hyperglycemia or hypokalemia.

Theophylline Derivatives

With theophylline derivatives the choice is far simpler. In mild cases, any of the oral preparations can be used, and if intravenous access is a problem, a rectal retention enema (but not suppositories, which are erratically absorbed) can be used. However, in most circumstances intravenous aminophylline is the best choice. Unfortunately, the simplicity of the routine use of intravenous aminophylline is more than counterbalanced by the subtleties in its clinical pharmacology. Clinically, the most important step is an estimate of liver function, because

Table 13.5
Drug Therapy of Acute Asthma

Severity of attack	β-Agonist	Theophylline derivative	Steroid
Mild	Salbutamol, 0.5% solution (nebulize 0.5 ml/2 ml saline)	*Or* aminophylline 6 mg/kg IV over 20 min	—
Moderate	Salbutamol as above and continue q4h	Aminophylline as above and continue IV 0.6 mg/kg/hr	± Prednisone 15–40 mg PO, bid.
Severe	Salbutamol, 0.5% solution, 1 ml/2 ml saline × 1–2 and continue q2h-q3h or IV salbutamol (5–15 μg/min)	As for moderate	Hydrocortisone (or equivalent) 5 mg/kg IV and continue 3 mg/kg IV q4h
Very severe	As for severe, plus bicarbonate if pH <7.25	As for moderate	Methylprednisolone 0.5–1.0 gm IV and continue 2 mg/kg IV q6h

85% of the theophylline clearance is by hepatic metabolism (and indeed anephric patients have near-normal clearance). The therapeutic goal is to generate serum levels required for useful bronchodilation (10–20 μg/ml). The problem, however, is the small toxic-therapeutic ratio, as indicated by the serum levels potentially associated with side effects: >15 μg/ml→gastrointestinal upset and minor CNS effects, >40 μg/ml→life-threatening side effects, such as cardiac arrhythmia, convulsions, and coma. Aminophylline is partly bound to serum albumin, and in the presence of hypoalbuminemia the effect of a given drug level is increased and the drug is cleared more rapidly. Finally even in apparently normal individuals there is about a fivefold variation in clearance. In acute severe asthma, there is almost always a reduced clearance due to right ventricular strain leading to hepatic congestion, but clearance may rapidly improve as the asthma is corrected, requiring an increased dose of aminophylline to maintain therapeutic levels. Hence, serum theophylline levels should be done frequently to optimize aminophylline dosage.

Method

1. Loading dose: aminophylline 6 mg/kg, IV, in 250 ml 5% dextrose/0.2 normal saline, run in over 20 minutes. If previous oral therapy: draw theophylline level before loading; halve dose if erratic or subtherapeutic oral therapy, and omit loading dose if adequate oral dosage.
2. Maintenance dose: aminophylline 0.2–1.2 mg/kg/hr (average adult dose 0.6 mg/kg/hr). Calculate maintenance dose on basis of ideal weight. Use higher dose for children (0.7–1.1 mg/kg/hr); lower for elderly (0.4–0.6 mg/kg/hr). Reduce if there is right-heart strain (0.3–0.5 mg/kg/hr). Drastically reduce dose if there is overt liver disease (0.1–0.3 mg/kg/hr). Use serum levels to guide therapy.

Steroids

Steroid administration is mandatory in all cases of severe acute asthma, and one of the commonest clinical errors is belated and inadequate steroid dosage. The fact that direct effects of steroids are usually not seen for at least 2–3 hours and peak much later (6–10 hours) is not a logical reason for delaying their administration. In addition, however, one action of steroids—the potentiation of β-agonist-induced bronchoconstriction—is rapid and may be clinically relevant, particularly in the situation of partial β-blockade caused by inhaler abuse. Additional benefits of using high-dose steroid regimens (e.g., methylprednisolone 0.5 gm IV q12h), rather than medium-dose regimens, have not yet been established. If high-dose regimens are employed, the risks can be minimized by prompt reduction of dosage if a response is achieved.

Assisted Ventilation

If the patient with acute asthma receives appropriate therapy promptly, there should rarely be a need for intubation and assisted ventilation. Further, because intubation with assisted ventilation often stimulates additional reflex bronchoconstriction, bypasses several mechanical lines of defense against lung infection, and carries its own risks (barotrauma, cardiac impairment, renal impairment), it should only be used when necessary. Nevertheless, in the severe attack this intervention may be required to save the patient's life. Although common indications for ventilation are summarized in Table 13.6, a decision to ventilate should be based on the overall clinical picture. Thus the patient who is obviously exhausted may need ventilation even if the arterial blood gases are near normal, whereas if the patient is improving by other criteria but has mild hypercapnia, it may be reasonable to defer ventilation, provided that very close observation in a critical care setting is continued. If ventilation is required, a volume-cycled ventilator is preferred, using a relatively slow respiratory rate to circumvent the greatly increased viscous resistance imposed by the patient's narrowed airways.

After the patient is intubated and ventilated, it is reasonable to provide sedation (e.g., diazepam 5–10 mg IV prn) to allow the patient to relax and recover. If the patient is initially hypercapneic the $PaCO_2$ should be reduced gradually. Paralysis with pancuronium bromide should only occasionally be necessary, and rarely, halothane anesthesia has been used in patients in whom ventilation is difficult, even with a volume-cycled respirator. Weaning from ventilatory support is not usually a problem because when the asthma improves it is usually quite clear that support is no longer needed.

Method

1. Use guidelines outlined in Table 13.6.
2. Use a volume-cycled respirator.
3. Use fully humidified gas mixture with an FiO_2 sufficient to maintain $PaO_2 > 60$ mm Hg.
4. Set at slow rate (e.g., 10–12/min) with tidal volume 10–15 ml/kg. Avoid high peak inspiratory pressures, e.g., >60 cm water. Use sedation to permit relaxation once ventilatory support is established.

Miscellaneous

In addition to the above methods, adjunctive modalities of treatment are sometimes indicated. An antibiotic with an appropriate antimicrobial spectrum (e.g., ampicillin, erythromycin, tetracycline) should be used if there is evidence of infection, remembering that there is often a mild leukocytosis due to stress and steroids and that sputum purulence may reflect the acute inflammation of asthma and not necessarily a bacterial infection. Sodium bicarbonate may be required to correct severe metabolic aci-

Table 13.6
Indications for Ventilation

1. Clinical hypoxia unresponsive to increased FiO_2
2. Decreasing ventilation (rising $PaCO_2$, or single $PaCO_2 > 60$ mm Hg)
3. Exhaustion, including respiratory muscle fatigue
4. Extrapulmonary air, if severe

dosis, particularly because β-adrenergic responses may be blunted in acid conditions. However, the primary treatment of respiratory acidosis is to improve ventilation, and bicarbonate administration is properly viewed as a very temporary adjunct that should not deflect the clinician from definitive therapy.

Sedation is mentioned only to be dismissed: although sedation may benefit a mild asthmatic with considerable anxiety, there is a considerable risk of masking a dangerous deterioration and each year some deaths from asthma occur that can at least partly be attributed to injudicious use of sedatives. Hence, the safest policy is to use sedatives for acute asthma only if ventilatory support is already established. Finally, it should be mentioned that several drugs that may be useful for prophylaxis, (e.g., aerosol steroids, disodium cromoglycate (DSCG), antihistamines) are not useful in the treatment of acute asthma.

Method

1. Use antibiotics if there is clinical evidence of infection.
2. Use sodium bicarbonate 50–100 mEq as a temporary measure if $pH < 7.25$.
3. Never use sedatives.
4. Do not use aerosol steroids, DSCG, or antihistamines.

CONCLUSIONS

The mortality from acute asthma should approach zero. This goal can be achieved if the patient is quickly but carefully assessed, monitored closely (it may be necessary, for example, to obtain blood gases as often as every 10–15 minutes), and treated aggressively and appropriately. In general, it is better to err on the side of more intensive management in terms of monitoring, drug therapy, and anxillary measures, such as assisted ventilation. Having treated the acute severe asthmatic attack successfully, the clinician and the patient must examine together the reasons for the failure of the asthma prophylaxis and adjust the prophylactic treatment program to prevent a recurrence of this primary treatment failure.

Suggested Readings

Leffert F: The management of acute severe asthma. *J Pediatr* 96:1, 1980.

McFadden ER Jr: Clinical physiologic correlates in asthma. *J Allergy Clin Immunol* 77:1, 1986.

Rebuck AJ, Read J: Assessment and management of severe asthma. *Am J Med* 51:788, 1972.

Saunders NA: Recognition and management of severe asthma. *Sem Resp Med* 3:251, 1982.

Van Arsdel PP Jr, Paul GH: Drug therapy in the management of asthma. *Ann Intern Med* 87:78, 1977.

RENAL, FLUIDS & ELECTROLYTES

CHAPTER

14 Acute Renal Failure: Management

Adam L. Linton, M.D.

Acute renal failure (ARF) is a condition fraught with difficulties concerning definition, diagnosis, management, specific treatment, and prognosis. It is, therefore, appropriate to begin with a simple definition that is broad enough to encompass all possible conditions to be considered in the differential diagnosis. ARF is defined as a temporary (and usually reversible) failure of the kidneys to excrete the waste products of metabolism. This broad definition obviously includes some nonrenal causes of uremia, such as hypovolemia, but expanding the definition is justified by the convenience of having a single term to embrace all acute causes of uremia. With this definition a preliminary diagnosis of ARF can therefore be applied to all cases where there is oliguria accompanied by a rise in blood urea nitrogen (BUN) and serum creatinine from whatever cause. Indeed, in a number of cases even oliguria is not a prerequisite—so-called nonoliguric ARF.

MORTALITY

In the critically ill patient oliguria and uremia are very commonly observed, and it is from that starting point that the diagnostic procedures are taken. This group of patients includes those with acute renal failure due to reversible intrinsic renal disease—the condition that used to be called tubular necrosis, but is now perhaps better called acute reversible intrinsic renal failure or vasomotor nephropathy. There is little doubt that this condition still carries a very high mortality, despite all of the modern improvements in resuscitation, nutrition, and surgical and dialysis techniques. Mortality rates in various published reports continue to fluctuate around 50% overall (Table 14.1), which is almost exactly Swann and Merrill's figure in an early series from Boston 1947–1953.

Comparison of individual series is hampered somewhat by differences in diagnostic criteria, type of patient population, and methods of expressing results, but confirmation of the continuing high mortality can be found in studies of relatively homogeneous groups of combat casualties. Mortality from posttraumatic ARF in World War II was 90%; with the availability of dialysis, the mortality fell to around 65% in Korea. Despite significant improvements in resuscitation and evacuation procedures, overall mortality in patients developing ARF in Vietnam remained around 65% from 1966–1970. It seems almost certain that the apparent failure to reduce mortality is due to counteracting effects of improved resuscitation and evacuation techniques—rapid resuscitation probably prevents ARF in the less severely injured, whereas rapid evacuation probably allows more of the severely injured to survive long enough to develop ARF. Similar considerations are likely relevant to mortality from ARF seen in civilian practice. In addition, simple and uncomplicated ARF from obstetric catastrophes now very seldom occurs, whereas ARF from multiple injuries and generalized sepsis and complicated by hepatic failure and cardiac failure is much more common.

Table 14.1
Mortality Rates in Acute Renal Failure

Series	Dates	Mortality (%)
Swann and Merrill	1947–53	50
Lunding	1955–62	58
Kirkland	1957–64	58
Kennedy	1960–70	44 (35–50)
Stott	1969–71	57
Kleinknecht	1966–70	34
Eliahou	1965–66	65

It is obvious, therefore, that the onset of ARF in the critically ill patient places him or her in a group with very high mortality, despite the fact that such patients seldom die simply of uremia now that dialysis treatment is readily available. Nevertheless, it is likely that uremia with all its complications may often contribute to the eventual outcome. It is possible also that, with the increased number of potent drugs available for use in the critically ill patient, iatrogenic renal damage is becoming more common, particularly as a result of the administration of diuretics and antibiotics.

PATHOPHYSIOLOGY

According to the definition given, acute renal failure is diagnosed in three major groups of patients: (1) those having prerenal uremia due to hypovolemia (which may be absolute or functional, as in shock); (2) those having obstruction of the urinary tract (postrenal uremia); and (3) those having acute reversible intrinsic renal disease or vasomotor nephropathy (Table 14.2). The pathophysiology of the first two groups is relatively simple. Dehydration, hypovolemia, and shock all result in a marked

Table 14.2
Categorization of Acute Renal Failure

Type of ARF	Cause
Hypovolemia (prerenal uremia)	↓ Renal perfusion → oliguria
Obstruction (postrenal uremia)	Obstruction → ↑ hydrostatic pressure in glomeruli
Vasomotor nephropathy (intrinsic renal disease), including some cases that are nonoliguric	Preglomerular vasoconstriction, glomerular capillary damage, necrosis of tubular cells

reduction in renal perfusion, which in turn leads to oliguria and a progressive increase in BUN and creatinine. The kidneys in this condition remain normal, and the principal problem rests in differential diagnosis. In obstructive uropathy, obstruction of the urinary passages leads to increased hydrostatic pressure in the glomeruli opposing filtration, and again, uremia results. At least in the early stages the kidneys are not irreversibly damaged, and identification of the problem followed by relief of the obstruction will result in restoration of function.

The principal renal cause of acute renal failure—vasomotor nephropathy—is a relatively common complication in the critically ill, and despite many years of investigation the pathophysiology of this condition has not yet been elucidated. In most of the situations in which vasomotor nephropathy occurs, "shock" has occurred at least temporarily. However, vasomotor nephropathy is often also complicated by tissue damage, acidosis, poor tissue perfusion, and the administration of potentially nephrotoxic drugs. It is not possible here to discuss the mass of conflicting evidence relating to the precise pathophysiology of vasomotor nephropathy. Two major points of view have emerged, one emphasizing necrosis of tubular cells (and/or back diffusion of filtrate) and the other, preglomerular vasoconstriction as the principal cause of the renal failure. Because histologic tubular necrosis is not a prominent feature of vasomotor nephropathy in humans, attention has been focused on the vascular hypothesis.

The fact that the condition almost always presents with oliguria, despite convincing evidence of continuing renal blood flow, defied explanation for some time, because reduction of renal blood flow in chronic renal failure is normally accompanied by a diuresis. Some change in glomerular dynamics, therefore, had to be postulated. It has been shown that glomerular filtration rate can virtually stop, despite continuing renal blood flow, when there is vasoconstriction of the afferent arteriole to the glomerulus (Fig. 14.1). This hypothesis is not yet proven, and it may be that vasomotor nephropathy in humans is not a homogeneous condition, but is rather one in which vasoconstriction, tubular damage, and even direct damage to glomerular capillaries all participate to a variable degree.

DIAGNOSIS

When a patient develops oliguria and uremia the physician is immediately faced with a primary differential diagnosis between prerenal uremia (hypovolemia), intrinsic renal damage (vasomotor nephropathy), and postrenal uremia (obstruction). The first step in the early diagnosis of ARF is, therefore, to be aware of situations in which it is likely to occur. Careful monitoring of fluid status and urine volume is required in all seriously ill patients, as well as serial measurements of electrolytes, BUN, and creatinine. The first sign of impending ARF is usually oliguria, which has been variously defined as a urine volume less than 720 ml/day to a urine volume of less than 400 ml/day. In critically ill patients it is probably better to record hourly urine volumes and to define oliguria as a urine output of less than 30 ml/hour. Doing so allows early recognition that a problem exists, and although this criterion suggested for a diagnosis of oliguria will in-

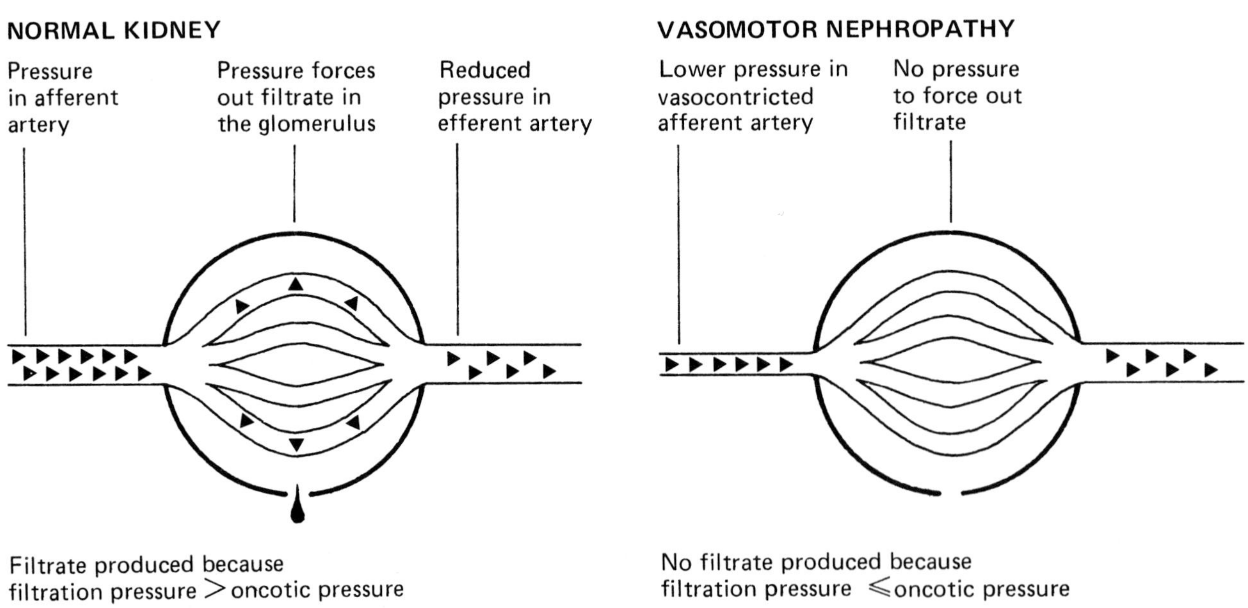

Figure 14.1. Preglomerular vasoconstriction in vasomotor nephropathy.

clude many patients who have nothing other than minor drops in perfusion pressure (which is rapidly reversible), it will activate other diagnostic measures quickly and promote rapid treatment. Routine monitoring of the critically ill often includes collection of urine for 2- to 4-hour periods for estimation of creatinine clearance and urinary indices.

At this point the history should be comprehensively reviewed with particular reference to recent surgery, trauma, blood pressure, previous renal disease, and drugs being administered. Physical examination should concentrate on the state of hydration (edema, neck veins, presence or absence of postural drop in blood pressure, external genitalia, bladder, rectal and vaginal examination). Following these simple guidelines often identifies simple problems that can readily be missed after a formal diagnosis of ARF is made.

Once the development of oliguria and uremia is established, the possibility that the patient has urinary tract obstruction should be actively considered in every case. This is particularly important if oliguria progresses to total anuria. Clues may be found from the history or the physical examination, but if any doubt exists as to the patency of the urinary tracts then further investigation must be undertaken. Ultrasound examination of the kidneys or retrograde pyelograms are required and should not be too long delayed. Further investigation and management of obstructive uropathy when found consist essentially of relief or bypassing of the obstruction and are not within the scope of this text.

Once the obstruction has been ruled out, the primary diagnostic problem in unexplained oliguria and uremia is whether the patient has prerenal ARF as a result of hypotension and hypovolemia or whether he or she has an intrinsic renal cause of ARF. The further diagnostic steps and their interpretation are outlined in the diagram on management (Fig. 14.2). Patients with ARF usually have complicated and severe illnesses, and the normal indices of dehydration, such as hemoglobin levels, are frequently unreliable. The demonstration that, in face of oliguria and a rising BUN, urinary concentrating power is maintained (as evidenced by urine osmolality in excess of 500 mOsm/liter) is a strong indication that there is no intrinsic renal damage. Further evidence that the kidneys are behaving appropriately is obtained from low urine sodium levels (less than 10 mEq/liter); this value shows that the kidneys can still retain sodium in response to volume contraction. In the oliguric patient, therefore, high urine osmolality and low urine sodium indicate that the ARF is due to hypovolemia, so rapid fluid replacement can safely be undertaken (see Chapter 5).

In contrast, the presence of isomolar urine and plasma in the oliguric patient indicates the presence of renal damage, which is confirmed if the urinary sodium excretion is high (usually greater than 50 mEq/liter). Renal damage may be due to pre-existing chronic renal disease, but is most commonly due in this situation to the onset of vasomotor nephropathy (acute tubular necrosis). Nevertheless, the possibility of pre-existing chronic renal disease should be considered and is often suggested if a flat plate of the abdomen or an IVP reveals the presence

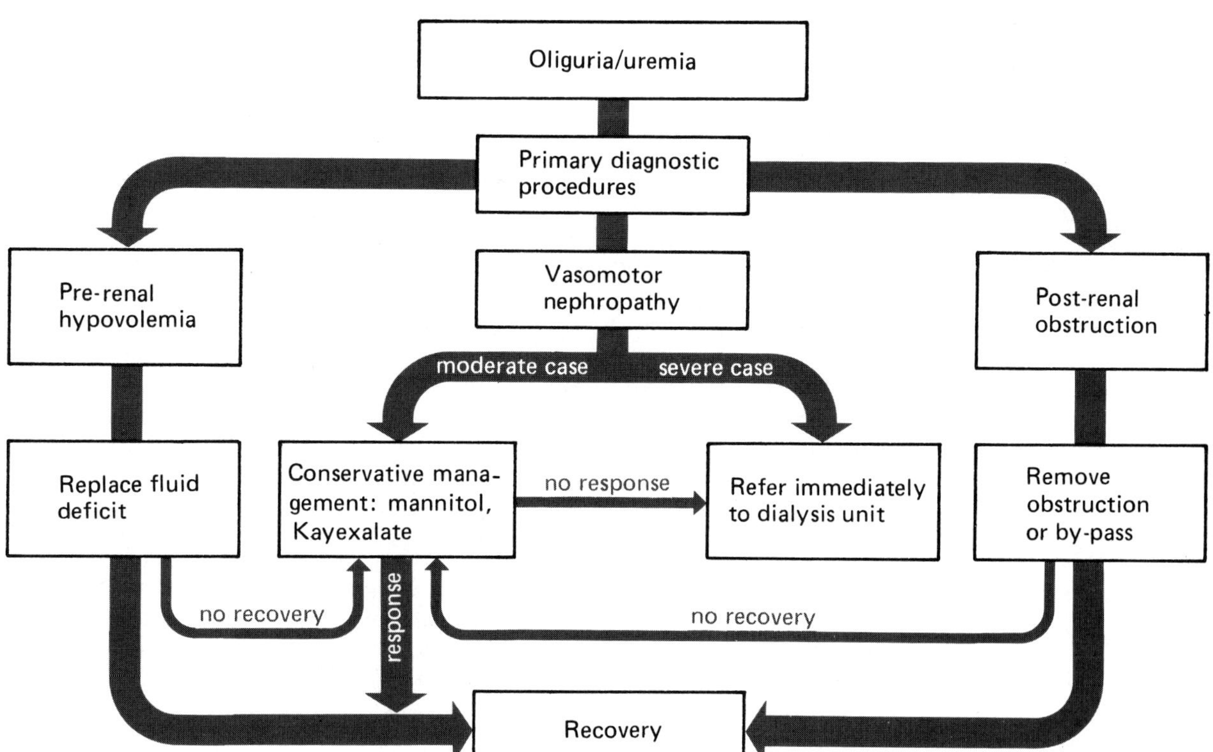

Figure 14.2. Management of acute renal failure.

of small or scarred kidneys. Acute glomerular disease, such as glomerulonephritis, may also mimic vasomotor nephropathy, but this diagnosis is suggested by the finding of red blood cells and red blood cell casts in the urinary sediment. Further elucidation of these two conditions depends upon renal biopsy.

The distinction between prerenal oliguria and vasomotor nephropathy is, therefore, usually made by the simple measurement of urine and serum osmolality and determination of urine sodium. In some patients, however, these values may be borderline or even misleading, particularly in complicated situations in which organs other than the kidney are impaired or when various drugs have been given. In the complex case, therefore, many attempts have been made to develop more reliable criteria. These have, in the main, consisted of mathematical functions derived from the basic measurements of urine and plasma osmolalities, urine sodium, and urine and plasma creatinine values. They have added little in terms of accuracy of diagnosis, probably because the reliability of the basic data is not altered. Additional measures may, therefore, have to be taken to ensure that the physician is not missing a fluid deficit that might, if restored, result in recovery of renal function. They usually involve monitoring of the pulmonary capillary wedge pressure with a Swan-Ganz catheter and measurement of cardiac output before and after a fluid challenge.

The condition of nonoliguric renal failure also presents a diagnostic problem. Oliguria is usually considered a cardinal sign of ARF and is part of the broad definition given earlier. Nevertheless, the existence of patients with reversible renal damage in the presence of continuing high urine volumes is recognized and indeed may account for up to 30% of all cases of ARF due to renal causes. The definition of this type of ARF is simply the occurrence of transient, reversible renal impairment in the absence of oliguria or evidence of the other conditions already discussed. The urinary diagnostic indices (osmolality and sodium), which are the cornerstone of the diagnosis of ARF, fall in the gray area between the values found in oliguric ARF due to vasomotor nephropathy and the values that would be taken to indicate the presence of prerenal uremia. Antibiotic nephrotoxicity or renal damage due to anesthetic agents seems to be the commonest causes of nonoliguric ARF. It is likely that nonoliguric ARF is simply a milder variant of vasomotor nephropathy, and it carries the same implications for management as full-blown oliguric vasomotor nephropathy. Patients who exhibit this type of renal impairment must be very carefully monitored, because they may progress rapidly to oliguric ARF.

TREATMENT

Treatment of ARF obviously depends on the primary diagnosis, which must be clearly established as early as possible.

Once identified, oliguria and uremia due to hypovolemia and reduced perfusion readily respond to replacement of the deficit. In individual patients the deficit may be of blood, plasma, saline, or simply water; rapid replacement is safe provided the diagnosis is established, and the vast majority of the patients will respond with an increased urine output and reduction in uremia. It should be remembered, however, that hypovolemia and hyperperfusion can themselves progress to intrinsic renal damage and vasomotor nephropathy. If a response is not obtained, the diagnosis should be reviewed.

If the preliminary investigations reveal obstruction of the urinary tract, then removal or bypassing of this obstruction will again, in virtually all cases, result in remission of oliguria and uremia. Occasionally, however, particularly if the obstruction has been of prolonged duration, intrinsic renal damage may have been produced. Such patients may also develop vasomotor nephropathy that will maintain the oliguria after relief of the obstruction.

Because the development of vasomotor nephropathy (acute tubular necrosis) in a critially ill patient indicates a very poor prognosis, it is appropriate to consider management of these patients at all stages beginning before the onset of the condition. However, prevention of vasomotor nephropathy is very difficult because of the varying and complex causative factors of the condition. The situation is compounded by the fact that the pathophysiology remains uncertain.

PREVENTION

Avoidance

Perhaps the best method of prevention currently available is avoidance. It is possible that a significant number of cases of ARF develop either because of failure to observe proper precautions or as a result of the administration of known nephrotoxic agents. In the area of treatment of trauma and shock there is now ample evidence to indicate that rapid and complete replacement of fluids, electrolytes, or blood as indicated will significantly reduce the incidence of vasomotor nephropathy. The fact that many cases of renal failure are iatrogenic and follow the administration of nephrotoxic drugs is not well enough known. In particular, drugs that should be used only with care include the nephrotoxic antibiotics, particularly the aminoglycosides. Iodinated contrast media are perhaps the second most common cause of drug-induced renal failure, and radiologic examinations utilizing these materials should be done only if urgently indicated and only after the patient has been adequately rehydrated. The abuse of potent diuretics is another common cause of temporary reduction in renal function, sometimes purely because of volume contraction, but occasionally resulting from potassium depletion or an allergic nephritis induced by furosemide or hydrochlorothiazide. Finally, nonsteroidal anti-inflammatory agents produce acute deterioration in renal function, most often in the elderly or in patients with pre-existing renal impairment.

Prophylaxis

Prophylaxis is the second element of prevention. In a patient scheduled for any of the major surgical procedures that are known to be associated with a high incidence of postoperative renal failure (e.g., major aortic surgery or operations on the gall bladder and bile ducts), valid evidence suggests that preoperative sodium loading has a prophylactic effect in preventing subsequent renal damage. There is no doubt that preoperative dehydration is still often practiced when a patient has oral fluids stopped before surgery; intravenous fluids must be started at this point.

Early Diagnosis

The third aspect of prevention relates to the possibility of reversing the early stages of ARF once its onset is recognized. In the critically ill patient it is mandatory to establish as quickly as possible the volume and electrolyte status of the patient. If vasomotor nephropathy is detected early, clinical and experimental evidence suggests that the administration of mannitol may sometimes abort the development of full-fledged renal failure. This remains a controversial point because there has never been a well-controlled trial, but certainly the administration of 100 ml of 20% mannitol and the observation of its effect on urine volume are worthwhile in the first 48 hours. Many other drugs have been tried in an attempt to correct the abnormalities in renal blood supply that characterize the early phases of vasomotor nephropathy. In the main, these drugs have been given because of their theoretical effect in reversing the preglomerular vasoconstriction that is thought to be one of the major factors in the development of the condition; for example, dopamine has been shown to increase renal cortical blood flow and glomerular filtration rate, but its use has been disappointing in ARF. Perhaps the most commonly used drug in this situation is furosemide, which is commonly given to anyone with reduction in urine volume. There is absolutely no evidence to support its use in this situation, and indeed it is likely that renal damage may be made more severe by ill-considered administration of this drug.

VASOMOTOR NEPHROPATHY

Conservative Therapy

The conservative management of patients with vasomotor nephropathy is undergoing considerable change. Conservative therapy can still be utilized temporarily and is aimed at maintaining the patient in as good condition as possible for as long as possible in order to delay the need for dialysis. Management consists largely of restricting intake to prevent accumulation of fluid or toxic substances for as long as possible. The principles of the regimen are as follows:

1. Water/fluid intake restricted to approximately 600 ml/day plus a volume equal to the previous day's urine output and additions for any excess losses from vomiting or sweating;
2. Protein intake reduced to approximately 20 gm daily, which in the uncomplicated patient is enough to prevent significant catabolism, but delays the accumulation of toxic products of protein metabolism;
3. Reduction of potassium in the diet to the lowest possible level to prevent hyperkalemia;
4. When hyperkalemia does ensue, it can be temporarily reduced with the use of insulin or sodium bicarbonate. On a longer-term basis, the potassium may often be held below 6 mEq/liter with the daily administration of 15–45 gm of sodium polystyrene sulfonate (Kayexalate), which is a cation-exchange resin exchanging sodium for potassium in the gut.

Recent Advances

In the past few years there has been a significant change in orientation with regard to management, particularly in the critically ill patient. It is increasingly recognized that these patients require adequate nutrition if they are to survive their underlying illness or injury; adequate nutrition has been made possible with the ready availability of frequent dialysis. In the majority of patients with renal failure, therefore, conservative management now consists of attempts to provide at least the essential amino acids in adequate amounts from the outset. Studies have suggested that oral or intravenous feeding that provides these amino acids improves nitrogen balance and produces symptomatic relief in uremic patients. Furthermore, the provision of sufficient calories to meet the metabolic expenditure spares endogenous protein with further benefit. The overall orientation of the management of vasomotor nephropathy has changed toward emphasis on continued feeding, even though this may mean an earlier requirement for dialysis.

A suggested plan for the management of patients developing oliguria and uremia is discussed in the section on treatment. Once the primary diagnosis has been established, those patients with prerenal uremia can readily be managed in any hospital with the facilities to administer blood and other intravenous fluids. If a diagnosis of obstructive uropathy is made, then the patient must be managed with the assistance of either a urologist or a general surgeon. If the patient seems to have developed vasomotor nephropathy, standard conservative measures can be implemented temporarily and the effects of mannitol assessed. In some cases these measures are effective in reversing the oliguria, and in others the oliguria remits spontaneously after a relatively short period. Nevertheless, the majority of these patients will have to be referred to a center with dialysis facilities, and this decision should not be too long delayed. Absolute indications for urgent transfer include fluid overload (which cannot of course be reversed in the patient with renal impairment without dialysis), serum potassium level over 6 mEq/liter despite the use of exchange resins, continuing hypotension, evidence of cardiac or hepatic damage, and the presence of severe underlying illness or injury. If in doubt, refer the patient to an intensive care renal unit, rather than delay.

Once the patient has been transferred to an ICU, dialysis may be required for variable periods of time. If fluid balance is the major problem, a new technique—continuous arteriovenous hemofiltration (CAVH)—is now available. This procedure uses a device that continuously filters water out of the blood, which is circulating through it from an arteriovenous shunt. It enables the patient to receive large amounts of intravenous feeding without becoming overloaded with fluid. CAVH, however, does not remove the need for repeated dialysis treatments.

Suggested Readings

Anderson RJ, Linas SL, Berns AS et al: Nonoliguric acute renal failure. *N Engl J Med* 296:1134–1137, 1977.

Bartlett RH, Mault JR, Dechert RE, Palmer J, Swartz RD, Port FK: Continuous arteriovenous hemofiltration: improved survival in surgical acute renal failure. *Surgery* 100:400–408, 1986.

Corwin HL, Bonventre JV: Acute renal Failure. *Med Clin North Am* 70:1037–1054, 1986.

Cronin RE: Drug therapy in the management of acute renal failure. *Am J Med Sci* 292:112–119, 1986.

Dixon BS, Anderson RJ: Nonoliguric acute renal failure. *Am J Kidney Dis* 6:71–80, 1985.

Golper TA: Continuous arteriovenous hemofiltration in acute renal failure. *Am J Kidney Dis* 6:373–386, 1985.

Levinsky NG: Pathophysiology of acute renal failure. *N Engl J Med* 296:1453–1458, 1977.

Linton AL: Acute renal failure. *Can Med Assoc J* 110:949–952, 1974.

Myers BD, Moran SM: Hemodynamically mediated acute renal failure. *N Engl J Med* 314:97–105, 1986.

Oken DE: Local mechanisms of the pathogenesis of acute renal failure. *Kidney Int* 10:94–99, 1976.

CHAPTER

15 Drug Dosage in Renal Failure

William F. Clark, M.D., and J. David Spence, M.D.

In patients with renal failure, conventional dosage schedules of drugs that are ordinarily eliminated by the kidneys often require alteration in order to avoid toxicity due to accumulation of the drug or metabolite of the drug. Pharmacokinetic principles are useful in establishing guidelines for dose adjustment in such patients. It should be understood that such guidelines are subordinate to the aphorism, "Treat the patient, not the numbers."

As soon as the drug enters the body its elimination begins, either by excretion and/or metabolism. The volume in which the drug is distributed can be likened to a leaky bucket where the level of fluid is constantly maintained by input from a water tap (Fig. 15.1).

The concentration of the drug is always halved in the same unit of time as long as the peaks (processes of elimination) are constant. This chapter considers only adjustment of drug therapy in patients with assumed normal hepatic and impaired renal function. Most important are drugs with a narrow therapeutic index that have the renal route as the major route of elimination from the body.

The management goal of physicians using drugs is usually to achieve a steady-state plasma concentration without toxic peaks or subtherapeutic troughs. Drugs are usually given at regular intervals that reflect the elimination half-life. A steady-state or plateau condition, at which the rate of drug elimination equals the rate of drug administration, is achieved for all drugs after four to five half-lives (Fig. 15.2).

For drugs with predominant renal excretion, the prolongation of the elimination half-life is proportional to the degree of renal impairment. Thus, if the drug is given at the same dose and interval in a patient with a 50% decrement in renal function there will be an approximate doubling of the half-life, with a consequent lengthening of the time required to achieve the steady state plasma concentration, which will be much higher than the desired level. If doses are reduced proportionally and administered as a maintenance dose, an undue delay may occur in achievement of therapeutic drug levels. Therefore, a loading dose may be required, particularly where drug effect is needed immediately, such as with antibiotics or antiarrhythmics. Because renal failure mainly affects drug elimination, the usual loading dose can be given in most cases of patients with renal impairment. Thus, the loading dose offsets the delay in time required to achieve a steady state concentration. However, maintenance doses will have to be reduced or dosing intervals lengthened to prevent the toxic peaks that would occur.

This chapter discusses three methods of dose adjustment in patients with renal impairment for drugs with a

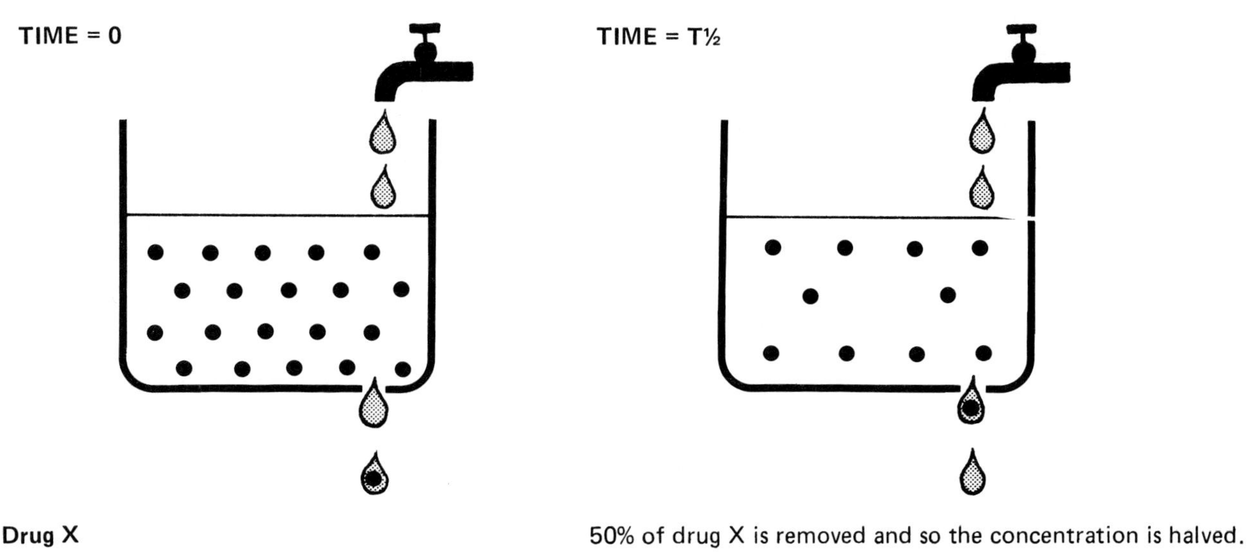

Figure 15.1. The law of first-order kinetics. If the leaks are constant and the bucket size is unchanged, then the time taken to halve any concentration is constant (T½). Leaks = renal excretion + thepatic metabolism; bucket size = volume of distribution.

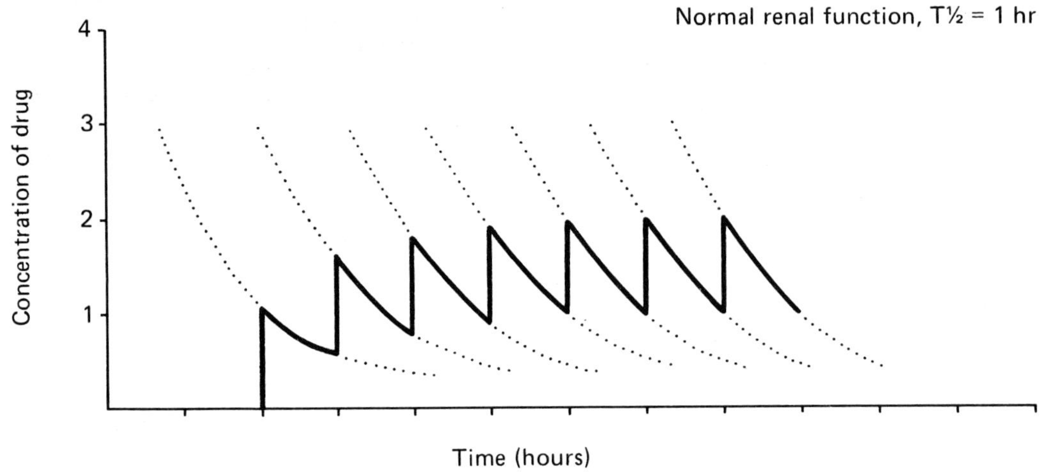

Figure 15.2. Steady state or plateau concentration. In normal renal function, T½ = 1 hour.

narrow therapeutic margin that are largely excreted by the kidney: (1) lengthening the dosing interval while administering the normal or recommended maintenance dose; (2) decreasing the dose, leaving the interval unchanged; or (3) decreasing the dose and lengthening the dosing interval. By lengthening the dosing interval proportionate to the decrement in renal function, the average plateau concentration will be achieved, with greater oscillations between peak and trough levels than if the dose is reduced and given at the usual intervals. The latter method, however, produces more constant blood levels. The choice of which method to use is controversial in most cases. However, because aminoglycoside toxicity relates to the trough rather than peak levels, a combination of interval and dose alteration may be preferable for this group of drugs.

For patients with renal impairment, two guidelines are provided for alteration of doses of drugs largely excreted by the kidney: (1) provide a loading dose to offset the delay in achievement of therapeutic levels (because of prolongation of half-life) and (2) provide maintenance doses in proportion to the decrement in renal function by changes in dosing interval, dose, or a combination of these alterations. An accurate assessment of renal function is necessary in order to calculate the appropriate dose adjustment.

Creatinine clearance corresponds to drug half-life, not only for aminoglycosides that are predominantly filtered but also for penicillins that are excreted by the tubules. In patients with unstable renal function the only accurate method is a 24-hour urine assessment for creatinine clearance (Cr_{c1}). However, this method does not permit dose adjustment over the first 24–36 hours. It is suggested that a creatinine clearance of <0.16 ml/second be assumed in the patient with unstable renal function who has developed isomolar oliguria (acute renal failure). In patients with stable chronic renal failure or in older age groups, there are several formulas for determining creatinine clearance from serum creatinine measurements. The formula of Cockcroft and Gault is both simple and accurate for estimating creatinine clearance in patients with stable chronic renal impairment:

$$\text{Male } Cr_{cl} \text{ (mL/sec)} = \frac{(140 - \text{age}) \times \text{weight in kg}}{50 \times \text{Cr (uM/liter)}}$$

$$\text{Female } Cr_{cl} = \text{Male } Cr_{cl} \times 85\%$$

Having obtained an accurate assessment of renal function, we can express this as a fraction of normal, the lower limit being 1.3 mL/sec.

Example

A 68-year-old 50-kg woman with a creatinine of 177 μM/L requires digoxin therapy.

Loading Dose

It is not affected by renal impairment, except in end-stage renal disease where the loading dose should be reduced by 50%; 0.01 mg/kg body weight in first 24 hours. Therefore, for a 50-kg female, loading dose of digoxin = $50 \times 0.01 = 0.5$ mg.

Maintenance Dose:

$$Cr_{CL} = \frac{[(140 - \text{age}) \times \text{weight (kg)}]}{50 \times \text{Scr (uM/liter)}} \times 85\%$$

$$= \frac{(140-68) \times 50 \text{ kg}}{50 \text{ (177 uM/liter)}} \times 85\%$$

$$= 0.35 \text{ ml/sec}$$

Therefore, approximate remaining renal function is

$$\frac{0.35 \text{ ml/sec}}{1.3 \text{ ml/sec}} \approx \tfrac{1}{4} \text{ of normal}$$

Thus, the dosing adjustment factor is ¼ times the usual maintenance dose (MD):

$$MD = 0.25 \text{ mg} \times \tfrac{1}{4} = 0.0625 \text{ mg q24h, or } 0.125 \text{ mg q48h.}$$

Having provided a loading and a maintenance dose relative to the decrement in renal function, blood levels should be measured, where possible, for drugs with a narrow therapeutic index to avoid serious over- or underdosage.

The timing of the levels around a given dose is dependent on the drug, the method of administration, and the dosage form employed. Generally, however, peak serum levels are drawn 30 minutes to 1 hour after an intravenous dose, and trough levels should be measured just before the next dose. For drugs with altered binding to plasma proteins in uremia (e.g., phenytoin), therapeutic levels may be much lower than in normals.

Tables 15.1–15.5 list drugs commonly used in a critical care trauma unit setting. These groups are subdivided into drugs mainly excreted by the kidney versus those with less than 30% renal elimination that require no dose adjustment in patients with renal impairment. Drug toxicity and, where appropriate, loading doses are given in the tables.

TOXICITY

Potential toxicity should not interfere with the choice of the best available drug in a patient with renal insufficiency. However, for drugs of equal efficacy, it is prudent to select the one with the least toxicity (at the required dosage). Table 15.1 suggests the avoidance of cephaloridine, urinary antiseptics, and tetracyclines (except doxycycline). The reason for general avoidance of the urinary antiseptics in patients with either acute or chronic stable renal impairment is that no therapeutic effect will be achieved by these agents in patients with reduced glomerular filtration rate (GFR), because these drugs require an adequate filtration rate to act as urinary antiseptics. Furthermore, nitrofurantoin and its metabolites are neurotoxic and can result in a peripheral neuropathy, particularly in patients with renal impairment. Cephaloridine should be avoided in patients with renal insufficiency because it has dose-dependent nephrotoxicity with a narrow therapeutic margin, unlike many other cephalosporins. The tetracyclines (except for doxycycline) are to be avoided in patients with renal impairment because they have been associated with both reversible and irreversible renal failure. Their antianabolic action (except for doxycycline) results in an increased plasma urea that causes an osmotic diuresis with subsequent further compromise of renal perfusion in patients with renal impairment. In addition, at high levels there is a direct tubular toxicity that interferes with the action of antidiuretic hormone and a subsequent loss of the ability to concentrate the urine. Therefore, the use of cephaloridine, nitrofurantoin, other urinary antiseptics, and tetracyclines (except for doxycycline) are not recommended when treating patients with impaired renal function.

Several of the drugs, in particular the aminoglycosides, have narrow therapeutic margins and a reported high incidence of nephrotoxicity. This high incidence is often attributed to inappropriate doses in patients with impaired renal function, but it may also reflect the heightened toxicity of combination antimicrobial therapy. Although combinations of antimicrobials in patients with sepsis are more frequently associated with nephrotoxicity, combinations of drugs are often given in the treatment of septicemia of undetermined etiology in order to increase the likelihood of success. The institution of specific antimicrobial therapy and the discontinuance of combination therapy, as soon as blood cultures have identified the appropriate organism, will not only result in decreased nephrotoxicity but will also reduce the risk of superinfection.

Table 15.1
Antimicrobial Agents

<30% renal elimination—no change in renal failure	
Cefoperazone	Chloramphenicol
Erythromycin	Amphotericin B
Clindamycin	Rifampin

<50% renal elimination

Drug	Loading dose	Toxicity
Penicillins	Usual first dose	Platelet and CNS dysfunction
Cephalosporins (except cefoperazone)	Usual first dose	Renal: avoid cephaloridine
Aminoglyclosides[a,b]		
Gentamicin	1.5 mg/kg	Vestibulo-ototoxic Nephrotoxic Neuromuscular blockage
Tobramycin	1.5 mg/kg	
Amikacin	7.5 mg/kg	
Kanamycin	7.5 mg/kg	
Streptomycin	10–15 mg/kg	
Tetracyclines	Avoid (except doxycyline)	Nephrotoxic
Urinary antiseptics		
Methenamine	Avoid	Nitrofurantoin—nephrotoxic
Nitrofurantoin	Avoid	
Nalidixic acid	Avoid	
Sulfonamides	Usual first dose	Nephrotoxic
Vancomycin[a]	Adults: 500 mg Children: 44 mg/kg	Ototoxic and nephrotoxic
Isoniazid	5 mg/kg	CNS dysfunction in slow acetylators
Metronidazole	Usual first dose	Seizures, vestibular toxicity
Acylovir	Usual first dose (in end-stage renal disease, decrease loading dose to 37% of normal)	Renal failure

[a] Narrow therapeutic level: monitor serum level.
[b] Concurrent penicillins may result in subtherapeutic levels of some aminoglycosides.

SUMMARY

The management of drug dosage in renal failure follows five steps.

1. Recognition of the agents that have a narrow therapeutic margin and are largely excreted by the kidney;
2. Provision of a loading dose for the patient with renal impairment, either acute or chronic, to overcome the lag time to achieve therapeutic concentration;
3. Alteration of the dose, interval, or a combination of both relative to the decrement in renal function;
4. Determination of an accurate assessment of renal function

Table 15.2
Cardiovascular Drugs

< 30% renal elimination—no change in renal failure		
Lidocaine Minoxidil Theophylline	Labetalol Verapamil Nifedipine	Diltiazem Quinidine Prazosin Nitroglycerin (renal blood flow may drop if mean arterial pressure is decreased excessively)

> 50% renal elimination		
Drug	**Loading dose**	**Toxicity**
Bretylium	Usual first dose	Hypotension
Hydralazine	Usual small initial doses, according to effect	Headaches, flushing, tachycardia, ↑ myocardial O_2 consumption, SLE[a] syndrome
Methyldopa	No change	Drowsiness, postural hypotension, hepatotoxicity, hemolytic anemia, drug fever
Procainamide (*N*-acetyl PA[a,b] accumulation)	No change	Hypotension, conduction defects, prolonged QT, QRS, and P-R intervals; SLE syndrome
Diazoxide	Use smaller doses (e.g., 50 mg repeated as needed)	Hypotension, fluid retention, diabetes
Propranolol (4-OH metabolite accumulation)	No change	Bronchospasm, bradycardia, congestive heart failure
Nadolol	No change	(As for propranolol)
Sodium nitroprusside (thiocyanate accumulation)	Usual small initial doses, titrate by effect	Thiocyanate-metabolite may accumulate, producing seizures and coma. Monitor thiocyanate level to keep <1.7 mM/liter. Cyanide poisoning may occur, impairing cytochrome pathways causing acidosis, hypotension
Digoxin[b]	0.01 mg/kg (usual) Decrease dose by 50% in ESRD[a]	Nausea, fatigue, arrhythmias, hallucinations, confusion. Radioimmunoassay may overestimate serum levels in ESRD

[a] The abbreviations used are SLE, systemic lupus erythematosus; PA, pulmonary-arterial pressure; ESRD end stage renal disease
[b] Narrow therapeutic margin—monitor serum level.

Table 15.3
Anticonvulsants

<30% renal elimination—no dose adjustment in renal failure

Phenytoin (but therapeutic level 11–20 μM/liter (normal therapeutic range 40–80 μM/liter) because of ↓ binding)

Valproic acid

Note: phenytoin clearance is increased because the unbound drug is metabolized by the liver; half-life of phenytoin is reduced to one-third of normal; therefore, although the therapeutic level is lower in uremia, the dose required is not lower and may even increase.

>50% renal elimination		
Drug	**Loading dose**	**Toxicity**
Diazepam (active metabolites)	No change	Respiratory depression, ↓ level of consciousness.
Phenobarbital	No change	Ataxia, nystagmus, drowsiness, ↓ level of consciousness, respiratory depression.

Table 15.4
Analgesics

<30% renal elimination—no change in renal failure		
	Fentanyl Acetaminophen Morphine Codeine	
	>50% renal excretion	
Drug	**Loading dose**	**Toxicity**
Aspirin[a] (at high doses)	No change	Tinnitus, hyperventilation, acidosis, pulmonary edema, bleeding
Meperidine (metabolites)	Avoid use	Respiratory depression, CNS dysfunction. Active metabolite accumulates to cause seizures.

[a] Narrow therapeutic margin—monitor serum level.

a. In stable renal failure by using the formulas for serum creatinine or a 24-hour creatinine clearance measurement,

b. In the patient with acute renal failure with iso-osmolar oliguria, by assuming a creatinine clearance of <0.16 ml/sec;

5. Measurement of peak and trough levels of agents with a narrow therapeutic index.

Table 15.5
Neuromuscular Blocking Agents

<30% renal elimination—no change in renal failure
Atracurium Vecuronium
>50% renal elimination
Pancuronium

Suggested Readings

Anderson RJ, Gambertaglio JG, Schrier RW: *Clinical Use of Drugs in Renal Failure*. Springfield, IL, Charles C Thomas, 1976.

Bennet WM: *Drugs and Renal Disease*, ed 2. New York, Churchill Livingstone, 1986, pp 26–66.

Bochner F, Carruthers G, Kampmann J, Steiner J: *Handbook of Clinical Pharmacology*. Boston, Little, Brown, 1978.

Cockroft DW, Gault MH: Prediction of creatinine clearance from serum creatinine. *Nephron* 16:31–41, 1976.

Knober JE, Anderson PO: *Handbook of Clinical Drug Data*, ed 5. Illinois, Hamilton Press, 1983.

Reiderberg MM: *Renal Function and Drug Action*. Toronto, LB Saunders, 1971.

Bennett WM: Approach to drug use in the azotemic patient. In Schrier RW: *Manual of Nephrology: Diagnosis and Therapy*. Boston, Little, Brown, 1981, pp 185–200.

CHAPTER

16 Electrolyte Disturbances

Adam L. Linton, M.D.

Fluid, electrolyte, and acid-base homeostasis disturbances are common problems facing the practicing physician and are encountered in almost all specialties. The understanding of the pathophysiology of these abnormalities, the recognition of their clinical manifestations and laboratory findings, and the ability to manage them appropriately are of critical importance. Because in many cases the symptoms of electrolyte disturbance are vague, the diagnosis depends upon the awareness that electrolyte abnormalities may occur in a variety of situations. The vast majority of these conditions are reversible with simple treatment, and failure to recognize them may lead to an unnecessary catastrophe.

SODIUM AND WATER BALANCE

Pathophysiology

The concentration of serum sodium is regulated within a narrow range, and levels below 134 mEq/liter or above 150 mEq/liter define hyponatremic or hypernatremic states, respectively. Serum sodium concentration is determined by the external balance of water; the intake of water is adjusted by the variations in the thirst mechanism, unless the patient is unable to ingest water. The excretion of water, on the other hand, depends upon release of antidiuretic hormone (ADH) by the hypothalamo-hypophyseal system and an intact intrarenal mechanism that is capable of responding to the hormone. A simplified scheme of the control of water and sodium status is shown in Figure 16.1.

A reduction in extracellular fluid volume for any reason activates two mechanisms that operate to restore extracellular volume:

1. Loss of water from the extracellular fluid results in a slight increase in the serum osmolality, which then activates the thirst mechanism. This of course promotes the ingestion of water, provided that it is available. Slight increases in serum osmolality simultaneously stimulate the production of ADH, probably both directly and via a reduction in left atrial pressure. This results in increased free water reabsorption from the distal tubular fluid, thereby preventing further undesirable loss.
2. Reduction in extracellular fluid volume also slightly reduces the glomerular filtration rate, which stimulates the production of renin. Renin then produces angiotensin, which, in turn, stimulates the production of aldosterone. One of the actions of aldosterone is to stimulate sodium reabsorption in the tubules, which will also serve to restore extracellular fluid volume.

In addition to the basic factors described above that operate in the control of water and sodium status, many other factors operate directly on sodium excretion. These include an increase in arterial pressure, which increases sodium loss in the kidney, whereas an increase in venous pressure reduces sodium loss. These factors are both important in the retention of sodium that occurs in congestive cardiac failure when the arterial pressure is reduced and the venous pressure is raised. Stimulation of the sympathetic nervous system decreases sodium loss as do increases in colloid osmotic pressure of the plasma. The precise role of renin and the still mysterious "third factor" in control of sodium excretion is not clearly defined.

Dehydration/Hypernatremia

Causes

Elevation in the serum sodium level over 150 mEq/liter constitutes hypernatremia and is usually due to the effect of water loss, not to sodium excess. It should be noted that few electrolyte disturbances involve just the electrolytes. Hypernatremia is most commonly observed in conditions where both sodium and water have been lost to the body, but the water loss has been quantitatively greater. The dehydration/hypernatremia syndrome is often the result of water deficit, either due to excess loss or lack of intake. Reduction of water in the extracellular fluid produces a rise in serum osmolality. This in turn draws water from the intracellular space and stimulates ADH with a consequent reduction in urine volume. The common causes of dehydration/hypernatremia are listed in Table 16.1.

Table 16.1
Causes of Dehydration/Hypernatremia

Failure of water intake (elderly, infants, postoperative)
Chronic renal failure
Diabetes mellitus
Sweating
Gastrointestinal losses
Acute renal failure (recovery phase)
Diabetes insipidus (central, nephrogenic)

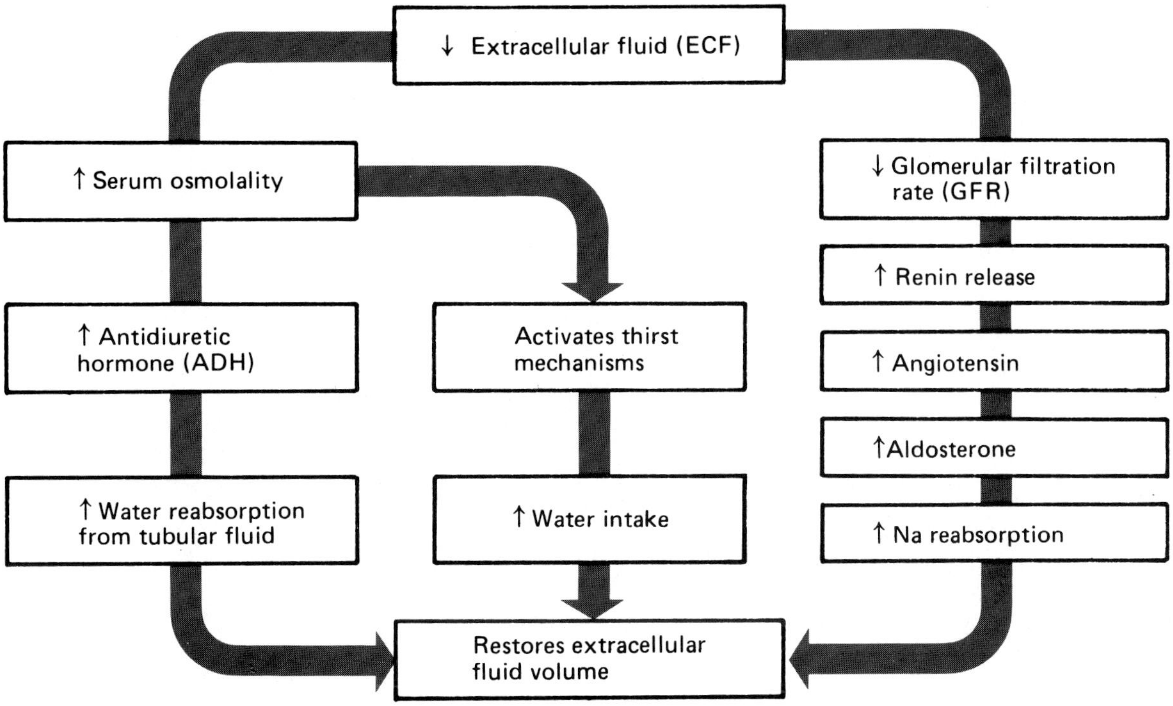

Figure 16.1. Sodium and water balance mechanism.

Dehydration/hypernatremia may be an extremely insidious condition, particularly in the elderly or the postoperative patient whose water intake is not perceived to be inadequate. Patients with chronic renal failure are unable to respond to volume contraction by reducing urine volume and consequently are particularly liable to become dehydrated. In diabetes mellitus, particularly when control is poor, the continuing osmotic diuresis produced by high serum glucose levels can readily lead to hypernatremia. Fluid lost in sweat is relatively hypotonic to serum. Substantial volumes of fluid may be lost by a patient with even a relatively mild elevation of temperature; if this is not recognized and the fluid replaced, dehydration will ensue. Progressive and unrecognized dehydration eventually leads to reduction in the jugular venous pressure, clinical symptoms of thirst and fever, and progression to confusion, seizures, and coma. Dehydration should not, of course, ever be allowed to progress this far, and it is usually easily diagnosed, provided that the possibility is considered.

Elevation in hematocrit or serum protein concentrations may be noted, and the serum sodium level will exceed 150 mEq/liter. Provided the patient has normal renal function, the urine osmolality will be high (usually in excess of 500 mOsm/liter) and the urinary sodium concentration will be low (less than 20 mEq/liter). Because the rise in the osmolality of the extracellular fluid draws water from the intracellular space, the total fluid deficit in dehydration/hypernatremia is distributed across the total body water; this means that considerable total body deficits may occur before the syndrome is clinically recognized.

Treatment

Treatment is very simple; the patient requires the administration of water, usually intravenously and commonly given as 5% dextrose solution. How rapidly hypernatremia should be corrected is not well established, although it is recommended that replacement fluid should be given over a period of at least 48 hours. Cases of fatal cerebral edema or permanent cerebral damage have been described in which correction of hypernatremia was completed too rapidly.

Hyponatremia

Causes

Reduction in serum sodium levels below 134 mEq/liter constitutes hyponatremia. A reduction in the serum sodium concentration may result from two primary mechanisms: sodium loss or water excess. Hyponatremia due to sodium loss is referred to as *depletional* hyponatremia, whereas that due to water excess is called *dilutional* hyponatremia. This primary distinction is of critical importance in determining therapy, because in depletional hyponatremia the patient is hypovolemic, whereas in dilutional hyponatremia the extracellular fluid is expanded. In addition to these two primary causes of hyponatremia, a reduction in serum sodium levels is occasionally seen when elevated plasma levels of glucose increase blood osmolality and enhance water movement from the intracellular space to the extracellular compartment. Furthermore, in patients with very marked hyperlipidemia or hyperproteinemia, the presence of these substances of high molecular weight reduces the percent-

Table 16.2
Causes of Hyponatremia

Depletional hyponatremia (due to Na loss)	
Diuretics	GI losses
Adrenal insufficiency	Sweat loss
Renal salt loss	Third-space loss
Vomiting	
Dilutional hyponatremia (due to H_2O excess)	
Cardiac failure	Excess ADH—drugs (chlorpropamide), SIADH
Hepatic disease	Excess IV fluids (iatrogenic)
Nephrotic syndrome	
Others	
Hyperglycemia (osmotic shifts)	
Pseudohyponatremia	

age of water contained in the plasma; this produces an apparent or "pseudohyponatremia" in which the concentration of sodium in the aqueous phase of the plasma remains normal and the patient remains asymptomatic with a normal serum osmolality. This condition is sometimes referred to as factitious hyponatremia. The common causes of hyponatremia are listed in Table 16.2.

Depletional hyponatremia may result from the administration of diuretics, from excess gastrointestinal fluid losses, or from salt loss from the kidney. Salt loss may be due to renal disease with impaired ability to conserve salt when necessary or from adrenal insufficiency (Addison's disease). Depletional hyponatremia may also occur if losses of sodium and water in the sweat are replaced by water only, in the severely ill or injured patient water and salt may be lost from the plasma into extracellular fluid, the peritoneum, the pleura, etc.

Dilutional hyponatremia is commonly seen in cardiac failure, hepatic insufficiency, and nephrotic syndrome. Water retention in these patients is due to a complex disturbance involving an inability to excrete free water, secondary hyperaldosteronism, and other factors. It may also be caused by the excessive administration of hypotonic fluids to the postoperative patient who, for some hours after operation, is usually unable to excrete large water loads. A separate and distinct form of dilutional hyponatremia occurs in the syndrome of inappropriate ADH secretion (SIADH). This is increasingly recognized as a fairly common complication of head injury, infections, respiratory diseases, and administration of such drugs as chlorpropamide. The inappropriate elevation in blood levels of ADH may be due to increased secretion from the hypothalamo-hypophyseal system stimulated by nonosmotic factors or to ectopic secretion of ADH by tumors.

The mechanism of depletional hyponatremia is important and is shown in Figure 16.2. Sodium deficit, either due to excess loss or failure of intake, leads to a reduction in serum osmolality, which suppresses ADH production and gives rise to polyuria. At the same time, the reduction in extracellular fluid (ECF) osmolality allows further water to escape from the ECF into the intracellular space. Serum sodium levels are therefore initially maintained, but at the expense of a fairly acute reduction in ECF volume. Eventually, however, the reduction in ECF volume leads to a reduction in glomerular filtration rate (GFR) and stimulation of ADH, both of which lead to oliguria. However, this is a late phase in the development of depletional hyponatremia, and unlike the situation pertaining in primary water loss, the volume deficit is borne entirely by the extracellular fluid.

Clinical Manifestations

The clinical manifestations of hyponatremia depend upon its cause. Hyponatremia due to hyperglycemia or to elevated plasma lipid levels is asymptomatic. Dilutional hyponatremia commonly presents as an edematous state in cardiac failure, hepatic disease, and the nephrotic syndrome. Dilutional hyponatremia due to the syndrome of inappropriate ADH secretion is usually diagnosed on the basis of a low serum sodium level in the absence of any other obvious causes of hyponatremia. The diagnosis of SIADH is confirmed by the demonstration that, despite the presence of hyponatremia and reduced serum osmolality, the urine osmolality is inappropriately high—usually in excess of 500 mOsm/liter while the urine sodium is high (greater than 20 mEq/liter).

Depletional hyponatremia is one of the most dangerous electrolyte disturbances. Because the body's original response to loss of sodium is to maintain serum sodium levels at the expense of extracellular fluid volume, estimation of serum electrolytes may not reveal much early reduction in the sodium level. Patients commonly complain of vague symptoms including headache, nausea, vomiting, lethargy, and cramps; they may often simply become confused for no obvious reason. As the condition progresses they develop asterixis, myoclonus, changes in reflexes, delirium, seizures, and coma. When the serum sodium falls below 110 mEq/liter, mortality is about 50%. The mortality rate is influenced by the rate of fall, but the high rate emphasizes the dangerous nature of the disturbance.

The distinction between depletional and dilutional hyponatremia can usually be made fairly readily on the basis of five diagnostic criteria (Table 16.3). Clinical examination of the patient with depletional hyponatremia usually reveals evidence of volume contraction; jugular venous pressure is low, and there is usually hypotension or at least a significant postural drop in blood pressure on standing. The patient with dilutional hyponatremia usually exhibits evidence of fluid overload in the form of edema, elevated jugular venous pressure, and no postural blood pressure fall. As noted above, these clinical signs are absent if the dilutional hyponatremia is due to SIADH.

Measurement of serum sodium may be misleading in terms of determining the severity and type of the hyponatremia. The serum sodium level in states of salt depletion falls slowly until the condition is fairly severe; in dilutional hyponatremia, on the other hand, the fall in serum sodium is more pronounced. In depletional states the urine sodium is low (less than 20 mEq/liter) because the volume contraction is stimulating sodium retention.

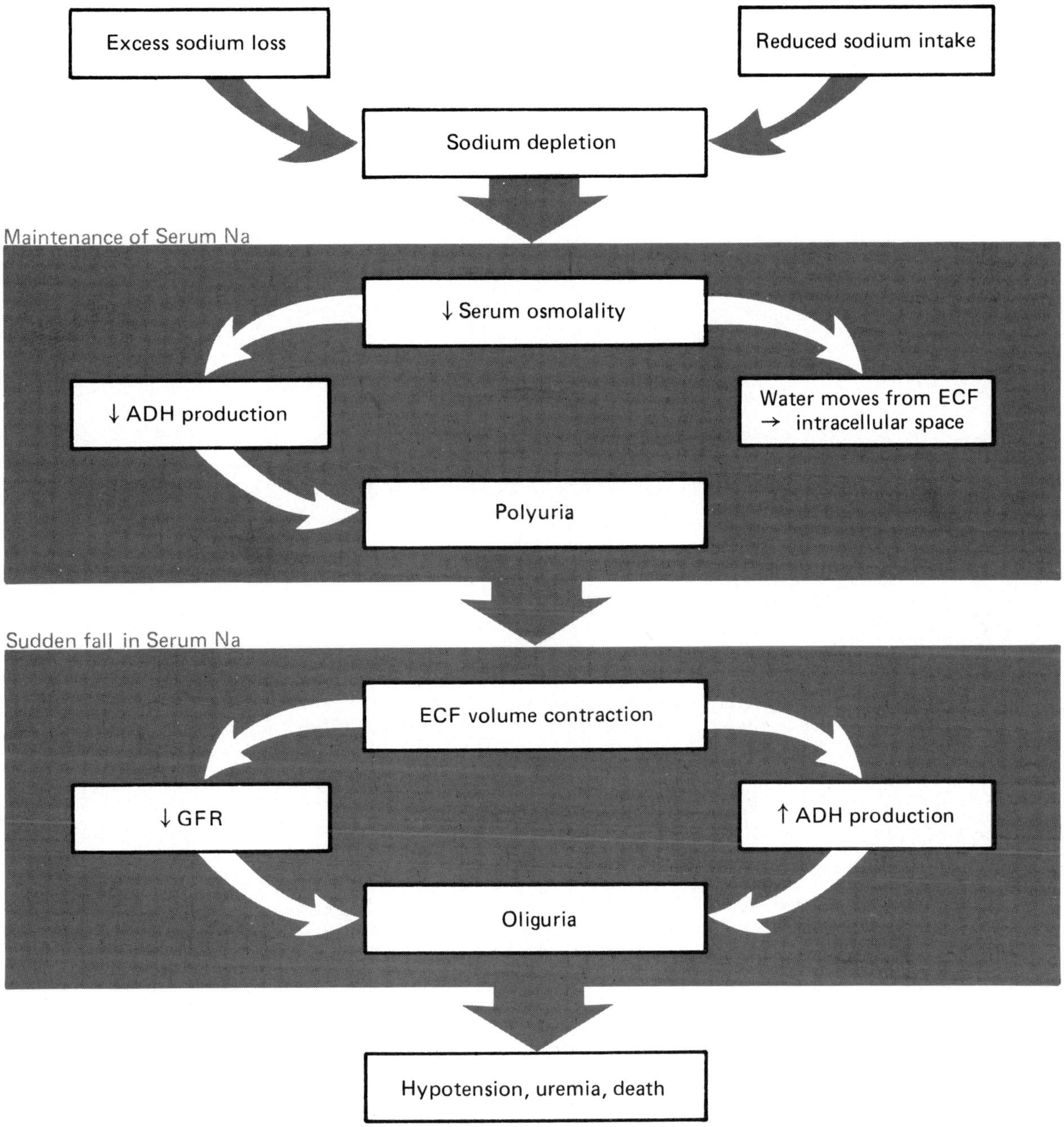

Figure 16.2. Mechanism of depletional hyponatremia.

This is not the case, of course, if the depletional hyponatremia is the result of sodium loss from the kidneys, either on the basis of renal disease or Addison's disease. In dilutional hyponatremia the volume expansion that accompanies the condition may result in high levels of sodium in the urine (usually more than 30 mEq/liter), unless the picture is complicated by secondary hyperaldosteronism, as in cardiac failure. Finally, the serum osmolality in depletional hyponatremia does not fall markedly until fairly late in the process. In contrast, in dilutional hyponatremia the serum osmolality is markedly reduced from the outset.

Treatment

The treatment of hyponatremia obviously depends upon the cause. The cause should be identified and the relevant measures taken to correct the sodium loss or the water retention. In depletional hyponatremia normal saline should be administered, but as with most electrolyte upsets, undue haste to correct the abnormality should be avoided. In patients with dilutional hyponatremia other than that due to SIADH, correction of the abnormality is not as urgent as in depletional states—indeed improvement often only results once the underlying cardiac, he-

Table 16.3
Diagnosis and Treatment of Hyponatremia

Hyponatremia = serum Na <134 mEq/l	Depletional	Dilutional: Cardiac, hepatic, renal disease	Dilutional: SIADH
Cause	Sodium loss	Water excess	Water excess due to excess ADH
Diagnostic criteria	1. ↓ Volume 2. ↓ Jugular venous pressure 3. Hypotension, or postural BP drop 4. Urine Na <20 mEq/liter (unless depletion due to primary renal Na loss) 5. Delayed fall in serum osmolality	↑ Volume (edema) ↑ Jugular venous pressure No postural BP fall Urine Na variable (depends on degree of secondary aldosteronism) Serum osmolality markedly reduced	↑ Volume (no edema) Jugular venous pressure usually normal No postural BP fall Urine Na >30 mEq/liter Serum osmolality markedly reduced
Treatment	Normal saline IV	Loop diuretics	Reduce water intake (<700 ml/day); saline and furosemide

patic, or renal disease has been corrected. Loop diuretics, such as furosemide, are usually prescribed, often in combination with spironolactone, in order to reverse the secondary hyperaldosteronism. Dilutional hyponatremia due to SIADH may respond simply to reduction in water intake below 700 ml/day, but usually requires the combined administration of saline and furosemide. The latter drug increases free water clearance, and this combination has been shown to be very effective. The patient can be given 20 mg of furosemide IV every 4 hours; urinary fluid losses should be replaced hourly with 0.9% saline. Finally, in very severe disturbances of sodium and water balance, either peritoneal dialysis or hemodialysis is occasionally required in order to correct the situation temporarily.

POTASSIUM DISTURBANCES

Potassium balance in the body is controlled for the most part by the kidneys and gastrointestinal tract. Of these two organs, the kidneys are the more important as they excrete 90% of the potassium that must be removed from the body for steady state conditions to be maintained. A normal diet contains approximately 100 mEq of potassium/day, 10 mEq of which is normally excreted in the stool and about 90 mEq in the urine. It is now clear that the majority of urinary potassium is derived from secretion in the distal nephron. In the proximal convoluted tubule the potassium concentration in the fluid is approximately equal to that of plasma; little is known about the nature of potassium transport in the loop of Henle, but the tubular fluid obtained from the bend of the loop shows that the quantity of potassium present is equal to that filtered. The majority of the potassium excreted in the urine is actively secreted in the distal convoluted tubule and collecting tubules. A number of factors have a major effect on renal potassium excretion, some of which are of clinical importance. Renal potassium excretion is increased by increased dietary intake, aldosterone, alkalosis, and diuretics and is decreased by sodium deficiency, acidosis, and spironolactone.

Increases in total body potassium from high potassium intake result in an increased potassium excretion in the distal nephron. In sodium-deficient states, a decrease in potassium excretion occurs that may be related to a diminished flow rate of tubular fluid or to a reduced availability of sodium in the lumen for exchange. Mineralocorticoid hormones, particularly aldosterone, enhance potassium excretion probably through effects on the permeability of the tubule to potassium. Finally, acid-base balance can have profound effects on renal potassium excretion: alkalosis enhances and acidosis diminishes the rate of potassium excretion. The vast majority of total body potassium, unlike sodium, is in the intracellular fluid, rather than the extracellular. This is of importance in considering disturbances of potassium balance, but it must be remembered that it is the *serum* concentration of potassium that influences cardiac conduction and the occurrence of arrhythmias—the most serious effect of disturbance in potassium metabolism.

Hypokalemia

Causes

Hypokalemia is defined as a fall in serum potassium level below 3.8 mEq/liter. The causes of hypokalemia are listed in Table 16.4. Inadequate dietary intake of potassium is rarely the only cause of potassium depletion, but it may be an important factor in determining the magnitude of the deficit in patients with other causes of potassium depletion. Various gastrointestinal disturbances may lead to hypokalemia; direct potassium loss may occur as, for example, in cases of persistent diarrhea, laxative abuse, or in the rare condition of villous adenoma of the colon.

Table 16.4
Causes of Hypokalemia

Inadequate dietary intake—contributory only
GI losses
Alkalosis → ↑ urine K loss
Diarrhea → direct K loss
Villous adenoma, laxative abuse
Renal losses
Diuretics
Aldosteronism
Accelerated hypertension/renal artery stenosis (↑ aldosterone)
Renal tubular acidosis (chronic and acute renal failure)
Antibiotics (carbenicillin)
Diabetic ketoacidosis (treated)
Some rare conditions, such as Bartter's or Liddle's syndrome

More commonly, however, persistent vomiting causes marked increases in urine losses of potassium as a result of the metabolic alkalosis produced.

Increased losses of potassium in the urine are caused by the administration of most diuretics. Yet, hypokalemia is a relatively infrequent complication of diuretic therapy, and indeed the degree of potassium deficiency induced by diuretics is very modest. Hypokalemia may occur as a result of hyperaldosteronism, either primary or secondary. Primary hyperaldosteronism (Conn's syndrome) is a rare condition in which an aldosterone-secreting tumor produces hypertension and hypokalemia; secondary hyperaldosteronism is, on the other hand, very common and may complicate cardiac, renal, or hepatic disease. Secondary hyperaldosteronism may also occur in patients with accelerated hypertension due to renal artery stenosis. Hypokalemia from increased urinary losses may occur in patients with impaired tubular function, either as part of chronic renal failure or in the diuretic phase after acute renal failure.

A number of drugs may induce hypokalemia, notably carbenicillin, which increases potassium excretion by behaving as a nonreabsorbable anion in the distal tubule. Gentamicin also increases the urinary loss of potassium, although the mechanism is unclear. Diabetic ketoacidosis normally produces hyperkalemia in the untreated phase as a result of the acidemia, but as treatment progresses total body potassium depletion is commonly revealed. Finally, there are various rare disturbances of metabolism, such as Bartter's syndrome and Liddle's syndrome, in which the mechanism of hypokalemia is not fully understood.

Clinical Manifestations

Hypokalemia is a serious condition, and its diagnosis depends to a large extent on an awareness of situations in which potassium loss may occur (Table 16.4). Part of the reason for its seriousness is that, although the total body potassium amounts to about 3000 mEq, only 60 mEq is in the extracellular fluid. Consequently, a reduction in the serum level usually conceals a very significant deficit. The principal manifestation of developing hypokalemia is a reduction in muscle tone, which in turn leads to abdominal distension, constipation, and eventual paralytic ileus, together with reduction in respiratory excursion and impairment in respiratory function. When hypokalemia becomes severe, cardiac arrhythmias are liable to occur. Patients who are hypokalemic are unusually sensitive to digoxin and may develop severe digoxin toxicity with doses not usually associated with toxicity. Finally, progressive hypokalemia leads to loss of renal concentrating power and a metabolic alkalosis.

Treatment

Once hypokalemia is found the treatment is usually fairly simple. The cause of potassium losses should be identified and corrected if possible. Although, as noted in Table 16.5, if the total body potassium deficit is usually large, it is important to *correct the deficit slowly.* With lesser potassium deficits (serum potassium levels between 2.5 and 3.8 mEq/liter) the oral administration of potassium is usually adequate unless associated complications of hypokalemia (arrhythmias) dictate more rapid replacement; oral potassium is often given as Slow-K, each tablet of which contains 8 mEq of potassium. With larger deficits or in patients who are unable to take oral medications, intravenous potassium chloride should be given. The concentration should not exceed 40 mEq/liter, and it should be given at a rate not exceeding 40 mEq/hour in the adult. Occasionally it may be necessary to give IV

Table 16.5
Diagnosis and Treatment of Hypokalemia

Hypokalemia = serum K <3.8 mEq/liter	**Moderate case: serum K = 2.5–3.8 mEq/liter**	**Severe case: serum K <2.5 mEq/liter**
Diagnostic criteria	↓ Muscle tone, which leads to Abdominal distension Constipation/paralytic ileus ↓ Respiratory excursion ↓ Respiratory function	Same as in moderate case plus Hypotension Cardiac arrythmias
Treatment (K replacement must be done gradually)	Oral Slow-K: 1 tab = 8 mEq K	IV potassium chloride: concentration not exceeding 40 mEq/liter, rate not exceeding 40 mEq/hr

potassium while restricting IV fluid intake: 10–20 mEq of potassium may be given by buretrol over a period of 1 hour. The rate must be reduced in children. In the course of potassium replacement it is vital to monitor renal function and follow the serum potassium levels closely; even minor reduction in renal function may result in very high serum potassium levels.

Hyperkalemia

Causes

An elevation in the serum potassium level over 5.0 mEq/liter constitutes hyperkalemia. Causes of hyperkalemia are listed in Table 16.6. In late-stage chronic renal failure or acute renal failure with oliguria, failure of the kidneys to excrete potassium (often associated with concomitant increased catabolism) leads to a rapid rise in the serum potassium levels. In chronic renal failure some adaptive mechanisms develop, notably an increased excretion of potassium from the gut; indeed, although the patient with chronic renal failure still has a high urine output he or she is more at risk from hypokalemia. Nevertheless, in the late stages, hyperkalemia develops.

Because the majority of potassium is located in the intracellular space, anything that impairs the integrity of cells or affects the cell membrane may allow potassium to escape into the extracellular fluid. Clinically this is most often seen in patients who have suffered muscle necrosis or who have developed severe acidosis. Hyperkalemia may complicate the administration of spironolactone or triamterene—both diuretics that promote the excretion of sodium but increase reabsorption of potassium. Hyperkalemia occurs in Addison's disease as a result of the deficiency of steroid hormones.

As mentioned above, excessive potassium replacement, usually by the intravenous route, may produce dangerous hyperkalemia. Finally, a factitious hyperkalemia may be defined if the blood being tested has undergone hemolysis of the red cells or if there is a very marked thrombocytosis with platelet counts around 900,000/mm^3; rupture of red cells or of increased numbers of platelets causes the detected increase in potassium levels.

Clinical Manifestations

There are virtually no symptoms that are diagnostic or even suggestive of hyperkalemia. The diagnosis, therefore, depends on a high index of suspicion and frequent measurements of serum potassium levels in patients at risk. Hyperkalemia is perhaps the most dangerous of the common electrolyte disturbances because once the serum potassium reaches 7 mEq/liter, cardiac arrhythmias or arrest is imminent. Hyperkalemia does produce recognizable electrocardiographic changes, particularly a widened QRS complex, various degrees of heart block, and high peaked T waves (Fig. 16.3). However, the appearance of ECG changes of hyperkalemia does not correlate well with the serum level of potassium and is a poor guide to the seriousness of the situation.

Table 16.6
Causes of Hyperkalemia

Chronic or acute renal failure
Shifts of potassium from cells (muscle necrosis, acidosis, digitalis intoxication)
Potassium-sparing diuretics (spironolactone, triamterene)
Addison's disease
Iatrogenic
Factitious

Treatment (Table 16.7)

Hyperkalemia is a medical emergency. In patients with less severe degrees of hyperkalemia (up to a serum potassium level of 6.5 mEq/liter) and when renal function remains adequate, the administration of cation exchange resins may be sufficient; sodium polystyrene sulfonate (Kayexalate) in a dose of 15–30 gm should be given either orally or by retention enema two to three times daily. If the serum potassium level is higher or if renal function is severely impaired, emergency measures that have a quicker action must be taken. First, a calcium infusion should be given to reverse the cardiotoxic effects of hyperkalemia. One to three ampoules of 10% calcium gluconate should be infused intravenously over 3–5 minutes during ECG monitoring. The onset of action of calcium is within 1–5 minutes, but is relatively transient so other more long-lasting agents must also be used. These should include the administration of glucose and insulin; a solution of 500 ml of 10% glucose with 10 units of regular insulin may be given over 30 minutes and then administered at a reduced rate. Alternatively, 2–3 ampoules of sodium bicarbonate, each ampoule containing 44 mEq of sodium bicarbonate, should be added to 1 liter of glucose

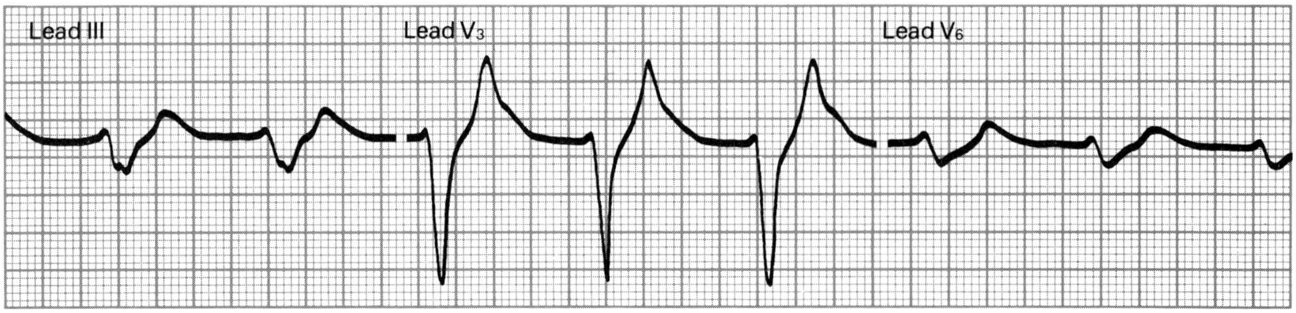

Figure 16.3. Electrocardiographic manifestations in severe hyperkalemia: tall peaked T waves, decrease in R-wave amplitude, widened QRS complex, and disappearance of the P wave.

Table 16.7
Diagnosis and Treatment of Hyperkalemia

Hyperkalemia = serum K > 5.0 mEq/liter	Moderate case: serum K 5–6.5 mEq/liter with adequate renal function	Severe case: serum K > 6.5 mEq/liter
Diagnostic criteria	Virtually none ECG abnormalities are poor guide	
Treatment	Sodium polystyrene sulfonate (Kayexalate) 15–30 gm orally or by enema two to three times daily	1. 1–3 amps 10% Ca gluconate IV over 3–5 min (ECG monitoring) 2. 500 ml 10% glucose with 10 units regular insulin IV over 30 min 3. 2–3 amps Na bicarbonate in 5% glucose given IV over 1–2 hours 4. Kayexalate as above 5. Dialysis

and infused over 1–2 hours. With the rise in blood pH, potassium moves into the cells, decreasing the hyperkalemia within about an hour. This effect may persist for several hours if the blood pH is maintained and if the patient is not too hypercatabolic. The administration of sodium polystyrene sulfonate should be initiated as indicated previously. Finally, in the presence of adequate renal function, such diuretics as furosemide may be of benefit by enhancing urinary potassium excretion. Where renal function is impaired it is very often necessary to proceed to either peritoneal dialysis or hemodialysis to reduce the potassium levels.

CALCIUM AND PHOSPHATE DISTURBANCES

Calcium metabolism is a major topic that is beyond the scope of this text because, in essence, calcium does not function as an electrolyte. In the past few years, however, there has been increasing interest in the role of phosphate in various electrolyte disturbances, quite apart from considerations related to bone metabolism. Hyperphosphatemia occurs in renal impairment and is a particular problem in chronic renal failure. The problems of hyperphosphatemia, however, again are in the realm of renal osteodystrophy and disturbances in parathyroid function and are not considered further.

Hypophosphatemia is now being recognized increasingly frequently. It is defined as a reduction in the serum phosphate below 2.5 mg/100 ml and is seen in a number of clinical situations, including patients receiving intravenous feeding, in the nutritional recovery syndrome, in treated diabetic ketoacidosis, alcohol withdrawal, hypothermia, sepsis, and after antacid abuse. A reduction in serum phosphate levels may impair function of red blood cells, white blood cells, platelets, and neurologic and muscular function (Table 16.8).

Table 16.8
Consequences of Hypophosphatemia

↓ Leukocyte chemotaxis
Shift of oxyhemoglobin dissociation curve to left
↓ Cardiac contractility
Respiratory failure
Obtundation and coma
Platelet dysfunction

Treatment

In the critically ill patient it is probably important to identify the development of hypophosphatemia and to replace phosphate intravenously as KPO_4 10–20 mM over 2–4 hours.

DISTURBANCES IN MAGNESIUM BALANCE

Magnesium is also a subject of increasing interest, particularly in the critically ill patient. As is potassium ion, magnesium is largely an intracellular cation, and the normal serum level lies between 1.5 and 2 mEq/liter.

Hypomagnesemia

As with potassium, a fall in the serum level indicates the presence of quite a large deficit. Hypomagnesemia is being identified in patients with malabsorption, those with long-continued gastric suction, in severe diarrhea, after diuretic administration, and in patients with diabetic ketoacidosis or pancreatitis secondary to alcoholism. The clinical signs are fairly similar to those of hypokalemia, consisting of vague nausea, apathy, muscular fibrillation, and ataxia. They may progress to full-blown hypomagnesemic tetany and psychotic behavior. It is important to consider the possibility that hypomagnesemia may be occurring in the above situations.

Treatment consists of the intravenous or intramuscular administration of magnesium sulphate in a dose of 50 mEq given over 6 hours. In the patient who is unable to eat, deficiency of magnesium can be prevented by the administration of about 10 mEq/day.

Hypermagnesemia

Hypermagnesemia may be seen in patients with renal failure or in those abusing magnesium-containing purgatives. Early clinical signs of hypermagnesemia are muscle weakness and hyporeflexia and appear at serum levels around 6 mEq/liter. More severe effects, including hypotension and arrhythmias, occur when the serum level reaches 10 mEq/liter. Hypermagnesemia is treated by correcting the underlying problem and administering intravenous calcium gluconate; occasionally dialysis may be required.

Suggested Readings

Bear RA, Byck RF: Review article: clinical approach to the diagnosis of acid-base disorders. *Can Med Assoc J* 120:173–182, 1979.

Massry SG (ed): Clinical pathophysiology of electrolyte and acid-base metabolism, 1. *Clin Nephrol 4:7,* 1977.

Oh MS, Carroll HJ: Current concepts: the anion gap. *N Engl J Med* 297:814–817, 1977.

CHAPTER

17 Acid/Base Balance

Trevor R. Lobb, M.D. and David G. Cunningham, M.D.

Evaluation of acid/base balance requires an appreciation of normal biochemistry, interpretation of laboratory-derived data, and application of clinical reasoning. Only by combining these elements can a rational approach to acid/base disorders be achieved. In this chapter, basic biochemistry and acid/base disturbances are presented, as well as rules for determining more complex mixed disorders.

BIOCHEMICAL BACKGROUND

The presence of any acid (a hydrogen ion donor) in solution influences the acidity or free hydrogen ion concentration of that solution. In biologic systems this acidity must be strictly regulated in order to (1) optimize enzymatic function and (2) control the ionization of salts crucial to nerve conduction, synaptic transmission, and muscle contraction alike. Because acids are continually generated in both normal and abnormal metabolism, the organism must excrete these acid by-products at the same rate as they are generated if acidity is to remain optimal. Acidity occurs when acids "dissociate," according to their chemical character, to liberate a free hydrogen ion $[H^+]$, as well as the conjugate base.

$$\underset{\text{(acid)}}{HA} \rightleftharpoons H^+ + \underset{\text{(base)}}{A^-}$$

It is important to understand that acids can only contribute to acidity by dissociating (i.e., a shift to the right) to produce free hydrogen ions in solution. Conversely, should excess base accumulate (e.g., as a sodium salt) then the free hydrogen ion would be forced to associate (i.e., shift to the left) to form the parent acid, thereby *reducing* the solution's acidity by removing free hydrogen ion. This activity of excess base is called *buffering*. The presence of buffers, such as hemoglobin and proteins, limits the acid's tendency to dissociate during times of acute disequilibrium, thereby further protecting acidity levels.

There are in fact several acid/base systems in human physiochemistry, but one stands out because of its sheer magnitude and importance—the *carbonic acid/bicarbonate* system. Its rate of turnover exceeds 200-fold that of all other systems combined. Its parent, carbon dioxide (CO_2), is the preferred end-product of all energy metabolism as it possesses a unique but highly adaptable form of excretion—pulmonary ventilation. It is the "respiratory" acid/base system, and its unique mode of excretion allows it to *compensate* acutely through overexcretion, should another acid accumulate to dangerous levels and threaten acidity control.

All other acid/base systems are lumped together under the title of "metabolic" acid/base systems because of their dependence for excretion on hepatic metabolism and/or renal elimination. It is also possible for this metabolic system to overexcrete in order to *compensate* for those times when the respiratory system is in imbalance; but this metabolic compensation takes longer to develop.

Compensation, like buffering, is a temporary or limited means of absorbing the shock of sudden changes in acid load. It is never as effective as the normal maintenance of acid load through effective production/excretion management.

ASSESSMENT OF ACID/BASE BALANCE

To assess a patient's acid/base status, electrolytes and blood gases must be secured and interpreted. A knowledge of what these values represent is mandatory to ascertain the type of acid/base disorder present. Only then can one entertain a differential diagnosis to determine treatment.

Interpretation of Laboratory Data

To assess the patient's acid/base status one would have to assess each individual system if it were not for the absolute predominance of the carbonic acid/bicarbonate or respiratory system, the reaction of which is stated below.

$$\underset{\text{(carbonic acid)}}{H_2CO_3} \rightleftharpoons H^+ + \underset{\text{(bicarbonate)}}{HCO_3^-}$$

Carbonic acid is not readily detectable, but is directly related to the amount of carbon dioxide (CO_2) in solution, which in turn is measured by its partial pressure ($PaCO_2$).

$$PaCO_2 \rightleftharpoons H^+ + HCO_3^-$$

This reaction is generally weighed on the "right" side by renal retention of excessive bicarbonate as a sodium buffer salt (having excreted the hydrogen ion in the urine).

$$\begin{array}{lll} PaCO_2 \rightleftharpoons H^+ + & HCO_3^- & \text{(pulmonary)} \\ \quad Na^+ + & HCO_3^- & \text{(renal)} \\ & \text{"actual" bicarbonate} & \end{array}$$

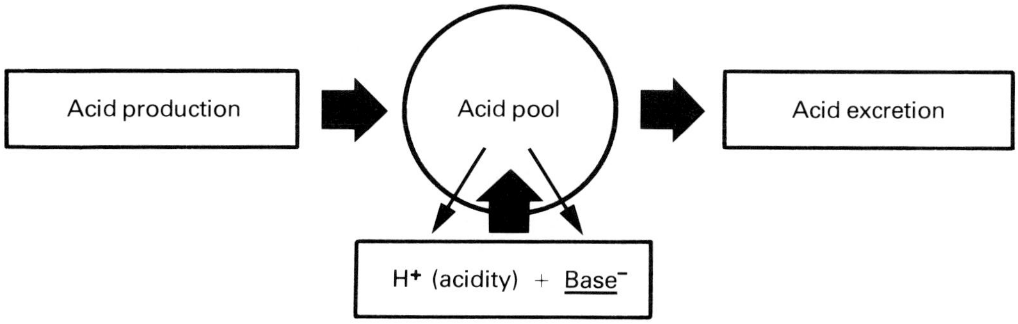

Figure 17.1. Determinants of acid pool—buffering.

The renal bicarbonate portion is regulated by the kidney as necessary in performing its function in metabolic compensation. The resultant "actual" bicarbonate level, therefore, is a combination of two sources: (1) CO_2 dissociation and (2) buffer retention by the kidney.

It is at this juncture that most problems in acid/base understanding begin. Total acidity can be measured by determining the total free hydrogen ion concentration (activity) in the solution; the relative interplay of the respiratory and metabolic contributions to the total acidity can be noted by the levels of $PaCO_2$ and the *buffer* portion of bicarbonate, respectively. The use of $PaCO_2$ to assess the respiratory component presents no problem, but acidity terminology and the isolation of the buffer component of bicarbonate are two very contentious areas.

Acidity

As mentioned earlier, acidity relates directly to free hydrogen ion concentration $[H^+]$ and can be reported in the same manner as any other electrolyte (i.e., moles/liter), which is feasible in medicine considering the fine range of acidity tolerated by the living organism. The small absolute amount would necessitate the usage of nanomoles/liter, as is presently recommended by Systéme International (SI) terminology. However, in the absolute chemical possibility, the range of acidity is infinite by physiologic comparison, and a different terminology was instituted by Sorensen, a pioneer in this area at the turn of the century. This terminology was based on the exponential (base 10) of the hydrogen ion concentration that easily encompassed the potential range of 1 (10^0) to 0.000,000,000,000,01 (10^{-14}) mol/liter—the negative aspect of the "power" (p) was ignored and the term $(p)H^+$ or pH was born. The reciprocal nature that allows acidity to increase while the pH declines is a frequent point of confusion.

However, it is useful to remember that a pH change of 0.3 is equal to a twofold change in hydrogen ion concentration. Table 17.1 is a conversion table for pH to hydrogen ion concentration.

Bicarbonate

Finally, one needs to quantitate the magnitude of metabolic acid/base disturbance. In fact, only carbon dioxide tension ($PaCO_2$) and acidity (pH) are actually measured in any blood gas sample, whereas the bicarbonate value

Table 17.1
Conversion of pH to Hydrogen Ion Concentration

	pH	H^+	
		(nmol/liter)	
	6.0	1,000	
	6.5	316	
	6.8	158	
	6.9	126	
	7.0	100	ACIDOSIS
	7.1	79	
normal 7.35	7.2	63	
range 7.45	7.3	50	
	7.4	40	
	7.5	32	
	7.6	25	
	8.0	10	ALKALOSIS

is arrived at via mathematical calculation and is termed the *actual* bicarbonate. Unfortunately, this bicarbonate value includes both "CO_2 dissociative" and "renally retained" bicarbonate forms. Yet, it is only the latter form that acts effectively as a buffer in reacting to metabolic acid/base disturbance.

Many formulas have been advocated to divest an *actual* bicarbonate of its useless part in order to leave some quantitative idea of metabolic buffering activity. Some laboratories already provide the finished product in the form of a *standard* bicarbonate determination, i.e., any deviation in *standard* bicarbonate is due solely to buffering activity. Confusion may result, in that proponents of one method rarely inform their students that the other method exists (for the sake of simplicity), and the "correction" may be applied to a *standard* bicarbonate or an actual bicarbonate may be left "uncorrected."

Base Excess

Clinicians may argue about the purity of methods, but it must be remembered that all techniques rely on calculations based on assumptions. All have error and are best considered roughly accurate and only indicators of trend. Therefore, rather than purity, simplicity of usage should be of prime importance, such as is found with *base excess* estimations. The calculation, again performed by the reporting laboratory, simply states whether buffer is (1) available at normal levels ("zero" base line) indicating balanced metabolic activity, (2) in deficit ("negative" value) indicating metabolic acidosis, or (3) in excess ("positive" value) indicating metabolic alkalosis. The absolute numerical value of *base excess* represents millimoles/liter (mmol/liter) of buffer; its range through 0-5-10-15 can roughly be equated with normal-mild-moderate-severe disturbances, respectively. This number is immediately useful in calculating dosage of buffer (sodium bicarbonate) administration should that become necessary.

In summary, the ultimate acidity of the patient is determined by the pH or $[H^+]$ and the interplay of respiratory with metabolic acid/base balance by $PaCO_2$ and *base excess* determinations. Respiratory status can be manipulated through ventilation and the use of respiratory adjuncts (see Chapter 6), whereas metabolic acid/base status requires further elucidation as to its exact cause for treatment to be effective. In general, "common things are common," and one proceeds down a prescribed list ruling out likely possibilities in view of the patient's history.

METABOLIC ACID/BASE DISTURBANCES

Metabolic Acidosis

Metabolic acidosis results from a gain in H^+ or a loss of HCO_3^-, both of which result in a decreased pH and a base deficit (negative base excess). Normally, the $PaCO_2$ should be decreased as compensation.

Differentiation between these two types can be made through calculation of the anion gap ($Na^+-(Cl^-+HCO_3^-)$) as those disorders resulting in HCO_3^- loss have a normal value (10–23 mEq/liter). With the accumulation or addition of acid, HCO_3^- is consumed as buffer, which results in an increased anion gap (Table 17.2). The overall clinical picture combined with laboratory determinations determines the course of treatment.

Sodium Bicarbonate Therapy

Sodium bicarbonate has long been used as a therapy in metabolic acidosis, but too often inappropriately. A metabolic acidosis is caused by the abnormal generation of acid, which is indicative of a disease process. Whereas bicarbonate administration may temporarily alleviate an acidity complication, it does little to correct the disease process. In addition, acidity is usually compensated by spontaneous pulmonary hyperventilation (respiratory alkalosis) or can be ensured by mechanical ventilation. The proper treatment of a metabolic acidosis necessitates detecting the causative source (e.g., hypovolemic shock leading to lactic acidosis) and instituting treatment to stop further acid generation, e.g., fluid resuscitation. If the patient can be stabilized through that treatment, any metabolic acidosis will be nicely handled along normal physiologic pathways without the long-term complications of bicarbonate therapy. Bicarbonate therapy is necessary only with certain prescribed routines (cardiac arrest resuscitation), when acid accumulation continues despite a known cause (renal failure), or when the patient fails to stabilize with basic resuscitation (see Appendix A).

Table 17.2
Metabolic Acidosis

Increased anion gap
Endogenous acids
Ketoacids
Lactic acidosis
Chronic renal failure
Exogenous acids
Salicylate ingestion
Ethylene glycol ingestion
Methyl alcohol ingestion
Normal anion gap
Renal tubular acidosis
GI loss—diarrhea, ileostomy, ureterosigmoidostomy
Carbonic anhydrase inhibitors

Metabolic Alkalosis

This is a very common though less life-threatening clinical condition characterized by an increased pH, positive base excess, and usually increased $PaCO_2$ as compensation. It results from a gain of bicarbonate or loss of nonvolatile acid (Table 17.3).

Therapy is usually aimed at correction of the underlying disorder and only in severe derangement involves the administration of exogenous acids.

Mixed Disturbances

Nothing is purely uncomplicated in medicine, and acid/base disturbances prove no exception to the rule. Much has been made of exact meshing of the systems in order to determine an acute or chronic nature, or primary versus secondary. Mixed problems do undoubtably occur frequently enough to make estimations of chronicity and primacy grossly misleading with respect to patient management. For example, consider the chronic CO_2-retainer who loses metabolic compensation through buffering a sudden metabolic acidosis induced by poor circulation (e.g., myocardial ischemia): the base excess that would have properly labeled the chronic pulmonary condition is missing, and the patient is mislabeled "acute," which means the recent metabolic acidosis is ignored while attempts are made to wean him or her from a ventilator to normal $PaCO_2$ values. Complicated as this may sound, it is not an uncommon example in real critical care practice.

Rules predicting expected compensatory changes (Appendix B), when taken in light of the patient's clinical

Table 17.3
Metabolic Alkalosis

Gastrointestinal loss
Vomiting/nasogastric suction
Urinary loss
Diuretics
Volume contraction
Exogenous base
Bicarbonate
Acetate (hyperalimentation)
Citrate (transfusions)

picture, may often uncover mixed disturbances. Mixed conditions, such as an acute metabolic acidosis on a chronic metabolic alkalosis (no apparent change in base excess) do exist and are readily perceived by a mind open to the possibilities as suggested by history and examination.

SUMMARY

A basic understanding of acid/base physiology, combined with measurement of pH and $PaCO_2$ and calculation of base excess, should make interpretation of acid/base problems easier. For those who must work with actual bicarbonate determinations, we would recommend selecting one formula for "correction" and staying with it alone (two such protocols are found in Appendix A and B). Finally, but most importantly, the treatment of acid/base disturbance lies primarily in intelligently ferretting out the cause and arresting further imbalance, not in depending on ventilatory compensation or added bicarbonate buffering.

Appendix A

SODIUM BICARBONATE ADMINISTRATION

Should sodium bicarbonate administration become necessary, then variations of the following formula are universally used.

$$NaHCO_3 \text{ dosage} = \frac{0.2 \times \text{body wt (kg)} \times \text{base deficit}}{2}$$

The base deficit (negative base excess) represents the buffer consumed in mmol/liter and, therefore, the amount of buffer theoretically needed to be replaced in the extracellular fluid compartment represented by 20–30% of the total (lean?) body weight. Because this formula involves certain assumptions and no one has any idea of what is going on in the intracellular compartment, most clinicians give half the calculated amount—one can always give more if subsequent acid/base analysis suggests that more is necessary.

Appendix B

METABOLIC ACID/BASE DETERMINATIONS USING *ACTUAL* BICARBONATE

I. ANNUAL REFRESHER COURSE 1979 (American Society of Anesthesiologists) W. E. Bernards, M.D.

Based on detailed observations of in vivo bicarbonate *(actual)* changes during graded degrees of hypo- or hypercapnia (both acute and chronic), assumed values can be ascribed to respiratory bicarbonate changes that, when added to "normal" bicarbonate (24 mmol/liter), would give the actual bicarbonate value to be expected for the given $PaCO_2$ if it were a purely respiratory disorder. Any variation between this "calculation" and the actual bicarbonate as reported would then be attributed to buffering action of a metabolic component; this difference in mmol/liter would be inflated by 25% to account for other buffers in the system (bicarbonate is responsible for 80% of all metabolic buffering!)

Rules

1. Acute respiratory *acidosis* is associated with a rise in bicarbonate of 1 mmol/liter for every $PaCO_2$ rise of 10 mm Hg.
2. Acute respiratory *alkalosis* is associated with a fall in bicarbonate of 2 mmol/liter for every $PaCO_2$ drop of 10 mm Hg.
3. *Chronic* respiratory acidosis is associated with a rise in bicarbonate of 4 mmol/liter for every $PaCO_2$ rise of 10 mm Hg.

Example

Male comatose diabetic with suspected chronic obstructive pulmonary disease.

	pH	7.08
	$PaCO_2$	60 mm Hg
(ACTUAL)	HCO_3	23 mmol/liter

Solution

A chronic respiratory acidosis would be expected to increase bicarbonate by 4 mmol/liter for every 10 mm Hg rise in $PaCO_2$ (20 mm Hg in this instance, for a bicarbonate rise of 8 mmol/liter).

His bicarbonate should be 32 mmol/liter (24 + 8) for his respiratory condition. In fact, it is measured at 23 mmol/liter, which represents a decline of 9 mmol/liter (23–32) due to buffering of a metabolic acidosis, presumed to be ketoacidosis in this instance (confirmed by urinary ketones).

Total buffering activity is probably around 11–12 mmol/liter (+ 25%) when all buffers are considered.

This is moderately severe metabolic acidosis.

II. ADVANCED CARDIAC LIFE SUPPORT 1975 (American Heart Association) Arnold Sladen, M.D.

This system (the "purest" of them all) ignores even actual bicarbonate because it, too, is only a calculation and works from "knowns" associated with pH and $PaCO_2$. These "knowns" or "Golden Rules" are stated below.

Rules

1. A $PaCO_2$ change of 10 mm Hg (up or down) is associated with a pH change of 0.08 in the opposite direction.
2. A pH change of 0.15 is equivalent to a buffer base change of 10 mmol/liter.

Example

Male comatose diabetic with suspected chronic obstructive pulmonary disease.

pH	7.08
$PaCO_2$	60 mm Hg

Solution

A rise of 20 mm Hg $PaCO_2$ (40–60) would decrease pH by 0.16, resulting in a pH of 7.24 (7.4–0.16)—Rule 1.

However, 7.08 is actually measured, which represents a further decline of 0.16 (7.24–7.08). This decline of 0.16 in pH would equate with a buffer base deficit of just over 10 mmol/liter due to the buffering of metabolic acidosis (compared with 11–12 mmol/liter by the previous method)—Rule 2.

This is a relatively complicated means of arriving at approximately the same value of metabolic acidosis, when a laboratory determination of base excess would have reported −13 mmol/liter (i.e., 13 mmol/liter of base deficit)! All different to be sure, but all in the same neighborhood and equally useful in the management of the problem.

NEUROLOGICAL SCIENCES

CHAPTER

18 Acute Disturbances of Consciousness

John D. Brown, M.D.

Conditions that may cause impaired consciousness or coma are commonly found in any busy general hospital. Alterations in consciousness indicate significant brain dysfunction, either from diffusely acting metabolic causes, local or widespread structural lesions, or both. Urgent attention is required to prevent further damage to the brain due to the primary cause or, as is now becoming more widely recognized, due to secondary events stemming from those primary causes.

PATHOPHYSIOLOGY (FIG. 18.1)

Consciousness is a state of awareness of self and environment, and coma is unarousable unresponsiveness. Consciousness is divided into two components: (1) arousal, which is behaviorally reflected in wakefulness and is located anatomically in the upper brainstem and diencephalon (thalamus and hypothalamus) and (2) content, which reflects total mental capabilities and is located in the cerebral hemisphere.

The arousal, alerting, or wakeful component of consciousness is subserved physiologically, in large measure, by the ascending reticular activating system. This system is composed, in part, of the brainstem reticular formation with connections to certain thalamic and other nuclei, and from there it connects via projection fibers to most areas of the cerebral cortex. The ascending reticular activating system is closely related to the midline ventricular system. The reticular formation is a complex system of polysynaptically interconnected neuronal clusters stretching throughout the tegmentum or floor of the brainstem from the cervicomedullary junction to the diencephalon. Functionally, the reticular formation may be divided into two areas: (1) lateral receptive areas in which sensory and other modifying neuronal influences are received from ascending sensory systems, cranial nerve nuclei, cerebellum, basal ganglia, hypothalamus, and cerebral cortex; and (2) a more medial, somewhat diffuse, projection area that influences activity of the cerebral cortex through the ascending reticular activating system. The reticular formation can also modify somatic and visceral motor activity via descending connections to the lower brainstem and spinal cord. Through its many interconnections, the reticular formation may integrate

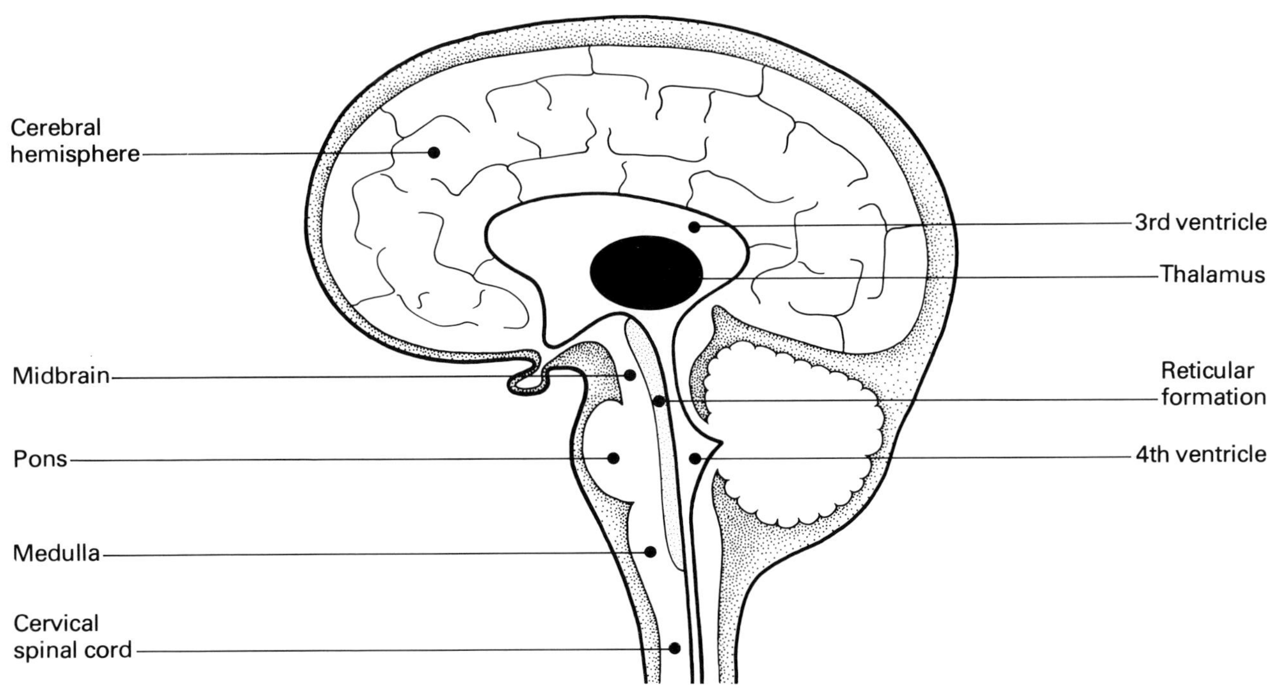

Figure 18.1. The structural components of consciousness.

sensory input and modify cerebral cortical and other activities. In terms of disturbances of consciousness, the most important portion of the ascending reticular activating system is that contained medially in the middle and upper thirds of the pontine tegmentum, the tegmentum and tectum of the midbrain, and connections to the posterior diencephalon. Stimulation of these areas in animals produces arousal or wakening, whereas bilateral destructive lesions in animals and humans have produced unresponsive states or coma. Intrinsic lesions below this level do not produce coma.

Although many areas of the cerebral cortex are concerned with specific motor and sensory functions, no single area is responsible for the content portion of consciousness. Rather, it is the interaction between areas of the cortex activated by the ascending reticular activating system that generates attention and other mental capabilities. Consciousness then, depends upon an interaction between arousal mechanisms originating in the upper brainstem and diencephalon and a relatively intact cerebral cortex. There can be arousal without content, but not content without arousal.

STRUCTURAL CAUSES

When considering a state of altered consciousness, the first question is whether it is due to a structural lesion. If so, the next question is whether the effect is primarily on the arousal mechanism of the brainstem and diencephalon, or whether it is the cerebral hemispheres that are directly involved. Lesions involving the cerebral hemispheres, unless diffuse or multifocal, rarely primarily alter consciousness, but they may through mass effects implicate deep midline structures associated with the arousal mechanism. The rate at which cerebral hemisphere lesions develop is important. Slowly progressing lesions may not significantly alter consciousness, but rapidly developing lesions almost certainly will. In contrast, discrete or focal structural lesions involving the upper brainstem, particularly in the medial portion of the reticular formation, can quickly cause coma. If such structural lesions can be excluded, then a search for the third and largest group of conditions causing alterations in consciousness can be pursued. These are the metabolic disorders acting either through their diffuse depressant effect on cerebral hemisphere neural function, on brainstem neural function, or both.

Certain clinical observations discussed in detail by Plum and Posner provide a useful basis for determining the anatomic location of structural lesions that may cause coma. These observations include the general state of consciousness and arousability; respiratory patterns; pupil size and light responsiveness; eye movement, either spontaneous or reflexly elicited; and skeletal motor activity.

General State of Consciousness

Between the two extremes of alert, wakeful awareness (consciousness) and unarousable unresponsiveness (coma) there is a continuum of states that has been the subject of many semantic battles. It is more useful to relate the stimuli used to the responses elicited when describing the individual's conscious condition. This practice allows for more accurate assessment by different observers, who may have different understandings of such terms as confusion, lethargy, stupor, obtundation, semicoma, delirium, etc.

Respiratory Patterns

Normal breathing is regulated by an interplay of metabolic and neural factors. Structural lesions and metabolic disturbances that cause coma frequently affect the pattern of respiration, and particular patterns may have localizing features or at least signify change in the patient's status. Only some of the more common patterns are discussed below.

One of the most common abnormal patterns of breathing is Cheyne-Stokes respirations in which respiratory excursion waxes and wanes and alternates regularly with periods of apnea. As cerebral activity, which normally regulates rhythmic breathing, decreases, there is an increase in ventilatory response to CO_2 stimulation. During the hyperpneic period, the CO_2 stimulus is reduced and apnea results. The stimulus to respiration does not return until there is sufficient accumulation of CO_2 to trigger the chemoreceptors and regenerate the cycle. This respiratory abnormality is seen most frequently with bilateral deep hemispheric or diencephalic lesions, although occasionally lesions as low as the upper pons produce a similar pattern. It may be seen in threatened transtentorial herniation because of increasing pressure on deep diencephalic structures or with metabolic abnormalities that diffusely affect cerebral function.

Central neurogenic hyperventilation is a respiratory abnormality in which persistent regular, fast, deep hyperpnea accompanies lesions in the low midbrain and pontine tegmentum, affecting the medial reticular formation. The respiratory threshold and CO_2 tensions are low, whereas O_2 tensions are normal or elevated, thereby excluding hypoxia as the respiratory stimulus. This respiratory abnormality often accompanies transtentorial herniation in which midbrain compression occurs, but it can be seen in metabolic disturbances.

Ataxic or Biot's respirations have a pattern in which the depth and rate of respirations are completely irregular, random, and often slow and at times decrease to apnea. They are seen with lesions in the dorsomedial medullary reticular formation that affect the reciprocal interaction between the inspiratory and expiratory neuronal clusters found there. An associated reduced chemical drive to these neuronal clusters is also present. In contrast, drugs and other metabolic factors insidiously depress the medullary respiratory centers to the point of apnea.

The occurrence of yawning, vomiting, and hiccups suggests lesions involving interacting neuronal systems in the lower pons and medulla. Because the cardiovascular system can retain its rhythm when released from neural

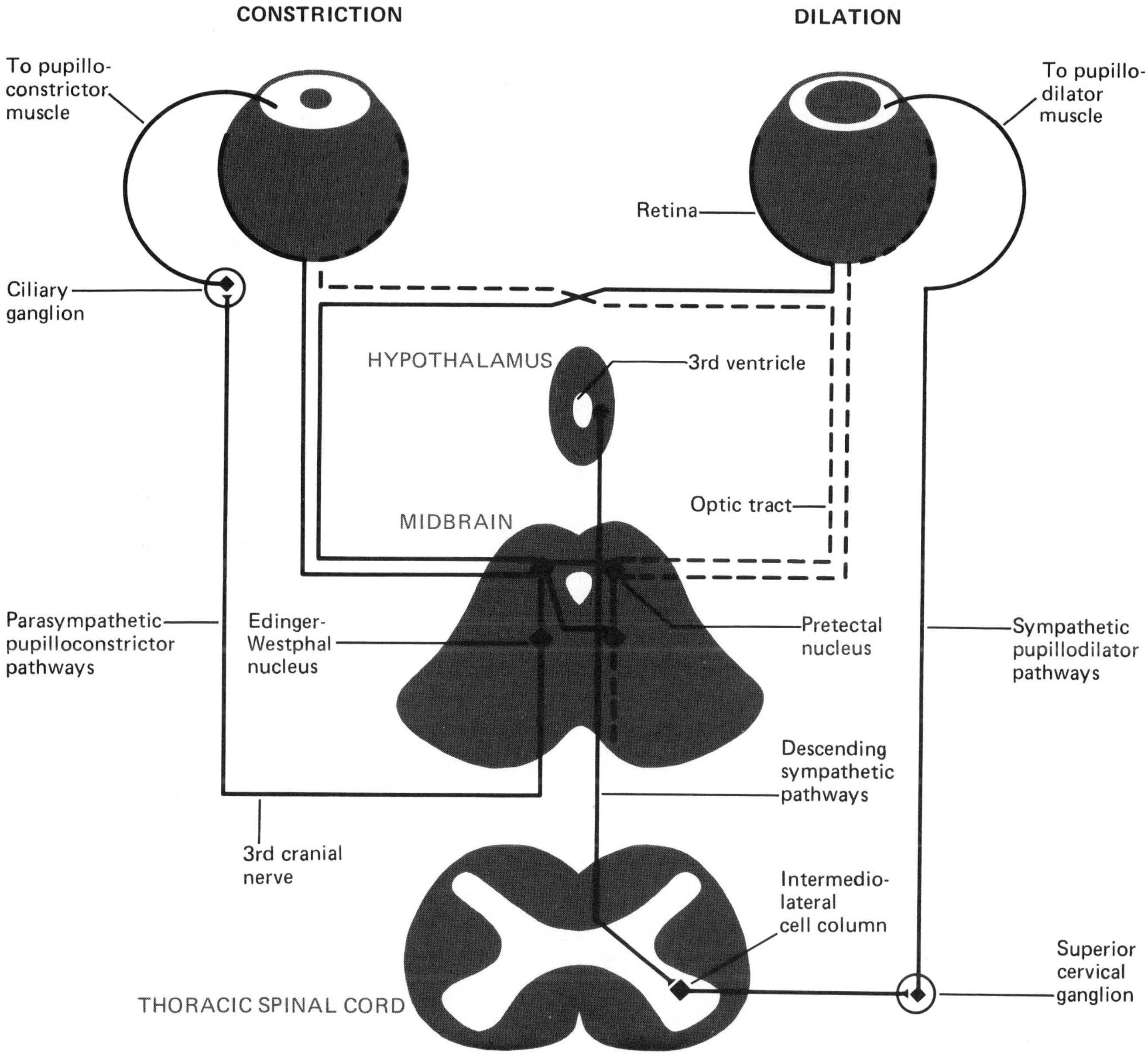

Figure 18.2. Pupillary control.

control, observations on this system provide few localizing clues in the diagnosis of coma.

Pupil Size and Light Responsiveness

Pupillary size and light responsiveness hold the key to structural disturbances involving the pontine tegmentum, midbrain, and diencephalon, i.e., the anatomic locus of the arousal mechanism. The autonomic nervous system strongly affects pupillary size and reactivity: parasympathetic activity contracts the pupil, and sympathetic stimulation dilates it. As both systems are continually active, the resulting pupillary size reflects their relative degree of ongoing activity. If either system is blocked there will be near maximum expression of the remaining system's unopposed tonic activity, resulting either in marked constriction or wide dilation of the pupil. If both systems are affected, the pupil will be midsized and poorly reactive or unreactive to light (Fig. 18.2).

Light striking the retina ultimately excites ganglion cells whose axons course through both optic tracts to synapse with the pretectal nuclei of the midbrain. Pretectal nuclear fibers pass to both Edinger-Westphal nuclei directly or through dorsal and ventral tracts around the aqueduct. As decussation of the light pathway occurs both at chiasmatic and pretectal levels, there is a sound anatomic basis for direct and consensual pupillary responses. The existence of cerebral parasympathetic preganglionic fibers is unknown. The major source of preganglionic fibers is thought to be the Edinger-Westphal nuclei of the midbrain tegmentum closely associated with the third nerve nuclei. Parasympathetic fibers pass with the third nerve through the brainstem and to the orbit, synapsing in the ciliary ganglion, which sends nerve fibers to the pupilloconstrictor muscle of the iris.

Although the sympathetic system may have cerebral representation, its presence in the hypothalamus is better recognized. The descending sympathetic system probably passes through the dorsal tegmentum of the midbrain while taking a more dorsolateral position in the pons, medulla, and cervical spinal cord before synapsing with preganglionic nerve cells in the intermediolateral cell column of the upper three thoracic, and possibly lower, cervical spine segments. Preganglionic fibers then pass to the superior cervical ganglion, and postganglionic fibers travel with the internal carotid artery. Ultimately, they enter the orbit with the oculomotor nerves and ophthalmic branch of the trigeminal nerve to innervate the pupillodilator fibers of the iris and Mueller's palpebral muscle.

In their excellent monograph on stupor and coma, Plum and Posner make the following observations on the localizing value of pupillary abnormalities in comatose patients:

1. Cerebral effects have no localizing value.
2. Injury to the ventrolateral and posterior portions of the hypothalamus result in an ipsilateral Horner's syndrome including ptosis and miosis. This may be the first sign of impending transtentorial herniation. The pupils may be symmetrically small when the diencephalon is bilaterally involved during rostrocaudal deterioration, but reaction to light is retained.
3. Midbrain dorsal tectal or pretectal lesions that interrupt the light reflex pathways produce midposition or slightly widened pupils that are light fixed but react to accommodation and may spontaneously fluctuate in size.
4. Nuclear midbrain damage from local lesions or with transtentorial herniation that interrupts both sympathetic and parasympathetic pathways results in light fixed midposition or unequal irregular pupils.
5. Lesions of the third nerve nucleus and intraparenchymal fibers result in widely dilated pupils and oculomotor paralysis that may be frequently bilateral, whereas peripheral third nerve lesions result in unilateral signs of a similar nature. When compressive lesions involve the third nerve peripherally, pupillary dilation may be the first sign of impingement on the nerve and of uncal herniation.
6. Pontine tegmentum lesions affect the descending sympathetic pathways and produce very small but light-responsive pupils.
7. Lateral medullary and cervical spinal cord lesions cause ipsilateral mild Horner's syndrome.
8. Optic nerve lesions result in decreased or lost direct light reflex and preservation of the consensual response in the same eye.

Local eye disease, many drugs, and some metabolic disturbances can affect pupillary responsiveness and size. Atropine and related compounds can cause dilated, fixed pupils, whereas glutethimide may give fixed mid- to moderately dilated and unequal pupils. Opiates may give pinpoint but light-responsive pupils, whereas drugs used in glaucoma treatment give very small unreactive pupils. Barbiturate intoxication may cause fixed, small pupils.

Anoxia, ischemia, or circulatory arrest usually causes widely dilated fixed pupils, but at times pupillary constriction may be seen until asystole occurs or cardiac output is reduced significantly. Anoxic pupillary dilation lasting longer than a few minutes is an ominous sign suggesting severe and usually irreversible brain damage, but in younger patients recovery may occur. Hypothermia can give fixed pupils, and anisocoria has been reported transiently during or following seizures.

As pointed out by Plum and Posner, with the above metabolic and pharmacologic exceptions, small pupils may accompany many metabolic encephalopathies. However, the light reflex is preserved and can serve as an important differentiating point between structural lesions of the midbrain and metabolic disturbances causing coma.

Eye Movement

There are three main areas of the central nervous system that affect conjugate or yoked eye movements; that is, where both eyes move together in the same direction (Fig. 18.3). These areas are in the frontal and occipital lobes and the labyrinthine vestibular system associated with the brainstem. Each area is a paired system with left- and right-sided tonically active components. The left-sided structures tend to push the eyes to the right and vice versa. The resulting eye position depends on the balance between relative degrees of activity in the paired systems. Stimulation of one side will drive the eyes to the opposite side, and if one side's activity is reduced or inhibited, then the relatively unopposed ongoing or tonic activity of the uninfluenced side will drive the eyes to the inhibited or less active side.

Brodmann's area 8, or the frontal gaze center, influences rapid voluntary eye movements. Stimulation of this area, including focal seizure activity, drives the eyes to the opposite side; bilateral stimulation produces upward movement. Destructive lesions may impair voluntary eye movement away from the side of the lesion or result in the tonic or ongoing activity of the intact side, driving the eyes toward the injured side. Brodmann's area 18, the so-called occipital gaze center, influences tracking or pursuit eye movements. Fibers from both areas 8 and 18 ultimately descend to the midbrain and pontine medial reticular formation where the final neural interconnections subserving vertical and lateral conjugate eye movements are found. Eye movements are strongly influenced by the labyrinthine vestibular system, but this influence is normally suppressed by activity in the frontal and occipital lobes. With reduction of such cerebral activity, stimulation of the labyrinthine system in the presence of

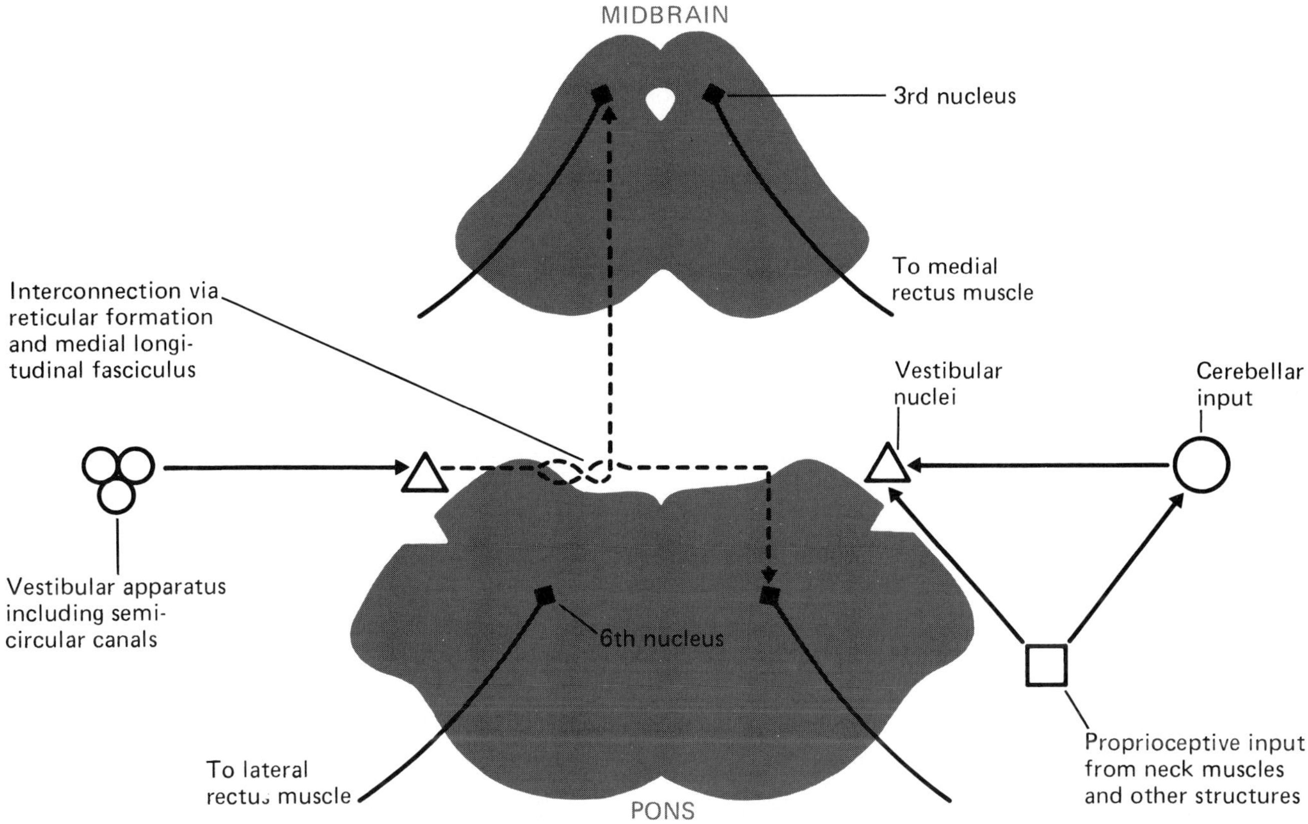

Figure 18.3. Control of lateral eye movement.

an intact midbrain and pontine tegmentum results in conjugate eye movement to the side opposite the stimulation. Also, proprioceptive activity from the joints, ligaments, and muscles of the neck passes at least through the lower portion of the medial longitudinal fasciculus and under certain circumstances may influence eye movement.

The ultimate connections between the cranial nerve nuclei that act as the final common pathway for vertical and horizontal conjugate or paired eye movement (i.e., the interconnections between the sixth nerve nuclei of the pontine tegmentum and the third and fourth nerve nuclei of the midbrain periaqueductal grey matter) are via the pontine and midbrain paramedian reticular formation and the medial longitudinal fasciculus. These internuclear connections lie adjacent to or pass near the medial portion of the reticular formation, which plays an integral part in the arousal mechanism of consciousness. If these pathways can be shown to be intact, then in all likelihood, the anatomic structures adjacent to them subserving arousal are also likely to be intact, and causes other than brainstem structural lesions must be sought to explain the alteration in consciousness.

There are many ways of examining ocular motility, either voluntarily or reflexly, but in the patient with an alteration in consciousness, the most valuable methods are by observing the oculocephalic or doll's head responses and the oculovestibular or caloric responses. These are brainstem responses: they do not involve the frontal or occipital gaze centers and do not occur in patients who are awake unless they voluntarily fixate or their frontopontine pathways are interrupted bilaterally.

Doll's Head Response

The doll's head response is elicited by holding the eyelids open and rotating the head quickly from side to side. With intact pathways, the eyes deviate to the left when the head is rotated to the right, and vice versa. The eyes deviate upward when the neck is flexed and downward when it is extended. The eyes rapidly return to the resting position after head movement, even if the head position is maintained. This maneuver should not be done where neck injury is suspected; rather, caloric stimulation should be performed then.

The oculocephalic response acts either through the vestibular system or through proprioceptive stimuli from the neck carried through the medial longitudinal fasciculus and reticular formation. Head turning produces currents in the endolymph of the semicircular canal that flow toward and stimulate receptors in the ampulla on the side toward which the head is turned. At the same time, currents flow away from the ampulla and its receptors in the semicircular canal of the opposite side, producing relative inhibition on that side. Stimulation of the ampullar receptors produces tonic deviation of the eyes to the side opposite the stimulation or toward the relatively inhibited side.

Caloric Stimulation

When performing this procedure, be sure the external ear canal is clear and the tympanic membrane is intact. Then, with the patient supine, raise the head 30° from the horizontal so that the horizontal semicircular canal is vertical. Place a small catheter in the external canal, slowly run ice water against the tympanic membrane, and watch for eye movement. Plum and Posner recommend that 120 ml of ice water be used before considering the response to be absent in comatose patients. With decreased consciousness, the eyes are tonically carried toward the side irrigated with ice water. Nystagmus may be seen, but usually the eyes tonically deviate for 2–3 minutes and then assume their original position. Wait 5 minutes before testing the opposite side to allow for stabilization of the system. Bilateral simultaneous ice water irrigation deviates the eyes downward, whereas warm water deviates the eyes upward when the brainstem and vestibular connections are intact.

Warm water produces convection currents in the endolymph of the semicircular canal toward the ampulla and results in tonic deviation of the eyes to the opposite side. Cold water results in relative inhibition or decrease in activity on the side irrigated. As the vestibular system is tonically active at rest, any decrease in activity on one side will result in the tonically active side driving the eyes to the opposite side. Stimulation of the horizontal semicircular canal excites the contralateral lateral rectus and ipsilateral medial rectus muscles via medial longitudinal fasciculus and medial reticular formation interconnections, resulting in conjugate deviation of the eyes to the side opposite the stimulation. Ice water has the opposite effect, as noted above. As it is a more potent stimulus in comatose patients, caloric testing is more likely to evoke a response than the doll's head maneuver.

Abnormalities of Eye Movement

Again, Plum and Posner have organized the important observations on abnormalities of ocular movement and position in patients with alterations in consciousness. Their monograph should be consulted for a detailed description of these abnormalities, which are summarized below.

1. In normal awake or in hysterical patients, the eyes usually look straight ahead at rest. Doll's head responses are usually absent, and caloric stimulation produces nystagmus, rather than tonic deviation.
2. With bihemispheric cerebral or basal ganglia dysfunction, cortical influences may be lost, and the eyes may be straight ahead, slightly divergent, or roving slowly and randomly. Doll's head responses are present, and caloric testing produces tonic lateral deviation of the eyes. Irritative hemispheric lesions, such as seizure activity, drive the eyes to the opposite side, whereas destructive hemispheric lesions allow the eyes to be driven to the side of the lesion by the tonically active intact side. Doll's head movement or caloric stimulation may overcome these deviations.
3. Spontaneous nystagmus is uncommon in coma because it requires cerebral cortical influences, but some forms of nystagmoid eye movements do occur spontaneously or with stimulation and may have localizing value. For example, retractory nystagmus in which the eyes irregularly jerk back into the orbit may be seen in midbrain tegmental lesions, presumably as a result of the simultaneous contraction of all the ocular muscles along with convergence nystagmus.
4. With lesions of the pretectal or midbrain tectotegmental area, the eyes are immobile and rest straight ahead. Reflex upward gaze is abolished. Downward eye deviation suggests midbrain compression, rather than destruction.
5. Oculomotor nerve or nuclear involvement affects all ipsilateral doll's head and caloric reflexes except those of the external rectus muscle.
6. Midbrain or pontine lesions involving the medial longitudinal fasciculus yield an internuclear ophthalmoplegia in which the eye ipsilateral to the lesion fails to adduct when the other eye abducts. Both eyes may fail to adduct. Medial longitudinal fasciculus dysfunction is seen with structural lesions, rather than metabolic disturbances, except perhaps with barbiturate intoxication.
7. Skew or vertical deviation is seen with dorsolaterally placed pontine lesions and with lesions of the medial longitudinal fasciculus.
8. Ocular bobbing, a term introduced by Fisher, describes episodes of intermittent quick downward eye movement with a slow return to the primary position. It is usually seen with severe lower pontine tegmental lesions.
9. Lesions in the area of the abducens nucleus produce lateral conjugate gaze paralysis that is unresponsive to doll's head or caloric testing. Laterally placed unilateral pontine lesions may cause the eyes to deviate conjugately away from the lesion. Failure of abduction of the one eye with adduction of the other suggests a lesion of the abducens nerve below its nucleus.
10. In bilateral brainstem lesions involving the vestibular nuclei or with streptomycin toxicity, caloric responses are absent, but oculocephalic reflexes may be retained because of proprioceptive afferent impulses from the neck traveling in the medial longitudinal fasciculus.

Motor Response

As the structures subserving motor function and consciousness are anatomically separate, they can be affected independently at different levels of the neuraxis. Nevertheless, the motor examination gives information about neurologic dysfunction that may reveal clues about the site, progression, or nature of lesions causing alterations of consciousness. Many patterns of motor dysfunction have limited localizing value, some may signify change in the patient's status or allow better localization.

Cerebral hemispheric dysfunction may produce alterations in tone, such as gegenhalten, and primitive motor responses, such as sucking, snouting, rooting, and grasping. Usually the responses are bilateral, but if they are unilateral they probably still signify bilateral cerebral dysfunction. They may be an early sign of a hemispheric mass and may reflect raised intracranial pressure or metabolic disturbance.

Motor and sensory interactions can be appreciated by noting the patient's motor response to noxious stimuli. One-sided loss of response suggests cortical spinal tract dysfunction anywhere along its course or loss of sensation on that side. Bilateral loss suggests bilateral cortical spinal tract involvement in the brainstem, involvement of the pontomedullary descending reticular formation and associated motor or sensory pathways, or psychogenic causes. Decorticate rigidity describes flexion of the arm, wrist, and fingers; upper limb adduction with extension internal rotation; and plantar flexion of the lower limb. In humans, this posture may be seen with lesions of the high cerebral peduncle, internal capsule, or cerebral hemisphere interrupting the cortical spinal pathways. Vigorous stimuli may be required to elicit the response, but it may occur spontaneously in acute hemispheric destructive and expanding lesions. Decerebrate rigidity describes opisthotonus, teeth clenching, stiffly extended adducted pronated arms, and stiffly extended legs with plantar flexed feet. Decerebration suggests at least partial and bilateral separation of midbrain-pontine structures from higher influences. It is seen in midbrain transections, such as infarction or hemorrhage, that spare the vestibular nuclei and adjacent pontine reticular formation. Decerebration may also be seen during rostrocaudal deterioration involving the midbrain, with posterior fossa lesions that affect the midbrain and upper pons, or with severe metabolic derangements, such as hepatic coma, hypoglycemia, anoxia, or drug intoxication affecting similar areas. Plum and Posner suggest it is preferable to use the terms "abnormal flexor," "abnormal extensor," or "absent response" and describe the limbs in which it is seen. Such a practice allows for more consistency in observation between examiners and reduces the need to assign to the findings precise localizing significance. Similar notation is used in the Glasgow coma scale, which is discussed later.

Decerebrate posturing in the upper limbs, with flaccid or weak flexor responses in the lower limbs, signifies extensive brainstem damage down to or across the pons at the trigeminal level and probable removal of descending vestibular nuclear influences.

Other observations, including plantar responses and tendon, corneal, nasal tickle, gag, or cough reflexes, help assess the patient's responsiveness and determine the structural integrity of different levels of the brainstem. In patients with alterations of consciousness the eyes are usually closed, and if lifted and released, will gradually close—an action impossible to duplicate voluntarily.

Failure to close the eyes suggests facial weakness, and resistance to opening suggests psychological causes, but reflex blepharospasm seen in structural or metabolic diseases may cause a similar response. Blinking to threat or sound suggests that brainstem pathways (particularly the pontine reticular formation) are functioning, as does an upward deviation of the eyes (so-called Bell's phenomenon) in response to corneal stimulation.

It is important to consider what constitutes appropriate noxious stimuli. There is no excuse for using tissue-destructive procedures, such as nipple twisting or testicular pressure, when pressure applied to the periosteum of the supraorbital region or to finger or toenail is almost invariably more than sufficient to elicit motor responses.

Conditions Confused with Coma

Certain clinical conditions superficially appear to alter consciousness, but accurate clinical evaluation will reveal the true anatomic and behavioral situation. In the locked-in syndrome or de-efferented state, paralysis of all four extremities and lower cranial nerves occurs without necessarily altering consciousness. The lesion in the basis pontis affects all descending motor influences, except for vertical eye movement through which the patient may be able to communicate. Mind and intellect are preserved.

The persistent vegetative state (and usually akinetic mutism) is seen in patients who survive severe bihemispheric brain injury without recovery of the content portion of consciousness. Many, but not all, of these patients are akinetic. No matter how severe hemispheric damage is, all patients begin to show sleep and awake cycles within 2–4 weeks, but they are left in a persistent mindless state even though brainstem activity governing arousal and other functions appears to be intact.

It is unclear whether acute lesions involving the dominant hemisphere resulting in global aphasia will reduce alertness, but such patients may seem harder to arouse than expected. Slowly progressive degenerative conditions, such as Alzheimer's disease, will gradually but inexorably affect the content portion of consciousness and may ultimately result in motor and other signs of neurologic dysfunction. Seizure activity, either focal or generalized, may result in postictal signs, including alterations in consciousness and sensory-motor findings that may initially be confusing, but reflect underlying cerebral abnormalities, as noted earlier.

One must also be concerned about the coexistence of structural and metabolic disturbances. A superimposed metabolic disturbance may make a structural lesion appear worse than it is. Or, there may be primary metabolic disturbances superimposed on a long-standing structural lesion that had shown adequate functional compensation, with the old signs manifesting only when the depression of neuronal function caused by the metabolic disturbance allows their expression. After a metabolic disturbance has been corrected it may be several hours before appropriate functional neural activity can be appreciated.

Psychogenic unresponsiveness is uncommon, and such

a diagnosis can be made only after a careful search has ruled out structural or metabolic causes that may not be readily apparent. Such a condition does not usually last long, and pupillary and caloric responses and respirations are usually normal. Eyelid opening may be resisted, and the slow eyelid closure and roving eye movements seen in truly comatose individuals are not present. Generally, deep tendon, plantar, and abdominal reflexes are normal, but the first two can be voluntarily suppressed. The EEG is similar to that seen in an awake patient.

Grouping of Structural Lesions

Alterations in consciousness or coma occur because of structural lesions, metabolic disturbances, or a combination of both. Structural lesions can be separated usefully into two groups, the anatomic demarcation being the folds of dura known as the tentorium cerebelli that divide the posterior fossa (infratentorial compartment and its contents of brainstem and cerebellum) from the anterior and middle fossa (supratentorial compartment with its contents of cerebral hemispheres, basal ganglia, and diencephalon). The two compartments are connected through an opening in the tentorium known as the incisura or tentorial notch (see Figs. 19.1 and 19.2 in Chapter 19). In pathologic states, which result in downward displacement of the supratentorial contents through this opening, the phenomenon of transtentorial herniation occurs. The accompanying changes in the neurologic examination and other physical parameters that show progressive dysfunction from hemispheric through diencephalic to upper brainstem levels are known as rostrocaudal deterioration.

Discrete unilateral hemispheric lesions do not alter consciousness. Rather, consciousness can be altered by diffuse and widespread bilateral involvement of the cortex or underlying white matter. Tissue edema, vascular compression or spasm, an expanding mass of tissue or blood, or obstruction of CSF pathways may cause hemispheric lesions to cross the midline secondarily, compress the contralateral hemisphere, or affect deep midline or diencephalic structures associated with the arousal mechanism and cause coma.

Structural lesions within the brainstem directly affect the arousal mechanism by destroying the reticular formation; if they arise in or about other posterior fossa structures through pressure, vascular, or other phenomena, they may secondarily affect the brainstem reticular formation. Upward herniation of the cerebellum and midbrain through the tentorial notch may compress the midbrain tegmentum; downward herniation of the cerebellar tonsils through the foramen magnum may directly compress the medulla oblongata, which contains the cardiovascular and respiratory control mechanisms.

In all the above situations the rate of change is important: large, rapidly expanding lesions are more likely to produce change in consciousness than small, slowly developing ones, although small strategically placed upper brainstem lesions may rapidly produce coma.

Supratentorial Patterns

One of two patterns is seen with supratentorial lesions causing rostrocaudal deterioration. The first, the so-called central syndrome, occurs more commonly with medial or diffuse lesions that slowly and inexorably impinge upon the diencephalon and midbrain. Initially, changes in alertness, behavior, and respirations occur. Roving eye movements, impaired upward gaze, and small reactive pupils may be seen. A pre-existing hemiparesis is common, but bilateral corticospinal tract signs or primitive motor responses may develop. Decorticate responses followed by decerebration or decerebration alone may then appear. Subsequently, midbrain dysfunction occurs and shows sustained central neurogenic hyperventilation, moderately dilated or fixed midposition and irregular pupils, and caloric-induced dysconjugate eye movements. Progressive pontine dysfunction presents with rapid respirations, fixed and midposition pupils, absent caloric responses, and flaccid limbs. Ultimate medullary dysfunction is reflected in slow irregular respirations, dropping blood pressure, and pulse irregularities. Breathing finally stops, the pupils dilate, and the patient dies.

The second pattern, or so-called uncal hernation, (see Fig. 19.3 in Chapter 19), is usually seen with laterally placed or temporal lobe lesions and has as its earliest sign a unilateral dilating pupil that may be present for hours before subsequent signs of midbrain compression appear. Once other signs appear, progressive deterioration may be alarmingly rapid. Pupillary dilation is followed by progressive third nerve paresis, progressive deterioration of consciousness, and disappearance of caloric responsiveness. As the opposite cerebral peduncle is pushed against the tentorial edge (Kernohan's notch) a hemiparesis or plegia ipsilateral to the lesion occurs, but ultimately bilateral motor abnormalities appear with decerebrate rather than decorticate responses manifesting spontaneously or with external stimuli. The opposite pupil may dilate, but ultimately both become fixed and in midposition as midbrain compression continues. Central neurogenic hyperventilation occurs, and from this point deterioration follows a similar course to that of the central syndrome noted above. The development of the uncal pattern occurs as the temporal lobe spills down over the tentorial edge and in so doing displaces vascular and brainstem structures compromising the third nerve. Occasionally a combination of both syndromes occurs more or less simultaneously, with progression usually as in the central syndrome.

Infratentorial Patterns

Posterior fossa lesions causing coma are either destructive or compressive and are accompanied by discrete pupillary and eye movement abnormalities that make anatomic localization relatively easy. Midbrain lesions frequently compromise the pupillary light reaction and third nerve functions; cerebral peduncle and other motor system involvement usually occurs bilaterally. Lesions of the upper pons spare the pupillary and third nerve function, but damage the medial longitudinal fasciculus, resulting in unilateral or bilateral internuclear ophthalmoplegias. Sympathetic tract involvement yields small or pinpoint but light-reactive, pupils. Facial motor and sensory impairment may be present. Lesions of the lower pons may give pinpoint pupils, absent lateral gaze, ocular bobbing, and quadriplegia or other motor abnormalities, including decerebrate posturing or decerebration of upper limbs with flexion of lower limbs. With posterior fossa lesions, vomiting and hiccuping and other cranial nerve abnormalities may occur.

Occasionally false localizing signs may occur that affect the correct interpretation of discrete neurologic signs accompanying alternations in consciousness. These occur particularly with slowly developing lesions or where significant hydrocephalus or raised intracranial pressure occurs. Through pressure, ischemia, or traction, cranial nerve, brainstem, or cerebellar function may be indirectly affected.

Specific Lesions Causing Coma

Lesions causing coma may be supra- or infratentorial, intra- or extraparenchymal, and may include neoplasms, infections, trauma, and vascular causes. The vascular causes may be secondary to trauma, vascular malformations or aneurysms, or occlusive, embolic, or hemorrhagic cerebrovascular disease. Alteration in consciousness secondary to head injury is dealt with in detail in Chapter 19. It is beyond the scope of this chapter to consider individual structural causes of coma; rather it is more important to recognize when a structural abnormality exists and how to attempt preliminary clinical localization. Contrast and other diagnostic procedures will soon reveal the anatomic correctness, as well as the etiology of these structural abnormalities. It is sufficient to say that vascular causes are frequently sudden, apoplectic, or catastrophic; neoplasms tend to be more insidious and slowly progressive, with the rate of the neurologic deterioration increasing dramatically only when intratumor bleeding occurs or the brain substance and cerebrospinal fluid content can no longer accommodate tumor expansion.

METABOLIC CAUSES

If structural causes of coma can be ruled out, then the third and largest group of causes of alteration in consciousness—the metabolic abnormalities—can be considered.

No characteristic clinical features distinguish one variety of metabolic coma from another. Generally speaking, the conscious level will improve when the metabolic disturbance is corrected, although there may be some delay in the return of appropriate neuronal function. Structural lesions associated with a metabolic defect can often only be assessed in retrospect. Generalized, multifocal, or myoclonic convulsions are common, as are primitive motor signs, tremors, and disorders of postural maintenance, such as asterixis.

Historical information, usually gained from relatives or friends, is important, particularly regarding such disorders as diabetes mellitus, thyroid dysfunction, or possible drug ingestion. Clinical examination may also suggest etiologic possibilities, such as hepatocellular disease, hypothyroidism, and diabetic ketoacidosis.

Pathophysiology

Metabolic encephalopathy may be associated with cardiac, respiratory, hepatic, or renal failure and with endocrine imbalance. The pathophysiologic mechanisms of the resulting cerebral dysfunction are complex, but some important factors to be considered diagnostically or therapeutically are discussed below.

Energy Supply to the Brain

Virtually all the brain's considerable energy requirements must be derived from the oxidative metabolism of glucose. Because there is no reserve oxygen in the brain and only small glucose reserves are present, the supply of these substrates in cerebral blood must be plentiful and constant. The brain uses about 60 mg of glucose and 45 ml of oxygen per minute; these rates account for a quarter and a fifth, respectively, of whole body glucose and oxygen utilization. Failure of energy metabolism may occur as a consequence of a reduction in cerebral blood flow (decreased cardiac output or increased cerebral vascular resistance), lowered blood oxygen tension (respiratory failure), reduced oxygen-carrying capacity of the blood (anemia, carboxy- or methemoglobinemia), and hypoglycemia (insulin overdose, pancreatic adenoma, liver failure).

Acid/Base Disturbance

There is a complex relationship between brain and cerebrospinal fluid (CSF) pH and plasma pH. The pH of the brain is probably more accurately reflected by the pH of the CSF than by that of the plasma. There is at most only a slight reduction in the CSF pH in a metabolic acidosis because the blood-brain barrier has a fairly low permeability to hydrogen ion and bicarbonate. On the other hand, in acute respiratory acidosis or alkalosis, changes in CSF pH follow the changes in plasma pH because the blood-brain barrier is highly permeable to carbon dioxide. These contrasting permeability rates must be kept in mind when treating acidosis. For example, both carbon dioxide and bicarbonate increase in plasma during the treatment of a metabolic acidosis with intravenous bicarbonate administration. However, only the carbon dioxide readily diffuses into the CSF, and as a result the CSF pH may actually fall as the plasma pH rises. This change may be accompanied by the worsening of the neurologic state, so a slow correction of metabolic acidosis is obviously desirable.

Osmolality

Metabolic encephalopathy, or coma, results from an increase in brain water that may occur with both serum hypo-osmolar and hyperosmolar states. The normal serum osmolality is approximately 290 mOsm/kg. Neurologic disturbances generally occur when the serum osmolality is less than 260 mOsm/kg or greater than 325 mOsm/kg, especially when these changes have developed rapidly. Hypo-osmolality results from abnormal water retention, as in the syndrome of inappropriate antidiuretic hormone (ADH) secretion (SIADH) (see Chapter 15) or when there is a state of relative salt loss seen when extracellular fluid volume deficits are enthusiastically replaced with 5% dextrose in water (DWS). Hyperosmolar states occur in dehydration, uremia, and hyperglycemia with or without ketoacidosis. In hyperglycemic coma, the increase in serum osmolality may be accompanied by an even greater increase in brain osmolality that occurs as a compensatory attempt to prevent brain intracellular dehydration. This situation occurs with the formation and accumulation in the brain of "idiogenic osmoles," such as polyols, free amino acids, and glucose. Their movement is very slow through both the brain cell membrane and the blood-brain barrier. Thus, the rapid lowering of serum osmolality during fluid replacement in the hyperglycemic individual will not be accompanied by a concomitant decrease of brain osmolality, and worsening brain edema can occur. The very slow correction of hyperosmolar states is therefore recommended. Similar problems with osmotic shifts are believed to be a factor in the development of the acute encephalopathy that is occasionally associated with coma observed during the rapid hemodialysis of an individual with very high retention of small molecules, such as BUN, creatinine etc. The term "dialysis disequilibrium" has been applied to this phenomenon.

Electrolyte Imbalance

The blood-brain barrier effectively maintains ionic equilibrium in the brain in the presence of acute changes of serum electrolytes. Where chronic electrolyte disturbances exist, then similar alterations will occur in the brain and may lead to functional difficulties. Profound hypocalcemia (as seen in advanced uremia, hyperphosphatemia, severe metabolic acidosis, and osteomalacia) can be associated with an encephalopathy. This condition can be improved by dialysis, together with the administration of large amounts of intravenous calcium. Marked hypophosphatemia, which may be a complication of intravenous hyperalimentation, can be associated with a progressive alteration in consciousness; reduced caloric load and phosphate repletion usually lead to neurologic improvement.

Toxic Metabolites

The effects of the endogenous toxic metabolic products that accumulate in renal and hepatic failure are poorly understood. Uremia is frequently associated with coma, but the patient's neurologic state often correlates poorly with the level of azotemia. Hemodialysis may improve consciousness even when the concentration of urea or creatinine in the dialysate is kept high. Correlation between the neurologic state and the serum ammonia level in cases of hepatic disease may be better, but not invariably so; at times hepatic encephalopathy may be difficult to recognize because evidence of hepatocellular dysfunction need not be profound.

Exogenous toxins accrued by drug and/or alcohol ingestion account for the majority of cases of metabolic coma; they generally act by depressing brain cell function. In some cases there may be more complex interactions, such as the acid/base changes associated with salicylate overdose.

Specific Metabolic Disorders

Postanoxic Encephalopathy

The neurologic sequelae after survival of an episode of acute brain hypoxia range from mild behavioral disturbances, severe intellectual and motor impairment, cortical blindness, and disabling myoclonus to a persistent vegetative state. Postanoxic encephalopathy has become an increasingly common problem in the era of intensive care units, and recent studies suggest that the presence of coma carries a grave prognosis. In one series of 284 patients who survived cardiac arrest, 122 were comatose, and of those only 20% lived and were able to be discharged from hospital. Nearly one-half of those discharged had permanent neurologic defects.

Myxedema Coma

Thyroid hormone has a profound effect on the metabolic rates of many processes in living organisms. Most tissues manifest increased consumption of oxygen in response to T_3 or T_4 administration, and thyroid hormone probably also affects cellular ion transport. In most mammalian cells, the maintenance of normal levels of intracellular ions (sodium, potassium, chloride, and bicarbonate being quantitatively the most important) requires 10–30% of the total energy expended by the cells. Animal studies have shown that the sodium-potassium-activated ATPase system varies according to the availability of active thyroid hormones. Thyroid hormones have many other effects on cellular regulatory functions, in addition to influencing the mitochondria and the cytochrome system. In the absence of active thyroid hormone, all cellular functions become depressed.

Severe hypothyroidism manifests primarily by progressive stupor ending in coma and hypothermia—the so-called myxedema coma. Also, the patient may have CO_2 narcosis with respiratory acidosis, hypoglycemia, hyponatremia, and hypotension. Myxedema coma can occur in both primary or secondary hypothyroidism and generalized pituitary dysfunction. Because emergency treatment is mandatory and it is difficult to exclude associated ACTH deficiency, it is best to use adrenal steroids in the initial therapeutic regime.

All ancillary features of the disease must be treated independently. The hypothermia is corrected by gradual warming; care must be taken to avoid too rapid warming as cardiovascular collapse may occur. Proper hemodynamic monitoring must be performed and any fluid and electrolyte abnormality slowly corrected. Hypercapnia may require treatment by ventilation, and any infection should be treated with the appropriate antibiotic.

Myxedema coma carries a high mortality and usually

affects elderly females. It may be precipitated by infection, cold exposure, or the administration of phenothiazines or other drugs that depress respiratory function. Although the administration of relatively large doses of thyroid hormone to hypothyroid patients may cause cardiovascular complications, it seems that the risk of withholding adequate therapy in myxedema coma is even greater. The administration of up to 40 μg of T_3 followed by 5 μg every 6 hours is therefore appropriate initial therapy for this condition.

Hypoglycemic Coma

Hypoglycemic coma may result in extensive cerebral cortical destruction; all patients with unexplained coma require prompt blood glucose determination and concomitant or immediate intravenous infusion of glucose. Hypothermia is an important clue to hypoglycemia. Although most patients with hypoglycemia experience lightheadedness, dizziness, headache, nausea, palpitations, anxiety, or sweating, the chronic diabetic with sympathetic dysfunction may not have these symptoms and yet may be profoundly hypoglycemic following insulin overdosage.

Hyperosmolar Nonketotic Coma

Hyperosmolar nonketotic coma is a rare syndrome usually found in the noninsulin-dependent elderly diabetic who lives alone. It is often precipitated by an infection or by a cerebrovascular event that leaves the patient uncared for and ultimately markedly dehydrated. Because the thirst mechanism is inhibited or the patient is immobile and cannot obtain fluid, water is usually lost in excess of salt. Profound hypernatremia may then accompany the extremely high blood glucose levels. The condition carries a very high mortality, and few patients with serum sodiums in excess of 160 mEq/liter survive. Water replacement is required and may be achieved by the administration of half-strength saline or dextrose and water. More hypotonic fluids will cause hemolysis and must not be given. Patients are very sensitive to insulin administration, and rapid falls in blood sugar may occur that may lead to the development of cerebral edema. Cerebral edema may be avoided if insulin therapy is stopped when glucose levels have fallen to around 300 mg/100 ml. Slow correction of hypernatremia and hyperglycemia may be best effected by peritoneal dialysis while the volume deficits are corrected under appropriate hemodynamic monitoring.

Pulmonary Disease

The encephalopathy of chronic lung disease probably results from a combination of hypoxemia and hypercarbia. Symptoms may be precipitated acutely in patients with marginal pulmonary function who develop a respiratory infection or take sedatives. In some, hypercarbia may lead to increased intracranial pressure, headache, vomiting, papilledema, and progressive deterioration in consciousness. The occurrence of asterixis and myoclonic jerks, the preservation of pupillary responses, and the absence of other focal neurologic signs, however, suggest the diagnosis of metabolic coma; the etiology is confirmed by the finding of abnormal blood gases.

Liver Disease

Encephalopathy may accompany acute hepatic failure from hepatitis or toxic cellular damage, or it may complicate chronic liver disease. In the latter situation, repeated bouts of acute hepatic coma may be precipitated by factors that increase the production of ammonia (gastrointestinal bleeding, excessive protein intake, uremia), by alkalosis that enhances the penetration of ammonia into the brain, or by less specific factors, such as fever, sedation, and electrolyte imbalances. Incipient hepatic coma may be accompanied by EEG abnormalities, which consist of diffuse theta rhythms during the confusional stage, progressing to synchronous triphasic delta waves as the encephalopathy worsens. The clinical and EEG changes are generally reversible, but occasionally permanent neurologic sequelae develop. Approaches to therapy emphasize protein restriction, gut cleansing, and induction of intestinal bacterial stasis. Lactulose, a synthetic disaccharide useful in the management of hepatic encephalopathy, is degraded in the colon by bacterial lactulases, thereby acidifying the colon and producing an osmotic diarrhea. Attempts to remove the toxins causing hepatic encephalopathy (including ammonia, methionine derivatives, and biogenic amines) have been made using charcoal and resin hemoperfusion, by dialysis using an acrylonitrile membrane, or by plasma exchange. There is no convincing evidence that any of these latter modalities work (for further details, see Chapter 30).

Reye's Syndrome

Reye's syndrome is an acute hepatic disorder of uncertain cause that occurs in children, often after a viral illness. The clinical features are protracted vomiting and diffuse encephalopathic manifestations, and hypoglycemia and hyperammonemia are frequent. Characteristic changes found on liver biopsy include abnormal mitochondria and widespread infiltration with small droplets of fat. Mitochondrial enzyme activity is decreased. Death usually results from increased intracranial pressure. Probably the most important aspect in the management of the child with this syndrome is careful monitoring of the intracranial pressure. If this is elevated, then the use of steroids and osmotic dehydrating agents, such as mannitol, is of value. Barbiturate coma as a means of decreasing intracranial pressure has been used in Reye's syndrome and might offer the most promise for survival. The administration of citrulline has been suggested because this agent allows the urea cycle to proceed via an extramitochondrial pathway and thereby reduces ammonia formation. Other measures to remove ammonia and other toxic metabolites include peritoneal dialysis, charcoal hemoperfusion, and plasma exchange, but their value is debatable.

Uremia

An encephalopathy may result from the metabolic disorders associated with uremia, but as previously mentioned, there is very poor correlation between the degree of encephalopathy and the concentration of currently measured uremic toxins. The neurologic syndrome has no characteristic features, and it is often difficult to distinguish uremic from hypertensive encephalopathy, a condition that often occurs in the individual with advanced renal failure. The presence of papilledema and focal neurologic signs is more typical, however, of the hypertensive state. Furthermore, the clinical picture may be complicated by subdural hematomas, Wernicke's encephalopathy, electrolyte imbalances, and hyperosmolar states. All of these must be considered and corrected if found. Encephalopathy may, indeed, result from the correction of uremia and its associated disorders by dialysis, i.e., the dialysis disequilibrium syndrome previously mentioned.

A progressively fatal encephalopathy associated with chronic dialysis treatment was recently described as dialysis dementia. It is associated with progressive confusion, psychosis, cognitive defects, aphasia or mutism, focal neurologic signs, and myoclonus. Eventually, the patients become comatose and die. There appear to be no specific neuropathologic findings at autopsy, but in some series excessive concentrations of aluminum were found in the brains of patients who died from this disorder. There may be a correlation between the aluminum content of dialysate and this syndrome, as the use of pure water (treated by reverse osmosis and deionization) seems to prevent its occurrence in dialysis units. Whether aluminum hydroxide agents, used as phosphate binders in uremia, can influence the development of this syndrome is unclear. As yet there is no treatment for this encephalopathy once it has occurred.

Drug Overdose

Drug overdose remains the commonest cause of metabolic coma and, therefore, must always be excluded. The management of patients with severe drug intoxications is so important that a separate chapter, Acute Poisonings (Chapter 32), deals with this subject.

INVESTIGATION AND MANAGEMENT

A flow diagram for the investigation and management of the patient with alteration in consciousness is shown in Figure 18.4. First, ensure that the patient's airway and respiratory status are secure, then evaluate and as far as possible control the hemodynamic system. When cardiopulmonary function has at least been temporarily stabilized, blood should be drawn for the assessment of metabolic factors, including drug excess that may be contributing to the pathologic state. In any situation of concern, a bolus of glucose should be given intravenously to correct a potential hypoglycemic state, and at the same time intravenous thiamine should be given to correct or prevent the development of Wernicke's encephalopathy. Seizures, if present, should be treated with intravenous diazepam, phenytoin, or phenobarbital.

Patients in coma suspected of having an underlying metabolic cause should particularly be observed for evidence of trauma, prior venipunctures (such sites as the saphenous vein, popliteal fossa, dorsal vein of the penis, sublingual veins, and neck veins should be examined closely), peristaltic activity, and signs of pre-existing cardiovascular, respiratory, hepatic, or renal disease. Erythematous and bullus skin lesions, especially at the sites of pressure or agitation-related trauma, are characteristic of drug-induced coma. Assuming a drug-induced coma, it is important to determine the agent used and the doses taken at the time of ingestion (information in the patient's wallet or purse may provide useful clues, as may gastric contents).

Toxicology services are valuable in identifying drugs and poisons and in guiding therapy. Appropriate clinical and biochemical leads should be followed for further investigation and management.

Once these preliminary maneuvers have been carried out, the nervous system may be assessed in the following manner. Assess or reaffirm spontaneous respiratory patterns and evaluate pupillary reactivity and size, as well as doll's head or caloric responses. Record the best motor response to noxious stimuli, and observe any asymmetries suggesting sensory or descending motor tract dysfunction. As outlined previously, these observations for the most part will allow the division of causes of coma into structural or metabolic categories. If structural abnormalities are suspected or present, they can be divided usually into supra- and infratentorial causes on the basis of these observations, and special investigations should be arranged where available. These investigations include skull x-rays, computed tomography, isotope brain scanning, or cerebral angiography. If such studies are not available and a space-taking lesion (be it tumor or of infectious or of vascular origin) is suspected, then consultation with a neurologic or neurosurgical service with option for transfer is mandatory.

Where available, the EEG may provide useful diagnostic, management, and prognostic clues in the comatose patient. Its current value may be greatest in assessing patients with metabolic abnormalities or where such therapeutic measures as barbiturate coma, hypothermia, and neuromuscular paralysis have been instituted.

Lumbar puncture can be dangerous in patients with masses or expanding intracranial lesions. Transtentorial or foramen magnum herniation may occur due to potential pressure gradients between different compartments of the intracranial cavity and the lumbar subarachnoid space. When evidence or concern about raised intracranial pressure is present, no lumbar puncture should be performed. The only exception should be where infection is strongly suspected and only after the presence of an intracranial space-taking lesion has been ruled out. Complications usually arise within 12 hours of lumbar puncture, and so the procedure should be carried out at such a time as to allow for careful monitoring during that critical period.

Current Concepts of Treatment

Injury to the CNS is in part related to primary events, such as trauma, ischemia, anoxia, tumor, infections, or

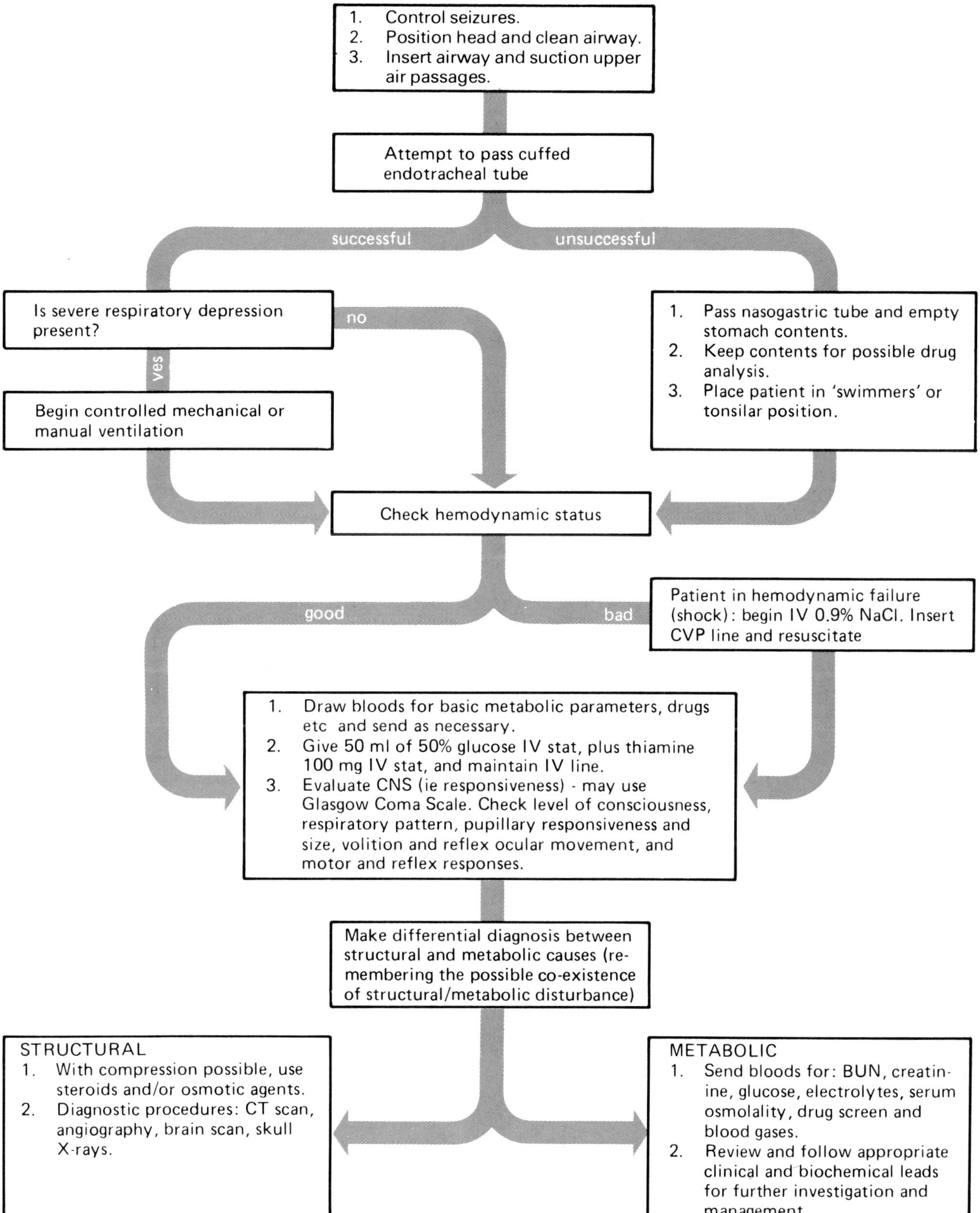

Figure 18.4. Investigation and management of the comatose patient.

toxins, and in part to secondary events occurring as a result of such insults. Cellular membrane changes, intracellular organelle and biochemical dysfunction, and the role of free radicals are assuming more importance in the understanding of these secondary events. Damage may be fixed and irreversible, or functional and potentially reversible. Not only must therapy be directed toward correcting or ameliorating the primary cause but also toward preventing or correcting the secondary events. These efforts may prevent or reduce the extent and severity of the potential neurologic deficit.

Protection may be afforded before the event occurs, as when hypothermia or barbiturates are used before elective surgical procedures requiring circulatory arrest, or possibly after the event has occurred, particularly in situations of anoxia, ischemia, and raised intracranial pressure. These efforts may include general measures, such as improvement in cardiopulmonary, hepatic, or renal function; correction of metabolic or endocrine disorders; treatment of infection; and the like. Raised intracranial pressure may occur early and incipiently in many conditions; its effect is frequently deleterious and at times irreversible and fatal. Its early detection and treatment before secondary events occur are appropriate, but require precise monitoring that may be beyond the capabilities of many units. Methods to control raised intracranial pressure include hyperventilation and curarization; cerebrospinal fluid drainage; steroids; dehydration with such agents as mannitol, glycerol, and diuretics; barbiturate narcosis; hypothermia; and, at times, surgical decompression.

Large doses of steroids, particularly dexamethasone, (20–100 mg daily), have been used with particular success in the reduction of brain swelling resulting from primary or secondary brain tumors and at times after trauma. Similar benefit in ischemic and hemorrhagic brain disease is not well established. Large doses of steroids may stabilize cellular membranes, reduce edema, scavenge free radicals, decrease CSF production, and possibly increase the seizure threshold.

Mannitol and glycerol, as well as dextran and albumin, act in part by raising serum osmolality and so attract water from the intracellular and interstitial regions into the vascular compartment. Because water but not sodium is removed, these agents only reduce tissue edema as long as the osmotic gradient favors the intravascular compartment. They may also improve cerebral blood flow through a mechanism that is not dependent upon their effects on intracranial pressure, but they do not improve cellular membrane integrity and are not effective in areas where the blood-brain barrier is damaged. Ultimately, rebound swelling occurs when the extravascular osmolality increases. Diuretics, such as ethacrynic acid, furosemide, and acetazolamide, may reduce intracranial pressure by decreasing CSF formation and by reduction of interstitial edema. If possible such therapies should be titrated by monitoring intracranial pressure and serum osmolalities. It is well to remember that brain shrinkage may promote the occurrence of subdural bleeding.

Increased body temperature increases cerebral metabolism, and permanent neurologic injury may occur at elevated temperatures. Hypothermia may protect the brain before or during ischemia or from other insults through the retardation of ATP depletion and lactacidemia. Also, it may decrease brain metabolism generally, reduce edema formation, and protect enzyme activity. Nevertheless, the benefits of cooling are not entirely accepted; in fact it may be deleterious because of its effect on other organ systems, such as the myocardium. Control is difficult, and if shivering and vasoconstriction occur, the intracranial pressure and oxygen consumption may be increased. It is potentially arrhythmogenic and may increase blood viscosity and reduce resistance to infection. Its value after an insult has occurred is still being debated.

Barbiturate Therapy

Barbiturate therapy or narcosis has been advocated to reduce ischemic brain damage after stroke or cardiac arrest and to reduce raised intracranial pressure resulting from a variety of conditions including head trauma, Reye's syndrome, subarachnoid and intracerebral hemorrhage, and encephalopathies of metabolic, viral, or hypoxic origins. The application of this technique requires the careful monitoring of intracranial pressure and cerebral electrical activity as the usual clinical reflections of deterioration are obscured by the therapy itself. The rationale for using barbiturates in patients with increased intracranial pressure is that they reduce the cerebral metabolic rate and cerebral blood flow. This results in a decrease in brain intravascular pressure and blood volume and thus a reduction in intracranial pressure. Also, a potential benefit is a decrease in vasogenic cerebral edema and the scavenging of free radicals known to injure cell membranes, including vascular endothelium. As such therapy is a major undertaking and the patient has to be anesthetized for a long period of time, it should be employed only when other simpler methods have proved ineffective. Such therapy subjects the patient to potentially dangerous arterial hypotension, and problems of pulmonary gas exchange arise. Too, its value is still being debated and trials on its use are continuing. Therefore, it should only be used where the patient's status can be strictly monitored and controlled.

GLASGOW COMA SCALE

Once the patient is in an intensive care or other unit and while the causes of alterations in consciousness are being investigated, some form of bedside testing should be established to estimate whether the patient's condition is deteriorating or improving. These tests should be reproducible, practical, and readily used by observers with different levels of sophistication and experience. A system known as the Glasgow Coma Scale has been devised by Teasdale and Jennett for the assessment of patients with head injury and is useful in the continued assessment of patients with other neurologic and metabolic conditions producing alterations in consciousness. Records should also be kept of pupil size and reactivity, eye movements, motor functions, body temperature, pulse and respiratory rate, arterial blood pressure, and other pertinent data so that changes may be recognized early and appropriate diagnostic and therapeutic measures instituted. Other continuously monitored parameters may include central venous pressure, hourly urine volumes, arterial blood gases, serum electrolyte levels, blood counts, liver function tests, serum creatinine, myocardial enzyme levels, and blood drug levels.

These records should be kept on a flow sheet, such as the observation chart here reproduced (Fig. 18.5), which includes the Glasgow scale. The following tests outline the use of the scale and how assessment is made. As noted before, it is difficult to define various levels of consciousness, and frequently methods of stimulation and recording of observations vary so considerably that they are of little value. The Glasgow Coma Scale uses observations on three behavioral parameters: eye opening, verbal response, and best motor response.

Eye opening may be graded as spontaneous opening, opening to speech, opening to pain, or no eye opening. Spontaneous eye opening implies that brainstem arousal mechanisms are functioning. One must take into account sleep-awake cycles and their reversal in some brain-damaged patients. Opening to speech requires spoken stimulus and nothing else, shouting may be required, and the patient's name may be used. Opening to pain is in response to physical stimuli, the best being simple nail-bed pressure using a pen or pencil for application. There is no practical value in other stimuli or grading. No eye opening implies a significant impairment of the arousal system.

Verbal responses may be graded as oriented, confused conversation, inappropriate words, incomprehensible sounds, or no verbal response. Orientation includes appropriate responses to questions relating to identification of self and place and a reasonable assessment of time, including month and year. Confused conversation indicates the patient is capable of producing language and even conversation, but is not oriented. Inappropriate words suggest the patient has occasional utterances, including swearing, which are usually obtained by physical rather than verbal stimuli. Incomprehensible sounds include groans, moans, or indistinct mumbling without any intelligible words. No verbal response indicates that repeated stimulation does not produce any phonation.

Best motor response includes obedience to commands and response to pain. Response to pain is divided as follows: flexion response, extension response, and no response to pain. Obedience to commands means the patient can appreciate instructions given verbally, by gesture or writing. Specific movements are requested after the patient has been maximally aroused. Simple finger squeezing is not an appropriate test for many reasons. If the patient does not respond to verbal exhortation, physical stimuli are applied. Localizing to pain requires the patient to move a limb in an appropriate attempt to remove the stimulus. A flexion response suggests the patient cannot localize the stimulus, but can at least flex the arm at the elbow when finger tip pressure is applied. An extension response is similar to decerebrate rigidity in which the shoulder inwardly rotates, the elbow extends, the wrist flexes, and the fingers extend. No response to pain indicates that repeated and varied stimuli evoke no apparent movement or limb tone change.

Limitations

Some practical problems may arise in using the Glasgow Coma Scale. The lids may remain open if drawn back in deeply comatose patients, and local pathology, such as swelling, may prevent eyelid opening. Aphasic patients may have an impaired verbal response and severe deafness; the presence of an endotracheal tube and lack of facility in the local language may provide further communicative barriers. Motor response means response in the arms and not the legs because a reflex withdrawal response in the legs may operate at a spinal level. Response may vary according to the site of stimulation, and a unilateral paresis should be noted separately. According to Teasdale, the finger-tip pressure method has proved to be the most reliable for eliciting such responses.

The use of such a scale, coupled with vital sign observations, pupillary responsiveness and size, and limb movement, allows for the ongoing assessment of a patient's neurologic status and can reflect early change in neurologic function. Importantly, it is easily standardized and can be readily reproduced by different examiners. In head injury it may also have predictive value, but studies regarding its usefulness in medical coma are still being assessed.

BRAIN DEATH

Any patient admitted to an ICU should be sustained until a primary diagnosis and the likely prognosis are determined. Potentially reversible conditions should be treated aggressively and CNS function assessed as previously outlined. Technically, life can be prolonged when there is no hope of cure and when return of useful cerebral function is not possible. Therefore, in situations of terminal illness and where brain death is evident, questions arise whether and when life-sustaining measures should be stopped. These questions have become critical with the advent of organ transplant and with the practical physical and financial constraints imposed on hospitals.

From the medical, and in most cases the legal, point of view, brain death is accepted as signifying death of the individual. Certain criteria that must be met have been the subject of much debate, but they all confirm that brain death is a condition of impending bodily and somatic death, as well as one of massive brain destruction. Consensus has been reached on the following points:

1. The basic cause of brain death must be fully established, and the patient must be deeply comatose.
2. All appropriate diagnostic and therapeutic procedures must be performed.
3. There should be no suspicion that the state is due to depressant drugs or primary hypothermia; other metabolic and endocrine disturbances must also be excluded.

Section	Subsection	Item	Score	Notes
DATE		MONTH/YEAR		
		DAY		
TIME				
LEVEL OF CONSCIOUS		ALERT		R = RESTLESS
		DROWSY		
		STUPOROUS		
		COMA		
GLASGOW COMA SCALE	Eyes Open	Spontaneously	4	S = Eyes swollen shut
		To Speech	3	
		To Pain	2	
		None	1	
	Best Verbal Response	Orientated	5	T = Endotracheal tube or tracheostomy
		Confused	4	
		Inappropriate	3	
		Incomprehensible	2	
		None	1	
	Best Motor Response	Obeys	6	Record the BEST limb response.
		Localizes	5	
		Withdraws	4	
		Abno.Flexion	3	
		Extension	2	
		Flaccid	1	
TOTAL SCORE				
LIMB MOVEMENT	ARMS	Normal Power		RECORD:
		Mild Weakness		R = RIGHT
		Severe Weakness		L = LEFT
		Spastic Flexion		E = IF EQUAL
		Extension		
		No Response		
	LEGS	Normal Power		
		Mild Weakness		
		Severe Weakness		
		Extension		
		No Response		
PUPILS	Right	Size		REACTION:
		Reaction		✓ = Brisk
	Left	Size		— = Sluggish
		Reaction		= = Fixed
				S = Swollen Shut
Pupil Scale (m.m.) 1, 2, 3, 4, 5, 6, 7, 8	BLOOD PRESSURE	220		
		210		
		200		
		190		
		180		
		170		
		160		
		150		
		140		
		130		
		120		
	PULSE RATE (in red)	110		
		100		
		90		
		80		
		70		
		60		
	Respiration	50		
		40		
		30		
		20		
		10		
TEMPERATURE °C				

Rev. 4/81 — 8460-2920-5

Figure 18.5. Neurologic record.

4. The patient has to be maintained on a ventilator because spontaneous respirations have become inadequate or ceased. Relaxants and other drugs must be excluded as a cause of respiratory failure.

Other diagnostic criteria for the confirmation of brain death include the following:

1. All brainstem reflexes must be absent. There is a consensus that a dead brainstem signifies brain death. The pupils must be fixed in diameter and unresponsive to light stimulation. Corneal, oculovestibular, and motor responses in a cranial nerve distribution should be absent. There should be no gag reflex or reflex responses to bronchial stimulation by a suction catheter passed down the trachea.
2. No respiratory movements should occur when the patient is disconnected from a respirator for long enough to ensure that the arterial carbon dioxide tension rises above the threshold for stimulation of respiration.
3. It is recognized that spinal cord function can persist after insults have irreversibly destroyed brainstem function. However, there should be no decerebrate or decorticate responses occurring spontaneously or following noxious or other stimuli, because these responses require brainstem activity for their production.

In some situations re-evaluation may be required, and the interval may be as long as 24 hours between test performance, but the criteria for brain death should be present for at least 30 minutes, 6 hours after the onset of coma and apnea.

Certain confirmatory investigations may be carried out, although they are not always needed. The use of these investigations will depend in part, upon local practice and medicolegal requirements. It is now becoming accepted that the EEG is not necessary for the diagnosis of brain death, but in situations where it is available, it should be used and strict technical criteria have been outlined. Cerebral angiography has been advocated to reveal the lack of cerebral blood flow and is used extensively in some European countries. Because it needs to be done to strict technical requirements, cerebral angiography, as with the EEG, may not be practical except in specialized centers.

Although practice varies, either a specialist in medical or surgical neurology or the opinion of two physicians is probably required for the diagnosis of brain death. This is especially true in situations where organ transplant is being considered; members of the transplant team should not be involved in assessing brain death.

It is obvious that the major factor determining the success of continued resuscitative measures is the state of the patient's brain. If it is not functioning, total bodily functions will eventually cease, despite continued measures to prolong cardiopulmonary function. Continuing such efforts only prolongs the anguish of relatives and friends and is a waste of limited health resources. Anyone concerned with establishing criteria for or diagnosing brain death should read the review by Peter McL. Black (1978), the letter to the *Lancet* (1981) by J. G. Robson regarding further recommendations from the United Kingdom Conference, and the Guidelines for the Determination of Death in the *Journal of the American Medical Association* (1981).

Suggested Readings

Black PMcL: Brain death. *N Engl J Med* 299:388–345, 393–401, 1978.

Guidelines for the determination of death. *JAMA* 246:2184, 1981.

Miller JD: Barbiturates and raised intracranial pressure. *Ann Neurol* 6:189–193, 1979.

Plum F, Posner JB: Diagnosis of stupor and coma. In *Contemporary Neurology Series,* ed 3. Philadelphia, FA Davis, 1980.

Robson, JG: Brain death. *Lancet* (letters) 2:365, 1981.

Teasdale G: Acute impairment of brain function: 1. assessing conscious level; 2. observation record chart. *Nurs Times* June 12 and 19, 1975.

CHAPTER 19

Traumatic Injuries of the Central Nervous System

A. Loren Amacher, M.D.

The central nervous system (CNS) is more protected by skeletal buttresses than any other system. Ironically, these very structures that have developed to afford such protection and the inability of neurons to regenerate are frequently the principal factors leading to neurologic catastrophe in traumatic and other insult to the brain and spinal cord.

After infancy, the skull acts as a closed, fixed container under acute conditions. Such a container has a constant volume and a negligible ability to expand—a feature that has been recognized in the Monro-Kellie doctrine that states that the intracranial volume is constant. Only one of the foramina in the skull—the foramen magnum at the craniocervical junction—is of sufficient size to allow for escape of volume (other than venous blood) from the skull. Within the skull cavity itself, the tentorium separates the posterior fossa from the supratentorial compartment; the latter, in turn, is partially divided by the falx cerebri. The cerebral hemispheres communicate across the midline below the falx, and the tentorial incisura permits the brainstem to join with the diencephalon. These openings also allow for blood vessel continuity and for passage of cerebrospinal fluid. Figure 19.1 illustrates some of these features. Such internal compartmentalization within the skull permits differential pressures to develop in some circumstances.

In physiologic conditions, the brain literally floats within the skull, immersed within cerebrospinal fluid. During violent movements of the head—acceleration, deceleration, rotational shearing motion—the skull and brain move at different velocities because they have different inertias. Certain anatomic features within the skull, such as the rough floor of the anterior fossa or the sharp edges of the sphenoid wings (Fig. 19.2), may induce brain injury at those times. Fragments of bone driven into the skull or the sharp edges of a linear skull fracture may lacerate the meninges and the brain surface. Cortical bruising may occur when the brain slaps against a skull

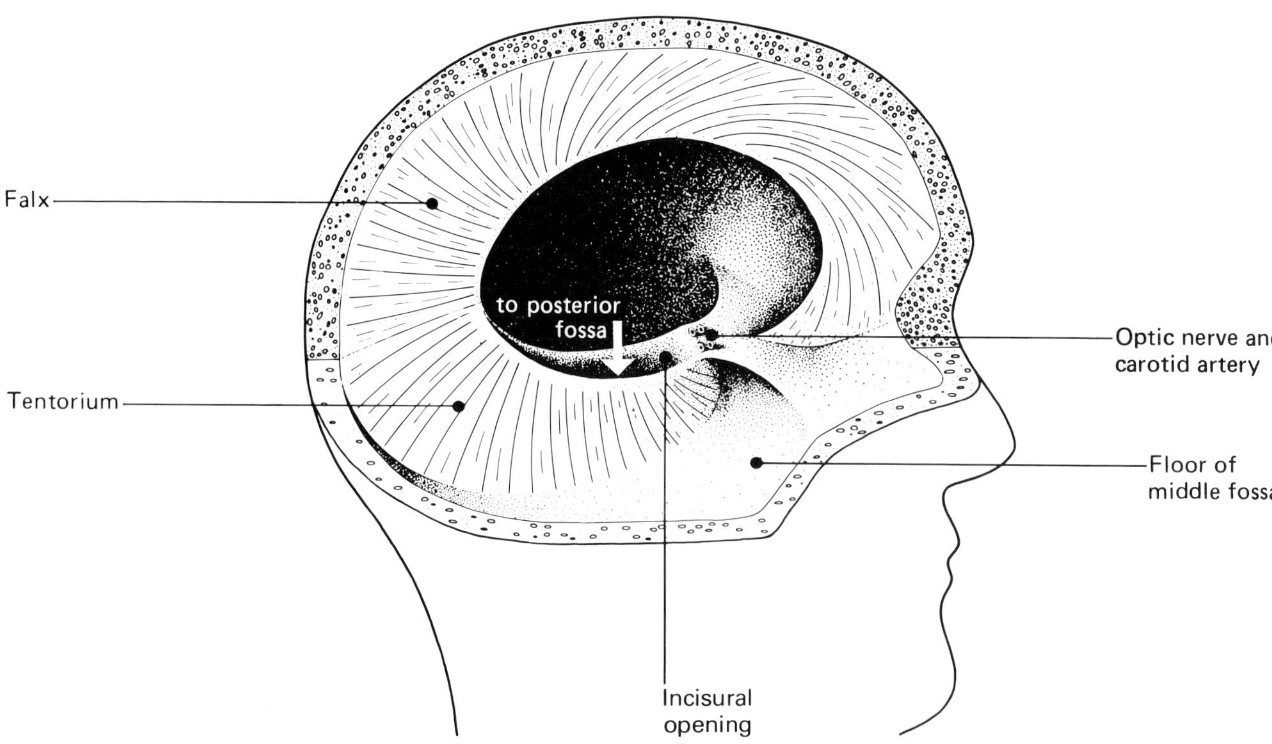

Figure 19.1. Skull interior showing the brain compartments.

surface that has suddenly stopped moving. The inherent instability of the spinal column when forcibly flexed, extended, or twisted beyond natural limits may allow for sudden mass movement of bone with resultant damage to the spinal cord. This is especially likely to occur in the cervical spine.

The shape of the brain resembles that of a mushroom. The heavy cap of the cerebral hemispheres sits upon a thin and compact brainstem. Rotational forces in particular may cause a concentration of kinetic energy in the upper brainstem that is capable of tearing tissue and blood vessels. In addition, the brainstem and the vessels attached to it are in a more fixed position than are the cerebral hemispheres. The spinal cord is tethered laterally by the dentate ligaments, which prevents displacement of the brainstem contents into the spinal canal.

Several vascular structures within the head are particularly susceptible to injury. The middle meningeal arteries, lying between the layers of the dura, may be cut by the scissors action of an overlying fracture at the moment of impact. To gain entrance to the great venous sinuses, the surface cerebral veins must cross the subarachnoid and subdural spaces, and being tethered at either end, they are liable to rupture with sudden violent movement.

The cerebrospinal fluid (CSF) system itself may contribute to intracranial disaster. Seventy percent of CSF is actively produced by the choroid plexuses in the ventricles. CSF absorption is passive and depends upon free passage to the region of the superior sagittal sinus. CSF is produced at a constant rate of 0.35 ml/min irrespective of a rising intracranial pressure (ICP). However, when ICP exceeds mean arterial pressure, intracranial blood flow ceases, and CSF production stops.

MECHANISMS OF CNS INJURY

Kinetic Energy

When the head strikes an object or vice versa, the usual laws of physics apply. Energy is absorbed by the scalp, the skull, and the meninges. Whatever energy remains must be dissipated within the cranial cavity. The brain moves within its cushion of fluid, and secondary impacts may occur. Whether functional or physical disruption of neuronal activity occurs depends upon the magnitude of the force applied and the time course of its activity. In general, the greater the force applied and the shorter the impact time, the more likely there are to be neurologic effects. Fracturing of the skull can be a protective mechanism for the brain because it dissipates energy. It is not uncommon to see patients with large open fractures, even with superficial brain lacerations, who are awake and alert shortly after the accident. But where significant force—particularly shearing or radially vectorized stress—is focused on the brainstem, neuronal tract and vascular disruption may occur, which may prove permanently incapacitating or even fatal. Diffuse axonal injury, a consequence of shearing forces within the brainstem and deep cerebral white matter, is the cause of much of the permanent damage wrought by the movement of the brain during the initial impact. Neuropathologic studies have shown that axons may be disrupted in large numbers even with so-called trivial concussions. Such damage is irreparable.

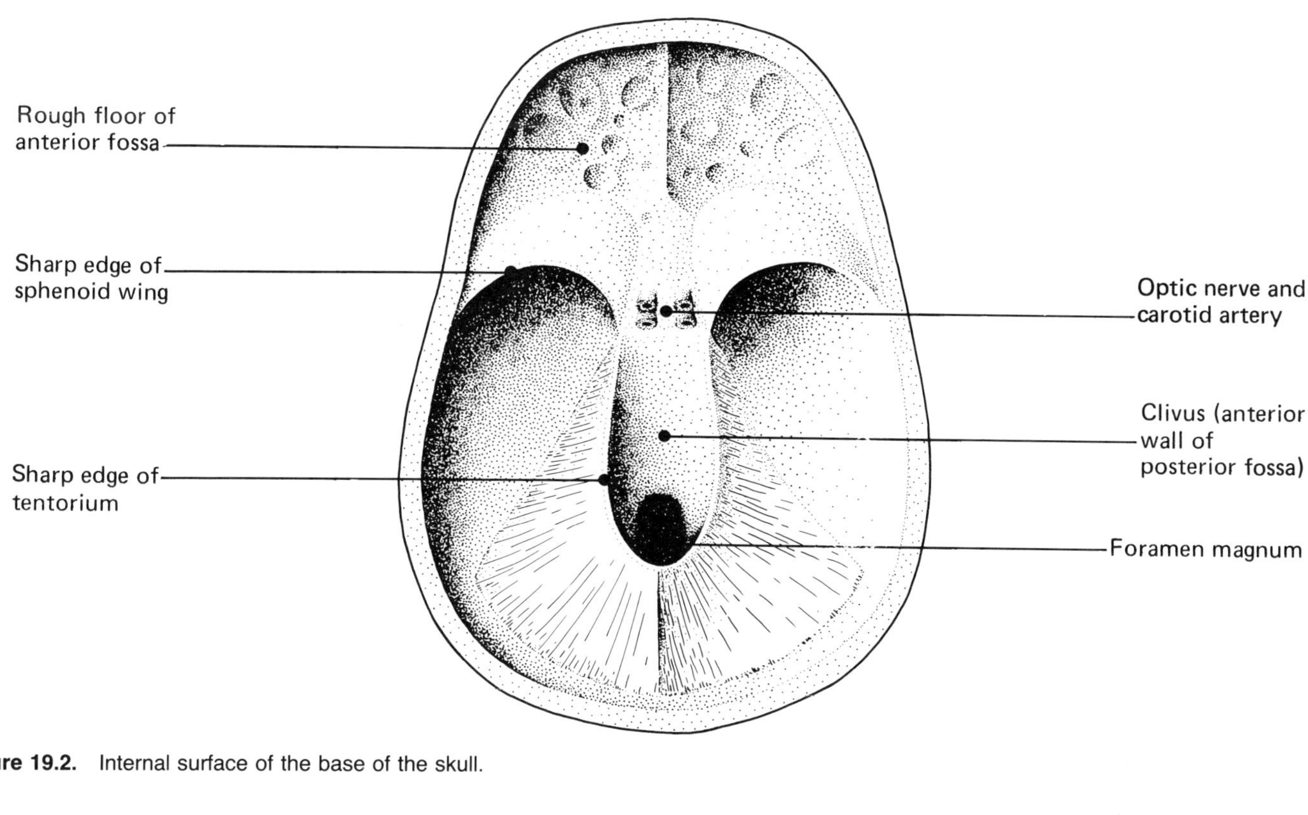

Figure 19.2. Internal surface of the base of the skull.

As suggested previously, the fact that the brain floats within the skull allows direct and rebound (contre-coup) injury to occur at the sites where brain slaps against bone. Cortical contusions at sites remote from the impact area often are caused by this mechanism. It is worth remembering that brain injury may occur without head impact; very sudden and violent extension-flexion-rotatory movements of the head upon the spinal column or strong forces transmitted up the spinal column to the cranium—as produced by a heavy fall onto the legs or spine—may cause brain injury. Penetrating injuries produce injury to the brain or cord by the direct action of the piercing object, be it bone fragment, knife blade, or bullet. Neural tissue is disrupted and blood vessels torn. With high speed projectiles, the effect is compounded by the radial velocity shock wave surrounding the object, which produces a much wider core of destruction.

Vascular Effects

Vascular damage, particularly tearing of venous structures, may occur during the original impact, causing extravasation of blood at low pressures. Likewise, arteries may be torn by direct laceration or by tissue movement when vascular channels are tethered at one or both ends—as in the case of the penetrating vessels arising from the basilar artery. Vascular arterial effects, however, are usually delayed. Torn arteries on the surface pump out blood under high pressure, thereby producing a secondary mass effect. Within the brain, a traumatic hematoma may develop. The shifting of brain tissue may catch an artery against a bony or dural buttress, producing arterial occlusion and distal infarction.

Delayed intracerebral bleeding may occur up to several days following injury. Almost always the hematoma develops in a volume of brain previously noted on CT scan to be edematous or contused. Not infrequently, an intracerebral hematoma of small volume seen on a CT scan done soon after injury will increase significantly in size over hours or days.

Secondary Effects

The consequences of expanding masses (hematomas) and infarctions and the development of cerebral edema are secondary effects. Expanding masses produce differential pressure gradients within the cranial compartments. The brain in acute situations is noncompressible, like a liquid. Because the cranial volume is fixed, any mass lesion expands at the expense of one of the normal components of intracranial volume—brain, blood, and water. To a point, the increasing mass volume is accommodated by the buffering effect of expelling CSF and venous blood from the head. Past that point, which varies with the rate of increase in mass size, the brain must shift. The medial temporal lobe may be pushed up against the midbrain and then down into the posterior fossa (Fig. 19.3). Such increasing pressure on the midbrain interferes with the function of the reticular formation, causing deterioration in the state of consciousness. The shift of the brainstem may cause disruption of the perforating arteries coming off the basilar artery, leading to secondary brainstem hemorrhages and permanent tissue damage. The cerebral peduncles are compressed, causing at first a contralateral hemiparesis and later decerebrate posturing as the brainstem motor nuclei are disconnected from the cerebral cortex. Not infrequently, the opposite cerebral peduncle is pushed onto the tentorial edge, becomes lacerated, and produces an ipsilateral hemiparesis. The posterior cerebral arteries are often caught up in this process, and if they become occluded, infarction within the thalamus, basal ganglia, medial temporal, and occipital lobe results.

Early in the process of tentorial herniation the third cranial nerve is stretched, causing pupillary dilation that almost always occurs first on the side of the expanding mass. This means disaster is imminent. Within the posterior fossa, tissue herniation may occur through the foramen magnum as the intracranial pressure increases. The cerebellar tonsils then become impacted against the lower

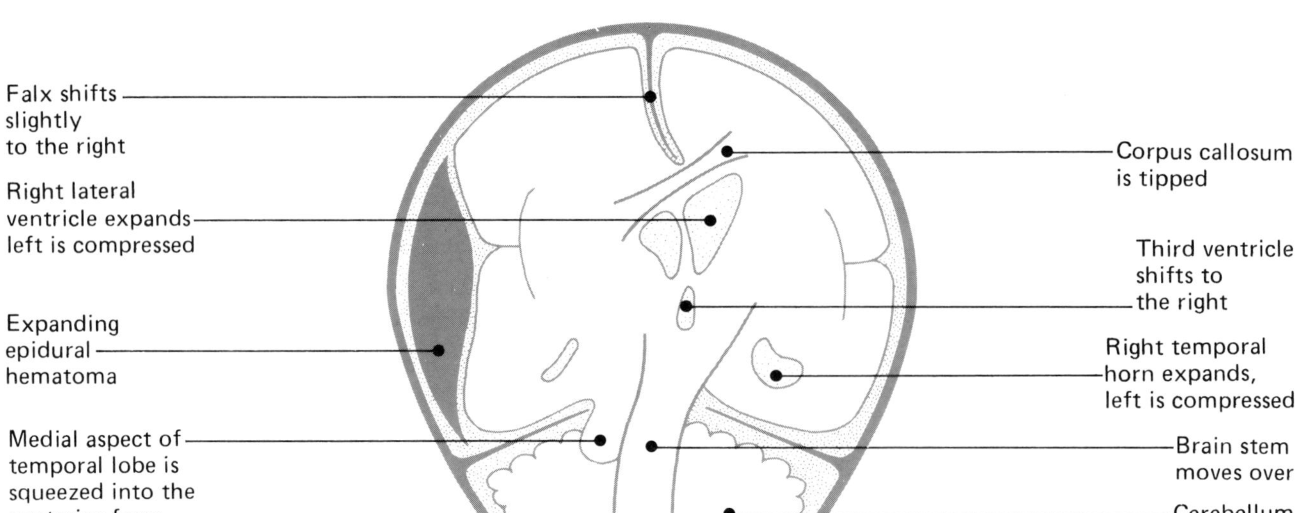

Figure 19.3. How the brain accommodates an expanding mass.

medulla and upper cervical cord, and respiratory arrest may occur.

Rising intracranial pressure may induce a reflex, centrally mediated elevation in mean systemic arterial pressure. This "Cushing reflex" is an attempt by the body to maintain blood flow to neurones. However, often the reflex does *not* occur until very late in the course of an imminent intracranial catastrophe. When mean intracranial pressure exceeds mean arterial pressure, cerebral blood flow stops and brain death ensues.

The term "cerebral perfusion pressure" refers to the hemodynamic driving force that ensures that the brain receives an adequate blood supply. In practical terms, it is the difference between mean arterial pressure and intracranial pressure, measured in torr (mm Hg). When cerebral perfusion pressure falls below 40 torr, cerebral blood flow declines drastically. Many of the therapeutic efforts directed against rising intracranial pressure are meant to preserve proper cerebral perfusion.

MANAGEMENT

The vast majority of head injuries have no permanent effects. However, evidence is accumulating that even the so-called trivial head injury is not innocuous. Interference with learning and short-term memory may last for at least 6 weeks. For example, the sports-related concussion in school-aged patients is a matter of some concern. Whether the concussed patient should be observed in hospital or at home depends upon several factors, including the ability and willingness of some responsible person to watch the patient and the presence or absence of dangerous fractures, concurrent injuries (especially of the chest and spine), or seizures.

Seizures that occur immediately or shortly after concussion seldom occur again. However, they are alarming to the relatives, and considerable reassurance is required. The secondary development of hematoma or severe edema following simple concussion is a rare event, occurring in less than 1 in 500 cases. All patients should be examined after any head injury, although most admissions prove to be unnecessary in retrospect. Where a neurologic deficit persists after an apparently simple head injury, a cerebral contusion or a Todd's postictal paralysis exists. The commonest such deficit is a mild hemiparesis with or without dysphasia. Occasionally, a depressed skull fracture will be discovered, accompanied by direct cortical bruising or laceration.

The following 12 points are intended to emphasize common pitfalls, early warning signs, and current management practices for the neurologically injured patient.

1. Head Injury and Shock. It is commonly taught that shock is not produced by head injury alone. But in certain situations a patient can be in shock from head injury alone: (1) the infant or young child with a scalp laceration involving a scalp artery, such as the superficial temporal or supraorbital, may bleed into shock; (2) the patient with shunt-controlled hydrocephalus loses the normal tamponade effect that quickly stops small bleeds from small surface vessels—in the young hydrocephalic, several hundred milliliters of blood may be lost into the head quite quickly in some circumstances; and (3) in the agonal stages following severe brain injury. In this situation there seems to be a direct depressant effect of brainstem compression on myocardial contractility. Therapy at this point often produces no results.

2. Multiple Injuries. Brain contusion combined with chest injury is particularly hazardous. Hypoxemia from any cause may turn a reversible injury into one that produces permanent sequelae. Such patients require close observation, and many benefit from intracranial and hemodynamic monitoring for exact control of total body volume and intracranial pressure. For example, excessive dehydration therapy in such patients may induce pulmonary arteriovenous shunting, producing hypoxemia that is reversible only by restoration of body volume. Similarly, positive end-expiratory pressure (PEEP) in patients with a combined head/chest injury, when used for treatment of intrapulmonary shunting, may be hazardous. PEEP above levels of 5 cm H_2O may increase the ICP, although clinical experience suggests that "stiff lungs" may protect the brain from the effects of PEEP.

3. Agitation. The agitated, irrational patient, picking at the bedclothes and IV lines, etc., may be on the verge of decompensation from the head injury, a chest injury, blood loss, or any combination thereof. In children, these clinical consequences of injury may take the form of listlessness and a very worried expression. The integrity of the vascular system and of the airway must be assured in such patients before they are transferred.

4. Fractures. Fractures that cross the middle meningeal artery or its two major branches, the great venous sinuses, or that extend into the foramen magnum are potentially dangerous. Fractures that are depressed more than half the width of the skull may require elevation. All patients with open cranial fractures should be started on broad spectrum antibiotics. It is quite permissible (and preferable) to suture clean lacerations loosely over fractures before transfer, but dirty wounds should be dressed only. Bleeders in the wound should be controlled, as a great deal of blood may be lost from scalp arteries.

Blood behind an ear drum or a blood-CSF mixture issuing from an external auditory canal is the hallmark of the basal-petrous skull fracture. Profuse arterial hemorrhage from the ears is usually caused by a ruptured carotid artery in the skull base. Antibiotics must not be given to patients with CSF rhinorrhea or otorrhea, as the overgrowth of resistant Gram negative flora may result in a fulminant meningitis that is difficult to treat.

5. Steroids. There is no acceptable evidence that steroids are of any value in the early management of head injury. In view of the immune system suppression exerted by corticosteroids, speculative administration of such agents to the head-injured patient is to be decried.

6. Brain-shrinking Agents. Brain-shrinking agents, such as mannitol, glycerol, or furosemide, should be started only after consultation with a neurosurgeon. Without doubt, such agents, when properly administered, can buy time for the brain in the face of an expanding mass. But they do allow an intracranial hematoma to enlarge and thus are not without hazard. Glycerol is best avoided, as it may contribute to acute tubular necrosis in some patients. Furosemide is now known to reduce CSF production, and this action, combined with its dehydration effect, makes it a useful agent in acute situations. The dose ranges from 5 mg IV for an infant to 40 mg IV for an adult.

Mannitol remains the most commonly used brain shrinker. It is given as a 20% solution, 1–4 mg/kg over 20–30 minutes. The initial diuresis produced is usually profound, and catheterization is usually necessary. There may be rebound cerebral swelling induced by the use of any osmotic agent.

One should remember that all of the osmotic and diuretic agents exert their actions throughout the body, not only in the head. Excessive use of these drugs may significantly lower total body volume with serious effects on cardiopulmonary dynamics and water and electrolyte balance.

7. On-the-spot Surgery. If a patient is rapidly deteriorating following head injury and there is no neurosurgeon available, a general surgeon should be called. On-the-spot surgery may be necessary to save neurologic function. The order of burr-hole placement to locate the blood clot is as follows: above and in front of the ear on the same side as the initially dilating pupil; same site on the opposite side; posterior parietal bos on the first side; comparable site on the opposite side; and frontal areas, 3–4 cm from the midline. Posterior fossa burr holes require the patient to be turned over—fortunately, they are very rarely necessary.

8. Neck Trauma. With such violent injuries as incurred by motor vehicle accidents or falls, neck trauma is a frequent accompaniment of head injury. Care must always be taken not to miss a spinal fracture in the unconscious patient or in the conscious one complaining of neck or lower spine pain. The commonest sites for inadequate radiologic examination are the occiput-C1–C2 area and the C7–T1 junction. When in doubt, transfer such patients in a cervical collar and on a fracture board with good supports. Intubation of a patient with a cervical fracture can be lethal if the situation is unappreciated. In-line cervical traction is required for safe intubation when neck injury may exist. Nasotracheal intubation usually obviates any risk of neck manipulation; severe midface trauma with an unstable maxilla is a relative contraindication to nasotracheal intubation.

Beware of the unconscious injured patient with a slow pulse, warm dry extremities, and hypotension. These findings usually indicate a sympathectomy effect from cervical cord injury and not some strange shock state.

9. Seizures. Persistent seizures following head injury are best treated with diazepam, 0.1–0.25 mg/kg. Such patients should be transferred to a neurosurgical unit. The onset of focal seizures may indicate cortical contusion or a slowly expanding mass. It is essential to establish the airway and check that pulmonary gas-exchange is adequate if seizures are persistent.

10. Secondary Deterioration. Following cerebral concussion, the usual pattern is recovery of normal consciousness over seconds, minutes, or hours. Persistence of a neurologic deficit in the face of an improving conscious state is the hallmark of focal cerebral contusion or a ictal paralysis. Persistence of an altered state of consciousness longer than 24 hours indicates diffuse cerebral contusion. Deterioration in the state of consciousness always indicates intracranial pathology, be it mass lesion, cerebral edema, metabolic encephalopathy, hypoxia-ischemia, or fat embolism. All such patients should be transferred to a neurosurgical unit.

11. Sequence of Rostrocaudal Deterioration. The most common pattern seen in the patient undergoing rostrocaudal deterioration is (a) deterioration in the level of consciousness; (b) appearance of hemiparesis and/or a dilating pupil; (c) appearance of stereotyped movement patterns (such as decerebrate posturing) shortly after the loss of protective, purposeful motor withdrawal patterns; (d) onset of abnormal and progressively inefficient breathing, in this order: neurogenic hyperventilation, periodic breathing, apneustic breathing (which resembles the pattern seen in chest-wall injury), and ataxic breathing (which is totally irregular and inefficient); and finally (e) agonal gasping.

12. Cautions. Most head-injured patients recover uneventfully, although all head injuries are potentially dangerous. Transfer patients when danger signs exist or when in doubt. Always call ahead. Beware of the patient with multiple injuries, especially with regard to airway and hemodynamic status. Never do a lumbar puncture on a neurologically injured patient. To do so may cause an intracranial disaster because of herniation of the brain.

OTHER CONCEPTS CONCERNING NEUROLOGIC INJURY

Intracranial Pressure

In acute situations, the terms "intracranial pressure" (ICP) and "intracranial volume" are synonymous. Intracranial pressure control seems to be related to prognosis. Patients with an intracranial pressure above 30 mm Hg, either consistently or in long-lasting waves, rarely do well; unfortunately, patients with consistently low pressures may do badly because of severe diffuse axonal injury. Present means of controlling a high intracranial pressure include controlled hyperventilation ($PaCO_2 = 25–30$ mm Hg), brain-shrinking agents, ventricular drainage, and barbiturate coma. Intracranial monitoring is essential for the proper control of intracranial pressure. The particular combination of monitoring and treatment procedures used depend upon the individual situation.

The Glasgow Coma Scale (Table 19.1) is the basis for assessment of the unconscious patient. If the score is 8 or less, the following measures are instituted: (1) intubate the patient to protect the airway; (2) obtain a CT head scan to rule out remediable surgical lesions while at the same time investigating and treating other associated injuries; (3) institute ICP monitoring, preferably using an intraventricular catheter; monitoring ICP from the

Table 19.1
Glasgow Coma Scale

Score[a]	Response category		
	Motor	Verbal	Eye opening
6	Obeys		
5	Localizes	Oriented	
4	Normal flexor (good withdrawal)	Confused	Spontaneously
3	Abnormal flexor (purposeless, random)	Inappropriate, but says words	To sound
2	Extensor (decerebrate)	Incomprehensible, but utters sounds	To pain
1	Nil	Nil	Nil

[a] Record best response, from best side. Any falloff in numerical score is a danger sign.

brain surface is an acceptable alternative; and (4) if the ICP exceeds 20 mm Hg, proceed as outlined below:

1. ***Hyperventilation.*** Control the $PaCO_2$ between 25–30 mm Hg and the PaO_2 above 80 mm Hg. If necessary, control the respiratory rate and keep the patient in phase with the respirator by using Pavulon or morphine. A $PaCO_2 < 22$ mm Hg is dangerous, due to rapidly increasing hemoglobin-O_2 binding. Hyperventilation is frequently sufficient, although it tends to become less effective with time. It works because hypocarbia causes cerebral vasoconstriction, reducing intracranial blood volume and thereby reducing ICP. Various combinations of the techniques described below may be necessary if ICP remains above 20 mm Hg.

2. ***Mannitol.*** Give 1–4 gm/kg run in over 20–30 minutes with other IV fluids shut off. The osmotic effect depends upon the intravascular/brain extracellular space osmotic pressure difference. Bladder catheterization is necessary. Osmotherapy is less useful and may be dangerous with repeated administration. Rebound cerebral edema may occur, as well as a chronic hyperosmolar state. Nevertheless, mannitol is a useful agent in a crisis.

Occasionally, children, less commonly adolescents, and rarely adults react to head injury with a sudden dilation of the vascular capacitance bed of the brain—the precapillary arterioles, the capillaries, and the postcapillary venules. This bed is large, and a significant increase in cerebral blood volume may occur. This hyperperfusion state will be worsened by the use of osmotic agents because they cause a transient increase in intravascular volume. The prompt institution of hyperventilation usually counteracts this potentially lethal form of brain swelling. It is generally true that hyperventilation therapy is the primary and safest initial therapy to combat traumatic brain swelling. There is one caveat: theoretically, at least, hyperventilation may reduce the amount of blood flowing through edematous brain. If such a reduction in local blood flow reaches critical levels, local ischemia could supervene.

3. ***Furosemide.*** The use of 1 mg/kg acts as a whole body dehydrator and as an inhibitor of CSF production. Repeated use requires very careful monitoring of water and electrolyte balance.

4. ***Ventricular drainage.*** This is especially useful when hydrocephalus is present. The risk is that the ventricles may collapse, making ICP monitoring difficult.

5. ***Barbiturate coma.*** Barbiturates reduce ICP by causing cerebral vasoconstriction and a fall in cerebral blood volume. They may also protect neurones by reducing brain oxygen demand and by acting as free radical scavengers. Dosage is titrated against ICP. Very high Pentothal or pentobarbital levels may cause myocardial depression. Continuous EEG monitoring is helpful, and the appearance of burst suppression correlates with a blood level of 5–7 mg/100 ml of Pentothal. If the ICP is uncontrollable by barbiturate therapy carried to the point of a flat EEG tracing, the situation is hopeless. In general, barbiturate coma is reserved as a last resort; early enthusiasm for its efficacy has proved illusory, and barbiturate coma may seriously affect white cell function.

Proper monitoring and control of total body volume, cardiorespiratory function, and general metabolism are essential while instituting the measures outlined above. The adjuncts to ICP monitoring are outlined in Table 19.2

Cerebral Edema

Cerebral edema may cause an increase in the ICP. After injury, it may be caused by diffuse contusion, nearby mass lesions, intravascular fat, hypoxia-ischemia, or the presence of oxygen-derived radicals, such as the superoxide anion or hydroxyl radicals. The latter agents are now known to be instrumental in inducing vascular permeability changes and intracellular dysfunction. Early on, traumatic cerebral edema is "vasogenic" in type. If hypoxia-ischemia becomes a factor or if the vasogenic edema becomes severe enough to interfere with interstitial diffusion of molecular oxygen, "cytotoxic" edema may set in as well. Combined hemodynamic and ICP monitoring is most useful in attempts to control cerebral edema.

Table 19.2
Adjuncts to Intracranial Pressure Monitoring

Pressures	Functions	Laboratory	New techniques
Systemic arterial	Continuous ECG	Blood gases	Brain water flux
Pulmonary arterial	Continuous EEG	U/S osmolalities	Membrane transport
Pulmonary wedge	Daily chest x-ray	Electrolytes	Cerebral blood flow (isotope tomography)
	Cardiac output	Urine sodium excretion	Free radical concentrations
	Renal		

Brain, Heart, and Lung Relationships

Certain neurogenic events, such as hypothalamic discharges, have direct and specific effects on pulmonary vasculature and cardiac conduction patterns. The result is neurogenic pulmonary edema, a form of the adult respiratory distress syndrome. Pulmonary and cardiovascular injury may have profound effects on the brain in the form of hypoxia and low perfusion pressures. Combined ICP and hemodynamic monitoring is helpful in defining these reciprocal influences and how to manage them.

Spinal Cord Injury

Useful recovery seldom occurs when motor and sensory function is totally absent at the first examination after cord injury. Valiant attempts to improve prognosis by early decompression, cord cooling and irrigation, or osmotic agents and steroids have been largely unfruitful. Prevention of further cord injury by recognition and immobilization of the injured spine remains the most important early aspect of cord injury care.

The spinal cord is easily damaged by compression by bone, bone fragments, arterial blood clot, and disrupted disk material. The flexion-extension and forced flexion injuries of the cervical spine remain the most common and potentially devastating causes of cord injury.

In addition to comments made earlier regarding cord injury, the following points should be stressed.

1. Deterioration in spinal cord function demands prompt investigation and therapy.
2. Initial treatment of patients with suspected cord injury must require as few patient movements as possible: sandbags, soft ruffs, or, preferably, Philadelphia-type collars should be used and there must be no flexion or extension movements of the spine.
3. Prompt treatment of cord injuries *may* restore function, but early improper care frequently destroys it.

Current opinion favors nonoperative treatment for total lesions or for situations where function is improving. Spinal stabilization by internal fixation is favored as an early measure in some cases, such as thoracolumbar dislocations. For unstable cervical fractures, skull tong or halo immobilization is used. The halo apparatus allows for early mobilization and rehabilitation.

Suggested Readings

Amacher AL: Critical head injuries. Part I. Pathophysiologic effects. *Emerg Care Q* 1: 48–61, 1985.

Amacher AL: Critical head injuries. Part II. Additional perspectives and principles. *Emerg Care Q* 1: 62–71, 1985.

Adams JH, Mitchell DE, Graham DI, Doyle D: Diffuse brain damage of immediate impact type. Its relationship to 'primary brainstem damage' in head injury. *Brain* 100: 489–502, 1977.

Jennett B: *An Introduction to Neurosurgery,* ed. 3. Chicago, Year Book Medical Publishers, 1977.

Plum F, Posner JB. Diagnosis of stupor and coma. *Contemporary Neurology Series 10,* ed. 2. Philadelphia, FA Davis, 1972.

TRAUMA

CHAPTER

20 Trauma: A Perspective on Management

Ronald L. Holliday, M.D. and William J. Sibbald, M.D.

Accidental injury is the fourth leading cause of death in North America and the leading cause of death in those under 40 years of age. In Canada there are approximately 6000 deaths a year due to accidental injury. The cost of accidental injury to society runs into the billions of dollars. Motor vehicle accidents cause the majority of accidental injuries and deaths. A typical Saturday emergency case might be a young male believing himself to be psychologically immortal—a state of mind reinforced by alcohol—who wraps his car around a lamppost or tree.

Prevention is obviously the answer. Driver education and the strict enforcement of alcohol abuse legislation are important. Reduction of speed limits and the enforcement of seat belt legislation have decreased the accidental injury rate slightly, but recent statistics show that the death rate is again on the increase. Therefore, all critical care units will continue to be presented with what is probably an irreducible minimum of accidental injuries.

ABCs OF TRAUMA CARE

The care of the traumatized patient begins at the scene of the accident. The ABCs of trauma care prevail here and throughout the patient's course in the medical system.

A. Airway. Ventilation must be secured. At the roadside, this may mean removal of fractured teeth, blood, and emesis. It may also mean mouth-to-mouth resuscitation and occasionally cardiopulmonary resuscitation.

B. Bleeding—control of hemorrhage. At the roadside, direct pressure is the easiest and most convenient way to control hemorrhage. The use of tourniquets is discouraged unless the risk of exsanguination is great.

C. Consciousness. The level of consciousness should be assessed at the roadside, when possible, and recorded so that any deterioration or improvement in the neurologic course of the patient's illness can be monitored.

Little can be done at the roadside for the assessment of:

D. Digestive or abdominal system,

E. Excretory or urogenital system, and

F. Fractures. Fractures should be stabilized to the best of one's ability with whatever is available. This may mean fashioning a splint with a ski pole, a piece of wood, or a magazine. Open wounds should be covered with the cleanest dressing available.

The next phase of resuscitation is delivery of the patient from the scene of the accident to the hospital. It is the responsibility of government and physicians to ensure that adequate ambulance care is provided. This means that a vehicle with adequate support systems is provided and that ambulance attendants are trained to a minimum of basic life support; training to the level of advanced trauma life support care is preferable if a systems approach to emergency health services is present in the community. Consideration must also be given to the appropriate utilization of air transport, by either helicopter or by fixed-wing aircraft for long distances, particularly in remote areas of the country. These vehicles must be manned with individuals trained in trauma resuscitation and with appropriate equipment so that safe, yet adequate, interventional care may be provided during transport.

The trauma patient must then be delivered to a facility that has a 24-hour physicians service interested and capable of taking care of this type of individual, a 24-hour laboratory service, and a 24-hour blood bank.

In the emergency department, injuries are sorted by triage. Injuries can be classified into those that are (1) an immediate threat to life; (2) severe injuries, but which allow stabilization and pose no immediate threat to life; and (3) injuries that may be significant, but are occult in nature. In the hospital, the ABCs must again be reviewed by a physician with expertise in the care of the traumatized patient and with meticulous attention to detail.

Hospitals responsible for the care of the trauma patient should follow the recommendations of the Committee on Trauma of the American College of Surgeons (see Suggested Readings). Optimization of facilities, personnel, and ancillary aids will result in increased survival from traumatic injury.

Airway

In initial resuscitation the airway is of primary concern. Signs of upper airway obstruction, such as stridor, crowing, and indrawing, should be noted. Certain patients are at particular risk of inadequately protecting the upper airway; for instance, the obtunded patient, the patient burned in a closed environment such as a motor vehicle, or those who have suffered severe maxillofacial or laryngeal injuries. The management in the emergency room includes sweeping of the mouth, removal of debris, suctioning, and simply pulling the mandible forward with

Table 20.1
Tubes and Blood Work for the Trauma Patient

Tubes used for trauma patients	
Essential	**Optional, depending on injuries**
Intravenous (12–14 Fr)	Chest tube
Bladder catheter	Peritoneal lavage catheter
Levin tube	Intracranial pressure monitor
	Pericardiocentesis
Baseline blood work for trauma patients	
Necessary	**May be helpful**
Hb, Hct	Serum amylase
Group and cross-match	Coagulogram (PT, PTT, platelets)
Blood gases	

slight hyperextension of the neck. Acutely, this protocol should reduce the risk of asphyxiation and aspiration of oropharyngeal contents. An oropharyngeal airway may be inserted, and the patient may be bagged with an Ambu bag with supplementary oxygen. Initial blood samples should then be drawn (Table 20.1).

Of importance in the management of ventilatory and other systemic problems is the passage of a nasogastric tube and subsequent aspiration of the stomach. Aspiration of gastric contents into the lung is the most common preventable cause of death in severely injured patients. The only group of patients who demand extra care in the passage of a Levin tube are those with severe maxillofacial injuries. The Levin tube in this situation should be passed under direct vision.

If, despite the aforementioned attention to the upper airway, signs and symptoms of inadequate protection of the airway or inadequate ventilation persist, intubation becomes a therapeutic imperative. Expertise is needed to perform this maneuver. Nasotracheal or orotracheal intubation can be performed. In patients with suspected cervical spine injuries, intubation by the nasotracheal route should be performed by a physician skilled in this procedure while in-line traction is performed by an assistant. Occasionally, a situation may arise where one is unable to intubate the patient. Coniotomy, or slitting the cricothyroid membrane, can establish an adequate airway. Alternatively, one or two 12- to 14-gauge needles can be inserted through the cricothyroid membrane and attached to a direct flow of oxygen; this method is considered to be less favorable because of the inadequate flows obtained.

If the airway is controlled but the patient fails to oxygenate, pleural collections of air or fluid, significant pulmonary parenchymal damage, aspiration, fat embolus, or mucous plugs in the distal airway should be considered. These should be dealt with by appropriate measures, which may include the early insertion of thoracostomy tubes.

Bleeding and Blood Restoration

At the same time as adequate ventilation is secured, intravenous portals must be sought to enable volume resuscitation to begin. It should be remembered that the traumatized patient in shock (i.e., blood pressure less than 90 mm Hg, heart rate greater than 100 min, or orthostatic hypotension) has most likely lost approximately 20–50% of his or her blood volume. The blood volume can be roughly estimated at 75 ml/kg body weight. Therefore, one must establish venous portals that will allow the rapid infusion of fluid. At least two large-bore catheters (12 or 14 gauge) should be inserted into central (i.e., subclavian, internal jugular, femoral) or peripheral veins. Intravenous solution lines should not be started in injured extremities or in lower extremities if there is suspicion of pelvic or intra-abdominal injury.

Although much has been written about the controversy between resuscitation with colloid or crystalloid, the most readily available solutions for administration to the volume-depleted shocked patient are Ringer's lactate or normal saline. These are excellent fluids with which to begin resuscitation. In cases of exsanguination hemorrhage, type-specific or O-negative blood may be indicated. It should be remembered that most blood banks take between 45–60 minutes to provide fully cross-matched blood. Therefore, the resuscitative regime will be dictated by the condition of the patient and the rapidity of delivery of the blood bank system. A simplified protocol for the emergent volume resuscitation of the traumatized patient is provided in Table 20.2, as adapted

Table 20.2
Clinical Signs of the Four Classes of Hemorrhagic Hypotension and Suggestions for Volume Replacement

Class	Blood pressure	Heart rate	Pulse pressure	Respiratory rate	Management
I	Normal	Slight ↑	Normal	Slight ↑	Crystalloid[a]
II	Normal	↑ (100–200)	Narrowed	↑	Crystalloid[a]
III	Decreased	↑ (120)	Narrowed	↑	Crystalloid[b] plus blood
IV	Decreased (mean BP < 50 mm Hg)	↑ (140)	Narrowed	>35/min	Crystalloid[b] plus blood

[a] Use Ringer's lactate or 0.9% NaCL in a ratio of 3 ml replaced for every 1 ml lost.
[b] Use Ringer's lactate or 0.9% NaCl, as above, until cross-matched blood is available. If life-threatening, use type-specific or 0 negative blood to maintain Hb > 10 gm/dl.

from the American College of Surgeons' trauma guidelines.

The success of the restoration of intravenous volume will be noted by monitoring the restoration of blood pressure, decrease in heart rate, evidence of capillary refill, a lightening in the level of consciousness, and an increase in urine output. Two to three liters of Ringer's lactate solution should be given rapidly to most hypotensive patients, i.e., in 30–45 minutes. Most hypotensive patients will respond to this infusion. If not, the physician should consider occult blood loss in the chest or abdomen or an underestimation of blood loss associated with fractures. Other rarer causes of failure to respond to adequate volume resuscitation include cardiac tamponade, a missed ventilatory problem (such as tension pneumothorax), the occasional acute gastric dilation, a significant myocardial contusion associated with trauma, or an endocrine problem, such as hypoadrenalism.

After the establishment of ventilation and circulation, a quick general systemic review of the patient can then be carried out at a more leisurely pace in most instances. The situation of course may occur where the patient will not resuscitate and is obviously exsanguinating. Rapid transport to a prepared operating room is essential for the proper management of the cranial, thoracic, or abdominal injury that often precipitates this catastrophe. However, when time is available, systemic review can be done as indicated in subsequent chapters, following the rest of the ABC trauma principles.

Suggested Readings

Hampton OP Jr: Categorization of hospital emergency capabilities: a progress report. *J Trauma* 16:21, 1976.

Optimal hospital resources for care of the seriously injured. *Am Coll Surg Bull* September, 1976.

CHAPTER

21 Abdominal Trauma

David P. Girvan, M.D.

Trauma and accidents are the fourth leading cause of death in the population as a whole and the leading cause of death in children. Abdominal trauma occurs less frequently than musculoskeletal trauma or head injuries, but the diagnosis can frequently be missed as the signs and symptoms of intra-abdominal injury may be more subtle. It is important to remember that externally the abdominal region can extend over an area from the nipple line to buttock crease. This means that the pelvic, retroperitoneal, and even lower intrathoracic regions may be involved with associated injuries, a fact that must be kept in mind when assessing patients.

PATHOPHYSIOLOGY

Abdominal trauma varies according to the nature of the wounding agent and the force with which it is applied. Two major types of abdominal trauma are seen: penetrating wounds, and nonpenetrating or blunt injuries. The penetrating wound may be due to a stabbing and is probably the least serious of the abdominal wounds. Any number of articles may enter the abdominal cavity, including knives, ice picks, or a variety of sharpened wooden or metal objects. The second major type of penetrating wounds, and one that is becoming more frequent, is the gunshot wound. These may be self-inflicted or homicide associated. With such gunshot wounds, multiple organ injury is frequent, and one must pay particular attention to the velocity of the missile. Low velocity missiles, such as a bullet from a .22, produce clean puncture wounds with little damage to surrounding tissue. In contrast, the high velocity projectile not only causes extensive destruction of the tissue that it comes in contact with but there is also a severe associated blast effect on the surrounding tissue. High velocity missiles (e.g., from a magnum pistol or military rifle,) produce a small entrance wound but an exit wound many times the size of the actual missile. The track of a missile is frequently less than straight, and one must be conscious of the position of the victim to the angle of bullet entry, as well as the possible effect of ricochet. The shotgun may result in minimal superficial lesions if fired from some distance. When discharged from a short range the injuries sustained are massive and frequently beyond the scope of the most valiant surgical efforts.

Blunt injuries may have little external evidence of their application, but the internal wounds are determined by the agent and force with which it is applied. The injury may be due to direct trauma, a severe crushing force between two fixed objects, acceleration/deceleration types of injury, or a shearing or twisting effect on organs with fixed points. The latter is especially true of small bowel injuries, with tears frequently being in the region of a fixed point, such as the ligament of Treitz or ileocecal valve. The severity and multiplicity of organ systems involved have a direct bearing on the ultimate outcome and survival. Single organ system involvement generally carries an excellent prognosis, whereas the involvement of each additional system increases mortality.

DIAGNOSIS

Penetrating Injuries

There is little difficulty diagnosing a penetrating injury of the abdomen, be it from a stabbing or a gunshot wound. However, all such injuries should be surgically explored to rule out penetration of the abdominal cavity. It is essential in gunshot wounds to examine the patient carefully for an exit wound that may give further information about the possible organ systems involved or body cavities entered and exited. However, in centers dealing with large numbers of penetrating injuries it is often physically impossible to explore all of these patients. Radiologic examinations of the missile tracks using contrast materials has been advocated to determine whether the peritoneal cavity has been violated.

Clinical abdominal examination is most important. Evidence of tenderness, muscular guarding, or increased intestinal activity all suggest entrance into the peritoneal cavity. Blood on rectal or pelvic examination or hematuria also suggests the need for laparotomy. In any center dealing with few penetrating wounds, laparotomy is the more conservative approach unless one is absolutely certain that the entry and exit wound have avoided the peritoneal cavity.

Blunt Trauma

Blunt abdominal trauma can pose a worrisome diagnostic challenge to the individual responsible for early management of these patients. Inspection of the abdominal wall may reveal bruising or other marks to suggest the site of injury or restraint by a seat belt, steering wheel, or dashboard. Physical examination and frequent reevaluation of the patient's clinical status are probably the most important factors in determining intra-abdominal pathology. A surgical abdomen manifested by diffuse tenderness, rigidity, guarding, or absence of peristaltic sounds should suggest a need for operation. If findings are minimal then re-examination in a few hours is indicated. As a general rule, narcotics and other analgesics should not be administered until a decision has been made regarding the need for operation. A rapidly expanding abdomen combined with failing vital signs is frequently an indication of ongoing intra-abdominal hemorrhage and the need for early laparotomy.

Vital signs, including pulse rate and blood pressure, should be monitored. More invasive techniques, such as central venous pressure lines and urinary catheters, may lead one to suspect ongoing hemorrhage when the clinical signs may be rather occult. Laboratory investigations, including a hemoglobin, hematocrit, serum amylase, and urinalysis, can be quickly obtained and may support the clinical diagnosis of significant injury. If the physical examination, vital signs, and laboratory investigations are all equivocal, then the patient must be closely observed until definite evidence of intra-abdominal pathology is present, or he or she has completely stabilized.

Paracentesis (Abdominal Tap)

This may be an especially helpful technique in the questionable abdomen or in the individual with a head injury or who is uncooperative, e.g., an inebriated individual. The author's method of choice is the insertion under sterile conditions of a peritoneal dialysis catheter just below the umbilicus. A small incision is made in the midline just below the umbilicus. The peritoneum is visualized and opened under direct vision before inserting the catheter. A liter of Ringer's lactate or saline is rapidly infused and then allowed to drain back into the bottle that has been placed below the patient. The patient may be rolled around or positioned to facilitate a lavage of most of the abdominal cavity. Frank blood may come out immediately, making infusion of fluid unnecessary. A pink color to the fluid is certainly suggestive of the need for laparotomy, and the inability to read newsprint through this fluid and the finding of greater than 100,000 RBCs/ml in the examined specimen of the lavage fluid are considered adequate indications for laparotomy. Peritoneal tap and lavage is felt to be contraindicated in an abdomen where there has been previous surgical procedures because of the risk of adhesions and entry of the catheter into bowel loops or other viscera. It is important that the bladder be emptied or a urinary catheter inserted before the dialysis catheter is used for the paracentesis (Fig. 21.1).

Radiographic Studies

Plain films of the abdomen, which usually include the lower chest, may show fractured ribs, directing suspicion toward the liver or spleen, or loss of the psoas shadows, suggesting retroperitoneal bleeding. Free air may be present in the case of a ruptured hollow viscus. Care must be taken to assess both diaphragms for the not-infrequent possibility of traumatic rupture of the diaphragm. In splenic injury, the spleen shadow may be enlarged or the gastric bubble deviated more medially than normally seen. Air in the retroperitoneal space is often suggestive of colonic or duodenal rupture. Intravenous pyelogram is

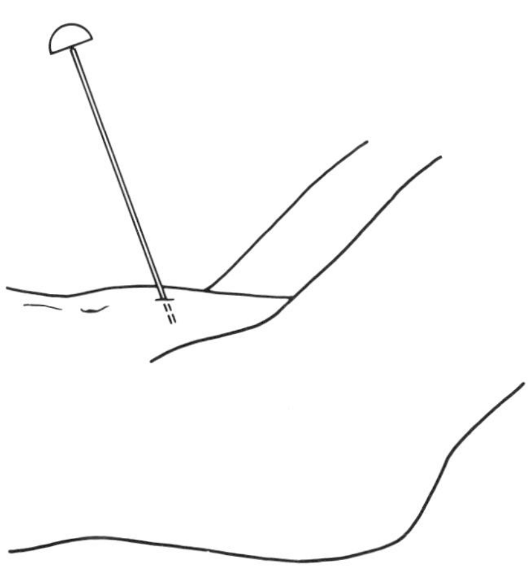

A midline incision is made in the skin 3–4 cm below the umbilicus, and the peritoneal dialysis catheter is inserted in the direction of the pelvic cavity after direct visualization and opening of the peritoneum. Bladder must be empty by voiding or catheter.

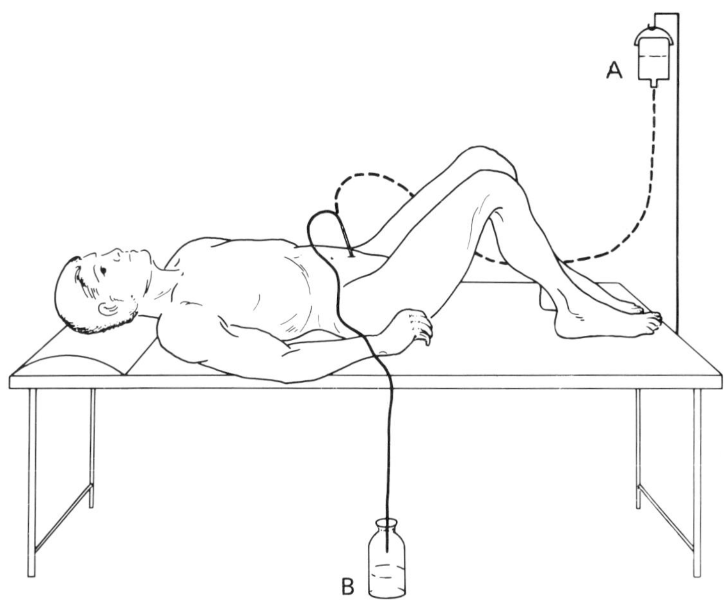

Lavage fluid is infused with bottle in position *A*. Bottle is then placed below the patient *(B)*, and siphon effect returns diagnostic fluid from peritoneal cavity.

Figure 21.1 Introduction of peritoneal dialysis catheter: infusion and retrieval of lavage fluid.

mandatory in cases where blood is found in the urine and may also assist in the diagnosis of other retroperitoneal injuries. As a general rule, barium studies are not done in the patient with acute abdominal trauma.

Computed tomography has been advocated in the initial assessment of the traumatized patient. It is most useful in assessing urologic or retroperitoneal injuries and solid viscus damage. It may also aid in the abdominal assessment of the comatose patient, but should not be done in the unstable patient.

Arteriography

Arteriography is most useful in those individuals with suspected pelvic injuries with evidence of rapidly increasing pelvic or perineal hematomas. These lesions are frequently impossible to deal with surgically and may benefit from an embolization if specific vessels can be shown to be leaking. Arteriography may be of value in selected cases of splenic, hepatic, or renal injuries.

Isotope Studies

Liver and spleen scans may be of some value in patients with minimal abdominal findings. As a general rule, the clinical course of the patient is far more important in establishing a diagnosis than are the radiologic findings.

MANAGEMENT

As with any trauma patient, the initial concern before diagnosing the exact injury is the stabilization of the patient's vital signs. Two important rules must be remembered:

1. One surgeon or physician must assume responsibility for the patient, particularly for the one with multiple system involvement who may be seen by many individuals.
2. No patient should go for x-ray or other investigations until his or her condition is stable with airway established and intravenous and nasogastric tubes in place.

Initial management involves establishment of an adequate airway, which may be as simple as clearing the oral cavity using an oral airway or, if necessary, nasal or endotracheal intubation. Careful stabilization of the cervical spine is essential until they have been cleared radiologically. Any obvious hemorrhage must be controlled by direct pressure. A tourniquet is rarely indicated. Large-bore intravenous portals must be established early. Ideally these should be in the upper extremity, particularly with abdominal or pelvic trauma, as intravenous portals in the lower extremity may simply add to bleeding in the abdominal cavity if the vena cava or aorta has been injured. Blood is drawn for laboratory investigations and cross-matching at the time the intravenous lines are started. Almost all patients, and particularly children, with abdominal injuries have some degree of gastric dilation and should have a nasogastric tube inserted. This tube can easily be removed at a later date if it turns out that there are no significant intra-abdominal injuries. Acute gastric dilation can lead to significant abdominal pain and discomfort and has been implicated in causing hemodynamic upset, possibly from obstruction to the vena cava and return of blood to the heart. Insertion of this tube can also prevent aspiration in the patient with neurologic injuries or a compromised respiratory system.

Once the above treatment priorities have been completed, a more thorough history and physical examination can be obtained and other less urgent procedures can be carried out, such as splinting fractures, inserting catheters, ordering radiology, and arranging for other investigations. Continuous close observation by the same responsible surgeon or physician and careful recording of pulse rate, respiratory rate, blood pressure, abdominal findings, and hemoglobin and hematocrit are the most valuable diagnostic aids in making a decision to explore the abdomen. Frequent re-evaluation of the clinical situation is the most valuable aid to early diagnosis.

It is important to remember that head injuries rarely produce shock; shock is usually due to thoracic or abdominal injuries and less frequently to fractures. If a patient is hypotensive or anemic and has no evidence of thoracic or major bony fractures, then he or she is considered to have intra-abdominal hemorrhage until proven otherwise.

Stomach

Penetrating injuries to the stomach are reasonably common and usually can be debrided and simply sutured. Blunt trauma injuries occurring after individuals have eaten may result in considerable peritoneal contamination with food stuffs. Simple repair up to a gastrectomy may be necessary.

Duodenum

Duodenal injuries are infrequent, but when they occur can be lethal. The duodenum is a retroperitoneal structure and usually is injured by compression against the vertebral column. Penetrating injuries may also occur. The finding of air or bile-stained fluid in the retroperitoneal space around the duodenum demands full kocherization of the duodenum and inspection of both the anterior and posterior aspects. Management may involve simple suturing, exteriorization of transected ends, or occasionally radical resectional procedures, such as a Whipple's procedure. Hematoma of the duodenal wall may present a diagnostic challenge and may require operation because of obstruction. Conservative management will frequently result in complete recovery, although evacuation of the hematoma has also been advocated.

Pancreas

Pancreatic injuries, like those of the duodenum, tend to be infrequent, but when they do occur they are a major challenge to the surgeon. The injury is frequently a crushing type, particularly a compression injury against the vertebral column. This injury may result in severe hemorrhagic pancreatitis with subsequent development of a pseudocyst or massive necrosis of the pancreatic gland. Transection of the pancreas may result in peritonitis or pseudocyst formation. Simple contusions and pancreatitis should be treated by drainage. Transection of the pancreas is likely best dealt with by distal pancreatectomy, although use of Roux-en-Y anastomoses to the two open ends has been advocated. In massive injury to the entire gland or the associated duodenum, more radical resections may be indicated.

Small Intestine

Blunt injuries in the small intestine tend to occur about fixed points, in particular the area just beyond the ligament of Treitz or before the ileocecal valve. These are likely to be acceleration/deceleration injuries resulting in a series of shearing forces. The mesentery alone may be torn with subsequent bleeding, or the bowel itself may be entered.

Of particular interest in recent years has been the small bowel injury due to use of lap or shoulder-lap seat belts. Frequently contusion on the abdominal wall marks the position of the belt; injuries may be found anywhere in the small bowel. Injuries from simple tears in the mesentery to multiple lacerations or perforations of the small bowel have been caused by seat belts. Associated vertebral compression or fracture injuries must be carefully ruled out.

Penetrating injuries of the small bowel must be carefully sought. Shotgun injuries are frequently associated with multiple perforations. It is essential to check not only the antimesenteric border but also the mesenteric border for signs of perforation. Treatment of small bowel injuries is generally straightforward with resection and primary anastomosis. Small bowel content is not normally considered contaminated and does not lead to the problems of anastomosic leak as seen in the left colon.

Large Intestine

Blunt injuries to the colon are infrequent, and most of the injuries tend to be of the penetrating type. Delayed perforation of an area of colon is occasionally seen and is probably due to considerable contusion or damage to its blood supply caused by blunt abdominal trauma a number of days earlier. Delayed perforation usually is manifested by the sudden onset of abdominal pain and evidence of an acute surgical abdomen with the appropriate associated systemic response (fever, tachycardia, leukocytosis).

As a general rule, colon injuries are best managed by exteriorization or repair with defunctioning colostomy proximally. This procedure is mandatory in left colon injuries or any injury where there is massive contamination or high risk of infection. In isolated right colon injuries with a relatively empty bowel, primary anastomosis or repair can be carried out in some cases.

Liver

The liver is the largest of the intra-abdominal organs and is reasonably protected by the rib cage. It can, however, be injured in blunt abdominal trauma, particularly if lower ribs on the right side have been broken or extensively compressed. The liver is also a frequent organ of injury in penetrating wounds, both from stabbings and gunshots. Liver injuries can range from simple superficial capsule laceration or multiple clean parenchymal lacerations to massive pulping and deep intrahepatic hemorrhagic lesions. Treatment varies from simple suture or resectional debridement to the occasional formal lobectomy. In rare cases with uncontrollable bleeding, ligation of the hepatic artery has been advocated and is tolerated in the majority of cases, but ligation of individual bleeding points and leaking bile ducts is preferable. Packing for uncontrollable hepatic hemorrhage is an alternative method that is occasionally required in extreme circumstances. Less than adequate treatment of liver injuries may result in large areas of devitalized and necrotic liver tissue that subsequently will undergo abcess formation or cause recurrent hemorrhage with intra-abdominal catastrophes or hematobilia. The mortality of liver injury has decreased as our understanding of liver anatomy and treatment techniques have improved. Because these injuries are not often seen in smaller centers, these patients should be transferred to a center with experience in dealing with these types of injuries, provided the patient is stable.

Spleen

The spleen is the organ that is injured most frequently in blunt trauma. In centers dealing with large numbers of penetrating trauma, the spleen ranks behind the small bowel, liver, and large bowel as a moderately frequent organ of injury. Any patient who has sustained injury to the left upper quadrant and has peritoneal signs frequently associated with shoulder-tip pain should be suspected of splenic injury.

Views on management have changed in the last few years because of the small but definite risk of overwhelming postsplenectomy septicemia (OPSS). This is a more frequent complication in patients whose immune system is already depressed, such as cancer patients undergoing radiotherapy or chemotherapy. Patients who have their spleens removed for hematologic disorders are also at an increased risk for this condition. There have, however, been isolated cases of OPSS in posttraumatic splenectomy patients, and this is of special concern in the pediatric age group, particularly in children below the age of 5. Therefore, an attitude of conservatism prevails in managing splenic injuries. If the bleeding has stopped at the time of laparotomy or if there are simply a few small lacerations or tears that can be controlled by suture or hemostatic agents, such as Avitene, then the spleen should likely be left in place. Hemisplenectomy has been carried out successfully.

Good clinical judgment, however, should not be overshadowed by the desire to save the spleen. If the patient's condition is critical and if other major injuries demand further attention, then a bleeding spleen should probably be removed and the small risk of later infection accepted. Pneumococcal vaccine should be given following splenectomy, and patients should be instructed to seek early medical treatment of unexplained infections or fevers.

Diaphragm

Traumatic diaphragmatic hernia is infrequent, but it can cause major respiratory difficulties and at times can be difficult to diagnose in the individual with multiple system injuries. The left diaphragmatic area is most frequently involved as the liver protects the right diaphragmatic region. There is generally a shift of the mediastinal structures, with the apical beat felt and the heart sounds heard on the right side of the chest. Breath sounds are absent or diminished on the involved side, and movement of the chest on that side may be minimal. X-rays usually confirm the presence of a large air-filled structure or possibly loops of bowel in the chest. Frequently there is evidence of compressed lung in the apical region of the chest, which should help rule out a tension pneumothorax. The diaphragmatic margin is almost always absent. Insertion of a large nasogastric tube may frequently relieve many of the symptoms, and the appearance of the nasogastric tube in the chest on an x-ray may help confirm the diagnosis. If doubt still exists, then barium studies may be required. This injury occasionally can occur on a delayed basis and may be picked up a number of weeks or months later in a relatively asymptomatic patient who has a routine chest x-ray.

Pelvic Organs

The female pelvic organs are well protected by the bony pelvis and are rarely injured in blunt abdominal trauma. They are, however, at risk from penetrating injuries, and this area must be carefully evaluated in any laparotomy.

Major Vessels

Aortic or vena caval injury may not be readily evident at the time of laparotomy. Retroperitoneal hematoma is frequently found and will usually resolve without operative intervention. Renal injuries must be ruled out. When confronted with a rapidly enlarging retroperitoneal hematoma, the retroperitoneal area should be opened and the vena cava and aorta examined. However, as a general rule, the retroperitoneal area is best not opened if the hematoma appears to be stabilized. With major aortic or vena caval injuries, the vessels should be occluded while the patient's vital signs are stabilized. Suturing the injuries may be possible; occasionally prosthetic material may be required with aortic injuries to bridge an extensive area of injury. With penetrating injuries, particularly gunshot wounds, major vessels, such as the hepatic artery, splenic artery, renal arteries, or iliac arteries and veins, may be severely damaged and require either ligation, repair, or substitution with prosthetic material. Multiple or major vascular injuries frequently cause such massive hemorrhage that the patient does not survive the journey to hospital or cannot be resuscitated to allow for emergency laparotomy.

CONCLUSION

A number of points are essential in the management of any trauma patient:

1. Establish the priorities and management.
2. Designate a chief.
3. Don't forget tetanus coverage. If in doubt or there are severe associated lacerations or puncture wounds, then administer human tetanus globulin.
4. Antibiotics are generally not given prophylactically. Routine exceptions are compound fractures, colon injuries, and penetrating abdominal injuries.
5. All penetrating injuries of the abdomen should be explored in the operating room.
6. Remember that head injuries rarely produce shock.
7. Don't forget the relatives during the period of assessment and resuscitation. Normally someone in the medical team can find time to keep them informed about the patient's progress. This may frequently avoid misunderstanding and difficulties later on.

Suggested Readings

Fabian TC, Mangiante EC, et al: A prospective study of 91 patients undergoing both computerized tomography and peritoneal lavage following blunt abdominal trauma. *J Trauma* 26:602–608, 1986.

Federle MP: Abdominal trauma: the role and impact of computed tomography. *Invest Radiol* 16:260–268, 1981.

Feliciano DV, Mattox KL, Jordan GL: Packing for control of hepatic hemorrhage. *J Trauma* 26:738–743, 1986.

Flint LM, Mays ET, Aaron WS: Selectivity in management of hepatic trauma. *Ann Surg* 185:613–618, 1977.

Flancbaum L, Dauterive A, Cox EF: Splenic conservation after multiple trauma in adults. *Surg Gynecol Obstet* 162:469–473, 1986.

Freeark RJ: Penetrating wounds of the abdomen. *N Engl J Med* 291:185–188, 1974.

Jordan GL, Beall AC: Diagnosis and management of abdominal trauma. In *Current Problems in Surgery*. Chicago, Yearbook Medical Publishers, 1971.

Kingston ME, MacKenzie CR: The syndrome of pneumococcemia, disseminated intravascular coagulation and asplenia. *Can Med Assoc J* 121:57–61, 1979.

Krivit W, Giebinic GS, Leonard A: Overwhelming portosplenectomy infection. *Surg Clin N Am* 59:222–233, 1979.

Perry JF Jr, Strate RG: Diagnostic peritoneal lavage in blunt abdominal trauma: indications and results. *Surgery* 71:898–901, 1972.

Sherk JP, McCort JJ, Oakes DD: Computed tomography in thoracoabdominal trauma. *J Trauma* 24:1015-1021, 1984.

Wienceh RG, Wilson RF: Abdominal venous injuries. *J Trauma* 26:771–778, 1986.

CHAPTER

22 Chest Trauma: Lungs and Bony Structure

Ronald L. Holliday, M.D. and William J. Sibbald, M. D.

Increasing violence in our society and the millions of people traveling at high speeds have led to a phenomenal increase in chest injuries. Active surgical or multidisciplinary ICUs most likely have one or more patients suffering blunt or penetrating trauma to the chest at any one time. Complications of chest trauma involving the lungs and bony structures are shown in Table 22.1.

PENETRATING TRAUMA

Penetrating wounds of the chest are most often secondary to gunshot or knife wounds, but also may be caused by impalement with such objects as ski poles or tree branches. The wound itself usually suggests the possibility of underlying injury. During forced expiration, the diaphragm may rise as high as the fourth intercostal space; concomitant interabdominal injuries, therefore, may occur with any penetrating injury at this level or below.

Most wounds penetrating the thorax can be managed with closed tube thoracostomy drainage. The preferential position would be the fifth or sixth intercostal space in the midaxillary line. Occasionally, exsanguinating hemorrhage or persistent hemorrhage from a thoracostomy tube is an indication for early or early-delayed thoracotomy.

NONPENETRATING OR BLUNT TRAUMA

Thoracic trauma is responsible for 25% of deaths in patients with multiple injuries and is an associated factor in another 50% of deaths from blunt trauma. Motor vehicle trauma and falls account for the majority of thoracic injuries. By definition, blunt injury indicates that there is no communication with the outside environment. Injuries may occur to the ribs, lungs, and mediastinal structures. The significance of the injury is proportional to the trauma and to the respiratory reserve of the patient. For instance, an elderly man with chronic bronchitis may develop significant respiratory compromise with only one or two fractured ribs.

Table 22.1
Complications of Chest Trauma

Immediately life-threatening	Potentially life-threatening
Airway obstruction	Pulmonary contusion
Tension pneumothorax	Tracheobronchial tear
Open pneumothorax	Esophageal injury
Flail chest	Disruption of diaphragm
Massive hemothorax	

Management of Nonpenetrating Injury

General

The patient with chest injury receives high priority in the management of multiple trauma. Establishment of the airway is paramount. Once the airway is established, one can proceed through the other basic principles of trauma care, i.e., control of bleeding, assessment of the level of consciousness, examination of the abdomen and the excretory organs, and assessment of fractures. While resuscitation and treatment are proceeding, a history should be obtained from the patient (if possible), a relative, the police, or ambulance attendants. Reconstruction of the details of accidental injury, such as whether the victim was the driver, may indicate specific patterns of chest injury. The definition and severity of pre-existing lung disease are also important.

Diagnosis

The classical maneuvers of physical examination (inspection, palpation, percussion, and auscultation) often lead to accurate diagnosis. Ancillary aids, such as a chest x-ray, blood gases, an electrocardiogram, and needle aspiration of the chest and/or pericardium, may simplify the diagnostic problem.

The physical examination involves

1. *Inspection:* observe skin color, mental status, and the presence of collapsed or dilated peripheral veins, especially in the neck. Be aware of Kussmaul's sign (paradoxical filling of the jugular veins on inspiration, usually indicating pericardial tamponade), cyanosis, stridor, or deviation of the trachea.
2. *Palpation:* note the presence of subcutaneous emphysema, absence of tactile fremitus, an obvious flail segment. Examine the sternum for fracture, the trachea for position, and the larynx for crepitus against the vertebral column (a normal finding).
3. *Percussion:* test for loss of resonance due to air and fluid collections.
4. *Auscultation:* note absent breath sounds on the side of the suspected injury. Listen for bowel sounds in the chest, abnormal heart sounds, or murmurs not previ-

ously present. Listen for friction rubs, indicating pericardial involvement.

With hemodynamic and respiratory stabilization, supplemental x-rays can be taken to document rib fractures, air or fluid in the pleural cavity, the presence of a widened mediastinum (rupture of thoracic aorta), abnormal shadows above the diaphragm, air in the mediastinum, or subcutaneous emphysema.

Intubation and Assisted Ventilation in Chest Injury

During evaluation, specific attention is directed toward the need to consider assisted ventilation. Criteria for intubation and assisted ventilation have been detailed elsewhere (Chapter 7), but briefly include the following:

1. Inability to protect the airway, i.e., coma;
2. Inability to clear secretions, i.e., pain from multiply fractured ribs;
3. Inability to ensure adequate CO_2 excretion. With chest injuries, hypoventilation due to pain is common; if the pain is severe enough despite adequate analgesia and/or respiratory fatigue develops, intubation and assisted ventilation are required;
4. Hypoxemia resistant to correction by supplemental oxygen provided by face mask. With obvious cyanosis or a PaO_2 less than 50 mm Hg on mask oxygen of 40% or greater, intubation is carried out to allow administration of higher concentrations of oxygen and the application of PEEP.

Intubation, when necessary, should be done with a large diameter tube to allow vigorous chest suctioning. The use of positive pressure ventilation in the traumatized patient with chest injuries may be associated with a drop in the blood pressure if volume resuscitation has not been completed; aggressive volume replacement is then provided to restore ventricular preload, thereby restoring cardiac output and blood pressure.

SPECIFIC CHEST INJURIES

Minor Trauma

Minor trauma is defined as one or more rib fractures, with or without pneumothorax, and no flail segment or significant underlying parenchymal injury. Management depends on the patient's underlying pulmonary reserve. The injury may require admission and observation, with monitoring of vital signs and blood gases. Management may be aided by the use of intercostal nerve blocks and minimal doses of analgesic, oxygen by mask, vigorous chest physiotherapy, adequate hydration, and repeat chest x-ray.

Pneumothorax

After rib fractures, pneumothorax is next most common; it may be present in up to 40% of patients with chest injuries. The great majority of these pneumothoraces can be adequately treated with tube thoracostomy. Some may be managed by observation, providing that lung collapse is small (i.e., less than 10 to 15%), interference with respiratory function is minimal and re-expansion is progressive as documented by repeated x-rays.

Insertion of a chest tube for pneumothorax is done through the second intercostal space in the midclavicular line, two finger breadths from the lateral border of the sternum. However, in the patient with multiple injuries, often with an associated hemothorax, the chest tube should be inserted into the fifth or sixth interspace in the midaxillary line. Rapid expansion of the lung occurs in the majority of patients. Continuing air leaks suggest major bronchial or tracheal rupture.

Hemothorax

Blood in the pleural space results from either the rupture of pulmonary parenchymal vasculature or the rupture of the intercostal vessels. It is estimated that 500 ml of blood must accumulate in the pleural space before it is noticed in the chest x-ray. Therefore, significant hemothoraces may be missed when the acutely injured patient is examined only in the supine position. Consideration should be given, when possible, to obtaining a chest x-ray in either the lateral decubitus or sitting position.

Hemothorax is best managed with the insertion of a large chest tube (e.g., 38 or 40 French) through the fifth or sixth intercostal space in the midaxillary line. Careful monitoring of blood loss is mandatory. Most bleeding from pulmonary vasculature will stop with evacuation of the pleural cavity and re-expansion of the lung because of the low pulmonary vascular pressures. Continued bleeding may indicate major great vessel injury and/or disruption of an intercostal artery. Thoracotomy is indicated with persistent hemorrhage or obviously exsanguinating hemorrhage; the usual indications for a thoracotomy are the drainage of 1000–1500 ml of blood initially or a continued rate of bleeding that is greater than 200–300 ml/hr. Clotted hemothoraces should be managed with early thoracotomy to prevent fibrothorax and/or empyema.

Pulmonary Contusion

With deceleration or blast type of injuries, pulmonary contusion is a common occurrence. The influence of contusion on the picture of progressive posttraumatic hypoxemia has been ignored until recently. It is important to realize that the contusion itself may be as important as an overlying flail chest segment. Pulmonary contusion may be focal or may be massive with involvement of both lungs; the latter type may lead to respiratory death if not recognized and aggressively managed. The injury is usually seen on the initial chest x-ray, but it's evidence may be delayed for 48–72 hours. There may be significant hemorrhagic pulmonary edema associated with this injury, with progressive deterioration in respiratory function and blood gases due to the disruption of the alveolocapillary membrane (see adult respiratory distress syndrome (ARDS, Chapter 11).

The management of pulmonary contusion varies according to its severity. Uncomplicated small contusions will resolve in 7–10 days, returning to a completely normal chest x-ray picture. More severe contusions will require individual care. Experimental evidence suggests that aggressive crystalloid resuscitation may actually increase pulmonary abnormalities secondary to contusion. Therefore, the isolated contusion is best managed by fluid restriction (i.e., 75–100 ml of fluid per hour) if such resuscitation is compatible with maintenance of adequate hemodynamic stability as assessed by the blood pressure, urine output, heart rate, etc. Central venous pressure monitoring, with or without sequential monitoring of the cardiac output and the arterial and central venous blood gases, may be required in the patient with a severe contusion. If the pulmonary contusion is severe and results in a significant defect in oxygenation, intubation with the application of positive end-expiratory pressure (PEEP) may be required. Standard criteria for intubation and PEEP are employed (see Chapter 7) in such patients. The use of PEEP will not prevent the egress of fluid across the damaged or traumatized alveolocapillary barrier, but will improve oxygenation by "splinting" the small terminal airways open. The use of corticosteroids in severe pulmonary contusion remains controversial. On balance, we do not feel their use improves recovery to any greater degree than would be obtained by good attention to respiratory and fluid support.

The patient with a pulmonary contusion plus significant extrathoracic injury may require aggressive fluid resuscitation. One will then have to accept the potential increased morbidity of increased pulmonary dysfunction due to accelerated egress of fluid across the damaged pulmonary gas-exchanging membrane to avoid complications, such as renal failure, that might accrue with fluid restriction therapy.

Flail Chest

Flail chest occurs in 10–20% of patients with chest trauma. By definition, multiple ribs must be fractured in two locations. Should the fracture occur through the costochondral junction, only one fracture will be radiologically apparent. The flail chest injury may not be apparent on the initial physical examination in the emergency room due to the patient's ability to splint with his or her respiratory muscles. Repeated observation is frequently necessary to identify the injury. An underlying pulmonary contusion associated with flail chest injury is usually of considerable importance. Mediastinal flutter and "pendelluft" are probably insignificant factors in the pulmonary dysfunction associated with this injury. More important are the pain of the fractured ribs, which leads to splinting, secretion retention, and atelectasis, and the underlying contusion, which results in increased intrapulmonary shunting and hypoxemia.

The management of flail chest should be directed to each patient's needs. Historically, this injury has been treated with external supports, such as adhesive strapping; orthopedic devices, such as wires, hooks, screws, and clamps; early emergency tracheostomy; and most recently with individual care depending on concomitant injury and close monitoring of blood gases.

The isolated flail chest may be successfully managed without the need to use intubation and mechanical ventilation. This is accomplished with modest fluid restriction; frequent suctioning; adequate analgesia, both orally and in the form of intercostal nerve blocks; supplemental oxygen, and aggressive physiotherapy. Mechanical ventilation should be reserved for those patients unable to maintain a PaO_2 greater than 50 mm Hg on room air or those with increasing CO_2 retention (see indications for intubation and ventilation, Chapter 7).

Another addition to the therapeutic management of the patient with a flail chest is the use of demand analgesia. In this situation the patient can medicate for pain according to preadjusted amounts of analgesic in an intravenous drip chamber. In our experience, this has been very successful in the management of pain and maintenance of adequate ventilation in this group of patients.

The patient with major extrathoracic trauma may need endotracheal intubation and mechanical ventilation. Tracheostomy can be done electively if prolonged endotracheal intubation leads to vocal cord dysfunction, usually in the form of ulceration. The occasional patient with a massive flail segment and considerable overriding of rib segments might still be considered for open reduction and fixation of these segments to allow adequate re-expansion of underlying lung and prevent either empyema or lung abcess formation.

Tears of Bronchus and Trachea

Major lacerations of the tracheobronchial tree secondary to blunt trauma are not common. Clinically, they may present with subcutaneous emphysema, pneumomediastinum, and, often, tension peumothorax. Fractures of the first rib and hemoptysis may also alert one to this injury. Management includes confirmation of the diagnosis with laryngoscopy and bronchoscopy, and subsequent operative repair of major tears of the trachea and first order bronchi.

Ruptured Diaphragm

Rupture of the thoracic diaphragm is an uncommon injury. It occurs most frequently on the left side through the tendinous portion of the diaphragm. In addition to being present in blunt thoracic and abdominal injuries, this injury occurs in patients who fall from heights. The injury presents in one of three phases: acute, delayed, or latent. The latent period may go on for a long time, and diagnosis may be made years after the inciting injury. In the acute situation, the diagnosis is made by hearing bowel sounds in the chest or on a routine chest x-ray when a gas-filled viscus is seen above the left hemidiaphragm. Inability to pass a Levin tube or an x-ray of the Levin tube curled in the chest is also evidence of this injury. In some patients with blunt chest trauma, diagnosis may not be apparent until the patient is weaned from ventilation and the intra-abdominal organs make their way into the thoracic cavity.

Treatment of ruptured diaphragm consists of operation, reduction of the abdominal contents from the thoracic cavity, and repair of the defect. Acutely, repair is best accomplished through the abdominal approach. Latent repair may be done by either approach, but often, the thoracic approach may be necessary because of adhesions from long-standing displaced abdominal organs.

Suggested Readings

Daughty D (ed): *Thoracic Trauma.* Boston, Little, Brown and Co, 1980.

Dougall AM, Paul MG, Finley RJ, et al: Chest trauma—current morbidity and mortality. *J Trauma* 17:547, 1977.

McElwee TB, Myers RT: Diaphragmatic rupture from blunt trauma. *Am Surg* 50:143, 1984.

Richardson JD, Franz JL, et al: Pulmonary contusion and hemorrhage—crystalloid versus colloid replacement. *J Surg Res* 16:330, 1974.

Shcaal MA, Rischer RP, Perry JE: The unchanged mortality of flail chest injuries. *J Trauma* 19:492, 1979.

Shackford SR, Smith DE, et al: The management of flail chest. *Am J Surg* 132:759, 1976.

Trinkle JK, et al: Management of flail chest without mechanical ventilation. *Ann Thorac Surg* 19:355, 1975.

Trunkey DD, Lewis FR: Chest trauma. *Surg Clin North Am* 60:1541, 1980.

CHAPTER 23

Chest Trauma: Heart and Great Vessels

Martin M. Goldbach, M.D.

The increased incidence of traumatic injuries to the heart and great vessels mirrors the violence of our society. Modern concepts for the management of trauma were gleaned primarily from experiences in World Wars I and II and from the Vietnamese conflict.

TRAUMATIC INJURIES TO THE HEART

Cardiac trauma may be blunt or penetrating. The types of blunt trauma—direct, indirect, bidirectional, acceleration or deceleration, blast injury, and concussion—and their mechanisms are shown in Figure 23.1. Automobile accidents account for the vast majority of blunt trauma injuries, which may combine direct, indirect, bidirectional, acceleration, and/or deceleration injuries.

Penetrating injuries are usually due to stab or gunshot wounds. Formerly, stab wounds were far more common, but in the last decade guns have gained in popularity as a wounding modality. Other rare causes of penetrating heart injury include intracardiac perforation secondary to pacemaker lead wires, Swan-Ganz catheters, and other intracardiac catheters.

Injury to each cardiac chamber reflects its area of exposure in relationship to the geometry of the anterior chest wall. The incidence of each injury is illustrated in Table 23.1. Ventricular wounds are the most common, and injuries to the vena cava, atria, and great vessels are less common. The coronary arteries, cardiac valves, or septa are rarely injured.

Table 23.1
Incidence of Chamber Involvement

Right ventricle	55%
Left ventricle	20%
Right atrium	10%
Vena cava and great vessels	15%

Impaired cardiac function from penetrating trauma is unusual and is seen only in rare instances where trauma to heart valves,the conducting system, or coronary arteries occurs. However, in patients who survive penetrating injury to reach hospital, cardiac tamponade is usually the dominant initial physiologic injury. Tamponade can delay or stop bleeding from a cardiac laceration, allowing the patient to survive long enough for definitive therapy. However, it is a double-edged sword; although tamponade provides an early opportunity for survival, it also contributes to mortality if it goes unrecognized. The normal pericardial sac can acutely accommodate only 100–250 ml of blood. When more fluid is collected, the increased pressure restricts filling of both the right and left ventricles in diastole, and a depression in cardiac output with hypotension results.

Clinical Features

The clinical features of cardiac injury following trauma vary in severity from immediate death to the gradual de-

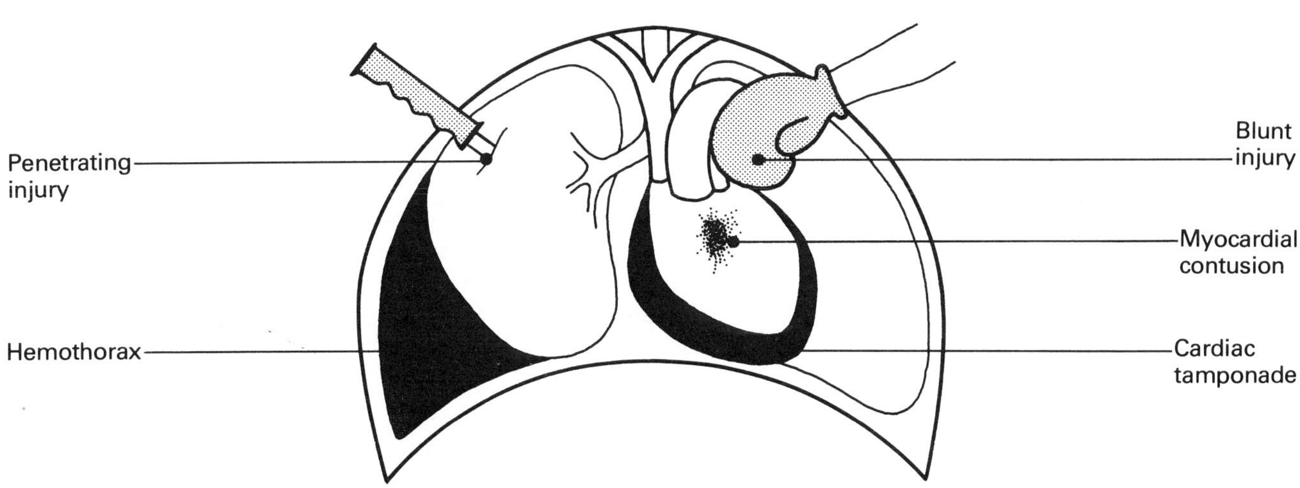

Figure 23.1. Assessment of chest trauma.

velopment of shock over several hours. Prompt recognition and treatment require a high index of suspicion that is derived from the history and nature of the mode of injury. In extreme cases, emergency measures are dictated by the history of trauma and history of signs of life from paramedical personnel and emergency room staff. An aggressive attitude is imperative if there is to be any hope for salvage.

Initial resuscitation should follow the principles of treatment for any shock patient. Hypovolemia should be treated intensively with a large central venous catheter and fluid replacement. Initial hypovolemia may mask the high central venous pressure secondary to tamponade.

Cardiac tamponade is a true medical-surgical emergency. Recognition, however, may at times be difficult. The classical signs of tamponade are faint, distant, muffled heart sounds; decreased arterial pressure with a paradoxical systolic pulse; and elevated central venous pressure. These three clinical signs are known as Beck's triad. Although these signs should be looked for, their absence does not rule out cardiac tamponade for the following reasons. Paradoxical blood pressure is difficult to ascertain without a continuous arterial monitor tracing. Central venous pressures are frequently altered by injury and hypovolemia, whereas the intensity of heart sounds varies with body build. It has been reported in large clinical series that only 50% of patients with acute pericardial tamponade secondary to trauma demonstrate this "classic" triad. Nevertheless, these clinical signs are of value and should be sought.

If the diagnosis of tamponade is unclear the following parameters should be assessed.

1. Central venous pressure: This is an essential measurement. If the central venous pressure is above 15 cm of water the test is virtually diagnostic. A false-positive reading may be due to straining, shivering, or, most commonly, malposition of the catheter. The catheter position should always be checked by radiography.
2. Chest x-ray: A chest x-ray usually does not show cardiac enlargement because the pericardium does not easily distend acutely.
3. Electrocardiogram (ECG) may demonstrate elevation of the ST segments and support the diagnosis.
4. Echocardiography may be diagnostic if it is easily available. One should not, however, take a shocked patient to an echo laboratory or delay treatment until this test is available.
5. Pericardiocentesis: Trinkle and his group in 1974 emphasized the limitations of pericardiocentesis. When they utilized pericardiocentesis in 18 patients, seven false-negatives and three false-positive results were obtained, for an error factor of greater than 50%. They, along with others, currently recommend a subxiphoid pericardial window rather than pericardiocentesis in any case where there is a high index of suspicion. If blood is found, the incision may be extended to a median sternotomy, which provides optimal exposure for treatment of the cardiac lesion (Fig. 23.2).

The diagnosis of myocardial contusion is difficult to make on clinical grounds alone. Typical clinical features may be an inappropriate tachycardia, a pericardial friction rub, or a cardiac murmur not previously known to have been present. "Unexplained" hypotension following trauma should also alert the clinician to the possibility of contusion. ECG features are insensitive, and classic changes indicative of an infarct may be misleading. Diagnosis based on an elevation of cardiac enzymes is likewise fraught with danger because the traumatized patient invariably manifests an elevation of these enzymes because of associated skeletal muscle or hepatic injuries. We have found the single most helpful test in the diag-

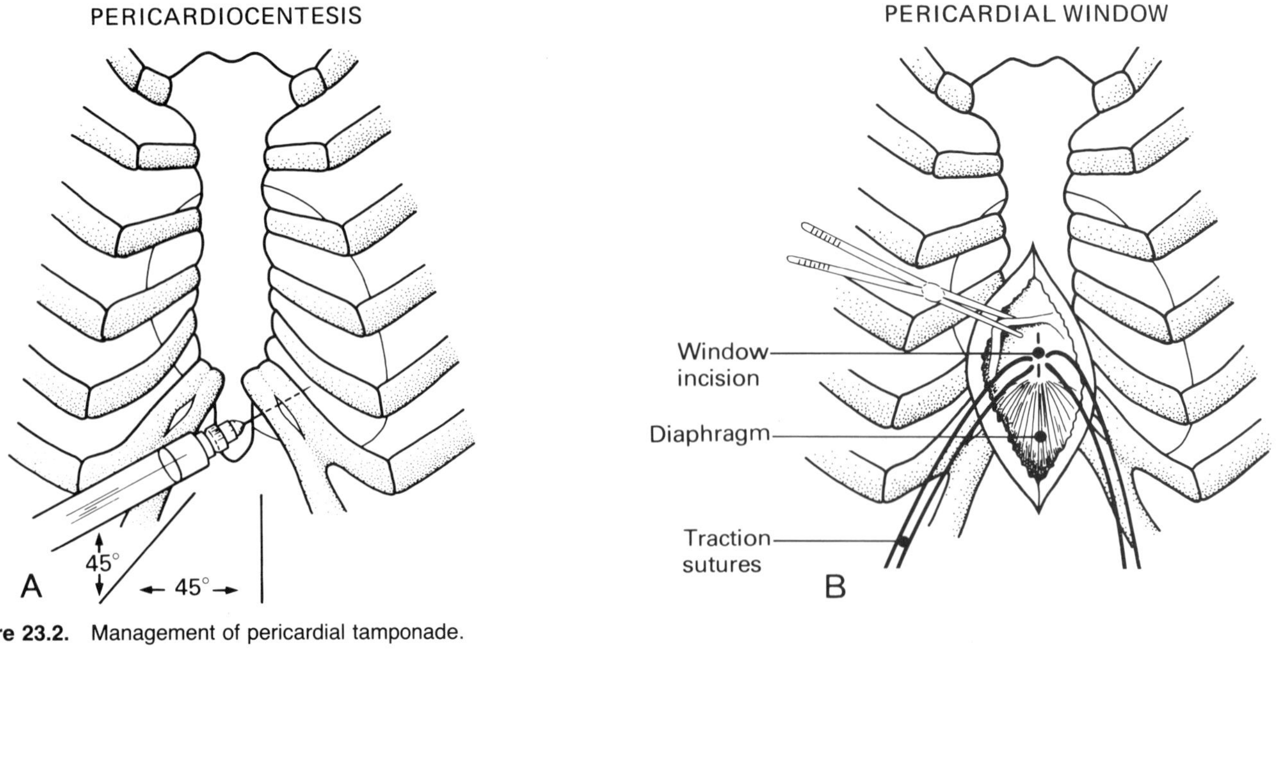

Figure 23.2. Management of pericardial tamponade.

nosis of myocardial contusion to be ECG-gated cardiac scintigraphy. With this examination, discrete areas of hypokinesis, akinesis, or dyskinesis strongly suggest contusion. Too, because this examination is noninvasive, it may be repeated sequentially to follow the course of the lesion. Occasionally, invasive cardiac studies are required to establish the anatomy of the lesion, particularly if there is clinical suspicion of traumatic valvular disruption.

Treatment

In the difficult group of patients in whom signs of life were present during the ambulance trip or on arrival to hospital but are no longer present, an immediate thoracotomy is recommended. Closed chest massage has no place in the presence of heart trauma as the cardiac wound will extend and the efforts of external massage will be buffered by the clot around the heart, thereby rendering massage ineffective.

In more elective cases, a thoracotomy or median sternotomy is performed in an operating room with a standby heart-lung machine. Most cardiac lacerations may be controlled with a finger or simple atraumatic clamp. Wounds are closed using simple suture techniques. Muscle injuries may be closed with the help of Teflon pledgets as bolsters. In the more unusual cases where dislocation of the heart is required, it may be necessary to support the circulation with the heart-lung machine. Injuries to the left ventricle, cardiac septa, or heart valves require cardiopulmonary bypass. Among the disadvantages of the pump are the need to give heparin to a recently traumatized patient who may have other bleeding foci. Absence of sophisticated cardiopulmonary bypass machinery should not be a deterrent to exploration if the situation is nonelective.

The surgical treatment results of two relatively large series are illustrated in Table 23.2. These findings included many instances in which the decision in the emergency department was to operate or pronounce the patient dead. The results support a continued aggressive approach.

Myocardial contusion, particularly of the right ventricle, is usually not a difficult therapeutic problem if suspected early. Occasionally, invasive hemodynamic monitoring is required to provide the objective data base needed to make a therapeutic decision about further volume (preload) expansion or the use of inotropic support (see Chapter 5). In our experience, myocardial contusion of either the left or right ventricle is a self-limiting injury with uniformly good recovery. However, in occasional cases, complete hemodynamic monitoring is required to establish therapeutic guidelines.

Table 23.2
Results of Surgical Treatment

Injury	Number of patients	Survivors	
		Number	Percentage
Mattox et al. series			
Stab wounds	11	9	82
Gunshot wounds	22	15	68
Blunt trauma	4	1	25
Total	37	25	67.5
Asfaw and Arbulu series			
Stab wounds	364		92
Gunshot wounds	36		98
Total	400		

TRAUMATIC INJURIES TO THE GREAT VESSELS

Traumatic injuries to the great vessels are usually secondary to decelerative forces of blunt trauma. Most commonly, the patient has been involved in an automobile accident and may or may not have associated injuries. Usually, the intima and media of the aorta tear just beyond the left subclavian artery, although tears above the aortic valve or in the neck vessels may occur. The thoracic aorta is fixed by the great vessels from a point just above the aortic valve to the area of the left subclavian artery. The area below the left subclavian artery is mobile, and when lateral and horizontal forces occur, the aorta flexes, resulting in tears in this area. Similarly, the heart is mobile and swings like a pendulum from its fixed position just above the aortic valve; thus often an aortic dissection tear occurs just above the aortic valve.

Continuity of the aortic adventitia determines the patient's initial survival because 60% of the strength of the thoracic aorta is provided by adventitia. About 80% of patients exsanguinate immediately at the scene of the accident. Of the 20% who reach hospital alive more than two-thirds will die within the first 2 weeks unless the aorta is repaired. Of the immediate survivors,only a very small percentage, about 2%, will live long enough to develop a chronic false aneurysm.

Diagnosis requires a high index of suspicion when a decelerative injury has occurred. A chest x-ray usually shows a widened mediastinum. In the presence of a widened mediastinum, an aortogram is absolutely vital.

It is important to know where the tear is and what vessels are involved. Aortography is performed using the Seldinger technique from the groin. Most trauma centers are aggressive with aortography when suspicion of a widened mediastinum is aroused. Aortography in experienced hands is associated with a very low complication rate.

Treatment

Treatment includes prophylaxis, resuscitation, usually intraoperative control of blood pressure, and repair (Table 23.3).

Repair of this lesion requires a left posterolateral thoracotomy incision. It is important to enter the chest at a high level to gain access to the proximal aorta and the subclavian artery. The aorta is resected, with aortic continuity re-established using a woven Dacron graft. On rare occasions, the aorta may be closed primarily. The pericardium should be explored at the time of thoracotomy as blood may trickle back into the pericardium and

Table 23.3
Treatment

Prophylaxis	
	Seat belts
	Low speeds
Resuscitation	
	IV, fluids, etc.
Intraoperative management	
	May be necessary to lower blood pressure pharmacologically
Surgery	
	Re-establish continuity (woven graft)

cause tamponade. It is also of value to look for contusion injuries to the right and left ventricle.

One of the great unsolved problems in cardiovascular surgery is paraplegia following injury to the thoracic aorta. Although the patient may arrive with normal neurologic function, he or she may be paraplegic at the end of an otherwise successful operative procedure. The incidence of paraplegia seems to be the same whether blood to the spinal cord is provided using cardiopulmonary bypass with an external shunt or the aorta is simply cross-clamped and continuity is re-established without perfusion of the lower thoracic aorta. Some believe that rapid performance of the anastomoses with aortic occlusion time under 30–40 minutes may be the essential factor in preventing this injury. At the present time this complication occurs in about 10% of cases.

Suggested Readings

Asfaw I, Arbula A: Penetrating wounds of the pericardium and heart. *Surg Clin North Am* 57:37, 1977.

Mattox KL, Beall AC Jr, Jordan GL, et al: Cardiorrhaphy in the emergency center. *J Thorac Cardiovasc Surg* 68:886, 1974.

Trinkle JK, Marcos J, Brover FL, et al: Management of the wounded heart. *Ann Thorac Surg* 17:230, 1974.

CHAPTER

24 Orthopedic Trauma

R. Baxter Willis, M.D.

The advent of seat belt legislation in the United States, Canada, and elsewhere in the world in response to high mortality rates from motor vehicle accidents has paradoxically led to increased numbers of multiply injured patients. These measures have resulted in lowered mortality but increased morbidity, because of the multisystem trauma sustained in motor vehicle accidents.

This chapter considers some basic principles of orthopedic trauma. Although the orthopedist has a rather low priority in the immediate management scheme, it is important that all the elements of a multidisciplinary approach be carried out systematically in the initial screening, investigation, and management of multiply injured individuals. This approach includes an assessment of the airway, investigation and restoration of loss of blood volume, and examination of the central nervous system, digestive system, genitourinary tract, and, finally, the musculoskeletal system. Often, major musculoskeletal injuries are the most clinically obvious, and it is possible to become so involved in the initial management of them that other, potentially more life-threatening injuries are overlooked. It is therefore imperative to stress the need for a total systematic approach to the examination and initial resuscitation of a multiply injured patient with musculoskeletal injuries. Key to this approach is the development of a dedicated team concept of individuals with multiple interests and capabilities interested in the care of the multiply traumatized patient.

FRACTURES

In recent years the surgical pendulum has swung to a more aggressive surgical approach in those patients sustaining multiple fractures (Table 24.1). Historically, these patients were often treated initially with traction, and subsequent surgical management of any fractures was delayed for several days until the general overall status of the patient permitted surgery. Paradoxically the status of the patient often deteriorated, precluding surgery in the first few weeks following injury. A number of recent critical care studies have suggested that early and aggressive surgical management of patients with more than two fractures in fact lowers the overall morbidity and mortality of these patients, especially from the adult respiratory distress syndrome (ARDS) (fat embolism syndrome). A team approach is therefore required, including general or trauma surgeons, neurosurgeons, and others, when the goals for initial management of the multiply injured patient are defined.

Table 24.1
Management of Multiple Fractures

Open fractures
Surgical debridement
Antibiotics
Tetanus prophylaxis
Rigid immobilization by means of external skeletal fixators
Multiple closed fractures
Early surgical approach
Open reduction, internal fixation if possible
Team approach to reduce anesthetic time
Rigid fixation lessens morbidity, facilitates nursing care
Rigid external fixation as an alternative to internal fixation

Following the initial definitive management of any chest or abdominal trauma, as well as neurosurgical stabilization, stabilization of long bone fractures is accomplished by closed or open technique if the general condition of the patient permits. This is best done in a team approach with several orthopedic surgeons working on different fractures simultaneously to lessen anesthetic time. If the fracture is open or compound or the general condition of the patient does not permit further prolonged anesthesia, then the use of external fixation is the technique of choice to immobilize fractures.

Unstable pelvic fractures can be stabilized to some degree by the application of an external fixator (Hoffman apparatus). This technique is particularly applicable when the pelvic fracture is associated with massive blood loss. Stabilization of the pelvis by an external fixator can aid in control of the hemodynamic state of the patient.

Early evidence suggests that the incidence and severity of fat embolism syndrome or ARDS can be decreased with an aggressive orthopedic approach. There is certainly no argument that this type of philosophy facilitates proper nursing care of patients in a critical care trauma unit, permitting easy turning and posturing of the patient for necessary chest physiotherapy, proper skin care, and the general well-being of the patient.

Open Fractures

One of the true orthopedic emergencies is the open fracture (previously termed compound) or open joint injury. There is a so-called golden period of approximately 8 hours after injury in which the wound should be surgically explored, debrided of devitalized tissue, and thoroughly irrigated with at least 10 liters of irrigating solution. The wound is then left open, to be closed on either a delayed primary basis or by secondary intent.

The initial emergency management of an open fracture should consist of proper tetanus prophylaxis and prophylactic intravenous antibiotics. If the patient has been actively immunized in the 10 years previous to the open injury, then a tetanus toxoid booster is adequate. If the patient's immunization is not up to these levels, then repeat primary immunization with tetanus immune globulin is necessary.

A broad spectrum intravenous antibiotic is used prophylactically for 48 hours in patients with open fractures or open joint injuries. This antibiotic should have coverage against Gram positive organisms, including *Staphylococcus* and *Streptococcus,* as well as against some of the common Gram negative organisms. Any one of the many available cephalosporins fills this role very well. If stronger Gram negative coverage is required, then one of the aminoglycosides is added to the regimen: gentamycin or tobramycin. The patient is then examined frequently, and in the absence of any clinical or biochemical evidence of established infection, prophylactic antibiotics are discontinued after 48 hours. It is important to emphasize that prolonged or excessive use of "prophylactic" antibiotics may indeed facilitate the development of hospital-acquired infections, particularly with Gram negative organisms. If, however, after 48 hours clinical evidence for sepsis exists, again a coordinated review of the patient with all consultants to the trauma team is necessary in order to identify potential sites of infection and establish therapeutic options. The multiply traumatized patient often manifests depressed host defense (see Chapter 38), and therefore is a particular risk of developing hospital-acquired infections.

The advent of numerous types of external fixators has permitted a more aggressive surgical approach to fracture management. The external fixators have the advantage of providing rigid fixation to the fracture, but without further violating the open wound with additional soft tissue devitalization. The external fixators are placed remote from the actual fracture site, thereby lessening the incidence of infection. They also allow easy access to the wound for dressing changes, wound closure, and for any skin grafts or rotational flaps in the case of more serious soft tissue injuries.

GAS GANGRENE

Gas gangrene is a life-threatening condition characterized by severe necrosis of soft tissues, especially muscle, due to the gas-forming anaerobic Gram positive bacilli, particularly *Clostridium welchii* (C. perfringens).

This condition is fortunately rare, but is most frequently encountered in the patient with an open fracture that has been inadequately debrided. The patient is acutely ill, febrile with tachycardia, and with profound hypotension and crepitus subcutaneously in the involved tissue—usually an extremity. A coagulopathy is common. If immediate and radical action is not taken, death is imminent from septic shock.

Prophylaxis is most important when considering gas gangrene. The greatest problem in prophylaxis is delay of effective treatment. Clostridial infections are not due to uniquely pathologic strains but the uniquely local circumstances. The most important step in prevention is early surgery that thoroughly removes all necrotic tissue.

Treatment (Table 24.2)

Once gas gangrene is found, success depends on prompt diagnosis and surgical debridement. Surgery consists of decompression of underlying muscle, radical excision of all nonviable tissue, and possible amputation in order to meet this objective.

Intravenous penicillin (3–4 million units every 3 hours) is the antibiotic of choice.

Hyperbaric oxygen may be a potential adjunct in treatment, but should *not* delay surgery. The patient is placed in a hyperbaric chamber for 60–90 minutes every 8–12 hours at three atmospheres of pressure. The hyperbaric oxygen profoundly decreases the action of clostridial histotoxins and inhibits the growth of the clostridial organisms.

The administration of polyvalent gas gangrene antitoxin for the treatment of gas gangrene is controversial. If employed, the polyvalent antitoxin is given in doses of 50,000 units q4–6h for 24–48 hours.

In summary, the successful treatment of gas gangrene depends on early diagnosis and prompt surgical debridement of devitalized tissue in conjunction with large doses of intravenous penicillin. Adjunctive measures include fluid and electrolyte replacement, hyperbaric oxygenation, and polyvalent antitoxin.

COMPARTMENT SYNDROMES

Compartment syndromes are a well-recognized complication of closed fracture and extensive soft tissue injury. With either a fracture or a crush injury, soft tissue swelling within an enclosed extremity compartment may occur. This swelling may be severe enough to occlude the arterioles to muscle, resulting in cloudy swelling, further inflammation, and circulatory compromise of both muscle and soft tissue (Fig. 24.1).

Table 24.2
Treatment of Gas Gangrene

Prevention
- Adequate debridement of all devitalized tissue

Definitive care
- Wide surgical excision of all devitalized tissue
- Penicillin G, intravenously
- Aggressive fluid resuscitation
  - Keep Hb >11 gm/100 ml
  - Keep serum albumin >3 gm/100 ml
- Maintain high urine output to prevent renal failure secondary to hemoglobinuria/myoglobinuria
- Controversial
  - Hyperbaric oxygenation
  - Polyvalent antitoxin

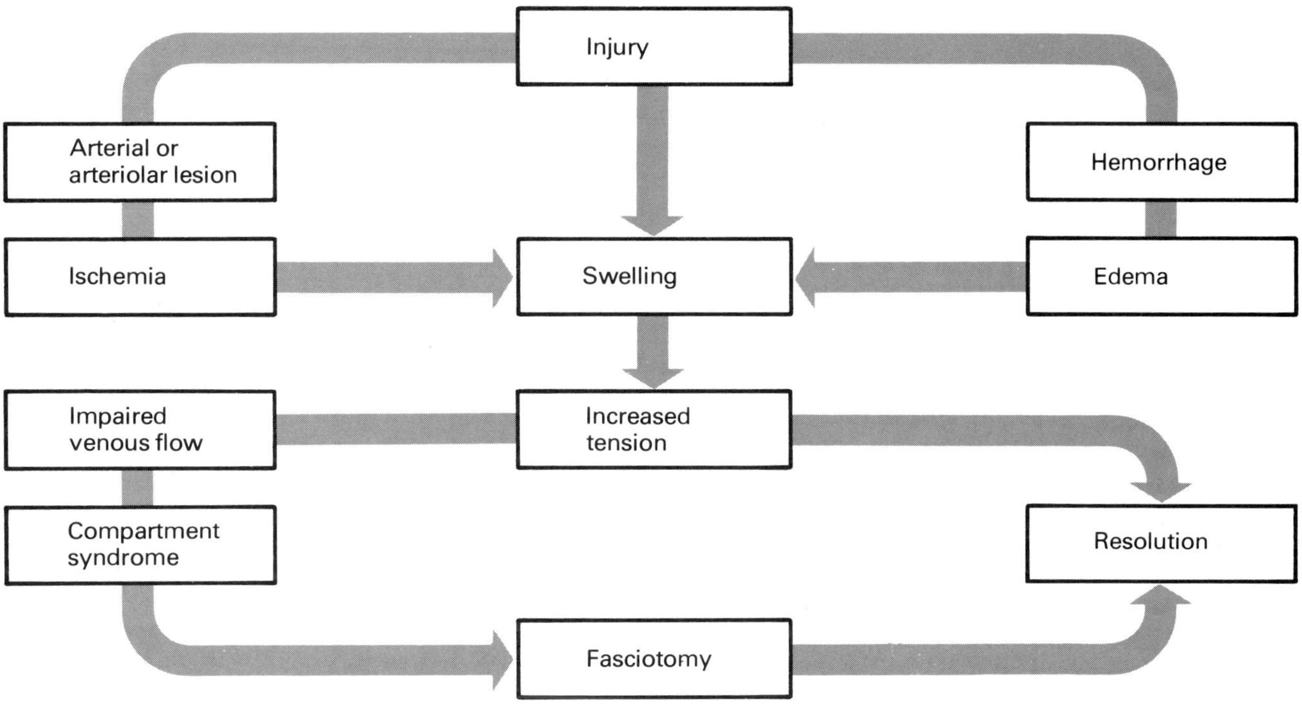

Figure 24.1 Pathophysiology of compartment syndromes.

The signs and symptoms of this syndrome are unrelenting pain, pallor, puffiness, paralysis and paresthesia (Table 24.3). Pulses are usually present. The compartments most commonly affected are the superficial and deep posterior compartments of the leg, the anterior compartment of the leg, and the volar compartment of the forearm. If severe pain is noted when the muscles of the affected compartment are put on the stretch, a strong suspicion of this clinical entity must exist, i.e., pain with passive dorsiflexion of toes implicates deep posterior compartment of the leg.

A strong index of suspicion for this injury is required in head-injured patients with associated extremity injuries. In addition, the condition is prevalent in drug overdose victims who develop compartment syndromes as a result of their body weight lying on an extremity for prolonged periods of unconsciousness. In these cases, objective confirmation of the condition is advisable by use of a special intracompartmental catheter in conjunction with an arterial pressure transducer. Normal compartment pressures are in the neighborhood of 12–20 mm Hg. When pressures exceed 30–35 mm Hg, a compartment syndrome exists and warrants fasciotomy to relieve the constricting pressure on the underlying muscle.

Table 24.3
Diagnosis of Compartment Syndromes

Pain on passive movement of involved muscle group
Pallor
Puffiness
Paresthesias
Paralysis
Pulses present
Pyrophosphate scanning
Intracompartmental pressure monitoring (wick or slit catheter)
Myoglobinuria (late)—signifies muscle necrosis

Although not a substitute for prompt diagnostic suspicion, pyrophosphate scanning can be an aid in location and severity of the compartment syndrome. If the compartment syndrome is early and not profound, the initial blood pool of the scan concentrates the pyrophosphate in the involved area, helping delineate the exact location of the compartment syndrome, either in the leg or the arm.

If, however, the condition is diagnosed late, then the pyrophosphate is not concentrated in the extremity as evidenced by a decreased blood pool in the particular muscle compartment.

Additional objective evidence can be ascertained by introducing a specialized catheter into the specific muscle compartment and measuring pressure by an arterial pressure transducer. This method is especially helpful in monitoring compartment pressures in the unconscious patient.

FAT EMBOLISM SYNDROME

Fat embolism syndrome is a clinical entity encountered in patients with massive trauma and usually with multiple fractures. It remains an important cause of morbidity and mortality in patients following such injuries. All age groups are equally at risk, and the incidence of this syndrome is higher in patients with closed fractures (30%) than with open fractures (2%).

This syndrome is not necessarily confined to patients after bony trauma. It has been reported following burns and after liver trauma, as well as in nontraumatic entities, such as diabetes, severe infection, neoplasms, blood transfusions, cardiopulmonary bypass, renal transplantation, hemoglobinopathies, and collagen-vascular diseases.

The fat embolism syndrome is but one of the many causes of the adult respiratory distress syndrome (see Chapter 11), a form of acute pulmonary insufficiency. With prompt recognition, appropriate treatment can be instituted, resulting in decreased morbidity and mortality from this complication of multiple trauma.

Pathogenesis

Fat embolism results when fat macroglobules, measuring approximately 20 μm in diameter, circulate through the pulmonary and systemic vasculature. The sites of origin of these macroglobules continue to be the source of considerable controversy. Fat globules in the pulmonary microcirculation cause pulmonary artery hypertension and increased microvascular permeability, as seen in ARDS. There are two theories as to the origin of these microemboli, mechanical and chemical. More than one possibility likely exists for the source of the fat emboli, and the causes discussed below are not mutually exclusive.

Mechanical Theory

The early German writers on this subject believed that fat droplets originated at the site of fracture or injury. Free fat was liberated into the general circulation by the increased interstitial pressure and collected in the pulmonary arteriolar circulation. These fat macroglobules are approximately 20 μm in diameter and are readily identified on histologic sections of the lung at autopsy.

Chemical Theory

There is also evidence that trauma and/or critical illness causes a physiologic change in circulating fat. These changes may allow for a coalescence of chylomicrons into fat globules.

Pathophysiology

Fat emboli pass into the pulmonary arterioles, producing a mechanical block in the pulmonary circulation and, if severe, right heart failure. The fat macroglobules attract platelets and red blood cells that eventually disintegrate, releasing serotonin, histamine, and other humoral substances. These humoral substances cause local vasoconstriction and bronchospasm. Many of the fat globules may also pass through the pulmonary microcirculation to other organs, such as the brain, kidney, and heart.

Blood-tinged sputum is a characteristic symptom of fat embolism syndrome. The fat in the lung is engulfed by macrophages and carried into the alveoli. Glycerol and free fatty acids are released as the triglycerides are broken down locally by tissue lipase. The free fatty acids cause a chemical pneumonitis, as well as a decrease in the amount of surfactant produced by the alveolar type 2 cell.

Clinical Manifestations

Manifestations of this condition range in severity from the very mild to very fulminant. This condition is usually found in a patient with one or more long bone fractures, but may also be seen in patients with relatively minor fractures.

The onset may be immediate, as in the fulminant form, or may not occur for 2–3 days after the traumatic incident. Sevitt found that, of 100 patients with fat embolism syndrome, 25 showed symptoms within the first 12 hours after an injury, 75 by 36 hours, and 85 patients by 48 hours.

In the fulminating and rapidly progressive form there is marked respiratory distress with severe arterial hypoxemia, the sudden onset of pulmonary hypertension with right ventricular strain, and, if unrecognized, coma due to anoxia, progressing to death.

In the subacute form, symptoms are shortness of breath, followed by restlessness and confusion. The clinical signs are fever to 39° or 40°C, tachypnea with rates of 30/min or higher, and tachycardia. There are often changing neurologic symptoms, with restlessness, disorientation, and confusion being the most common manifestations.

Petechiae may be seen characteristically across the chest, axillae, and base of the neck, as well as in the conjunctiva, on the second or third day after injury. The petechiae may be fleeting, lasting only a short time.

A chest x-ray reveals bilateral, fluffy infiltrates consistent with a diagnosis of pulmonary edema. Blood gases should be done early and repeated often. The patient will show hypoxemia on room air. More sophisticated studies reveal an increased pulmonary shunt fraction, and there may well be EEG and ECG abnormalities.

Diagnosis

The diagnosis is confirmed only by assimilation of the clinical picture in the patient at risk (Table 24.4). The only definitive signs of fat embolus are retinal fat globules, biopsies of kidney or skin lesions demonstrating embolic fat, or autopsy examination showing fat and bone marrow particles in lung and other viscera. The usual clinical picture of fat embolus may be associated with mortality because of protracted, progressive respiratory failure. The respiratory failure again is due to pulmonary edema, but without any associated signs or symptoms of a left ventricular failure (see diagnosis of ARDS, Chapter 11).

Table 24.4
Diagnosis of Fat Embolism

Clinical suspicion
Tachycardia
Tachypnea
↓ Hb
↓ Platelet count
Laboratory confirmation
Hypoxemia
Fat in sputum & urine
Infiltrate on X-ray
Definite diagnosis
Retinal fat globules
Fat in skin biopsy
Autopsy

Treatment

Treatment can be considered in two categories—general and specific measures. As with all patients who have sustained major trauma, the following priorities are established: airway maintenance, restoration of blood volume, restoration and maintenance of fluid and electrolyte balance, and immobilization of the injured part or parts. The extremities should be properly immobilized before any transport is carried out, and such immobilization is likely the major factor in decreasing the incidence of the syndrome in those patients who undergo immediate fixation of their fractures. Most importantly, close monitoring of the blood gases in patients with long bone fractures over the first 5 days will allow early diagnosis and treatment.

Specific Treatment (Table 24.5)

When routine blood gas determination reveals a $PaO_2 < 60$ mm Hg on room air, the patient is started on supplemental oxygen given by nasal cannulae or mask. Further deterioration of the lung picture, which may be accompanied by confusion, demands aggressive ventilatory support and other modalities for the treatment of the oxygenating defect of this syndrome. This situation usually requires transfer to a special care unit, where frequent monitoring and aggressive physiotherapy and respiratory care may be provided. The management of acute respiratory insufficiency is detailed in Chapter 7.

For resolution of the pulmonary injury by fat globules, the most specific therapy is immobilization of the fracture site(s). All other care is primarily supportive, because there is at this time no specific pharmacologic therapy proven to prevent the injurious effects of the fat globules in the pulmonary microcirculation.

There have been many suggested adjuvant treatments for fat embolism, but there is no specific therapy. Pharmacologic doses of steroids (e.g., 30 mg/kg Solu-Medrol q6h for 48 hours) have been reported of benefit in giving some protection to the lung from the damage associated with the chemical pneumonitis.

Other modes of treatment have been employed in an attempt to lower the plasma lipid content and to improve microcirculatory flow. Heparin has been suggested for this role because (1) it is a lipolytic agent that increases serum lipase activity and theoretically hastens the hydrolysis of fat and (2) it is an anticoagulant that prevents platelet aggregation. Low molecular weight dextran improves microcirculatory flow and decreases platelet adhesiveness. Intravenous alcohol has also been suggested as a therapeutic agent on the theory that it enhances emulsification and hydrolysis of fat.

Table 24.5
Treatment of Fat Embolism

Treatment of definite value
Supplemental oxygen
Ventilatory support
Immobilization of fractures
Treatment that may be of value (controversial)
Corticosteroids
Alcohol
Heparin
Hypertonic glucose
Aspirin

Yet, there is no prospective or randomized study that shows that any of the adjunctive pharmacologic therapies indicated above alter the mortality and morbidity of ARDS secondary to the fat embolism syndrome. A successful outcome depends mostly on early recognition, prompt fracture immobilization, and support of the defects in oxygenation and ventilation that may accrue if the syndrome becomes established.

Suggested Readings

Altameir WA, Fullen WD: Prevention and treatment of gas gangrene. *JAMA* 217:806–813, 1971.

Evarts CM: Complications in fractures. In Rockwood CA, Green DP: *Fractures*. Philadelphia, Lippincott, 1974, vol 1, pp 156–243.

Fowler PJ, Willis RB: Vascular compartment syndromes. *Can J Surg* 18:157–161, 1975.

Gossling HR, Ellison LH, Degraff AC: Fat embolism. *J Bone Joint Surg* 56A:1327, 1974.

Gustilo RB, Anderson JT: Prevention of infection in the treatment of 1025 open fractures of long bones. *J Bone Joint Surg* 58A:453, 1976.

Gurd AR: Fat embolism: an aid to diagnosis. *J Bone Joint Surg* 52B:732–737, 1970.

McMurtry R, Walton D, Dickinson D, Kellam J, Tile M: Pelvic disruption in the polytraumatized patient: a management protocol. *Clin Orthop* 151:1980.

Mears D, Fu FH: Modern concepts of external skeletal fixation of the pelvis. *Clin Orthop* 151:180

Peltier LF, Collins JA, Evarts CM, et al.: Fat embolism. *Arch Surg* 109:12, 1974.

Sevitt S: The significance and classification of fat-embolism. *Lancet* 2:825–828, 1960.

Trunkey DD, Chapman MW, Lim RC Jr, Dunphy E: Management of pelvic fractures in blunt trauma injury. *J Trauma* 14:912, 1974.

Wade PA, Campbell RD: Open versus closed methods in treating fractures of the leg. *Am J Surg* 95:599, 1958.

CHAPTER

25 Genitourinary Trauma

Robert R. Shepherd, M.D.

Potential genitourinary (GU) tract involvement must be excluded in all cases of major injury. The salient manifestations of GU trauma are hematuria and/or an inability to void. Less specific manifestations include lower abdominal pain, the presence of a flank mass, signs of ongoing blood loss without a well-defined site, suprapubic discomfort, and urethral bleeding. The immediate objectives of GU assessment following trauma are the localization of the injury and selection of conservative management or operative intervention.

The major mechanisms of GU trauma include the following (Fig. 25.1):

1. Penetration by bullet, knife, or impalement following a motor vehicle accident (MVA) or fall;
2. Blunt injury as seen with
   a. Direct force (from a fall, kick, blow, or MVA);
   b. Deceleration injury (from a fall, MVA) with stretch of a renal artery and an intimal tear, or division of the ureteropelvic junction, particularly in a child;
   c. Injury by a bony fragment (e.g., pelvic fracture) with subsequent bladder perforation or ureteral laceration;
   d. Ligamentous traction (e.g., bladder tear) as seen with a pelvic fracture.

Certain factors seem to predispose to major GU injury. For example, a bladder that is full at the time of the accident is more prone to rupture. The patient with an underlying primary renal abnormality, such as hydronephrosis, is more likely to suffer serious GU injury after blunt abdominal trauma. Youth predisposes to injury because the bladder in these patients is more intra-abdominal, and the kidneys are relatively larger and less protected by the rib cage and perinephric fat. Therefore, particularly close scrutiny is given to GU examination in the young patient.

The possibility of injury to the urinary tract should be considered in all cases of blunt abdominal trauma and/or pelvic fracture. Penetrating wounds ordinarily indicate directly where an injury is to be suspected. Yet, one must remember that multiple deflections of a missile within the body may result in injuries that might not be suspected if one were to assume a straight course between point of entry and that of arrest or exit.

Suspicion of an associated renal injury may be strengthened by a history of penetrating or blunt injury to the loin area or of severe generalized force to the abdomen associated with a fall or MVA. The presence of a puncture, contusion, mass, or swelling in the loins might support this suspicion. Fractures of the ribs or transverse processes of the vertebrae may be noted and, when associated with hematuria, may indicate an important renal injury.

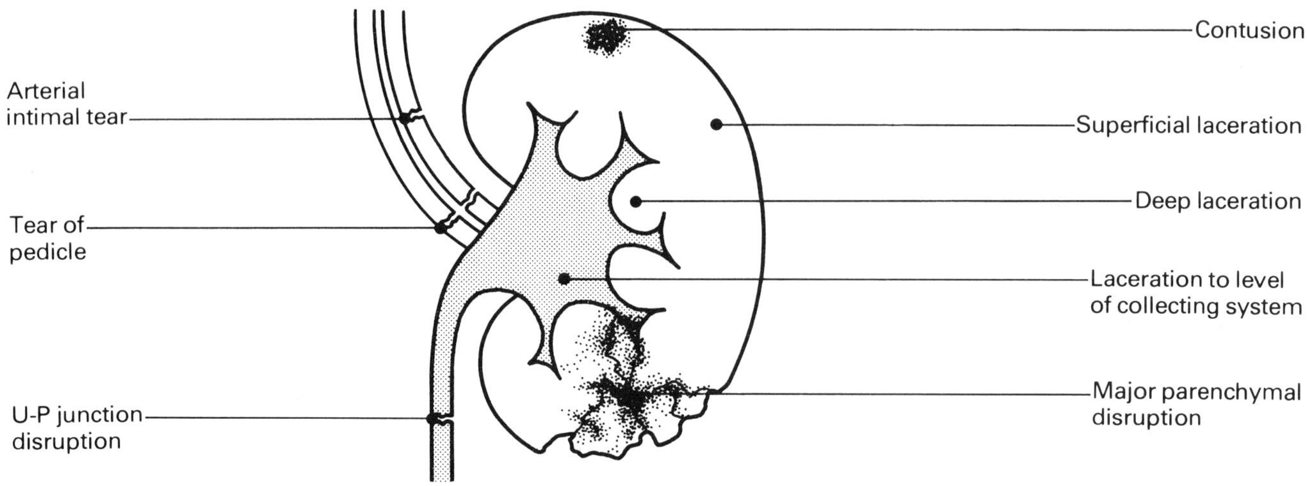

Figure 25.1 Major types of genitourinary trauma.

INVESTIGATION OF THE PATIENT WITH SUSPECTED GU TRAUMA

In all cases of multiple trauma where there is suspicion of renal injury, high-dose infusion pyelography is required early in the patient workup as the major investigative procedure to delineate renal injury. The renal factors assessed by pyelography include the number of kidneys and the presence of depression of function, extravasation of dye, polar nonfunction, or a perinephric collection of dye.

Ureteral visualization may be imperfect. However, good renal function accompanied by bladder filling and the absence of extravasation at least exclude ureteral obstruction or loss of ureteral continuity. The most effective means of clarification of any renal injury is renal angiography. It delineates accurately any renal pedicle injury (e.g., intimal tear), peripheral arterial lesions, parenchymal tears, or areas of infarction. At the same time, flush aortography and selective injections exclude or delineate other visceral injuries. Because of its anatomic accuracy, in most situations angiography has displaced retrograde pyelography, which may give a false suspicion of the degree of extravasation but without critical information concerning the vascular pattern.

Noninvasive techniques of evaluation, such as abdominal ultrasound, may be of use in assessing the presence of a mass (e.g., hematoma or urinoma) around the kidney. Where integrity of blood flow or renal functional evaluation is desired, isotope studies may be useful, but they do not provide the anatomic definition of angiography.

CT scanning with contrast enhancement provides definition of normal vascularized renal parenchyma, intrarenal and subcapsular collections, and perinephric hematoma or urinoma. Tissue disruption and loss of vascular supply may be delineated, as may areas of extravasation of contrast that are suggestive of disruption of the collecting system. In addition to clarifying renal morphology and function, CT scanning may be useful in identifying other visceral injuries in cases of multiorgan injury.

Clinical supervision consists of close monitoring of all vital signs and repeat clinical observation and measurement of any flank mass to detect expansion. Serial urine samples are kept in a rack in order to follow associated hematuria.

The patient with a normal pyelogram or minimal extravasation of dye may require nothing more than bed rest, observation, and possibly antibiotic prophylaxis.

A patient with an expanding flank mass, gross hematuria, circulatory instability, pedicle injury, segmental parenchymal separation, or total parenchymal disruption will likely require operative intervention.

Operation is indicated urgently when renal blood flow is occluded, if viability of renal tissue is to be preserved. Exploration of the artery may allow resection and anastomosis of the injured arterial segment or bypass grafting according to technical considerations.

Lesions with significant parenchymal disruptions are prone to complications from urinary extravasation, persisting hemorrhage, or secondary hemorrhage. For these reasons, debridement and repair are indicated to control hemorrhage, remove devitalized tissue, and obtain closure of the urinary collecting system. In certain cases nephrostomy drainage is added to decompress the collecting system, whereas protection by Penrose or other types of drain is routine.

There is considerable controversy about the ideal operative approach. Urologists, familiar with the flank approach, tend to favor it despite the fact that access to the pedicle may be difficult with resultant problems in the face of heavy bleeding. A transabdominal approach allows more direct access to the renal pedicle for early vascular control and is the incision of choice when vascular repair is required. It also could be of value where major disruption of parenchyma would likely allow heavy bleeding. This approach is less desirable, however, for the full exposure required for debridement and repair of lacerations or polar separation. Clearly, the operative approach depends on diagnosis and the experience and preference of the surgeon.

Injection of coils or microspheres by angiographic methods may provide another method for controlling bleeding where operative intervention is contraindicated.

URETERAL INJURY

Penetrating

Ninety-five percent of such injuries are the result of gunshot injuries. Low velocity missiles produce less blast effect, and high velocity missiles may produce a large exit wound. The course of the missile may be irregular within the body due to internal deflection.

Five percent of penetrating injuries result from impalement or perforating foreign bodies. After stabilization and general assessment, an intravenous pyelogram (IVP) should be performed. Retrograde pyelography may be helpful if a ureteral lesion is suspected, but abdominal exploration is mandatory. Methylene blue dye injected intravenously colors the urine and may aid in identification of the site of perforation intraoperatively.

Nonpenetrating

Nonpenetrating injuries occur with severe skeletal injury or with deceleration, as in a fall from a roof or the catapault type of injury seen in a cyclist who is thrown over the handlebars. Ureteropelvic junction disruption has an increased incidence in children. Suspicion of ureteral injury is raised by the appropriate history and pyelographic findings, and excretory studies may suggest this diagnosis. Retrograde studies are of preoperative confirmatory value. Anatomic repair is carried out with a technique appropriate to the site of injury.

BLADDER

Bladder perforation associated with trauma may be intraperitoneal (15%) or extraperitoneal (85%). Pelvic fractures are a common associated injury, although bladder rupture occurs in only about 10% of such fractures. The mechanisms of injury have been previously discussed.

Bladder rupture should be suspected where there is pelvic fracture or a history of a blow to the lower abdomen. Findings may include lower abdominal pain, shock, peritonitis, sepsis, inability to void, or hematuria.

Once suspected, the diagnosis is confirmed by a cystograph using IVP media in low concentration (~10–15%). To identify leaks that might have sealed with clot, gravity filling of the bladder of this media with contrast should be augmented by an additional 100 ml of contrast injected by syringe to a total volume of about 300 ml of contrast. Films should be taken in the control, full, and empty phases. Oblique or lateral views delineate extravasated contrast that might otherwise be considered as "residual" urine following the bladder evacuation. Before catheterization, urethral injury must be excluded if necessary by means of urethrography.

The unsafe assumption that the bladder is intact if a volume of fluid returns after instillation is mentioned only to be condemned. A situation in which the volume returned was, in fact, greater than the volume instilled due to free communication with the peritoneal cavity has been observed.

URETHRA

Urethral injury may occur above or below the urogenital (UG) diaphragm. Usually injuries above the UG diaphragm result from pelvic fracture, with major bone fragment displacement causing urethral tear or attenuation. Injury below the UG diaphragm may result from a fall astride a solid object with trapping of the urethra against the pubic arch. Injuries to the more distal aspect of the urethra are not common in traumatic situations, except in cases of genital avulsion from power equipment.

Urethral bleeding, penile or perineal swelling and discoloration, and inability to void are the common features of these injuries. In addition to local external findings, rectal examination is important to ascertain the normal position of the prostate; disruption of the urethra at the UG diaphragm will cause the prostate to be elevated by hematoma so that it is described as "floating" or riding high.

Evaluation requires urethrography using an aqueous contrast medium to confirm urethral integrity or to delineate a defect prior to catheterization. The identification of associated injury with skeletal views and IVP should be part of the preoperative evaluation. Urinary drainage is then established. It may be achieved by gentle urethral catheterization where no defect is identified or may require operative intervention to establish suprapubic drainage with associated evacuation of hematoma, debridement, and repair according to the surgeon's philosophy and experience. In urgent situations, suprapubic decompression by catheter or large bore tubing will enable urinary diversion, allowing for definitive management when conditions are more favorable.

Suggested Readings

Morrison, Gittes, Perlmutte, et al: In Hartwell J, et al: *Campbells Urology,* vol 4. Philadelphia, WB Saunders, 1979.

Peters PC(ed): *Urologic Clin North Am* 9:207–312, 1982.

Smith DR: *General Urology,* ed 9. Los Altos, CA, Lang Medical Publications, 1978.

CHAPTER

26 Upper Airway Trauma

Patrick J. Gullane, M.D. and Thomas E. Havas, M.D.

Injuries to the facial skeleton, oropharynx, larynx, and trachea frequently lead to upper airway obstruction. In the past, injuries to the face and neck were the result of fistfights and other expressions of man's inhumanity to man. Today, the automobile accident is by far the main cause of facial and neck injuries. After intracranial injuries, obstructive damage to the airway associated with trauma about the head and neck is the second most common cause of death (Table 26.1).

The site of injury causing upper airway obstruction should be thoroughly assessed once the patient is stabilized. Unrepaired injuries can result in airway compromise, altered vocal function, and disturbances in deglutition. Early diagnosis and surgical repair are mandatory if these complications are to be prevented.

FACIAL AND OROPHARYNGEAL TRAUMA

Open Injuries

With an increase in civilian crime, there has been an upsurge in the number of open and penetrating injuries to the face and neck. The damage caused by bullet wounds to the head and facial skeleton is largely dependent on the velocity of the missile. Because bone is of high specific gravity, it is more vulnerable to shattering and splintering than any other body tissue of lower specific gravity.

Early management of either penetrating or closed face and head wounds embodies basic principles of emergency care, with control of hemorrhage and the airway assuming priority.

There is no rationale for probing extracranial penetrating wounds as to do so may provoke massive hemorrhage. Radiographs are mandatory and usually show the location of the missile, with its path determined from residual metal and bone fragments. Radiographs may reveal a penetrating foreign body where none was expected, or conversely, they may fail to show a metallic foreign body despite an entrance wound and lack of exit. The latter situation may occur in three ways. First, the tract may be from a stab wound; second, a bullet upon entering the neck may strike the vertebral column and ricochet anteriorly to perforate into the nasopharynx or pharynx and then be swallowed; and finally, a bullet on piercing the soft tissue of the head and neck may enter a large blood vessel and embolize to a distant location. The treatment of open and penetrating wounds requires a thorough evaluation of the upper airway, facial skeleton, vascular tree, and cervical spine. Patients with penetrating injuries of the face usually have wounds similar to those with maxillofacial trauma except that vascular structures are more likely to be injured in the former group.

Table 26.1
Upper Airway Obstruction

Facial and oropharyngeal trauma
- Open injuries
- Closed injuries

Laryngotracheal trauma
- Open injuries
- Closed injuries
- Others
  - Endotracheal intubation
  - Laryngoscopy
  - Bronchoscopy
  - Foreign body inhalation

Closed Injuries

A significant reduction in the number of severe facial injuries has occurred with the introduction of mandatory seat belt legislation. When an occupant is not using a seat belt, injury and often death result with ejection from the vehicle. Frequently, with sudden deceleration, the individual is thrown forward and strikes his or her face and head against the windshield, dash board, or instrument panel, receiving facial lacerations and crushing facial injuries.

Closed facial injuries are often of secondary importance, and both their diagnosis and management can wait until more serious injuries are stabilized. If the patient is conscious, assessment includes the patient's bite, sites of tenderness or deformity on palpation, areas of anesthesia, or detection of diplopia. Associated injuries to the cervical spine and larynx should be remembered in the clinical examination. Suspicious facial fractures should be assessed radiologically when the patient's general physical condition permits. The most important general film in the diagnosis of facial fractures is the Waters view; it gives an excellent view of the zygoma, orbit, and maxillary sinuses.

CT scanning has to a large extent replaced conventional radiology in the assessment of facial fractures. CT scans provide an excellent three-dimensional representation of the facial skeleton with good resolution of fractures and deformities. Associated soft tissue problems, such as blow-out fractures of the orbit, are also well delineated.

Treatment

Patients who have sustained extensive facial and upper neck injuries must be evaluated and treated as a whole patient. In order of importance, the steps of evaluation should include:

1. Maintenance of the airway;
2. Control of hemorrhage;
3. Treatment of shock;
4. Determination of associated injuries;
5. Diagnosis of possible facial fractures.

Maintenance of the Airway

Blood, vomitus, or dentures can fully or partially obstruct the upper airway, and the obstruction should be cleared by suction or sweeping a finger deep into the mouth and oropharynx. Airway obstruction from uncontrolled hemorrhage can be dramatically improved by sitting the patient upright. Occasionally, extensive compound fractures of the midface and mandible require either intubation or tracheostomy. Peroral intubation can be performed occasionally, provided that prior laryngoscopy indicates that obstruction is secondary to mucosal swelling or hematoma. Blind intubation should be avoided. In difficult cases where no contraindication exists, intubation over a fiberoptic endoscope facilitates correct placement of the tube and minimizes tissue trauma. Many of these patients with compound fractures of the midface and mandible have difficulty in clearing secretions, and often posterior displacement of the tongue further limits the airway in injuries of this type. Aspirated foreign bodies or laryngeal edema from trauma may require prompt treatment with tracheostomy. If necessary, tracheostomy is best performed in an operating room.

It is important to suspect and recognize associated perforating injury of the lower respiratory tract. In such cases tracheostomy should be performed under local anesthesia. The use of positive end-expiratory pressure could lead to pneumothorax, pneumomediastinum, massive subcutaneous emphysema, or tension pneumothorax.

Control of Hemorrhage

Severe bleeding from facial injuries usually results from severance of the facial artery, the superficial temporal artery, or the angular artery. Control of the hemorrhage can usually be achieved by pressure, ligation of the vessel through the open wound, or reduction of a displaced fracture. If there is continued bleeding or an expanding hematoma, an arteriogram should be performed to determine the site and extent of the vascular injury.

Treatment of Shock

Facial injuries alone rarely cause shock. A patient with persistent hypotension should have other injuries sought and the cause and treatment appropriately instituted.

Determination of Associated Injuries

Patients rarely die of facial injuries, but do die from associated injuries to the skull, cervical spine, larynx, trachea, cardiopulmonary, and gastrointestinal systems.

Diagnosis of Possible Facial Fractures

After control of the airway, hemorrhage, shock, and associated injuries, the facial fractures can then be evaluated and treated. Diagnosis may be established by (1) observation, (2) palpation, and (3) radiologic examination. Suspicion of any facial asymmetry can, in the absence of severe edema, indicate underlying fractures. Palpation can elicit tenderness at the site of a facial fracture. Malar and zygomatic arch fractures are evident with periorbital ecchymosis, crepitus, depression, or angulation, and often limitation of mandibular excursion. Fractures of the maxilla reveal dental malocclusion, periorbital ecchymosis, a mobile maxilla, asymmetry of the dental arch, and often misplaced or fractured teeth. The cardinal signs of a mandibular fracture include asymmetry of mandibular contour, asymmetry of dental arch, dental malocclusion, limitation of mandibular excursion, abnormal motion, misplaced teeth, and anesthesia of the lower lip. Radiologic examination plays a definitive role in the evaluation of facial injuries. The most important views includes the Waters view, posteroanterior view of the facial bones, lateral view of the facial bones, and posteroanterior oblique and occlusal views of the mandible. Tomography and CT scans can help in evaluating the more subtle fractures.

Treatment of Facial Fractures

Definitive repair of facial fractures may be delayed for 7–10 days while more life-threatening conditions are treated. Soft tissue injuries amenable to repair under local anesthesia are taken care of as soon as possible. The main goal of mandibular and maxillary stabilization is to secure the unstable inferior facial skeleton to the superior facial skeleton or cranial vault with a combination of Erich arch bars and suspension wires. Restoration of proper dental occlusion is of paramount importance in management.

LARYNGOTRACHEAL TRAUMA

Open Injuries

With an increase in societal violence, stab wounds to the neck have become a common problem. Missile injuries, which are more frequent in military situations, result in more extensive tissue loss and a higher morbidity. Severe damage to associated structures, particularly the great vessels of the neck in stab wounds and the cervical spine in missile injuries, may occur.

The major problems encountered include hemorrhage, dyspnea, and occasionally a progressive neurologic deficit that suggests that increasing pressure is being placed on nerves in the neck by an expanding hematoma. Dyspnea with cyanosis, hemoptysis, subcutaneous emphysema, dysphagia, hoarseness, or bubbling air and blood from the wound all suggest laryngeal or tracheal injuries. Dyspnea may accompany an expanding hematoma of the neck and larynx, displaced cartilage segments into the airway, or increasing mediastinal emphysema.

Open wounds involving the laryngotracheal system require immediate exploration. A preoperative roentgenogram of the neck and chest is valuable because it discloses associated cervical spine injuries, subcutaneous emphysema, pneumothorax, pneumopericardium, pneumomediastinum, or hemothorax. The unpredictable course of a bullet or the downward thrust of a knife blade may lacerate subclavian vessels that bleed more into the chest than might be recognized by the external examination.

The basic principles of treatment are control of the hemorrhage and provision of an adequate airway, which often can be done through the open neck wound. With institution of hemorrhage and airway control, the appropriate exploration and repair can be performed in an orderly fashion. Major vessels may be ligated or repaired either with end-to-end anastomosis, or if necessary, autogenous vein grafts can be utilized.

Open wounds of the larynx should be immediately repaired to avoid infection, distortion of the cartilaginous framework, scar contraction of the lacerated mucosa, or stricture of the airway.

Closed Injuries

Blunt laryngotracheal trauma is frequently caused by motor vehicle accidents, but often occurs with sporting injuries, such as occur in basketball, hockey, and karate. In these sports the commonest injury is a fractured hyoid bone.

In motor vehicle accidents the type of injury sustained depends on whether seat belts are worn, the type of belts, the height of the individual, and length of the anterior cervical compartment. Sudden deceleration of a car causes the body to move forward and the neck backward. A person not wearing a seat belt is projected forward, striking the dash board, windshield, or steering wheel, with injury to the head, neck, and thorax (Fig. 26.1). Wearing a lap belt without the shoulder harness permits the individual to strike the dash board or steering wheel. If the distance is short he or she will suffer a facial injury, but with greater distance the neck becomes hyperextended and laryngotracheal injury is sustained. The relative paucity of laryngeal fractures in children may reflect the resilience of young elastic cartilage in children.

Classification of Closed Laryngotracheal Injuries

Soft Tissue Injuries

These can occur as superficial lacerations of the mucosa and hematoma formation of the epiglottis, aryepiglottic folds, and false and true cords.

Cartilaginous Injuries

Several classifications of laryngeal injury have been suggested. An anatomic classification groups laryngeal injuries into supraglottic, glottic, and subglottic. A second classification is based upon the severity of the injury: group I—minor injuries that require no surgical intervention; group II—injuries severe enough to require tracheostomy but no open repair; group III—fractures of the cartilage that require open repair; and group IV—injuries severe enough to require open repair and stenting. This classification fails to distinguish between cartilaginous and endolaryngeal injuries.

A fractured hyoid is the most common laryngeal fracture in sporting injuries. It results in severe odynophagia, with crepitus at the fracture site. Occasionally hematoma formation of the epiglottis accompanies the injury.

Fractures of the thyroid cartilage may be vertical, oblique, or horizontal depending on the force and its direction. There may be a posterior displacement of the base of the epiglottis, or the thyroepiglottic ligament may be lacerated, causing the epiglottis to be separated from the false cords and anterior commisure. The epiglottis may be displaced posteriorly into the laryngeal lumen; the vocal cords may be avulsed from the anterior attachments or vocal processes, or the arytenoids may become dislocated.

A cricoid cartilage fracture is often recognizable by loss of its prominence on palpation. This fracture may occur

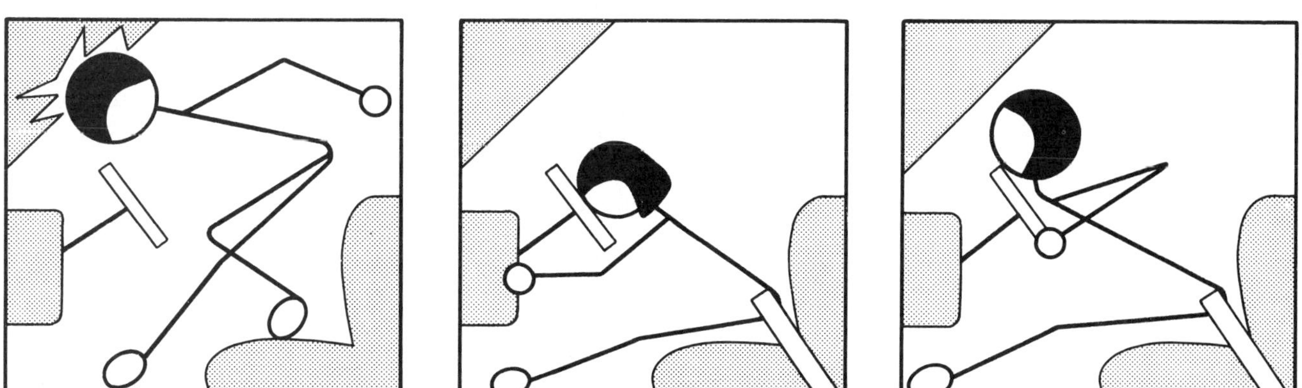

Injury to face, neck and thorax in person not wearing seatbelt. Facial injuries from sudden deceleration with 2-point seatbelt. Hyperextension of neck and laryngeal injury with 2-point seatbelt.

Figure 26.1. Mechanisms of facial injury.

in association with a thyroid cartilage fracture. A recurrent nerve injury should always be sought in this fracture type.

In severe trauma the trachea may be partially or completely transected. Total avulsion (Fig. 26.2) results in severe respiratory distress, and most patients die at the time of injury. Tracheal avulsion is usually accompanied by severance of the recurrent laryngeal nerves. The possibility of perforation of the pharynx or esophagus must be ruled out with a contrast study using a water-soluble radiopaque dye, such as gastrograffin.

Diagnosis

Early diagnosis and treatment of laryngeal trauma are absolutely vital to successful management.

The signs and symptoms of laryngeal injury include voice alteration, airway compromise, subcutaneous emphysema, crepitus, hemoptysis, dysphagia, and changes in normal neck anatomy with bruising, laceration, or flattening (Fig. 26.3).

The key element in the diagnosis of laryngeal trauma remains the physical examination. Palpation of the neck and visualization, either direct or indirect, of the upper respiratory passages are the simplest, least expensive, and most accurate means of establishing the diagnosis and severity of the injury. If the patient is unable to tolerate the use of a laryngeal mirror, flexible fibroptic endoscopes are available and can be inserted intranasally or intraorally to allow adequate visualization.

A helpful adjunct to the physical examination is radiographic assessment of the larynx. However, radiologic studies are performed only when the airway is secure. Anteroposterior and lateral radiographs may demonstrate endolaryngeal swelling, displacement of the epiglottis, and surgical emphysema with the possible association of a cervical spine fracture (Figs. 26.4 and 26.5). The radiologic study of choice is CT scanning. It provides information of high specificity and is particularly useful in patients with moderately severe injury, when the indications for surgery may be in doubt.

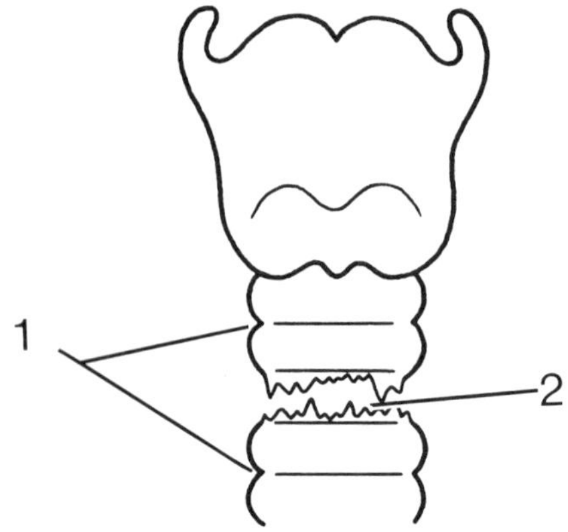

Figure 26.2. Tracheal avulsion. Note the associated injuries: *1,* severed recurrent laryngeal nerves; *2,* pharyngoesophageal laceration/perforation.

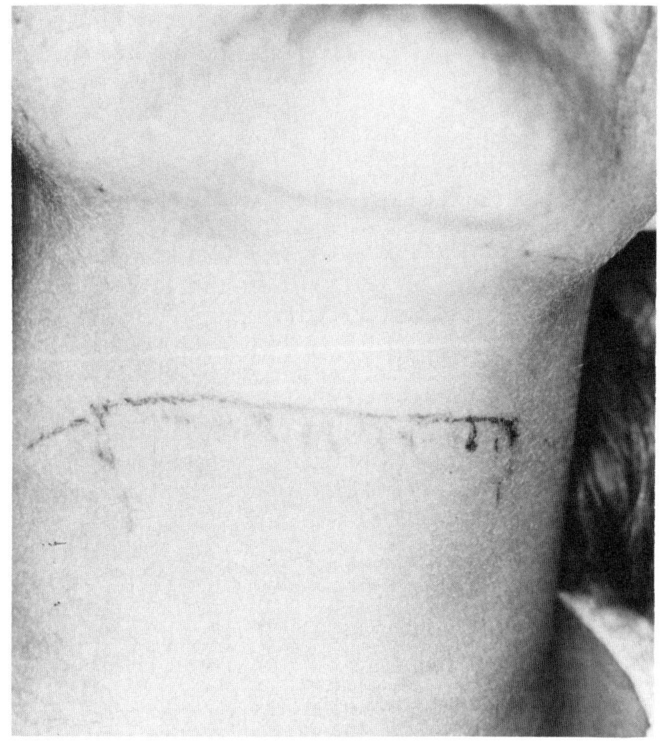

Figure 26.3. Abrasion and flattening of the neck.

Treatment

Patients with minor laryngeal injuries are usually treated conservatively without surgical intervention. Management consists of voice rest, soft diet, a high oxygen humidified atmosphere, possible use of antibiotics and steroids, and a daily examination of the larynx.

Patients with severe laryngotracheal injuries require tracheostomy with open surgical repair. The best functional results are obtained by early open reduction and

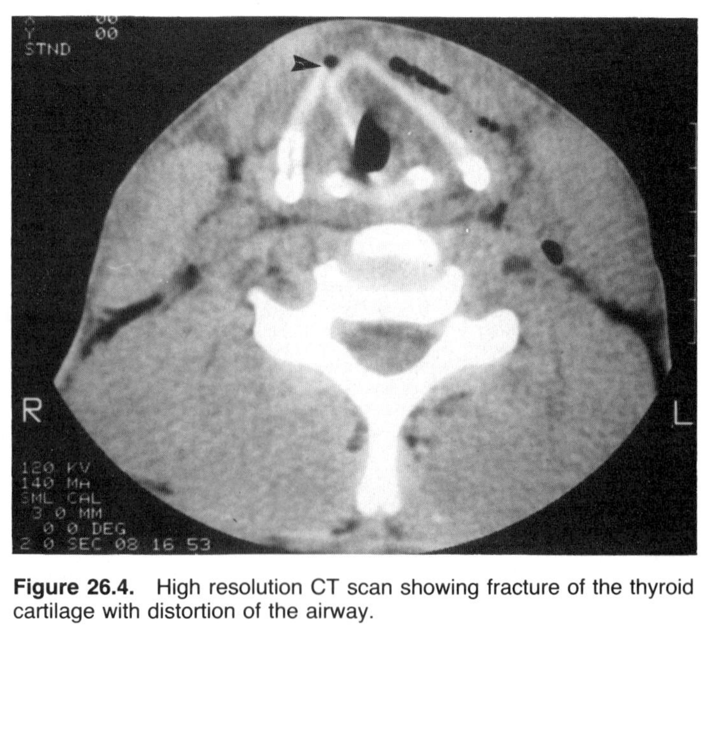

Figure 26.4. High resolution CT scan showing fracture of the thyroid cartilage with distortion of the airway.

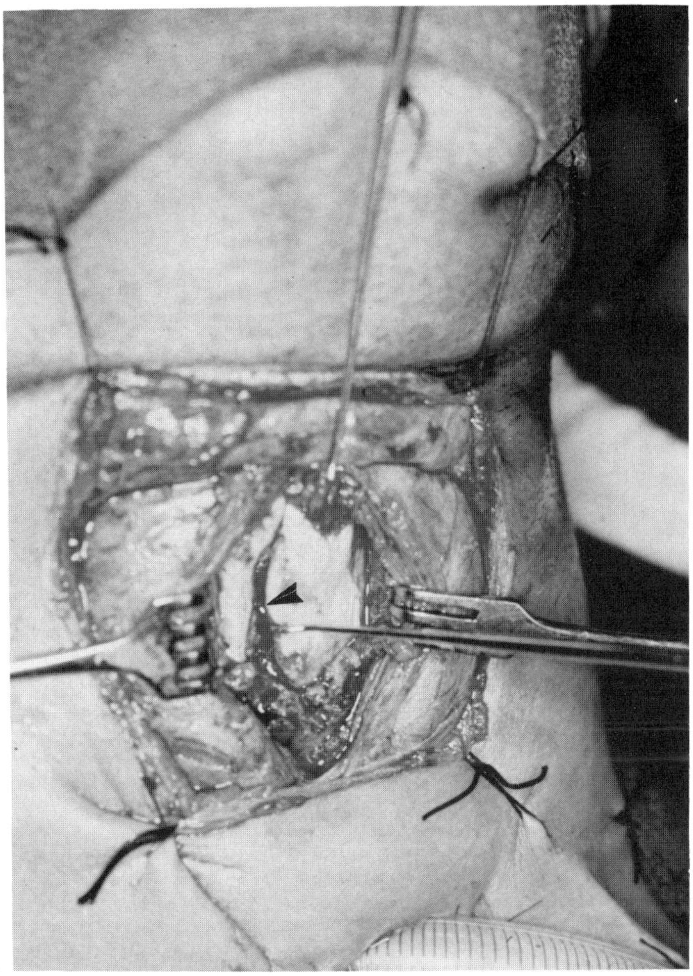

Figure 26.5. Intraoperative slide showing reduction and repair of the fractured cartilage and restoration of mucosal continuity.

simultaneous definitive surgical repair (Figs. 26.6–26.8). The ultimate goal of repair is to achieve an adequate airway with a functional larynx. Factors facilitating the achievement of this goal include early diagnosis and treatment, careful approximation of the mucous membrane and cartilage fragments, replacement of a dislocated arytenoid, and stenting when necessary. Delayed recognition of laryngeal trauma or delayed repair is associated with a high incidence of failure of decannulation, aspiration, and poor speech.

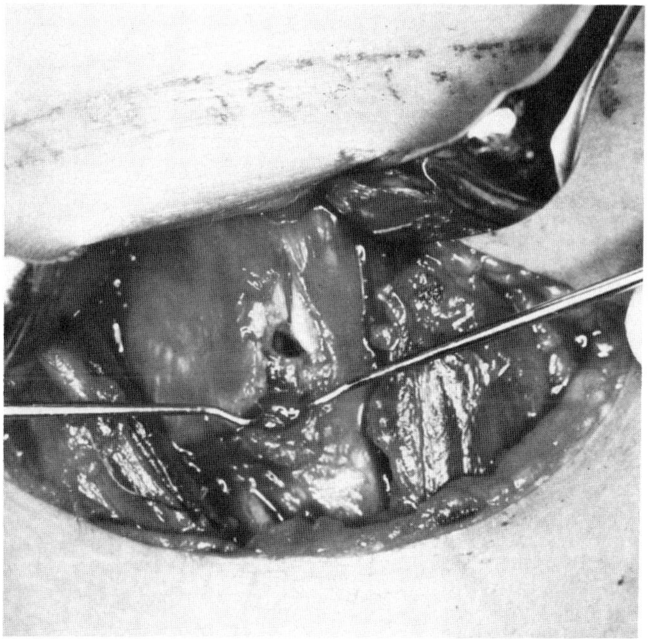

Figure 26.6. Thyroid cartilage fracture.

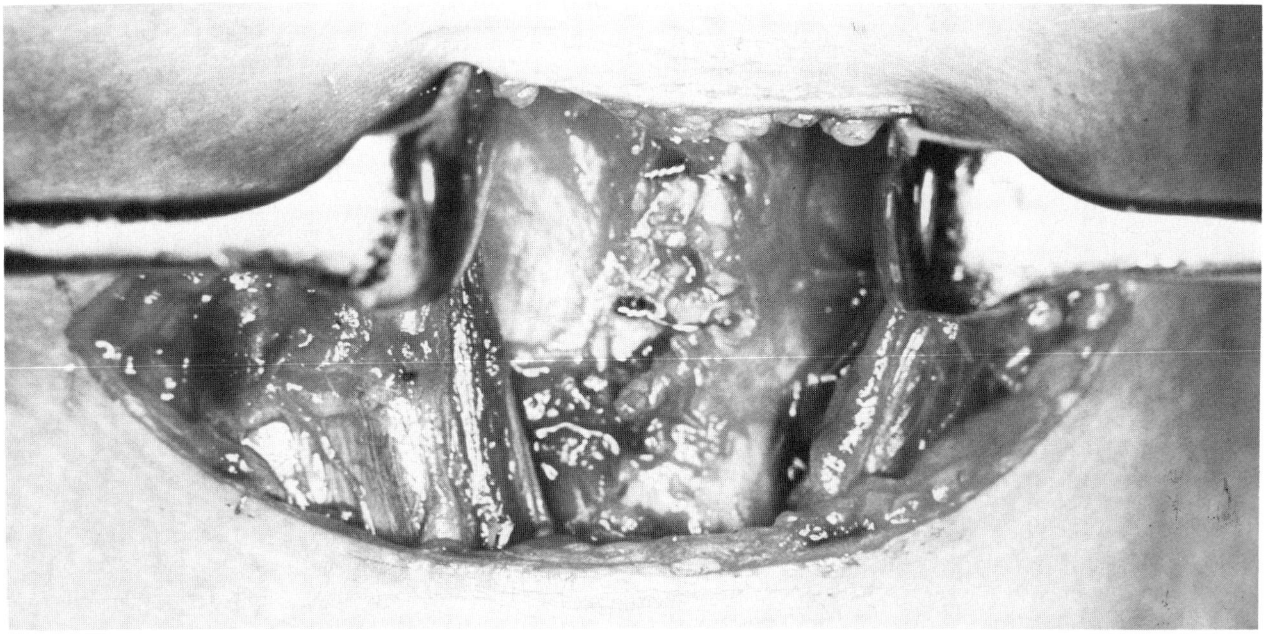

Figure 26.7. Repair with mucosal approximation and wiring of cartilaginous segments.

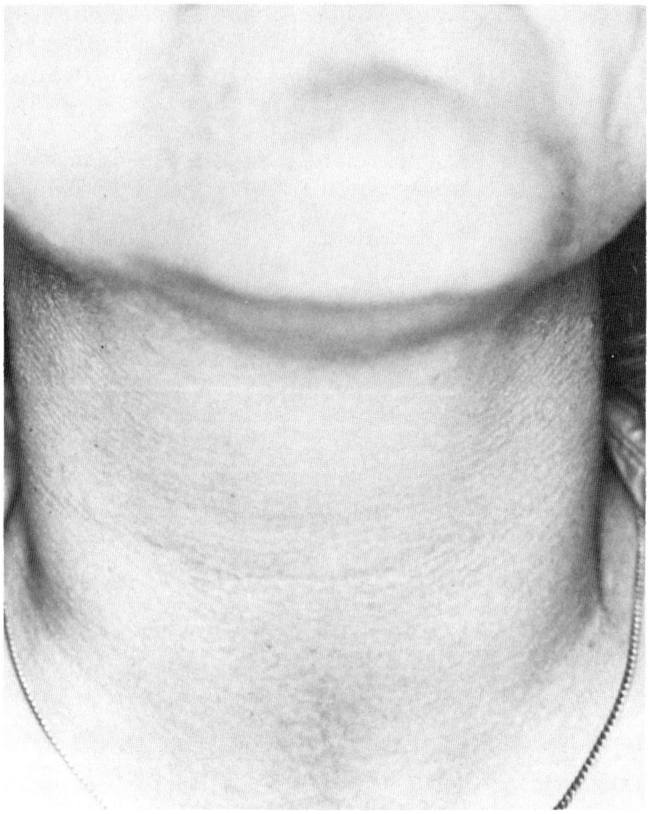

Figure 26.8. Result at 1 year.

Others

Ingestion of corrosives, inhalation of irritant fumes, or excessive or poorly designed radiotherapy to the upper airway can produce edema, perichondritis, cartilage necrosis, and airway collapse. Management will vary from intravenous fluids, antibiotics, and steroids in the mild cases to tracheostomy and eventful resection of the damaged structures.

Suggested Readings

Beahrs OH, Devine KD: Treatment of traumatic lesions of the head and neck. *Surg Clin North Am* 43:917–927, 1963.

Brandenberg JH: Management of acute blunt laryngeal injuries. *Otolaryngol Clin North Am* 12:741–751, 1979.

Fitchett VH, et al: Penetrating wounds of the neck. *Arch Surg* 99:307–314, 1969.

Gregor RT, et al: The management of laryngotracheal injury. *S Afr J Surg* 22:41–45, 1984.

Harris H, Tobin H: Acute injuries of the larynx and trachea in 49 patients. *Laryngoscope* 80:1376–1384, 1970.

Hortmann PK, et al: Diagnosis and primary management of laryngeal trauma. *Oral Surg, Oral Med, Oral Path* 60:252–257, 1985.

Larson DL, Cohn AM: Management of acute laryngeal injury: a critical review. *J Trauma* 16:858–862, 1972.

Leopold D: Laryngeal trauma. *Arch Otolaryngol* 109:106–111, 1982.

Manusco AA, Hanafee WN: Computed tomography of the injured larynx. *Radiology* 133:139–144, 1979.

Mintz DR, Gullane PJ, Thomson DH, et al.: Perichondritis of the larynx following radiation. *Otolaryngol Head Neck Surg* 89:550–554, 1981.

Nahum AM: Immediate care of acute blunt laryngeal trauma. *J Trauma* 9:112–125, 1969.

Narrod JA, et al: Initial management of penetrating neck wounds—a selective approach. *J Emerg Med* 1:17–22, 1984.

Pennington CL: External trauma of the larynx and trachea. *Ann Otol Rhinol Laryngol* 81:546–554, 1972.

Potter CR, Sessions DG, Ogura JH: Blunt laryngotracheal trauma. *Otolaryngology* 86:909–923, 1978.

Schaefer SD, et al: Selective application of CT in the management of laryngeal trauma. *Laryngoscope* 93:1473–1475, 1983.

Shaia FT, Cassady CL: Laryngeal trauma. *Arch Otolaryngol* 95:104–108, 1972.

Snow JB: Diagnosis and therapy for acute laryngeal and tracheal trauma. *Otolaryngol Clin North Am* 17:101–106, 1984.

Stein A, Seward P: Penetrating wounds of the neck. *J Trauma* 7:238–247, 1967.

CHAPTER

27 Acute Burn Care

Michael J. Halls, M.D., and Robert G. Colcleugh, M.D.

There are few traumatic events as totally devastating to an individual as a major burn injury. Burns not only produce profound derangements of physiologic and homeostatic mechanisms but can also cause catastrophic psychological effects on the patient and his or her family. The total care of major burn patients has therefore been organized into regional burn units where experienced personnel from all branches of medicine, nursing, and multiple support services are readily available. This chapter is not intended to be a complete synopsis of all facets of burn care but rather is aimed at giving interested health care workers an appreciation and an understanding of the basic requirements for proper treatment of the severely burned patient.

EPIDEMIOLOGY

Burns and fires are the third leading cause of accidental death in North America. Between 6,000 and 10,000 burn-related deaths occur in the United States each year, and approximately 70,000 burn patients require hospitalization annually. Only motor vehicle accidents cause more accidental deaths than burns.

As with other types of trauma, burn-related injury is primarily a problem of youth, with a peak incidence among children aged 1 to 5 and another peak among males aged 17 to 25. Young children are most frequently burned with scalding liquids. Accidents with inflammable liquids remain the major cause of burns in teenagers and adults. Structural fires account for less than 5% of burn admissions, but are responsible for 45% of burn-related deaths.

Improved care in burn units has reduced the mortality from major burn injuries over the past 20 years, although the mortality rate from 80% body surface area burns still exceeds 50%.

CLASSIFICATION

Many different classifications of burn trauma have been developed in an effort to predict the severity of the injury and the treatment necessary for a successful outcome:

1. Depth (Fig. 27.1). Although depth may be one of the

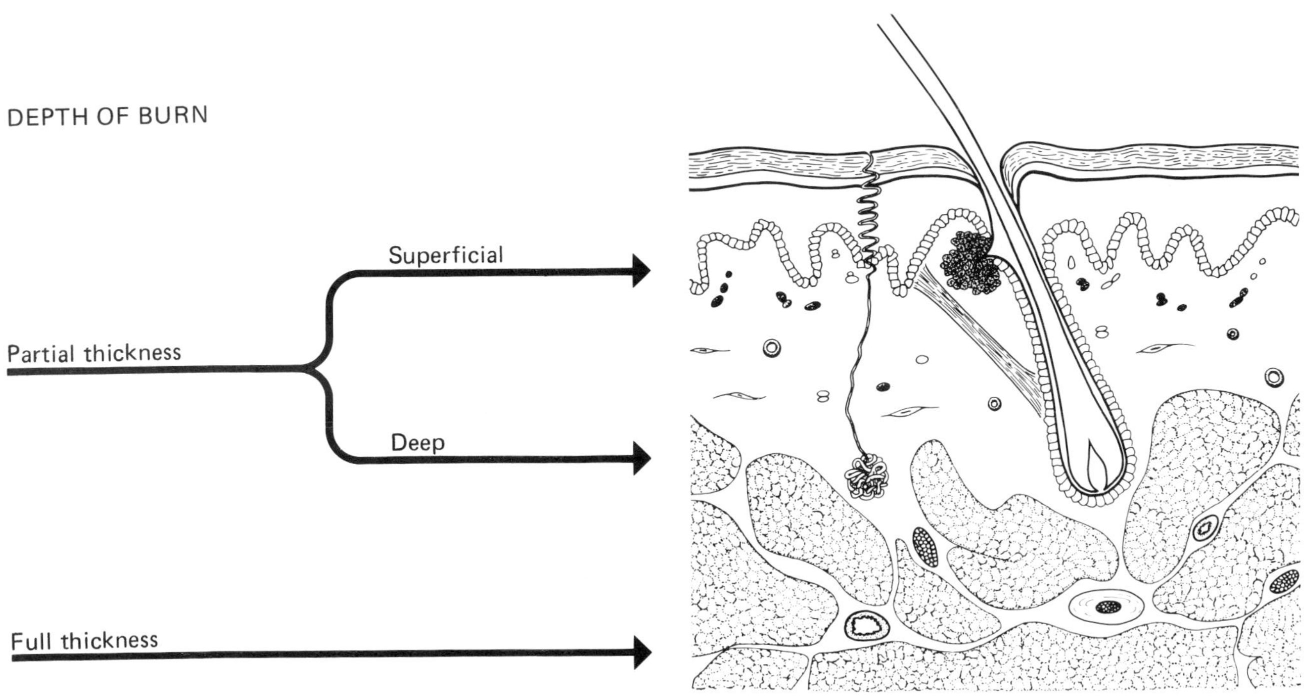

Figure 27.1. Classification of burns by depth.

most important aspects of a thermal injury it is often the most difficult to predict accurately immediately following injury. A superficial partial thickness injury (first degree) is usually painful and erythematous, blanches on pressure, and has little to no blistering. A full thickness injury (third degree) is often anesthetic, waxy yellow to black, and inelastic and has thrombosed vessels visible in the base. Most burns, however, are mid to deep partial thickness (second degree) and are quite variable in appearance, although blistering is a usual finding. The only reliable method of determining the exact depth of these injuries is to inspect the burn wound daily with an experienced eye. Another helpful test is to pull on a hair in the burned area; if no resistance is felt and the hair can be extracted without discomfort to the patient, the burn is probably deep partial to full thickness.

2. Extent (Fig. 27.2). Probably the most important determinant of the prognosis of burn injury is the body surface area (BSA) that has been affected. This factor affects the degree of physiologic and homeostatic derangement, the method of burn coverage to be used, and also the predicted mortality. The commonest and most easily remembered method for determining the extent of the burn injury is the "rule of nines." However, this is often an inexact method and is best used by actually mapping the patient's burns on a blank diagram. Charts are available that divide the areas of the body into smaller units so that estimations of patchy burns can be more accurate. Special burn charts should be used for infants and children to age 7 because the head and neck have a relatively larger surface area in these age groups. Another helpful method for determining the extent of diffuse patchy burns is to remember that the palm represents 1% of the body surface area. With a sterile glove the examiner can sequentially cover the burned area with his or her hand and add up the total number of "palm areas" to arrive at a quite accurate approximation of extent.

3. Etiology (Fig. 27.3). A careful history of the exact mechanism of injury is as important to the diagnosis and treatment of burns as it is to any other type of trauma.

I Thermal	a) Contact b) Scald c) Flash
II Electrical	a) High voltage b) Low Voltage
III Chemical	a) Acid b) Alkali
IV Radiation	a) Acute b) Chronic
V Friction	

Figure 27.3. Etiologic classification of burns.

Thermal injury is by far the commonest cause of major life-threatening burns. Various factors are important in determining the severity of thermal trauma, such as the temperature of the injuring agent, the duration of contact, and the anatomic location of the skin involved. In general, *contact burns* from hot objects or burning clothing tend to be deep. *Scald burns* can be quite extensive, and oil-based liquids often produce deeper injuries than aqueous solutions. *Flash burns* result from exposure to a brief cloud of flame, such as occurs when a barbeque is improperly lit, and are usually on exposed cutaneous surfaces and not very deep.

Electrical injuries must be considered under specific pathophysiologic problems and are discussed separately.

Chemical burns are usually industrial in origin and very often involve the hands and face. Alkalis tend to be more penetrating than acids; both should be treated by copious irrigation with physiologic solutions until the pH is normalized to testing with litmus paper.

Acute radiation injuries, such as sunburn, can be diagnosed and managed as if thermal in origin. The discussion of chronic radiation injury is beyond the scope of this chapter.

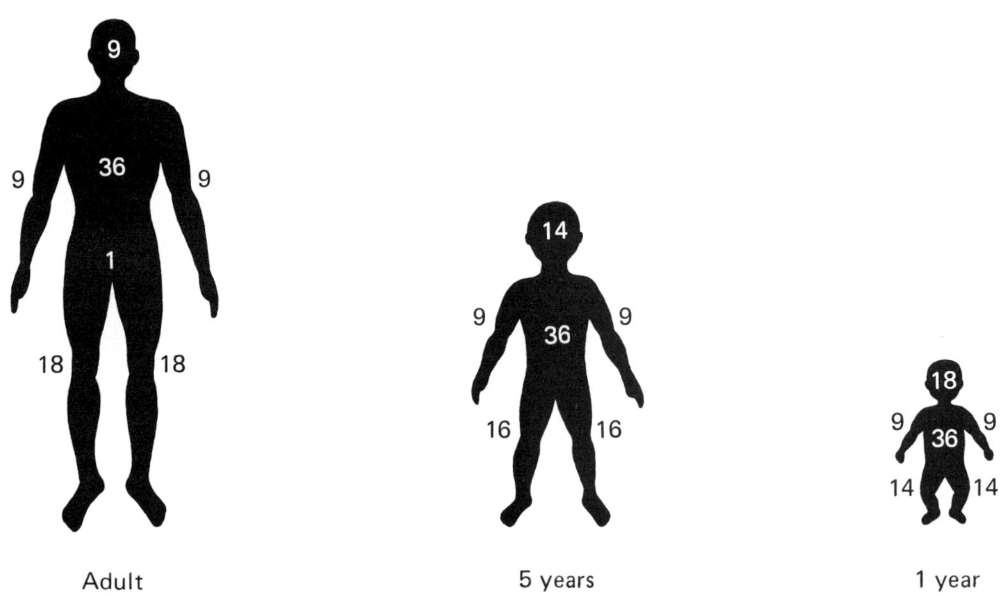

Figure 27.2. The "rule of nines."

Frictional burns are usually well localized and deep. They may often coexist with degloving-type cutaneous injuries.

4. Severity. Once a determination of depth and extent has been made, the burn may be classified as to the proposed treatment.

- *Minor Burns*—May be treated on an outpatient basis; are second-degree burns covering less than 15% BSA or third-degree burns of less than 2% BSA.
- *Moderate Burns*—Require hospitalization and may require resuscitation; are second-degree burns from 15–30% BSA or third-degree burns from 2–10% BSA. Burns of the feet, face, hands, and perineum often require hospitalization for optimal care, regardless of the extent.
- *Critical Burns*—Should be dealt with in regional burn units; are second-degree burns greater than 30% BSA or third-degree burns greater than 10% BSA.

These guidelines often need to be interpreted differently for each individual case as pre-existing disease, associated trauma or complications, and the extremes of age affect the severity of the burn-related injury.

RESUSCITATION

Severe burns are associated with dramatic shifts in body fluids and plasma proteins. The exact pathophysiology of these changes is the topic of intense research. Many factors seem to be involved in the development of "burn edema."

The transvascular flux of fluid and protein within burned tissue is due to an increased microvascular permeability, coupled with an increase in the interstitial osmotic pressure. The basement membrane seems to play a pivotal role in edema formation at this level. Vasoactive mediators that are released by burned tissue—prostaglandins, kinins, histamine, serotonin, and oxygen radicals—probably play some part in the edema formation process; however, attempts to remove these substances with exchange transfusions or specific inhibitors have only met with mixed success.

The development of edema at sites distant from the burn wound was thought to be the result of a generalized increase in microvascular permeability throughout the body. However, this altered protein permeability in nonburned tissues probably does not occur, and recent evidence suggests that the severe hypoproteinemic state of the burned patient is probably responsible for generalized edema formation. Early colloid infusions may therefore be indicated.

The goal of rescusitation then is to maintain the intravascular volume and tissue perfusion during this period of profound fluid disturbance. This goal is usually accomplished with some type of salt-containing fluid that is isotonic in nature. Various formulas have been developed to estimate the volume of fluid necessary to maintain hemodynamic stability in the immediate postburn period. The formula currently used at this center is 4 ml per kg/% burn of Ringer's solution, with one-half of this amount administered in the first 8 hours and the remainder over the next 16 hours. In burns over 50% BSA one unit of fresh frozen plasma is added every 6–8 hours.

It should be stressed that this and all other formulas are guidelines only, and modifications are often required according to the patient's clinical response. The routine administration of colloid during the first 24 hours would seem to be indicated if indeed it can be maintained in the intravascular space. Early colloid infusion can return cardiac output to normal more quickly and results in somewhat less of an increase in lung water. Those opposed to its use feel that colloid is less readily mobilized from the interstitium in the postburn period, thereby impeding the resolution of burn edema. No study to date has been able to show that early colloid infusion improves survival.

An alternative to isotonic crystalloid resuscitation is the use of hypertonic fluids, usually hypertonic saline of 250 mm/liter. An adequate salt load is provided with these regimens, and the necessary volume to maintain hemodynamic stability is derived from the intracellular space. This type of resuscitation usually reduces burn edema formation and can be useful for patients who cannot handle large volume loads, such as those with pre-existing cardiac disease. Intracellular dehydration and hypernatremia are consequences of hypertonic saline resuscitations, and the maximal limits of these parameters compatible with organ function will determine the limitation of this type of fluid management.

Hourly monitoring of the burn patient is mandatory during the first 24 hours. Such clinical parameters as blood pressure, pulse, and urine output should be followed. *Inadequate urine output during this period means inadequate fluid administration until proven otherwise.* Indwelling central catheters may be useful to determine central venous pressure, and in severely burned patients the insertion of Swan-Ganz catheters can be extremely helpful in following the cardiac output and its response to fluid administration. The cardiac index should be restored to normal as quickly as possible, and it can be expected to remain elevated for as long as it takes to achieve wound closure. Catheters should be placed through nonburned tissue if possible. With the exception of blood gas analysis, serum electrolytes, and serum/urine osmolality, laboratory investigations are not necessarily helpful in the early postburn period. A normal pH implies adequate tissue perfusion and alveolar ventilation; a low pH should be investigated as to its cause and treated.

Certain patients require volumes of fluids in excess of the calculated amounts in order to achieve hemodynamic stability. Patients with "incineration burns" of greater than 80% BSA usually need more than the calculated volumes and should also be watched for myoglobinuria and hemochromogenuria from deep tissue and red cell destruction. Patients with coexisting trauma, delayed resuscitation, and electrical burns may also require increased amounts of fluids.

In the second 24 hours postburn, large molecular weight substances can be maintained in the intravascular space, and colloid solutions are included in all formulas. We use a combination of fresh frozen plasma and albumin at 0.5 ml/kg/% burn. Further crystalloid administration should be based on urine output, clinical condition, associated injuries or disease, and the need to replace insensible losses through both respiration and the burn wound.

INHALATION INJURY

Many different types of postburn lung dysfunction may be encountered. The most immediate life-threatening pulmonary complication seen in closed space burns is carbon monoxide poisoning. Because carbon monoxide is taken up by hemoglobin preferentially over oxygen, hypoxia can result from exposure to the carbon monoxide generated by combustion. Carboxyhemoglobin concentrations should be measured in all victims from a fire environment, and empirical treatment with high levels (up to 100%) of inspired oxygen concentration may be warranted.

Smoke inhalation injury occurs in up to 20% of patients admitted to burn centers. The diagnosis should be entertained in any patient burned in a closed space or with facial and circumoral burns. Singed nasal hairs, upper airway erythema, and carbonaceous sputum can also be seen. Routine fiberoptic bronchoscopy and xenon ventilation-perfusion scanning in suspected cases have resulted in more frequent and earlier diagnosis of smoke inhalation injury. It is still, however, impossible to ascertain the magnitude of the injury with any method of diagnosis.

The pathophysiology of inhalation injury is explained by a complex chemical burn to the tracheobronchial mucosa and the resulting inflammatory reaction of the lining tissues. Lipid- and water-soluble gases found in the smoke react with water and carbon particles on the mucous membranes to produce strong acids and alkalis that impair ciliary function, induce bronchospasm, and also cause ulcerations. Alveolar macrophages add to the inflammation by releasing potent chemotoxins.

Even in severe injuries early symptoms are usually absent, with mucosal edema and bronchorrhea occurring 24 to 48 hours postburn. After this time x-ray changes will become evident as diffuse pulmonary edema and blood gas abnormalities can be detected.

Current management consists of protecting the airway from constricting edema in the early phases of injury. Endotracheal intubation and mechanical ventilation with positive end-expiratory pressure remain the treatments of choice for severe pulmonary injuries from smoke inhalation. Corticosteroids are no longer used as they may increase morbidity and mortality by increasing the risk of infection.

The long-term morbidity of inhalation injury is primarily related to the treatment of the injury. Sequelae are more frequent and severe after tracheotomy than after translaryngeal intubation. Tracheal stenosis and granuloma formation are the commonest lesions and are directly related to the presence of tracheal stoma and the duration of tube placement.

IMMUNOLOGY AND INFECTIONS

Sepsis and associated organ system failure are still the leading causes of death due to burns. In addition to the loss of normal barrier skin function in the burned areas, many alterations occur in both the cellular and humoral components of the immune system in burn patients.

Neutrophils and macrophages show impairments of chemotaxis, phagocytosis, and bacterial killing, which may precede the development of clinical sepsis by up to 48 hours. Phagocytic abnormalities may in part be due to a circulating inhibitory factor that is biochemically similar to collagen fragments released by burned skin.

Lymphocyte abnormalities include increased numbers of T suppressor cells. The reversal of normal T suppressor to T helper cell ratios may be another early indicator of impending sepsis. Many of the complex macrophage-lymphocyte interactions are also altered, and correction of these types of abnormalities with immunomodulators may hold promise in the future. Currently, most of the abnormalities in immunity disappear with burn excision and wound closure.

The result of this impaired immunity in burn patients is infection. The burn wound and the lungs are the most frequent sites of fatal infections; however, systemically absorbed endotoxin from the gastrointestinal tract may also produce sepsis. Suppurative thrombophlebitis and endocarditis may also result from improper care of indwelling intravascular catheters or lines that are not changed frequently. Intravenous sites should be routinely changed every 48 to 72 hours if possible and immediately if clinical signs of sepsis appear.

Virulent Gram negative organisms are usually responsible for most burn wound and associated infections. Burn eschar itself can also produce the same type of hyperdynamic state as sepsis, and attempts should be made to excise this tissue in cases of apparent systemic sepsis with negative cultures.

Prophylactic antibiotics are not recommended for burn patients as they lead to the development of resistant strains, as well as superinfections by such organisms as *Candida albicans* and other fungi. Systemic antibiotics are of use for documented invasive infections or perioperatively at the time of excision and burn wound closure. These agents should always be chosen on the basis of cultures and sensitivities when available.

Topical antibacterials, such as silver nitrate and silver sulfadiazine, remain the main method of burn wound infection control. Complications from these agents are rare. Silver nitrate is used in burn units that prefer a "dry eschar" type of treatment. In contrast, silver sulfadiazine cream must be removed at dressing changes by tubbing and produces a "wet eschar." Mafenide can be useful immediately preoperatively to help eradicate bacteria from burn eschar because it penetrates this tissue well, although it may be painful with continued use.

NUTRITION AND METABOLISM

It is often said that severe burn injury is the most extensive stress sustained by humans, and indeed no other trauma leads to the same increase in metabolic rate. This hypermetabolism is accompanied by protein catabolism, lipolysis, ureagenesis, and accelerated gluconeogenesis.

Skeletal muscle protein is broken down, providing amino acids for acute phase protein synthesis and hepatic glucose conversion. The burn wound converts glucose to lactate, which is again recycled in the liver to new glucose by means of the Cori cycle. Fat oxidation fuels these reactions.

Another important phenomenon of this stress response is a reset of the hypothalamic temperature center to 1 to 2 °C above normal. Unless the patient is kept in a warm, moist environment, the hypermetabolic response will be exaggerated to maintain this temperature. Steady core temperatures of 38 to 39°C are therefore normal for burn patients, rather than being evidence of sepsis, and should not be treated with measures aimed at reducing the temperature. Maintenance of burn patients in ambient temperatures at or above 30°C will decrease total energy expenditures and therefore caloric requirements.

The afferent mediators of this hypermetabolism are mainly the "anti-insulin" hormones. Levels of catecholamines, glucagon, and glucocorticoids are all elevated after severe burns. The growth hormone level is also elevated. Chemically and neurally modulated signals from the burn wound seem to initiate and maintain these hormonal imbalances. These afferent signals can also be accentuated by pain or anxiety.

Although certain measures can be used to minimize this hypermetabolic response, it persists until wound closure. Current management revolves around supplying sufficient calories to prevent muscle wasting and weight loss. Caloric requirements were often calculated by various formulas; however, recent studies have shown that providing two times the basal energy expenditure (BEE) is sufficient and possibly better than giving increased calories, which can lead to fatty infiltration of the liver and also increase carbon dioxide production.

Protein breakdown is minimized by providing 50% of the total caloric intake as glucose. Twenty percent is given as proteins or amino acids and the rest as fat. A calorie-to-nitrogen ratio of 100:1 is probably best.

THE BURN WOUND

Many complex biochemical and cellular events occur in the burn wound following cutaneous thermal trauma. The wound can be divided into three continuous zones (Fig. 27.4), the relative sizes of which depend on the degree of injury. The area of stasis seems to result from the production of thromboxane and related compounds, with subsequent fibrin deposition in initially patent blood vessels. The area of hyperemia develops in conjunction with the generalized hyperdynamic state and remains until wound closure.

After several days neutrophils and macrophages appear in the wound and release many potent vasoactive substances that act locally and can also cause detrimental systemic effects on pulmonary function. The macrophage plays a major role in wound healing, producing angiogenesis factor or growth factor depending upon the local partial pressure of oxygen. Angiogenesis factor, produced when oxygen concentrations are low, leads to the development of granulation tissue. Macrophage-derived growth factor is produced under higher oxygen concentrations and stimulates fibroblasts to divide, as well as to manufacture collagen and ground substance, the components of scar tissue. As the depth of the wound is evolving, epithelialization is progressing from the wound margins, from the uninjured hair follicles and sebaceous and sweat glands.

If re-epithelialization is complete by 2 weeks, as in a superficial burn, the underlying dermis will rapidly revert to near normal. The cosmetic and functional results under these circumstances are excellent. If the wound is still open after 2 weeks, contractile fibroblasts called myofibroblasts appear in large numbers within the wound, and wound contraction follows. The clinical results of wound contraction are joint contractures and severe cosmetic deformities. Mast cells appear in the wound that indirectly stimulate vasodilation and the accumulation of firm ground substance. This results in erythematous, hard, plaque-like scars.

Wound Management

Burns that will heal within 2 weeks should be allowed to do so, with protection against infection provided by topical antimicrobials. Deeper, extensive burn eschars and open wounds produce immune deficiency and hypermetabolism; there is general agreement that eschar should

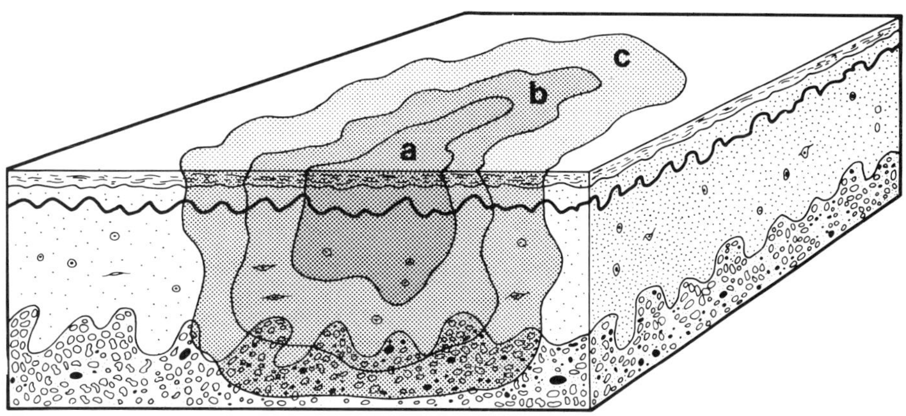

Figure 27.4. Cross-section of a burn wound: *a*, zone of coagulation; *b*, zone of stasis; *c*, zone of hyperemia.

be removed and the wound closed as quickly as possible. In large surface area burns this process is done in stages, beginning almost immediately after the patient has been resuscitated and stabilized. Successive areas representing about 15% of the BSA are excised and grafted at each operative procedure until wound closure is complete.

Skin Grafts

After wound excision, coverage of the excised wound must be provided. Currently, the only form of permanent coverage is autograft skin obtained from unburned areas of the patient's body. Skin grafts can be harvested from unburned areas many times and can also be meshed and expanded in order to cover large surface area burns.

Allografts obtained from cadavers can be used for temporary wound coverage. These grafts can be changed frequently to act as biologic dressings or can be allowed to "take." Allografts that have healed to the wound will eventually reject unless surgically removed; however, this rejection phenomenon is usually delayed due to the immune suppression caused by the thermal injury. Porcine skin can also provide temporary wound coverage to reduce pain and evaporative water losses, although these grafts do not establish vascular connections with the wound bed and therefore do not take.

Various synthetic skin substitutes have been developed and can be of benefit as temporary coverage until permanent autograft material is available.

Permanent Skin Substitutes

The persistent high mortality in patients with burns covering greater than 75% BSA is largely due to the lack of sufficient autografts to effect wound closure before infective sequelae develop. The solution of this problem is on the near horizon with the development of artificial skin and skin culture techniques.

Most artificial skin products consist of a bilamellar structure with a collagen-glycosaminoglycan dermal component and a synthetic epidermal layer. This synthetic layer must eventually be replaced by some type of autologous epidermal coverage. Recently a product that has both layers derived from cultures of the patient's own cells has been tested.

Cultured epidermal sheets have been used clinically at some burn centers. These are grown from small biopsies of the patient's unburned skin using sophisticated culture techniques. These grafts seem to provide permanent coverage when placed on excised wounds or granulation tissue; however, their cosmetic characteristics have the same drawbacks as very thin split-thickness grafts.

SPECIAL PROBLEMS

Infants

Infants with burns pose unique problems in management. Because the buffering capacity of infants is significantly less than that of older children or adults, their metabolic acidosis may be severe on admission. Because the surface area of an infant is greater per kilogram of body weight than in an adult, the greater quantities of fluids sometimes required are more apparent than real. Also, the large surface area of the young infant with burns may result in the rapid development of moderate-to-severe hypothermia, particularly when initial therapy is carried out in air-conditioned rooms with the patient exposed. Hypothermia results in severe vasoconstriction, which can significantly affect fluid therapy.

Finally, hypoglycemia may result from the limited glycogen stores in the liver. Frequent determination of blood sugar and the addition of small quantities of glucose to the isotonic resuscitation fluid may be necessary in a few severely burned children.

The Elderly

Elderly patients with burns present problems with resuscitation because of their limited capacity to compensate for hypovolemic shock. Atherosclerotic blood vessels fail to constrict, and myocardial blood flow is severely impaired. This group is characterized by bradycardia, arrhythmia and/or low voltage electrocardiograms and clinical shock. Intravenous fluid therapy must be given at a rate within the tolerance limits of the myocardium to allow it to maintain maximum cardiac output.

Electrical Injuries

Electrical trauma frequently produces devastating tissue destruction as the electrical current passes through the body searching for an electrical ground. Frequently there are both entrance and exit wounds of considerable proportions. Low voltage injuries, in contrast, may produce minimum amounts of surface burning as the current passes along tissue planes of least resistance. The latter form of trauma is often associated with ECG abnormalities because the path of the current may vary considerably as it passes through the body and may interfere with the conductive mechanism of the heart itself. The damage to deep tissues, particularly skeletal muscle, results in extensive intracellular and extracellular fluid losses, necessitating additional fluid requirements. Myoglobinuria is a sign of muscle damage, but does not predict the extent of fluid requirements.

Prevention of renal failure secondary to myoglobinuria is best done with a forced alkaline diuresis including (1) keeping the urine output greater than 75–100 ml/hr with appropriate intravenous replacement, (2) keeping the urine pH greater than 5 with intravenous bicarbonate, and (3) using mannitol, which will also maintain a high urine output, to reduce the adverse effects of myoglobin on the kidney.

Suggested Readings

Ruberg RL (ed): Advances in burn care. *Clin Plast Surg* 13:1986.

CHAPTER

28 Transport of the Critically Ill

Frank S. Rutledge, M.D. and Kenneth A. Boyle, R.R.T.

Transportation of a critically ill or traumatized patient between hospital centers is an important aspect of the patient's total medical care. The reality of economic limitations, a relative low frequency of need, and personnel and resource limitations dictate that all hospitals cannot provide care for all patients. For some patients, transport to an appropriate center for definitive care may be life saving. Improved survival for such patients is possible, but is dependent in part upon the availability of an effective transport system.

THE PHILOSPHY OF TRANSPORT

Although transport of a critically ill patient may be necessary, the actual process of moving the patient is not in his or her best interests and indeed runs the real risk of making the situation worse. Positive results are only achieved once the transport is complete and definitive care has been instituted in the receiving hospital. The safest place for a critically ill patient is in a hospital, with medical personnel in attendance—not in the confines of an ambulance, helicopter, or plane. The purpose of transport is therefore to move the patient as *safely* and as *rapidly* as possible to a setting that can provide the definitive care required for the patient's unique problem.

The goals of the transport team become

1. First, do no harm;
2. Worsen nothing;
3. Ensure stability;
4. Ensure safe and rapid transport.

WHO SHOULD BE TRANSPORTED?

The transport of patients from hospital to hospital should be considered when the care and treatment required for these patients exceed the referring hospital's capabilities in terms of space, diagnostic or therapeutic equipment, staffing, and/or medical expertise. In all instances, patients should be transfered from the care of one physician to the care of another physician, and this change in responsibility should be agreed upon in advance.

Myocardial infarction, complicated pregnancies or deliveries, postoperative complications, and trauma can occur anywhere, often in areas not equipped to deal with all of the potential complications. These patients should be considered for transport after consultation with a physician in a receiving hospital that can provide the specialized care required.

Guidelines for maternal transfer and guidelines for the transport of traumatized or injured patients are available (see Selected Readings) to assist in getting the right patient to the right hospital at the right time. These guidelines could be used for any center in North America. Examples of conditions that might require transport are included in Table 28.1. If there is any doubt about the need for transport, consultation and discussion by telephone would allow agreement among physicians on how best to meet the patient's needs.

TRANSPORT RESPONSIBILITIES

It is the responsibility of the transport team to provide the necessary care for the patient while en route. The referring and receiving physicians are important components of this transport process, with well-defined responsibilities. The *referring physician*

1. Initiates the process by contacting the receiving physician;
2. Continues with resuscitation of the patient;
3. Maintains availability for ongoing patient care and communication with the transport team;
4. Maintains communication with the receiving physician.

The *receiving physician's* responsibilities include the following:

1. Advising the referring physician;
2. Contacting the local ambulance (land or air) communications center;

Table 28.1
Examples of Conditions that might Require Critical Care Transport

Myocardial infarction with recurring arrythmias, ventricular septal defect, ruptured papillary muscle, or cardiogenic shock
Trauma with hemopneumothorax, wide mediastinum, lacerated liver, or ruptured spleen
Intracerebral bleed, subdural or epidural hematoma
Acute abdomen or trauma with pregnancy
Spontaneous rupture of the membranes with or without labor in preterm pregnancy (see Maternal Transfer Guidelines in Suggested Readings)
Surgical conditions of the newborn, e.g., tracheoesophageal, fistula, diaphragmatic hernia, congenital heart disease

3. Briefing the transport team about the case, patient needs, and anticipated complications;
4. Communicating with (a) the transport team throughout the transport, (b) the necessary support services at the receiving hospital, and (c) the referring physician regarding the patient's management and progress.

Continued and repeated communication between referring and receiving physicians is essential to ensure an effective transport.

DOES TRANSPORT MAKE A DIFFERENCE?

Experience indicates that rapid and safe transport of critically ill patients from hospital to hospital will improve survival by 30–60%; this has been demonstrated for neonates, high-risk pregnancies, as well as for patients suffering multiple trauma and myocardial infarction. The literature also strongly suggests that the time taken to arrive at definitive care is important; a two- to threefold increase in mortality occurs with every 30-minute delay in reaching definitive care. Thus, the goals of achieving patient stability and rapid transport are often in conflict.

One additional consideration is that up to 40% of patient transports develop complications that require immediate therapy. These complications cannot always be managed by a nurse or ambulance attendant and cannot always be predicted. For these transports, a medical or paramedical escort is necessary.

TYPE OF TRANSPORT

The type of transport is necessarily influenced by several interrelated factors: (1) the patient's disease and needs, (2) geographical considerations, (3) weather, (4) time of day, and (5) system availability. The natural history of certain medical problems can often be predicted, i.e., some conditions might require urgent attention and dictate air transport or a referring physician to accompany the patient with a local transport vehicle. Similarly, some problems might preclude the use of air transport, such as recent scuba diving or untreated pneumothorax.

At present, there are two primary modes of critical care transport commonly in use in North America: (1) land ambulance (dedicated critical care transport unit) and (2) air ambulance (dedicated helicopter, jet, or propeller-driven fixed wing aircraft) (Figs. 28.1–28.3). Each of these modes of transport is capable of providing full life support care, including assisted ventilation, hemodynamic monitoring, defibrillation, suction, and all potentially needed pharmacologic support. Each of these vehicles can be equipped with telemetry and communications equipment that will allow the transport team to be in contact with its base hospital at any time. Each vehicle can carry up to two stretchers and can be staffed by any combination of critical care attendants, emergency medical technicians, registered nurse, respiratory therapist, or physician, depending upon the need.

The advantages of air transport over land transport are that greater distances can be covered in a shorter time

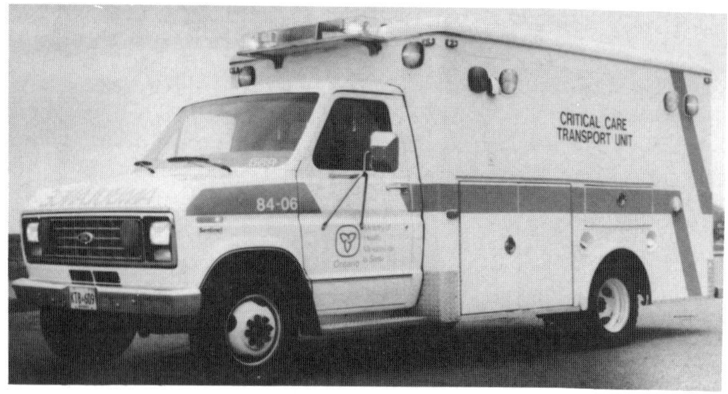

Figure 28.1. Critical care transport unit.

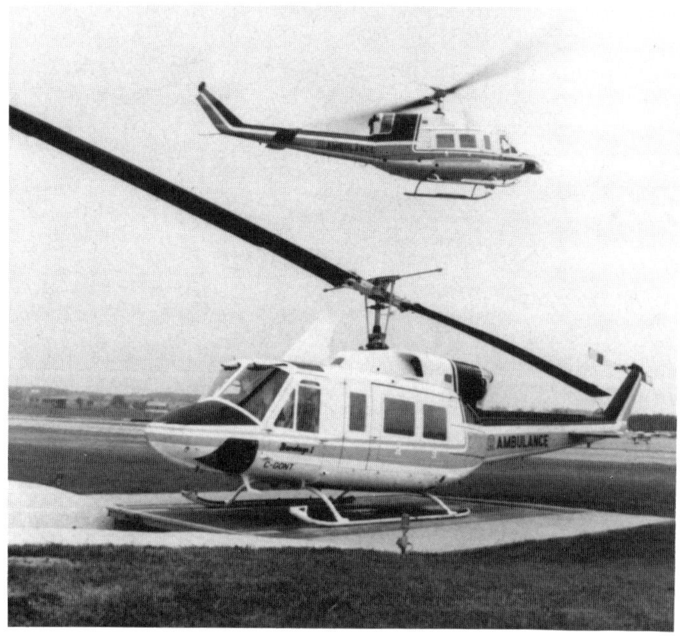

Figure 28.2. Bell 212 helicopters.

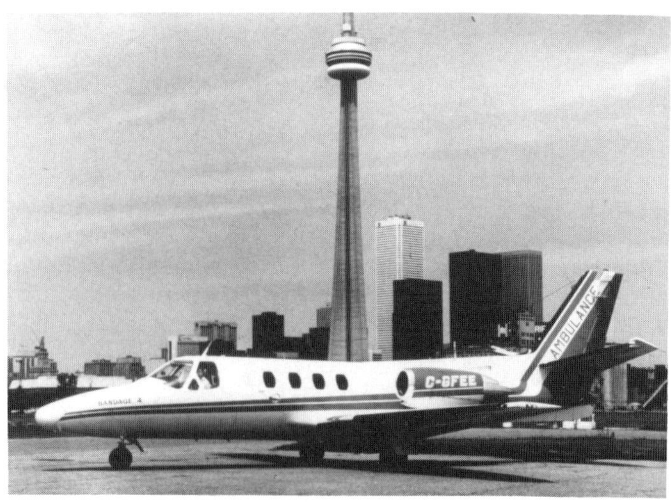

Figure 28.3. Citation I jet aircraft.

and the actual time in transport is decreased. However, there are major disadvantages to air transport: some geographic areas may not have easy access to air transport capability, and the patient frequently requires more transfers, i.e., from hospital bed to ambulance stretcher to aircraft stretcher to ambulance stretcher to hospital bed.

Aviation Physiology

With changes in altitude both the partial pressure (Dalton's law) and the volume of gases (Boyle's law) change. At an altitude of 8000 feet, without supplemental oxygen, the P_{ATM} is 565 mm Hg, and the alveolar PO_2 (PaO_2) is 69 mm Hg (Table 28.2). Obviously many patients could not tolerate this change in pressure without additional O_2. Similarly, at 8000 feet (commercial flights are pressurized to 6000–8000 feet equivalents), the volume of gas increases by a factor of 1.3 (Table 28.3). This has obvious implications for the patient with an untreated pneumothorax and the one who has air in the endotracheal (ET) tube cuff, GI tract, sinuses, and/or cranium. These considerations thereby affect (1) the choice of aircraft with different pressurization capabilities, (2) the suitability of certain patients for air transport, (3) anticipated changes in the patient's condition and physiology during the transport, and (4) necessary preparation or anticipation of the patient's needs before transport. When absolutely necessary, patients can be transported in pressurized aircraft at low altitudes and with proper mechanical and pharmacologic restraints (Table 28.4).

Table 28.2
Effect of Altitude on Partial Pressures[a]

FiO_2	Altitude	P_{ATM}	Alv PO_2
.21	0	760	110
.21	8,000	565	69
.21	18,000	380	30
.21	40,000	141	−20
1.00	40,000	141	48

[a] It is apparent from this table that many patients with borderline PaO_2s at sea level will not be able to tolerate an altitude of even 6000–8000 feet without supplemental O_2.

Table 28.3
Effect of Altitude on Gas Volumes

Altitude	Gas volume
0	1.0
5,000	1.2
8,000[a]	1.3
10,000	1.5
15,000	1.9
18,000	2.0
20,000	2.4

[a] At 8000 feet there is a 30% increase in gas volume.

Table 28.4
Contraindications to Air Transport

Absolute contraindications	Relative contraindications
Untreated pneumothorax	Recent scuba diving
Gas gangrene	Sickle cell anemia
Air trapped in cranium	Arterial hypoxemia
	Recent abdominal surgery
	Psychiatric conditions

PATIENT PREPARATION

As mentioned earlier, the goals of transport are to do no further harm, to ensure stability, and to ensure rapid safe transport. There may be a necessary trade-off between the desire to stabilize the patient and the desire to transport as soon as possible. *It is sometimes impossible to stabilize the patient without rapid transport to definitive care,* but there are certain requirements that must be met before moving the patient.

Respiratory Considerations

The airway must be secured. If the patient is unable to protect his or her airway or if ventilatory assistance is required, then endotracheal intubation is mandatory (nasal or oral). If air transport is used, sterile water should be used to inflate the ET tube cuff to prevent changes in cuff volume and pressure with changes in altitude. Supplemental oxygen should be used to maintain a $PaO_2 > 80$ mm Hg and a hemoglobin saturation of >90%. It may be delivered by mask or ET tube and may require high levels of inspired O_2 or the use of end-expiratory pressure.

The head-injured patient should be hyperventilated to a $PaCO_2$ of 25–30 mm Hg to reduce cerebral edema and intracranial pressure. The patient with chronic lung disease may require intubation for ventilation as hypoxic drive may be blunted with high levels of supplemental oxygen. A nasogastric tube should be inserted to minimize the possibility of aspiration. Suction and chest tubes should be used as needed.

Hemodynamic Considerations

When necessary, blood volume replacement should be initiated *before* moving the patient. A reliable, secure IV access with at least two large-bore catheters or insertion of a central line may be required. Medications and large volumes of IV fluids are often required en route, and the back of a moving vehicle is not the best setting in which to establish a lost IV access. Blood pressure should be maintained with fluid and/or vasopressors at a level sufficient to support cerebral and renal perfusion. Cardiac arrythmias should be treated with the appropriate antiarrhythmics; continuous ECG monitoring is therefore necessary. A urinary catheter connected to closed drainage is usually necessary and advisable for patient comfort and to monitor and contain urine output. All IV solutions should be administered from a plastic bag to avoid the possible breakage of glass containers.

Central Nervous System Considerations

Potential spinal injuries should be managed with spine boards, cervical collars, and immobilization. Known C-spine fractures should be treated with tong traction; if intubation is required, the nasal route is preferred. Patients with head injuries should be hyperventilated to a $PaCO_2$ of 25–30 mm Hg and, if not contraindicated (e.g., unstable thoracolumbar spine), nursed with the head of the bed elevated to 30°. Steroids and/or a mannitol loading dose might be suggested by the receiving institution; this therapy should be discussed, however, as there may be contraindications (e.g., pulmonary edema and acute renal failure) and the need for this therapy might indicate the need for other therapy, such as a Burr hole. A record of the initial neurologic examination, such as the Glasgow Coma Scale, is vitally important and should be made available to the receiving center before transport.

Fractures

All fractures should be immobilized. The cervical spine should be assessed radiologically, if possible, and should be secured with a soft cervical collar and sand bags before transport of any head-injured patient. Newly applied casts should be split before air transport, particularly if edema is present, because the edema may worsen and thereby compromise blood supply to the casted limb.

Gastrointestinal Considerations

As mentioned, a nasogastric tube helps prevent aspiration. It also assists in the removal of air from the abdominal cavity during air transport and thus helps prevent respiratory embarassment, abdominal pain, or dehiscence of abdominal wounds. Antiemetics may reduce motion sickness and assist with sedation. If jaws are wired before transport, one should consider replacing the wires with elastics. Ease of access to the airway remains a top priority.

PEDIATRIC TRANSPORT

Neonates, infants, and children differ from adults in many respects, and consequently their needs before and during transport are different. While awaiting the transport team, therapy should be directed toward the following goals:

1. *Correcting hypoxemia* (to a PaO_2 between 60 and 80 mm Hg)—If ventilation is inadequate, the infant should be intubated and bagged.
2. *Establishing normothermia*—Normothermia is particularly important in neonates or infants because of the relatively large surface area to volume ratio and because of their limited ability to generate heat and maintain body temperature. Normothermia decreases oxygen consumption, improves perfusion, and helps prevent the development of acidosis. Drying the infant after delivery and providing extra humidity will decrease heat loss by evaporation. Radiant warmers or incubators increase surrounding temperature. If unavailable, a single layer of Saran Wrap or aluminum foil, with warmed blankets, may prevent heat loss and insulate the infant. Hot water bottles should *not* be used.
3. *Prevention of hypoglycemia*—Dysmature infants, those with asphyxia at birth, and infants of diabetic mothers may become hypoglycemic. Ten percent dextrose and water should be provided at 4 cc/kg/hr.
4. *Correction of acidosis*—It is usually best to allow metabolic acidosis to correct itself by attending to hypoxemia, hypothermia, and hypoglycemia. A persistent metabolic acidosis may, however, require sodium bicarbonate administration.
5. *Frequent monitoring*—Blood gases, temperature, blood sugar, and heart rate should be monitored every 10 to 15 minutes. A chest x-ray may be helpful in identifying the cause of respiratory distress, e.g., aspiration, diaphragmatic hernia, pneumothorax.

Unique skills, experience, training, and equipment are necessary to transfer the neonate and infant safely. Attention to the factors mentioned above should substantially improve the patient's condition and thereby increase the chances for a favorable outcome.

DIAGNOSTIC STUDIES BEFORE TRANSPORT

If possible the following studies should be obtained before transport. They are often diagnostic, will often alter treatment when abnormal, and will help ensure adequate patient stabilization before commitment to transport.

- Hgb, hematocrit
- Blood gases
- Blood glucose
- Electrolytes
- ECG
- CXR
- Other x-rays, as indicated
- Urinalysis

If results are pending, they may be sent via radio to the transport team en route.

INFORMATION THAT MUST ACCOMPANY THE PATIENT

All available information that may be potentially pertinent to his or her management must accompany the patient. This includes the patient's name, age, address and next of kin; a complete history of injury or illness; a medication history; and a record of the initial physical and neurologic examination. In addition, a record of all vital signs (prehospital to time of transfer) and any treatment given (dose and route) should be provided. A sample of gastric or peritoneal lavage if available should be sent. Finally, the referring physician's name and referring institution and the contact physician's name at the receiving institution should be recorded by the transport team.

THE REALITIES

As one attempts to achieve the goals of transport, it becomes apparent that they cannot all be attained in a given

Table 28.5
"Golden Rules" of Transport[a]

1. Plan ahead.
2. Transports are palliative, not curative.
3. Any treatment can only be as good as the diagnosis for which it is administered.
4. Some hospitals are better than others. Any hospital is a better hospital than an airplane or ambulance.
5. If it is possible for a sick person to become sicker, he or she probably will.
6. Big problems are simply small problems that you have not anticipated.
7. Common things are common, and "probably" is good enough for common things to happen commonly.
8. No transport unit is ideal for every patient.
9. Nothing lasts forever, i.e., O_2, battery power.
10. Some days are better than others; no matter what you do, the outcome may be poor.

[a] Adapted from the Department of Critical Care Transport, Stanford University, Palo Alto, CA, 1984.

situation. The patient's problem may get worse despite one's efforts. Stability may be lost or may have to be sacrificed, in part, to ensure rapid transport if it is decided that this has greater priority. Sometimes operator errors and unavoidable transport delays or equipment malfunctions occur. An inaccurate assessment of the situation or of the problems of the patient that overemphasizes his or her stability or the need for rapid transport may cause difficulties. In addition, difficulties may arise if one does not take into account the different needs of children, i.e., blood volume, amount of blood loss, IV rates, drug dosages, position of subclavian vein, etc. Following the "Golden Rules" in Table 28.5 will help reduce the difficulties of transport.

What Can Go Wrong?

Most transports proceed uneventfully and do not require use of the capabilities of the transport team, critical care transport unit, or the air ambulance. A significant percentage, however, experience complications that require attention by experienced personnel with the appropriate equipment, medication, and supports. Often these complications can be anticipated and therefore avoided. The possibility that a relatively simple problem will become complicated is enhanced on a transport; it is for this reason that receiving institutions place what might be perceived as too much emphasis on stability and preparations. A patient's chance for survival is not improved if he or she arrives 2 hours earlier than otherwise with an ET in the right mainstem bronchus, having aspirated, and with IV fluids and medications running interstitially. Some of the common problems that are encountered with transport of a critically ill patient, despite attention to the Golden Rules, are now described.

Airway

Although the airway is secured before transport, stability can be lost. ET cuffs can leak, and ET tubes can be positioned too high or too low, e.g., in the right mainstem bronchus. The presence of adequate O_2 supplies needs to be ensured. Pneumothoraces may become a concern if the patient has suffered chest trauma or requires end-expiratory pressure. If the patient has required one chest tube before transport, he or she might require a second one on the other side during transport. This becomes a real possibility with changes in altitude (Boyle's law). For these reasons, a chest x-ray is advisable before transport.

Hemodynamics

As mentioned earlier, secure IV access is necessary. When IV fluids and medications are required, their infusion cannot be delayed while IV access is re-established. Arrhythmias may happen at any time and require appropriate recognition and treatment. Sudden unexpected hypotension will require appropriate administration of IV fluids and/or vasopressors. The patient who is stable at the start of transport may not remain so.

Medications

During transport, many medications may be required, and each carries with its use certain risks and side effects. Restless patients are more likely to injure themselves further, threaten the security of their IV access or airway, and make their overall care more difficult. Yet, needed sedation may compromise their ability to ventilate, an effect that should be anticipated. Morphine is frequently used for management of pain and anxiety, but can alter venous return, blood pressure, and ventilatory function.

Aminophylline can contribute to arrhythmogenic potential, and Dopamine can be disastrous if it is given interstitially. Lidocaine can contribute to seizures and should be used as indicated but cautiously.

Suggested Readings

Ehrenwerth J, Sorbo S, Hackel A: Transport of critically-ill adults. *Crit Care Med* 14:543–547, 1986.

Guide to Critical Care Transport in Ontario (Southwest Region). Ontario, Ministry of Health, Emergency Health Services, May 1986.

Hospital resources for optimal care of the injured patient. *Bull Am Coll Surg,* August 1979 (revised 1983).

Ontario Medical Association Committee on Perinatal Care: Emergency inter-hospital maternal transfer guidelines. *Ontario Med Rev,* December 1983.

Birnbaum ML, Robinson NE, Hunter-Handler DL, Krembs DA, Bose JH, Fryback DG: Comparison of ambulance and mobile critical care unit for patients with ischemic heart disease. *Crit Care Med* (Abstr). 3:240, 1984.

Donn SM: Neonatal transport. *Curr Probl Pediatr* 15:1985.

SPECIFIC SYNDROMES

CHAPTER

29 Acute Gastrointestinal Hemorrhage

David P. Girvan, M.D.

Gastrointestinal hemorrhage may be a manifestation of a variety of diseases occurring from the oral pharynx to the anus (Table 29.1). Hematemesis (vomiting of blood) may be fresh, clotted, or altered by gastric secretions (coffee grounds). Bleeding in hematemesis generally occurs at a site between the oral pharynx and the ligament of Treitz, but eventually melena will occur and may occasionally be the initial manifestation of upper gastrointestinal (GI) tract bleeding. Melena is the passage of a black, tarry stool and requires only about 50 ml of blood, which will present for some time after the bleeding has actually stopped. Distal colon bleeding tends to be red, whereas bleeding from the proximal colon or terminal ileum is often a burgundy color and mixed with the stool. Upper GI tract blood tends to be tarry, although massive hemorrhage can produce reasonably red-appearing blood due to rapid intestinal transit.

PATHOPHYSIOLOGY

Gastrointestinal bleeding occurs when the mucosal barrier is broken, which may be caused by acid pepsin digestion, pressure erosion, tumor necrosis, or direct mucosal trauma. The GI tract has a rich, submucosal blood supply. Major arteries or branches are near the principal areas of pathology and so can be readily eroded. In variceal bleeding the esophageal venous pressure is markedly elevated due to intrahepatic or portal vein obstruction and resulting portal hypertension.

Peptic ulcer disease can present as hemorrhage caused by a breakdown in the delicate balance between the aggressive acid pepsin factors and the defensive mucosal barrier. A prime requisite is the presence of acid: no acid, no ulcer is a true axiom. Acid pepsin destruction of the mucosal barrier may result in duodenal ulceration, gastric ulceration (where bile reflux may be a contributing factor), and esophageal bleeding, either from esophagitis or a breakdown of the thin-walled varices.

Table 29.1
Most Common Causes of Gastrointestinal Hemorrhage

Upper gastrointestinal bleeding	Lower gastrointestinal bleeding
Erosive gastritis	Diverticulitis
Peptic ulcer: gastric, duodenal	Neoplasm: carcinoma, polyp
Esophageal varices	Inflammatory bowel disease: ulcerative colitis, Crohn's disease
Mallory-Weiss syndrome	Ischemic colitis
Neoplasms: carcinoma, lymphoma, leiomyoma, polyps	AV malformation
Aorto-intestinal fistula	Angiodysplasia
	Meckel's diverticulum
	Hemorrhoids
	Aorto-intestinal fistula
	Upper GI lesion

Erosive gastritis usually combines the acid pepsin mechanism and some additional factor. Aspirin, indomethacin, and phenylbutazone may cause drug-induced lesions that not only may have a direct effect on increasing acid secretions but also may change the composition of the mucous layer. Stress situations, including trauma, burns, intracranial lesions, sepsis, and hypovolemic shock, can lead to a bleeding diathesis. This bleeding problem is probably due to ischemic cellular insult and the presence of a major defect in the defensive mucosal barrier causing inadequate neutralization of the back flux of hydrogen ion.

Variceal bleeding results from dilation of lower esophageal venous plexuses as an alternative pathway for portal venous drainage to the caval venous system. Obstruction at the liver interface causes portal vein hypertension. This opens up existing small collateral channels, which soon enlarge and become thin-walled veins that are easily eroded by acid pepsin reflux, direct trauma, or a sudden increase in pressure as seen with forceful vomiting. Forceful vomiting, frequently on a full stomach and with an excess of alcohol in the system, results in the traumatic tear of the lower esophageal or cardiac mucosa into the submucosa. (Mallory-Weiss syndrome). Portal hypertension and varices are not prerequisites for this condition.

Tumor growth, either in the upper or lower GI tract, may result in pressure necrosis and ulceration of the mucosa or else erosion into adjacent vessels. Tumor necrosis itself can lead to ulceration and hemorrhage.

Diverticular bleeding is secondary to inflammation or pressure necrosis due to inspissated feces in a small neck diverticulum. Each diverticulum occurs at the point of entry of a blood vessel through the bowel wall, and thus it takes little erosion to enter an adjacent vessel. Polypoid bleeding is a result of fecal trauma on a very friable and vascular polypoid mucosal covering. Arterial venous malformations are generally submucosal collections that may erode through the thin mucosal covering because of sheer size, growth of the lesion, or increase in intravascular pressure. Arteriosclerosis may result in more friable vessels, or rarely an aneurysm may form adjacent to a GI lumen. Erosion into the lumen can be caused by arterial pulsation and the increasing size of the aneurysm. In any patient who has had a major arterial reconstruction with a prosthetic graft, the presence of sudden unexpected GI hemorrhage is diagnostic of a graft to GI tract fistua until proven otherwise, e.g., aortoduodenal fistula following aortic aneurysm resection.

Hemorrhoidal bleeding is usually fairly obvious, but occasionally can be massive and unsuspected if there are no external signs. Increased venous pressure and distension, along with trauma from straining or a hard, constipated stool, can result in a bleeding episode. Colitis and other inflammatory bowel disorders may cause bleeding if mucosal ulceration occurs, but usually are suspected because of associated diarrhea with mucus and other systemic symptoms—cramps, weight loss, failure to thrive, anorexia, fever.

DIAGNOSIS

The site of presentation of the GI bleeding determines the type and order of various investigative procedures. Investigation of upper GI bleeding is somewhat different than that for lower GI bleeding. However, one must keep in mind at all times that lower GI hemorrhage may be a manifestation of bleeding that has occurred as high up as the esophagus, unless the bleeding has been sudden and massive and resulted in nausea and vomiting. All investigative procedures must take second place to stabilization of the patient's condition, which is the priority item in any GI hemorrhage (discussed more fully in the management section).

Upper Gastrointestinal Hemorrhage (Hematemesis)

Insertion of Nasogastric Tube

This simple maneuver very quickly confirms the presence of blood in the stomach, which indicates an upper GI site of bleeding. The presence of bright red blood confirms ongoing hemorrhage, whereas the presence of dark and clotted blood or coffee grounds is more indicative of earlier hemorrhage that may have since ceased. The presence of a nasogastric tube allows one to monitor ongoing hemorrhage and to irrigate blood out of the stomach. A clot-filled, distended stomach is far less likely to stop bleeding than one that is collapsed and can contract down. There is considerable controversy over the use of iced versus normal temperature solutions, but iced saline lavage is considered to be more efficient. Once all evidence of active bleeding has ceased, then the nasogastric tube may be removed, unless it is required for medication.

Endoscopy

With the advent of the flexible fiberoptic endoscope, early endoscopic evaluation of the esophagus, stomach, and duodenum has become the initial method of investigation. This procedure is particularly valuable in diagnosing erosive gastritis, which is a superficial lesion and is never evident on an upper GI series. Varices, ulcers, tumors, and Mallory-Weiss tears are all readily seen on endoscopy. Problems with endoscopy arise when massive continuous bleeding prevents adequate inspection, when there is a clot-filled stomach, or when the patient is agitated and uncooperative and will not tolerate the endoscope.

Upper GI Series

Barium examinations of the esophagus, stomach, and duodenum have now taken second place to the endoscope. They probably are of more use in the patient who has stopped bleeding or in the patient who has a history of upper GI symptoms that may be more indicative of chronic peptic ulcer disease or underlying GI malignancy. Esophageal varices often can be visualized with barium swallows. The presence of active bleeding can rarely be demonstrated, and very shallow erosions or clot-filled ulcers may readily be missed.

Angiography

If endoscopy and barium studies fail to reveal a bleeding point and the patient is continuing to hemorrhage actively, then selective arteriography of the celiac axis and its branches may identify the bleeding point. This technique is not routinely used and is reserved more often for the extremely poor risk patient who is unlikely to withstand a major surgical procedure and for whom one may wish to combine attempted treatment with embolization.

Lower Gastrointestinal Hemorrhage (Melena)

Nasogastric Tube

Even with lower GI hemorrhage it is frequently valuable to insert a nasogastric tube to rule out a gastric or duodenal cause for the patient's bleeding. A positive return of blood should lead to investigations of the upper GI tract as outlined above. If the stomach is clear of blood or coffee grounds then one can focus on the lower GI tract. However, duodenal lesions should not be completely excluded, as reflux of blood into the stomach does not always occur, particularly if bleeding is at a slow rate.

Sigmoidoscopy

Using the rigid 20-cm sigmoidoscope or the more recently available flexible sigmoidoscope that reaches up into the lower descending colon is a quick and easy way of ruling out lesions in the lower GI tract. The hemorrhoidal plexuses can be readily inspected and the viability of the bowel and mucosa assessed, particularly if ischemic bowel problems are suspected. A dusky or cyanotic mucosa is evidence of inferior mesenteric artery occlusion with poor or absent collateral supply from the superior mesenteric artery. Inflammatory bowel disease, such as ulcerative colitis, may be diagnosed, or the presence of bright red or dark blood coming from higher in the colon can be ascertained. Only rarely is a bleeding diverticulum seen. A colonic carcinoma or polyp may also be seen with these simple instruments. The major drawback to lower GI endoscopy is poor preparation of the bowel or the presence of ongoing bleeding that obscures any meaningful examination of the mucosa or bowel lumen.

Barium Enema

The advisability of barium enema versus angiography in lower GI bleeding is somewhat controversial. If ischemic bowel disease is unlikely, then barium enema is the next examination of choice to demonstrate diverticular disease, carcinoma, polyps, or a volvulus. Unsuspected ischemic bowel disease may be suggested by the characteristic thumb printing; inflammatory bowel disease, such as ulcerative colitis and regional enterocolitis, may be confirmed by the presence of ulcerations, edema, or loss of normal bowel patterns. The major drawback to a barium enema at this point in the investigation is the residual barium that may not be cleared and subsequently will prevent the use of angiography if bleeding should continue.

Angiography

A number of physicians do selective angiography of the superior mesenteric artery and inferior mesenteric artery before doing a barium enema. This technique, however, requires that the patient be actively bleeding in order to detect the point of hemorrhage. The use of labeled red cell scintigraphy to demonstrate active bleeding should aid in the selection of patients for angiography. Angiography may not be technically easy in older individuals with arteriosclerotic vessels, and there is certainly some risk of dislodging clots and causing subsequent embolization. However, angiography has proven to be particularly useful in picking up some of the more uncommon arteriovenous malformations and, in particular, the more recently described angiodysplasias that are frequently seen in the cecum and right colon and are responsible for a large number of undiagnosed lower GI hemorrhages in older patients.

Scintigraphy

Recent reports have renewed interest in the use of radiotracers to detect and localize the site of GI bleeding. Earlier studies were not generally accepted because of technical difficulties and unreliable results. Recently the use of technetium ^{99m} sulfur colloid has shown improved reliability, particularly as compared with angiography in the localization of GI bleeding sites that are not readily apparent. Newer techniques of labeling red cells also are being developed, and scintigraphy may prove to be a valuable tool when used in conjunction with existing diagnostic methods and clinical examination of the patient.

Colonoscopy

In order for the long flexible colonoscope to be most useful in diagnosis the bowel should be clean and well prepared. The colonoscope's use in the actively bleeding patient is limited because of the technical problems of advancing the instrument through a number of bends and curves that require rather accurate sight of the lumen ahead of the instrument. It has proven to be a useful instrument in the investigation and treatment of polyps, the diagnosis of some arteriovenous malformations, and in the diagnosis of inflammatory bowel disease involving the more proximal colonic segments.

MANAGEMENT (FIGURE 29.1)

Prevention

GI hemorrhage is frequently the first indication of GI pathology, so there is little chance of prophylaxis. Ulcerogenic anti-inflammatory drugs, such as aspirin, indomethacin, and phenylbutazone and the many newer nonsteroidal anti-inflammatory drugs, should be prescribed with caution, and the concomitant use of excessive alcohol or anticoagulants must be avoided by the patient. Rapid correction of stress situations, such as hypovolemia, sepsis, and hypoxic states, may help reduce the incidence of acute stress ulceration. The concomitant prophylactic use of antacids or cimetidine (Tagamet) in these high risk patients is frequently warranted.

Initial Management

In any patient with GI hemorrhage, the initial priority of management must be the stabilization of the patient's vital signs, which must take precedence over any investigative procedures outlined in the previous section. The patient should have at least one, and if the bleeding is excessive, multiple, large-bore intravenous lines inserted. Blood is immediately drawn for routine blood work, including hemoglobin, hematocrit, coagulation profiles (prothrombin time (PT), partial thromboplastin time (PTT), platelets) and blood for group and cross-matching. Initial stabilization of the blood pressure is obtained with the use of saline or Ringer's lactate in volumes sufficient to maintain blood pressure and correct any ongoing tachycardia. Albumin or plasma may be used until properly cross-matched blood is available. In the face of ongoing hemorrhage, stabilization must be obtained with the use of whole blood or packed cells that are now more readily available.

The patient must be monitored on a frequent and continuous basis until the bleeding has stopped or a decision to operate has been made. Monitoring of several single parameters, including blood pressure, pulse, urine output as measured with a urinary catheter, and central venous pressure, can easily be done. The use of a Swan-Ganz catheter is certainly valuable, but is not absolutely necessary and is usually reserved for those patients who require monitoring in an intensive care unit and who have underlying cardiopulmonary problems. Such problems may make assessment of fluid requirements more critical as these patients are less tolerant of sudden changes in intravascular volume.

Upper Gastrointestinal Lesions

The majority of upper GI lesions are initially managed in similar fashion. If there is evidence of continued bleeding, then insertion of a nasogastric tube and continuous iced saline lavage should be carried out until the return is clear. Intravenous cimetidine (Tagamet) 300 mg every 6 hours (q6h) should be started to reduce acid secretion. This is probably most efficiently administered with a continuous infusion of 600 mg in 1000 ml of 5% dextrose

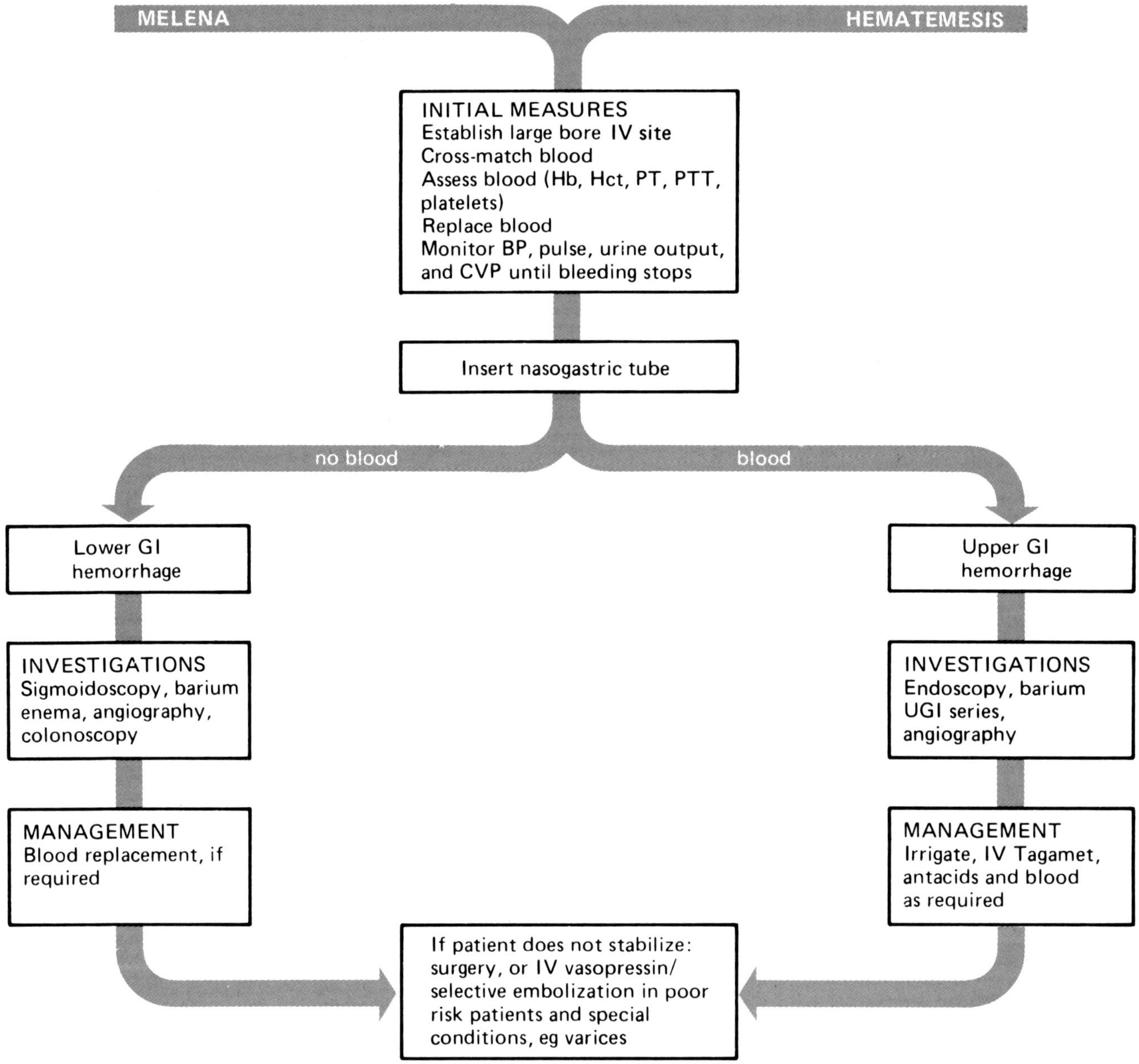

Figure 29.1. Management of gastrointestinal hemorrhage.

in water (D5W). Antacids can be administered (60–90 ml, q2h) using the nasogastric tube clamped for 30 minutes. Gastric acidity can best be monitored by testing the pH of the gastric return and attempting to keep the pH above 4.5.

Studies comparing Tagamet and antacids have shown that antacids are more effective in reducing acidity if administered in sufficient volumes to keep the pH above 4.5. Cimetidine is certainly easier to use, but occasionally it is necessary to combine both cimetidine and antacids to achieve adequate neutralization. In patients in whom neutralization cannot be achieved with antacids and even double-dose cimetidine, one should be very suspicious that occult or ongoing sepsis is preventing adequate neutralization. These patients are at particular risk for development of acute gastroduodenal mucosal lesions, with hemorrhage being the major complication. The majority of cases of erosive gastritis and peptic ulcer disease (which make up 80–90% of all upper GI hemorrhage) can usually be controlled by these measures and require no further treatment other than prevention of their recurrence.

Ranitidine, a newer H_2 antagonist, is equally effective, but appears to have fewer side effects, especially neuropsychiatric, hepatic, and endocrine than cimetidine. Other new therapies include omeprazole, a substituted benzimidazole that is a proton pump blocker and acts in the secretory membrane of the parietal cell. Prostaglandin derivatives not only inhibit acid production but also improve cytoprotection by stimulating gastric mucus production and increasing bicarbonate secretion in gastric and duodenal mucosa.

Endoscopic control of bleeding vessels is possible with lasers and photocoagulation. They are probably equally effective, but photocoagulation is cheaper and more portable.

Ongoing bleeding, which means initial failure to stabilize vital signs or requires the continued use of transfusion beyond 36–48 hours, will require surgical intervention. Vagotomy and pyloroplasty with oversewing of the bleeding vessel are usually adequate for a bleeding duodenal ulcer. Erosive gastritis and bleeding gastric ulcers are best managed by generous gastrectomy and, in the case of erosive gastritis, the addition of a vagotomy. If continued bleeding occurs in the residual gastric remnant in those cases of erosive gastritis, then a total gastrectomy may be required. Gastric malignancy will require resection if possible. Mallory-Weiss tears frequently will stop bleeding when treated by conservative management, blood replacement, and the occasional use of vasopressin. If continued bleeding occurs, then gastrotomy and suturing of the tear are usually adequate.

Treatment of bleeding esophageal varices secondary to alcoholic cirrhosis continues to be a controversial area, with an average mortality from variceal bleeding of about 50% in most large series. The presently available methods of treatment are less than ideal, primarily because of the underlying alcoholic cirrhosis. Following confirmation of the bleeding site by endoscopy, the initial measures for stabilization as outlined above should be started. If the patient fails to stop bleeding with nasogastric lavage and blood replacement, then vasopressin therapy is indicated. Intravenous and intra-arterial routes using selective catheterization are equally effective. An intravenous drip of vasopressin (0.4–0.5 units/min in D5W) is begun. The dose should be increased or decreased as necessary to control bleeding, and there should be continuous electrocardiographic monitoring, with the dose being lowered if ischemic changes occur in the ST segment of the tracing. If bleeding continues the Sengstaken-Blakemore tube should be used. Initially the gastric balloon is inflated and may control hemorrhage if cardiac varices are primarily involved. If this is unsuccessful then the esophageal balloon is inflated. The tube is left inflated for 24 hours after bleeding has stopped and then is removed. In continued bleeding, angiography may be useful to determine the site, and an attempt can be made to use intra-arterial infusions of vasopressin at the same rate given above. If continued bleeding occurs then emergency portosystemic shunting may be required. Ideally this is best done on an elective basis when the patient's general metabolic and liver function can be properly assessed. It is helpful to have documentation of portal hemodynamics to determine whether portal blood flow is hepatopetal (toward the liver) or hepatofugal (away from the liver). Child's classification of cirrhosis according to hepatic functional reserve looks at bilirubin and albumin levels, the presence or absence of ascites and encephalopathy, and the nutritional state. Operative risks varies from low in the A group to very high in the C group. A variety of shunting procedures have been devised, including portocaval, splenorenal, mesocaval, and the selective distal splenorenal shunt of Warren. Other nonshunting types of surgical approach include esophagogastric devascularization and transection, and transection and reanastomosis of the esophagus with the newer stapling guns. There has been a resurgence of interest in sclerosis of varices by injections with such substances as ethanolamine oleate using the flexible endoscope. In many centers this procedure is becoming the initial treatment of choice for bleeding varices. Results appear to be favorable, although some patients continue to require surgical procedures. In very high risk patients and Child's type C this may offer a useful alternative to shunting. Considerable debate continues as to whether shunting procedures result in increasing survival. There is no question that it may be easier to conservatively manage a patient who is dying of hepatic failure, rather than massive GI hemorrhage.

Lower Gastrointestinal Lesions

Most lower GI lesions are initially managed by careful monitoring of vital signs because, in the majority of cases, bleeding will cease spontaneously, and investigation can be carried out on a more elective basis. If bleeding continues and stabilization of vital signs is difficult or massive transfusion is required, then emergency laparotomy is indicated. If the individual lesion has been identified it may be dealt with readily, whereas occasionally, it is necessary to do a blind laparotomy in the hope of identifying the bleeding point. This is a procedure to be avoided if possible, because the bleeding point is not frequently self-evident.

Diverticular disease, tumors, arteriovenous malformations, and Meckel's diverticulum are all best dealt with by resection of the lesion and, depending on the state of bowel preparation, either primary anastomosis or a colostomy and mucous fistula with delayed closure. Severe forms of ulcerative colitis may require total colectomy and a permanent ileostomy. Significantly bleeding hemorrhoids may have to be dealt with by an emergency hemorrhoidectomy. During laparotomy for patients with still undiagnosed lesions, the use of a light source within the bowel, provided by the flexible colonoscope or on-table angiography, may facilitate finding the location and thus more exact treatment of the offending lesion. If no lesion can be found and the patient is elderly, a blind right colectomy or occasionally a total colectomy has been advocated because of the high incidence of angiodysplasia in these individuals. Other surgeons advocate doing a transverse colostomy and waiting to see from which half of the bowel further bleeding may occur. Occasionally in very poor risk patients, selective angiography can be used to locate the bleeding point. A small bleeding vessel can then be embolized with Gelfoam or other embolic materials.

Suggested Readings

Alavi A, Ring EJ: Localization of gastrointestinal bleeding: Superiority of ^{99m}Tc sulfur colloid compared with angiography. *AJR* 137:741–748, 1981.

Boley SJ, Sammartano R. Brandt LJ: Vascular ectasias of the colon. *Surg Gynecol Obstet* 149:353–359, 1979.

Debas HT, Mulholland MW: New horizons in the pharmacologic management of peptic ulceration. *Am J Surg* 151:422–430, 1986.

Dronfield MW, Langman MJS, et al: Outcome of endoscopy and barium radiography for acute upper gastrointestinal bleeding—controlled trial in 1037 patients. *Br Med J* 284:545–548, 1982.

Finkelstein W, Isselbacher KJ: Cimetidine. *N Engl J Med* 299:992–996, 1978.

Goff JS, Bipolar: Electrocoagulation versus Nd-Yag laser photocoagulation for upper gastrointestinal bleeding lesions. *Dig Dis Sci* 31:906–910, 1986.

Hanna SS, Warren WD, Galambos JT, et al.: Bleeding varices. *Can Med Assoc J* 29–47, 1981.

Hastings PR, Skillman JJ, Bushell LS, et al.: Antacid titration in the prevention of acute gastrointestinal bleeding. *N Engl J Med* 298:1041–1045, 1978.

Hunt RH: Rectal bleeding. *Clin Gastroenterol* 7:719–740 (colonoscopy), 1978.

Kivilaakso E, Silen W: Pathogensis of experimental gastric mucosal injury. *N Engl J Med* 301:364–369, 1979.

McCormack TT, Kennedy HJ, Salisbury J, Simms JM, Triger DR, Johnson AG: Implications of sclerotherapy program for the medical and surgical care of bleeding in portal hypertension. *Surg Gynecol Obstet* 161:557–562, 1985.

Richter JM, Hedbey SE, Athanasorilis CA, Shapiro RH: Angiodysplasia—clinical presentation and colonoscopic diagnosis. *Dig Dis Sci* 29:481–485, 1984.

Stothert JC, Simonowitz DA, Dellinger EP, et al.: Randomized prospective evaluation of cimetidine and antacid control of gastric pH in the critically ill. *Ann Surg* 169–174, 1980.

Veidenheimer MC, Corman ML, Coller JA: Colonic hemorrhage. *Surg Clin North Am* 58:581–595, 1978.

CHAPTER

30 Intestinal Ischemia

David P. Girvan, M.D.

A series of conditions make up the syndrome of intestinal ischemia, including acute occlusion of the superior mesenteric artery, nonocclusive mesenteric infarction, chronic mesenteric arterial insufficiency (intestinal angina), and mesenteric venous occlusion. Mesenteric artery occlusion may be complete and sudden due to embolus or thrombosis, or it may be partial and gradual due to obliterative disease. A combination of the above is also possible, leading to a complete and sudden occlusion. The majority of acute and chronic occlusions occur within the superior mesenteric artery (SMA). Inferior mesenteric artery occlusion is only symptomatic if the collateral blood supply from the superior mesenteric artery and iliac arteries has been interfered with or previously occluded.

Venous occlusion can also lead to intestinal ischemia and gut infarction. Although venous occlusion is usually thrombotic in origin, sudden, and complete, it may also occur in severe hyperosmolar states, e.g., nonketotic hyperglycemic coma. Intestinal ischemia in this latter situation is likely secondary to profound volume depletion and a concomitant low flow state in a patient with underlying small vessel disease.

PATHOPHYSIOLOGY

Acute superior mesenteric artery occlusion usually results from an embolus secondary to a mural thrombus in the postmyocardial infarction period or in a patient who has atrial fibrillation. Endocarditis may predispose to emboli, and cholesterol plaques in the aorta can be dislodged during arteriography. The embolus usually occludes at the first division after the take-off of the superior mesenteric artery from the aorta. This results in sparing of the first few inches of the jejunum, unless there is a pre-existing stenosis in the SMA, and then even this first part of jejunum may become infarcted. Thrombosis of the superior mesenteric artery usually completes occlusion already begun by arteriosclerosis and is a major cause of small bowel ischemia. Decreased cardiac output secondary to congestive heart failure or acute myocardial infarction may enhance the effects of thrombosis, because of poor mesenteric blood flow and possibly associated vasoconstriction. If previous stenosis has been present for some time, collateral circulation may exist to protect the gut from the effects of a complete occlusion secondary to thrombosis.

Nonocclusive infarction reveals no gross obvious occlusion of the artery and is likely secondary to a sustained low cardiac output as a result of profound circulatory collapse seen with sepsis, myocardial infarction, dysrhythmias, or hypovolemic shock. The prolonged splanchnic vasoconstriction associated with a low flow state may be further potentiated by the use of vasopressor drugs (e.g., dopamine) that, although capable of improving cardiac function and output, may in fact cause further splanchnic vasoconstriction if the doses used are in the alpha range (15 μg/kg/min).

Chronic mesenteric occlusion, often called intestinal angina, results from partial narrowing of the major mesenteric vessels—the celiac, superior, or inferior mesenteric arteries—due to arteriosclerosis; compression by adjacent structures, such as the celiac ganglion or arcuate ligament; involvement by an expanding aneurysm; or more rare diseases, such as thromboangiitis obliterans or periarteritis nodosa.

Mesenteric venous occlusion results from acute thrombosis that may be idiopathic in a significant percentage of cases or secondary to intra-abdominal suppuration (appendicitis, pelvic abscess), hypercoagulable states (polycythemia, carcinomatosis, postsplenectomy), or local venous congestion and stasis secondary to tumor mass or fibrosis (cirrhosis).

Sudden arterial occlusion results in an ischemic infarct with intense vasospasm, leading to a hypertonic and contracted bowel with mucosal ulceration. Within a period of several hours, spasm subsides and the bowel musculature fatigues because of its inability to receive essential nutrients and oxygen. Visceral veins thrombose and the bowel becomes inert, edematous, and cyanotic, usually with a large accumulation of intraluminal fluid. Finally, full thickness necrosis occurs, giving a picture of hemorrhagic infarction as seen with acute venous occlusion. As gangrenous changes advance and intraluminal pressure increases, perforation occurs, resulting in generalized peritonitis or localized abscess collection.

DIAGNOSIS (FIGURE 30.1)

There is a diagnostic triad for superior mesenteric artery embolization that should alert the physician to its possibility and lead to early treatment, which is the only chance the patient has of surviving. The triad includes (1) sudden severe abdominal pain; (2) a patient with a cardiac lesion that is likely to produce embolization (previous in-

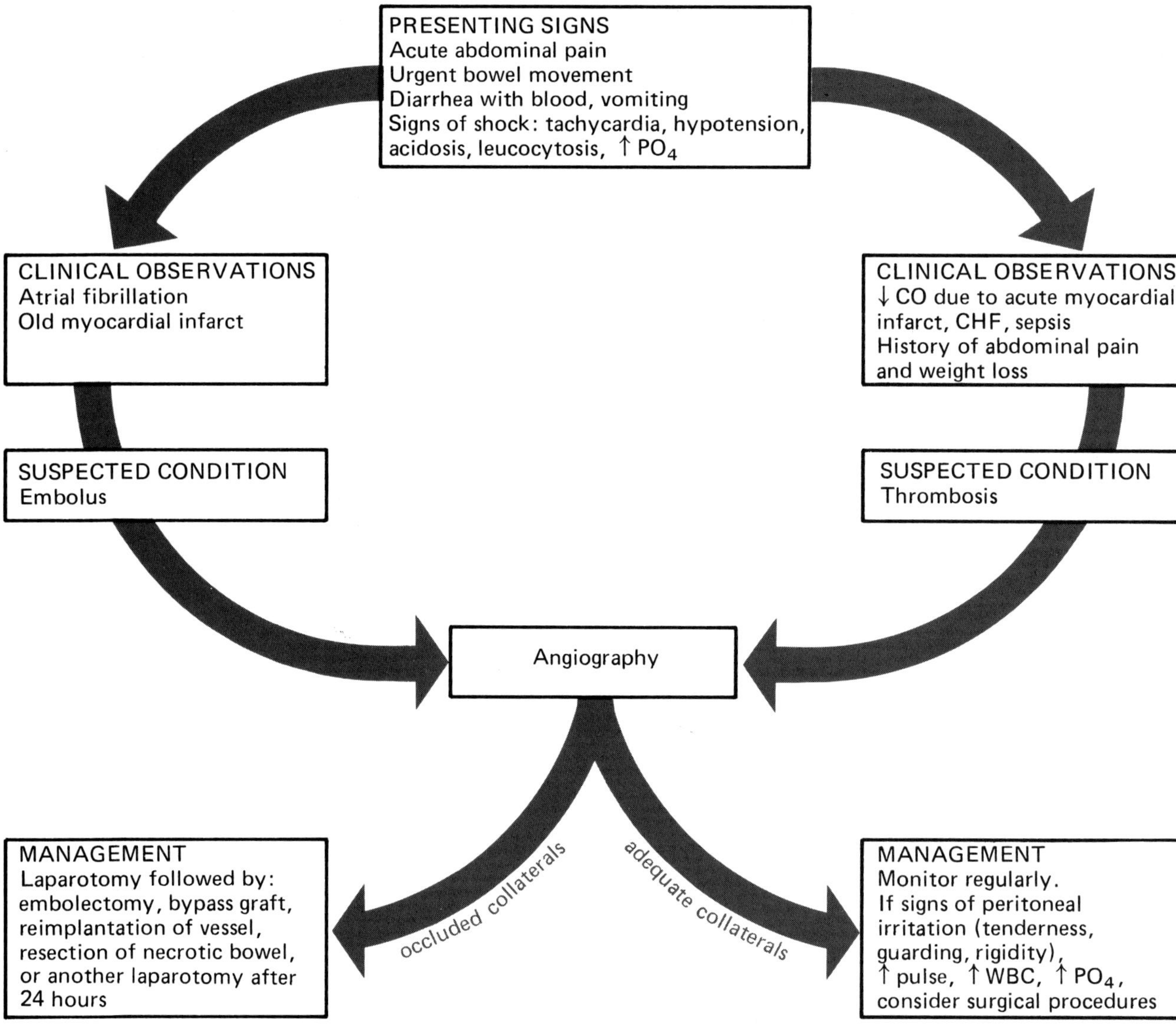

Figure 30.1. Diagnosis and management of mesenteric vascular insufficiency.

farct, atrial fibrillation, or rheumatic heart disease); and (3) urgent emptying of the bowel, possibly associated with bloody diarrhea and vomiting. Examination of the abdomen may reveal an acute surgical abdomen with marked peritoneal signs (tenderness, guarding, and rigidity) or, not infrequently, rather vague signs out of keeping with the patient's rather severe clinical condition, i.e., tachycardia, hypotension, fever, acidosis, and hemoconcentration.

A significant number of patients may have a history of previous embolic episodes. There is usually a severe leukocytosis, severe metabolic acidosis within the first few hours, and an elevation of the serum phosphate level. Peritoneal fluid and urine may also show elevated phosphate levels. The suspected diagnosis must be confirmed by emergent selective abdominal angiography followed by urgent laparotomy. Nonocclusive infarction with resulting vasoconstriction within the mesenteric arterial bed usually presents with abdominal pain due to gut spasm, and again, diarrhea, melena, and leukocytosis will likely ensue.

Chronic mesenteric occlusion may initially be relatively asymptomatic, or it may produce anoxic postprandial pain due to an inability to increase the blood flow required by the intestines to provide the increased oxygen delivery needed after eating. As motor activity increases and more forceful contractions occur, arterial flow is further reduced and severe intestinal spasm may result. This is often interpreted by the patient as rather diffuse and nonspecific abdominal pain. Frequently there is associated weight loss because the patient is afraid to eat a large meal and thus has a reduced calorie intake. Malabsorption may occur, but is not a prominent factor. Diarrhea and constipation can occasionally be present, as may occult blood in the stool. These patients often have evidence of atherosclerotic arterial occlusive disease elsewhere, such as angina or previous myocardial infarction, peripheral vascular disease, or previous history of strokes. Angiography again is essential for diagnosis, and all three major vessels should be studied. Careful attention should be paid to the presence of collateral circulation.

Acute thrombosis of the mesenteric veins also presents as an abdominal emergency with diffuse pain resulting from local inflammation, paralysis of the gut, and eventual venous gangrene. Signs of generalized peritonitis are frequently evident, along with blood in the bowel movements.

Mesenteric venous occlusion may present as an abdominal catastrophe with an acute onset as seen with arterial infarction. In other cases, a more gradual and progressive course is seen, with abdominal discomfort, anorexia, and change in bowel habits. Serosanguineous ascites is frequently seen. Abdominal findings are usually nonspecific. Diagnosis is made at laparotomy, and resection of the involved bowel is the only treatment.

In all cases of suspected mesenteric vascular occlusion, whether complete or partial, a strong index of suspicion is essential and is followed by urgent emergency selective angiography. Only if this attitude is adopted will any patient stand a chance of survival. Plain films of the abdomen may show distended loops of bowel with air fluid levels and thickening of the bowel wall due to edema or hemorrhage, but the bowel may also appear essentially normal. Barium enema examination may be useful in the more chronic forms of ischemia or in the patient who is not acutely ill. Thumb printing is a valuable diagnostic sign and may be associated with segmental spasm and other mucosal irregularities. Care must be taken not to preclude the use of angiography by having a colon filled with residual barium as a result of an earlier barium examination.

Sigmoidoscopy may reveal a dusky, ischemic bowel with early signs of mucosal damage, such as edema, loss of vascular pattern, and increased mucus production or blood. If the inferior mesenteric artery supply is adequate, a normal appearing mucosa will be present and is of little value in diagnosis.

MANAGEMENT

Vigorous correction of fluid deficits to compensate for plasma loss should include intravenous colloid solutions. Broad spectrum antibiotics against intestinal bacteria including anaerobic organisms should be instituted.

Early surgical management is the only treatment that will ensure survival in these patients. The pathology found at angiography determines the type of treatment to be offered. Early embolectomy with or without a venous patch graft may be all that is required in the case of acute superior mesenteric artery embolism. In acute thrombotic or chronic obstructive conditions, endarterectomy is usually of limited value, and some form of revascularization procedure using a vein graft, Dacron graft, or Gortex graft from the aorta to the postobstructed area can be carried out. Use of Fogarty catheters with removal of as much clot as possible is indicated. Following these procedures, careful inspection of the bowel should be carried out to determine what, if any, resection is required.

Other methods in addition to clinical judgment that have been used to assess blood flow include Doppler ultrasonic flow detection and fluorescein fluorescence. This latter method involves the injection of sodium fluorescein intravenously into the peripheral circulation and the examination of the bowel under ultraviolet light to see if it fluoresces, which would indicate adequate perfusion. This method is not in wide clinical use, but may prove to be helpful. A second laparotomy 24 hours later may be indicated in cases where the viability of the remaining bowel is questionable. Attempts should be made to control any underlying problem that may have accounted for a thrombotic episode. In the case of mesenteric venous thrombosis, the only accepted treatment is bowel resection.

These patients should be aggressively monitored, invasively in most instances. Gut ischemia may itself produce shock and a low flow state due to release of myocardial depressant factor from ischemic bowel and/or pancreas. An arterial line and Swan-Ganz catheter are helpful in the most critically ill patients. Their use permits sequential and constant monitoring of the pulmonary capillary wedge pressure (PCWP) and cardiac output (CO), and mean arterial pressure, respectively.

If the CO is low, and needs to be augmented, volume loading is utilized according to the PCWP as the method of first choice. Use of vasopressors may be required to augment CO after the preload has been pushed to the tolerable maximum, e.g., PCWP 12–16 mm Hg. However, vasopressors may also cause further splanchnic vasoconstriction, especially if used in α-agonist doses. If necessary, we utilize dopamine to maintain the mean blood pressure (BP) at levels commensurate with a cardiac index greater than 2.5 liter/min/m^2. Myocardial depression may also result from the metabolic acidosis that accompanies intestinal infarction, and therefore intravenous bicarbonate is utilized to keep the pH greater than 7.25.

These conditions carry a mortality of 60–80%. Only by maintaining a high index of suspicion combined with early angiography and immediate laparotomy can a small percentage of these cases be rescued. The majority of these patients are elderly, frequently have many other underlying problems, and may have other manifestations of their severe and generalized atherosclerotic disease process that may preclude a successful outcome.

Suggested Readings

Boley SJ, Brandt LJ, Veith FJ: Ischemic disorders of the intestines. *Curr Probl Surg* 1978.

Boley SJ, Sprayregan S, Siegelmann SS: Initial results from an aggressive roentgenological and surgical approach to acute mesenteric ischemia. *Surgery* 82:848–855, 1977.

Bulkely GB, Zuidema GD, Hamilton SR, et al.: Intraoperative determination of small intestinal viability following ischemic injury. *Ann Surg* 193:628–637, 1981.

Cooperman M, Martin EW, Carey LC: Evaluation of ischemic intestine by Doppler ultrasound. *Am J Surg* 139:73–77, 1980.

Jamieson WG, Taylor BM, Troster M, et al.: The significance of urine phosphate measurement in early diagnosis of intestinal infarction. *Surg Gynecol Obstet* 148:334–338, 1979.

Jaxheimer EC, Jewell ER, Persson AV: Chronic intestinal ischemia. *Surg Clin North Am* 64:123–130, 1985.

Saegesser F: Acute abdomen arising from vascular disorders in the elderly. *Clin Gastroenterol* 10:145–176, 1981.

Stoney RJ, Olcott C: Visceral artery syndromes and reconstructions. *Surg Clin North Am* 59:637–647, 1979.

CHAPTER

31 Septicemia

Thomas W. Austin, M.D.

Septicemia is a frequent reason for admission to the intensive care facility. It is, as well, a problem that often complicates the management of the critically ill patient. Certain major determinants of survival are beyond our ability to control: age, underlying disease, and infecting organisms. Nonetheless, initial vigorous supportive treatment, early appropriate antibiotic therapy, and timely surgical intervention all enhance recovery. This chapter examines the pathophysiology of sepsis and provides a practical approach to the problem of patient management for the intensive care worker.

CAUSES

The organisms most commonly isolated in blood cultures from septic patients in general hospitals are listed in Table 31.1. The predominance of *Escherichia coli* reflects the importance of the genitourinary tract as a major source of infection in both community and hospital-acquired (nosocomial) sepsis. Additional important sources of infection are the GI tract, lungs, and skin. The isolation of *Staphylococcus aureus* from patients with community-acquired disease should alert the clinician to the possibility of concomitant endocarditis because there is a strong association. About one-third of the patients with pneumococcal pneumonia have concomitant bacteremia. These patients are more often hypotensive and have a higher mortality rate than those with sterile blood cultures. *Pseudomonas aeruginosa* is most frequently isolated from patients who are leukopenic or have burn wound sepsis.

Table 31.1
Causes of Bacteremia A Typical Sample

Bacteria isolated	Percentage of patients affected
Aerobes (strict, facultative)	
Escherichi coli	32
Staphylococcus aureus	17
Klebs-enterobacter	6
Proteus species	6
Staphylococcus epidermidis	5
Streptococcus pneumoniae	5
Pseudomonas aeruginosa	5
Pseudomonas cepaciae	4
Others	10
Anaerobes (strict)	10
Polymicrobial	8%

Anaerobes account for approximately 10% of all isolates, primarily from patients with bowel disruption, gynecologic disease, or aspiration pneumonia. Although debate surrounds the relative importance of anaerobic bacteria as a cause of septic shock, it is apparent that these organisms are the major or only organism isolated in some patients. In particular, community-acquired aspiration pneumonia and gynecologic sepsis are frequently due to anaerobic organisms, whereas intra-abdominal sepsis is usually caused by a mixed aerobic-anaerobic infection. Polymicrobial bacteremia (more than one species of micro-organism in the blood) is in general an unfavorable prognostic factor, usually indicating a markedly compromised host or massive contamination, as in generalized bacterial peritonitis. However, in the ICU this finding may indicate an infected intravascular line.

PATHOGENESIS AND PATHOPHYSIOLOGY

We are continuously exposed to micro-organisms that can potentially result in life-threatening infection. This seldom occurs, due to our excellent and multifaceted host defense mechanisms—physical, humoral, and cellular. A defect in any or all of these may precipitate potentially fatal sepsis. The effect of micro-organisms and their products on the host is an area of active study.

The use of the Swan-Ganz catheter has permitted a delineation of cardiovascular events associated with sepsis. Early on, one sees a picture of relative hypovolemia characterized by hypotension and by a low systemic vascular resistance (Table 31.2). This phase appears to be mediated by vasoactive substances, such as the kinins

Table 31.2
Characteristic Features of Sepsis

Early sepsis	Late sepsis
Hyperdynamic—warm shock	Hypodynamic—cold shock
Low mortality	High mortality
↑ Cardiac output	↓ Cardiac output
↓ Peripheral resistance	↑ Peripheral resistance
↓ Pulmonary wedge pressure	↑ Pulmonary wedge pressure
↑ Pulmonary resistance	↑ ↑ Pulmonary resistance
↑ Oxygen consumption	↓ Oxygen consumption
↑ CO_2 production	↑ or ↓ CO_2 production
↓ $PaCO_2$ → respiratory alkalosis	↓ HCO_3 → metabolic acidosis

and prostaglandins. The release of these substances reflects an interaction between the host and the infecting micro-organism. Subsequently a picture of generalized, increased vascular permeability and multiple organ dysfunctions evolves. This stage of the septic process is believed to be mediated by activated complement, neutrophils, and platelets.

Throughout the course of septic shock, most patients demonstrate an enhanced cardiac index, low pulmonary wedge pressure, lowered peripheral resistance, and respiratory alkalosis (Table 31.2). Such findings, although more characteristic of Gram negative sepsis, are also seen with Gram positive organisms. Indeed, capillary flow studies utilizing xenon-^{133} clearance show clearly that enhanced tissue blood flow is a feature of septic shock. Some patients fail to demonstrate an increase of cardiac index, due either to a pre-existent heart problem or, on occasion, because of myocardial depression secondary to sepsis. It is apparent, however, that the previously held notion of arteriovenous shunting is erroneous; rather, the data suggest a defect at the cellular level, possibly mitochondrial failure with impaired ATP production (see Chapter 5).

Because alterations in blood flow do not likely account for changes in sepsis, metabolic derangements may be of some significance. The normal response to fasting is gluconeogenesis, glycogenolysis, and lipolysis mediated by insulin, glucagon, growth hormone, thyroid hormone, glucocorticoids, and catecholamines. Adaptive responses to prolonged fasting include a decrease in the breakdown of muscle protein as a source of carbohydrate intermediates for gluconeogenesis. This protective phenomenon apparently does not occur in sepsis. Protein catabolism continues, as evidenced by the disappearance of muscle mass.

These metabolic pathways are under hormonal control. Insulin is the major anabolic hormone inhibiting lypolysis, which promotes protein synthesis and glucose utilization and hence positive nitrogen balance. Antagonists include glucagon, which stimulates glycogenolysis and gluconeogenesis. Therefore, it has been suggested that alterations in insulin and glucagon play an important role in the metabolic response to septicemia. Hyperglucagonemia has been demonstrated in sepsis. The insulin-glucagon molar ratio is reversed toward the catabolic state. This presumably makes amino acids available for gluconeogenesis at the expense of protein synthesis, which may be beneficial for a short while but detrimental if prolonged. Noradrenaline and adrenaline also enhance catabolism. The increased blood level of glucagon may be secondary to increased catecholamine activity because catecholamines directly inhibit the release of insulin from the beta cell of the pancreas. Catecholamines are also lipolytic in both muscle and liver tissue. Glucocorticoids are probably also important catabolic factors, although their mechanism of action in altering gluconeogenesis is not firmly established in sepsis.

Studies have shown a marked elevation of the catabolic hormones in sepsis, along with hyperglycemia, hyperalanemia, and increased blood lactate. Interestingly, markedly increased phenylalanine levels are found in patients with severe sepsis. This amino acid is metabolized only in the liver, which suggests that subclinical liver failure may also be an important aspect of severe sepsis. Other evidence for liver dysfunction is the glucose intolerance associated with sepsis.

MANAGEMENT

Upon making a presumptive clinical diagnosis of septicemia one should establish the probable source of infection and the probable organism(s) involved. However, supportive therapy should be promptly initiated, and antibiotic treatment should not necessarily await identification of the infecting organism(s).

Laboratory Investigations (Table 31.3)

A Gram stain of any suspect material (pus from a wound, sputum if applicable, urine if the urinary tract is suspect) may give immediate tentative information about the primary source of sepsis, the most likely pathogen, and therefore the most reasonable antibiotic. Blood cultures are likewise necessary. Any patient likely to be salvagable by any therapeutic modality can tolerate withholding antibiotics long enough to obtain these cultures. Two sets of blood samples taken in the space of 1 hour is preferred. The second set will help increase the yield of positives and may, on occasion, clarify the significance of an isolate that could represent a skin contaminant.

Although leukocytosis is seen at some time in most septic patients, within the first hours the white blood cells (WBC) count may be normal or even low, particularly if the infectious organism is Gram negative. Additional hematologic tests include a platelet estimate, red cell morphology, prothrombin time, partial thromboplastin time, and assay for fibrin split products if disseminated intravascular coagulation is suspected. It is important to have an idea of the patient's renal function because most antimicrobials are excreted by the kidney and therefore may require dosage modification if azotemia is present. Further, renal function requires monitoring during therapy because it may deteriorate secondary to sepsis. Other indicated tests are serum electrolytes, serum phosphate, blood sugar, a chest x-ray, and, particularly in the elderly, an electrocardiogram. Hypophosphatemia sometimes accompanies severe sepsis. Its cause is unknown, but the effects can be severe (see Chapter 2). Initial sup-

Table 31.3
Laboratory Tests in Sepsis

Local cultures plus Gram stain examination
Blood cultures
Hb, WBC, and differential
Coagulation profile—platelet count, prothrombin time, partial thromboplastin time, fibrinogen level, fibrin monomers, and split product assays
Serum electrolytes, blood sugar, serum phosphate and calcium, serum creatinine
Blood gases—PaO_2, $PaCO_2$, HCO_3, pH, base excess or deficit
Chest x-ray, additional appropriate x-rays
Electrocardiogram

portive treatment of the hypotensive septic patient often requires aggressive fluid and electrolyte infusion (see Chapter 5).

Blood gas determinations are important to ascertain not only lung status and whether ventilatory support may be necessary but also to determine whether there is an associated pH abnormality. Hypoxemia ($\downarrow$ PaO_2 (arterial oxygen tension)) accompanies early sepsis because of ventilation/perfusion abnormalities in the lung that result in intrapulmonary shunting. Hence, the blood gas picture in early sepsis includes a low PaO_2 and a compensatory fall in $PaCO_2$ as the patient hyperventilates in response to the hypoxia. The picture also includes an early metabolic alkalosis. However, if metabolic acidosis subsequently develops, usually secondary to lactate accumulation, the prognosis is poor and justifies an attempt at correction with sodium bicarbonate.

Supportive Management

Whatever the triggering mechanism(s), it is apparent that multiple organ dysfunction (lungs, heart, liver, kidneys, CNS) is a feature of established sepsis. This provides the rationale for multisystem supportive care while attempting to deal with the underlying cause of sepsis. Volume infusion is important to the treatment of sepsis, but cardiac decompensation must be watched for, especially in the elderly or chronically ill patient. The Swan-Ganz catheter is of value to measure both capillary wedge and pulmonary artery pressure, in addition to the more commonly used measurement of central venous pressure and frequent clinical examination for evidence of cardiac decompensation. Monitoring of tissue perfusion is facilitated by frequent determinations of blood pressure and arterial lactate, as well as attention to the patient's sensorium and urine output. Electrolyte solutions, such as saline, are used in initial renal resuscitation; administration of plasma or albumin as colloid replacement may also be important. It is probably wise to maintain a relatively normal plasma oncotic pressure, because recent evidence suggests that the pulmonary edema frequently seen in septic patients correlates in part with low serum oncotic pressure and hence serum albumin. As respiratory failure is a common finding in sepsis, the question often arises as to the need for ventilatory support. Ventilatory support is recommended in the following situations: (1) to protect the airway and carry out tracheobronchial toilet; (2) to improve oxygenation if $PaO_2 < 60$ mm Hg on room air; (3) when respiratory acidosis is present, $PaCO_2 > 45$ mm Hg; (4) to apply positive end-expiratory pressure (PEEP); and (5) to decrease the effort of respiration.

Specific Management

In some clinical situations the history, physical examination, and Gram stain may strongly suggest the source of sepsis and the etiologic agent. Lobar pneumonia with hypotension in a previously well, nonhospitalized patient whose sputum contains largely Gram positive diplococci can safely be assumed to be due to *Streptococcus pneumoniae* and treated accordingly. Sepsis in the leukopenic patient is often secondary to *P. aeruginosa,* probably derived from the gut, and initial therapy should include combined tobramycin and pipercillin. Sepsis with bowel disruption is often associated with mixed aerobic-anaerobic infection; therefore initial antibiotic administration should reflect this fact. The preferred antibiotic coverage for anaerobes is either clindamycin or metronidazole.

Frequently one is faced with a patient whose source of sepsis is obscure, or alternatively, although the source may be apparent, the causative organism may be unknown. Initiation of antimicrobial therapy should not be delayed, particularly in the critically ill or compromised patient. Therefore, in most cases parenteral antibiotic treatment will need to be started before culture results or sensitivity data are available. The combination of an aminoglycoside plus a penicillinase-resistant penicillin or a cephalosporin is chosen for its broad coverage. Once the sensitivity of the causal agent is known, a less toxic, less cost, and easier to administer drug, or one with a narrower spectrum of activity, can be used. Antibiotics are given in uncomplicated cases for 7–10 days.

Antibiotics

With gentamicin or tobramycin a loading dose of 1.5–2 mg/kg can be given irrespective of renal function. The maintenance dose will require modification in the face of renal impairment. Various formulas can be used to calculate dosage; for instance in patients with stable renal insufficiency: loading dose = 1.5–2 mg/kg ideal weight; maintenance dose = 50% of loading dose every half-life ($T\frac{1}{2}$) of the antibiotic—$T\frac{1}{2}$ (hours) = 4 × serum creatinine (mg/100 ml). Maintenance dose for normal renal function is usually 1.5 mg/kg every 8 hours (q8h). Fever or burn wounds may be associated with lower serum levels and anemia with higher serum levels than predicted. Therefore an assay of serum levels should be obtained if possible. A measurement obtained 1 hour after injection should be less than 8 μg/ml, but greater than 4 μg/ml. Significant eighth-nerve toxicity is rare in patients without renal insufficiency or burn wounds; more often inadequate dosage is a problem. Tobramycin may be less nephrotoxic than gentamicin and should therefore be considered if renal insufficiency is present.

Although there is some debate over the best penicillinase-resistant penicillin, differences in the minimum inhibitory concentration for *S. aureus* of the various agents are largely offset by differences in protein binding. Therefore, one need be familiar with only one preparation for parenteral administration. The incidence of cross-hypersensitivity to cephalosporins in penicillin-allergic patients is low; nonetheless, if the patient has a history of a previous acute allergic reaction to penicillin, cephalosporins should be withheld. An alternative in this situation would be vancomycin or clindamycin.

Notwithstanding the associated GI toxicity, clindamycin seems to be an excellent drug for the treatment of suspect or proven nonneurologic anaerobic infections, with the exception of those due to clostridia where penicillin remains the drug of choice. Metronidazole (Flagyl) as an agent active against anaerobes is efficacious for bacteroides species; however, Gram positive nonsporulating anaerobes may be relatively resistant to it.

A variety of cephalosporins are available for clinical use. For infections due to *S. aureus* my preference is cephalothin, given the drug's relative resistance to cephalosporinase. Cefamandole has the advantage over cephalothin of expanded activity against the aerobic Gram negative rods. It is a useful drug to consider in the initial treatment of hospital-acquired pneumonia if *P. aeruginosa, Serratia marcesens,* and *Acinetobacter* are infrequent pathogens in your unit. Cefuroxime has a more limited Gram negative spectrum than cefamandole. However it is more active against the β-lactamase positive *H. influenzae* and can be administered less frequently. A number of new cephalosporins, active against even a wider range of aerobic Gram negative rods, including the *Pseudomonas* species, presently appear to be equivalent to the aminoglycosides in some situations.

Amphotericin-B remains the drug of choice in life-threatening fungicemias, despite its toxicity. Catheter-associated candidemia may be cured simply by removal of the catheter.

The major drugs frequently used in the treatment of sepsis in adults are listed in Table 31.4 along with their spectrum of activity, dosage, major toxicities, mode of ex-

Table 31.4
Antibiotics Commonly Used in the Treatment of Bacteremia

Antibiotic	Spectrum of activity	Dosage	Major toxicity or side effects	Excretion/ detoxication	Modification with renal impairment	Contraindications
Penicillin-G	Streptococci, penicillin sensitive staphylococci, clostridia	4×10^6 IU and up/day	Seizures with high doses	Kidney	Reduce dosage to 50% with moderate renal failure	History of allergy to penicillin
Cloxacillin	Gram positive cocci, fecal *Streptococcus* resistant	4–12 gm/day		Kidney	Reduce dosage to 50% with moderate renal failure	History of allergy to penicillin
Cephalothin	Like cloxacillin, but also limited Gram negative rod spectrum	4–12 gm/day	Phlebitis, sterile abscess if given IM. May be nephrotoxic when given with furosemide or gentamicin	Kidney and liver	May be cephalosporin of choice with impaired renal function because of greater nonrenal excretion	Use with caution if allergic to penicillin
Cefamandole	Like cephalothin but with expanded Gram negative rod spectrum	4–8 gm/day	Should be given intravenously. May be associated with hypoprothromidemia	Kidney	2–4 gm/day	Use with caution if allergic to penicillin
Cefotaxime	Inhibits most of the enterobacteriacae but not active against acinetobacter or *Pseudomonas* species. Moderately active against Gram positive organisms, except the enterococci.	4–8 gm/day	Like other cephalosporins	Kidney	2–4 gm/day	Like cephalothin
Clindamycin	Gram positive cocci, anaerobes with possible exception of *Clostridia*	600–1800 mg/day	Pseudomembranous colitis	Liver	None	History of allergy to lincomycin or clindamycin
Gentamicin or Tobramycin	Aerobic Gram negative rods, *S. aureus* and *S. albus* (limited data on efficacy)	1.5–2.0 mg/kg every 8 hrs	8th nerve damage (vestibular and/ or cochlear), may be nephrotoxic	Kidney	Yes (see text under Antibiotics)	Allergy to aminoglycosides
Pipercillin	*P. aeruginosa* (many other Gram negative rods are sensitive), streptococci and penicillin sensitive *S. aureus;* at high doses many anaerobes sensitive	3 gm every 4 hr (organisms other than *P. aeruginosa* 4–6 gm/day	Bleeding diathesis, hypokalemia	Kidney	Reduce dose to 4–5 gm/day with severe renal insufficiency ($C_{cr} < 10$ ml/min)	Allergy to penicillin

cretion or detoxication, need for dosage modifications with renal insufficiency, and contraindications.

In the final analysis, effective control of sepsis in the patient with intra-abdominal spillage of bowel content, pleural empyema, or pus accumulation anywhere must remain surgical. Indeed, persistent fever, particularly if associated with the continuing isolation of micro-organisms from the blood, should alert one to the probability of undrained pus. Many patients with intra-abdominal sepsis require more than one operation to sterilize the abdominal cavity effectively. If the patient persists in running a septic course, the possibility of suprainfection must be considered. This often arises from one of the many invasive devices used in supportive management and monitoring. In addition, abdominal ultrasound, abdominal CT scanning, and Indium white cell scanning may define a persistent focus of intra-abdominal infection. If the patient continues to deteriorate, exploratory or empirical laparatomy is strongly advised, in particular if prior abdominal surgery has been carried out.

Therapeutic Adjuncts

Additional supportive therapy includes dialysis for renal failure and continuous positive pressure ventilation for adult respiratory distress syndrome (ARDS). The use of hyperalimentation in sepsis to increase caloric intake appears justified, despite the risks and problems inherent in such therapy. Other adjuncts include the use of a β-adrenergic stimulator, such as dobutamine, for left ventricle failure and packed cell transfusion for anemia, where specifically indicated.

The role of pharmacologic doses of steroids in the treatment of septic shock has been clarified as most trials have found no benefit. The administration of naloxone has been shown to correct the hypotension of severe sepsis temporarily, presumedly through inhibition of the circulatory effect of endorphins; it does not appear, unfortunately, to alter survival. Passive immunization against endotoxin has been shown to improve the outcome with Gram negative septic shock.

Prevention is obviously the best form of treatment for sepsis. Use of the closed urinary catheter drainage system, avoidance of prolonged use of the same intravenous line, and properly cleaned respirators will all have a significant impact on reducing the incidence of hospital-acquired sepsis. Unfortunately we do not have the same control over the rest of the patient's environment.

Suggested Readings

Finley RJ: Pathophysiology of sepsis. *Ann Roy Coll Phys Surg Can* 9:133, 1974.
A good overview of the metabolic and hormonal changes associated with sepsis.

Jardin F, Sprotiche M, Bazin M, et al: Dobutamine: a hemodynamic evaluation in human septic shock. *Crit Care Med* 9:329–332, 1981.
Dobutamine appears useful when shock is complicated by myocardial failure or fluid overload.

McCabe WR, Treadwell TL, De Maria P: Pathophysiology of bacteremia. *Am J Med* 75:7–18, 1983.
A good, current overview of the pathophysiology of septicemia.

Peters WP, Friedman PA, Johnson MW, Mitch WE: The pressor effect of naloxone in septic shock. *Lancet* 1:529–532, 1981.
Naloxone, a beta-endorphin antagonist causes a transient increase in blood pressure in septic shock provided that adrenocortical function is intact.

Schumer W: Steroids in the treatment of clinical septic shock. *Ann Surg* 184:333–341, 1976.
A single dose of steroid was found to reduce immediate mortality significantly, as well as subsequent death attributable to continuing sepsis.

Spring CL, Caralis PV, Marsial EH, et al: The effects of high dose corticosteroids in patients with septic shock. *N Engl J Med* 311:1137–1143, 1984.
Although the early administration of steroids improved blood pressure and immediate mortality, overall mortality was the same as the placebo-treated group.

Ziegler EJ, McCutchan JA, Fierer J: Treatment of gram negative bacteremia and shock with anti-serum to mutant E coli. *N Engl J Med* 307:1225–1232, 1982.
Anti-serum against the common core antigens of endotoxin given at the outset of a Gram negative rod bacteremia reduced mortality significantly.

CHAPTER

32 Fulminant Hepatic Failure

Stephen M. Sullivan, M.D.

Fulminant hepatic failure (FHF) is a rare but frequently fatal disease that is defined as the development of encephalopathy within 8 weeks of the onset of symptoms in a person with previously normal liver function. It may result from viral, chemical, metabolic, or ischemic injury to the liver (Table 32.1). With expert care the survival rate has improved in recent years, but still averages only 40%. The major causes of death are cerebral edema, GI hemorrhage, sepsis, and renal failure. In a significant number of patients, only massive hepatic necrosis is found at autopsy and the exact cause of death cannot be identified.

PATHOPHYSIOLOGY (TABLE 32.2)

With severe hepatic necrosis there is loss of the synthetic and excretory functions of the liver. In addition there is secondary dysfunction of other organs, including the brain, lungs, kidneys, and pancreas.

The major clinical feature of hepatic failure is encephalopathy. The pathophysiology of the encephalopathy is unknown, but it is probably due to circulating "toxins" that are not adequately cleared from the blood by the damaged liver. These toxins are in some way related to the protein content of the diet and the bacterial flora of the colon. Many toxins have been suggested, and for a long time ammonia was the favored agent. However, the encephalopathy is not due only to ammonia because blood ammonia levels correlate poorly with the severity of coma and occasionally may even be normal. Elevated levels of short chained fatty acids, tryptophan, tyramine, and false neurotransmitters (octopamine) have also been proposed as the cause of coma. More recently, alterations in the ratio of branched chain to aromatic amino acids have been suggested but not proven to be the cause of the encephalopathy. In hepatic failure numerous neurobiochemical changes occur, and it is likely that the cause of the metabolic coma is multifactorial. There are also structural causes of coma. Cerebral edema is a frequent finding in the patient dying from FHF, and in extreme cases cerebral edema causes transtentorial herniation and compression of the brainstem. The pathogenesis of this cerebral edema is not known. Intracranial hemorrhage may also occur.

Table 32.1
Causes of Fulminant Hepatic Failure

- Viral hepatitis: hepatitis A, hepatitis B, "non A, non B" hepatitis, EB virus, herpes
- Drugs: acetaminophen, halothane, isoniazid, and rifampin are most common
- Toxins: alcohol, carbon tetrachloride, Amanita mushrooms
- Hepatic ischemia
- Acute fatty liver of pregnancy
- Wilson's disease
- Reye's syndrome

Table 32.2
Complications of Hepatic Failure

Encephalopathy	Sepsis
Cerebral edema	Pulmonary edema
Bleeding	Pancreatitis
Renal failure	

Bleeding may result from failure of synthesis of coagulation factors, reduced clearance of fibrinolysins, dysfibrinogenemia, thrombocytopenia, and platelet dysfunction. Bleeding occurs at the sites of venipuncture and occasionally results from the trauma of an endotracheal tube. Clinically significant bleeding usually occurs from gastric or duodenal erosions.

Renal failure is a common complication of FHF. The pathophysiology of this disorder is unknown, but the kidneys are morphologically normal and function normally when transplanted. The impairment of renal function may be due to circulating endotoxin or reduced production of vasodilatory PGI_2, which causes shunting of blood from the renal cortex to the renal medulla. The overall renal perfusion is reduced. As oliguria develops, the urinary osmolality increases, and the urine sodium concentration decreases. Eventually the urinary osmolality drops and approaches that of plasma, and the urinary sodium concentration then increases. If the patient survives, improvement in renal function parallels improvement in hepatic function.

Sepsis is also common. The white blood cell (WBC) count may be elevated in the absence of infection, but neutrophil function is impaired. Corticosteroids may aggravate the problem and are contraindicated. Hyperventilation and respiratory alkalosis occur early in FHF, but later ventilatory support may be needed, particularly if there is transtentorial herniation. Intrapulmonary microvascular shunts open, and ventilation/perfusion imbalance leads to hypoxia. Increased pulmonary extravascular water decreases lung compliance and occasionally causes pulmonary edema. The pulmonary edema is related to cerebral edema—not to volume overload, sepsis, renal failure, or hypoalbuminemia—and is, therefore, another form of "noncardiac" pulmonary edema (see Chapter 11). Acute pancreatitis develops in up to one-third of patients with FHF.

CLINICAL MANIFESTATIONS

Clinically FHF is characterized by jaundice, disturbances of intellect and sensorium, asterixis, and fetor hepaticus. Hyperventilation, vasodilation, tachycardia, and hypotension are common. Asterixis is not specific to hepatic failure, but may be found in all types of metabolic encephalopathy. Fetor hepaticus is a sweet musty odor due to mercaptans. If correctly identified it is pathognomonic of hepatic failure. Liver size is variable. Serial clinical measurement of liver size by the same observer is important in following the course of FHF, because a small liver is a sign of massive necrosis in viral hepatitis. Spider nevi and palmar erythema may develop within 2–3 weeks and do not necessarily signify pre-existing chronic liver disease. Mild ascites is common, but marked ascites usually only occurs in the Budd-Chiari syndrome or in alcoholic hepatitis.

Hepatic encephalopathy progresses from irritability or agitation and changes in intellect to stupor, deep coma, and finally death. The encephalopathy is graded I to IV (Table 32.3). Grade IV coma may be subdivided into A or B, depending on whether the patient responds to pain. In addition to the changes in sensorium, convulsions may occur, both hypo- and hyperreflexia may develop, and extensor plantar responses may be found. Decerebrate and decorticate posturing frequently occur. The pupillary response to light may be lost, and following transtentorial herniation brainstem reflexes are lost. Prognosis correlates with the severity of encephalopathy. EEG monitoring is the most reliable method of predicting outcome, whereas at the bedside the loss of the oculovestibular reflex means almost certain death. There is no correlation between the duration of grade IV coma, reflex changes, oculocephalic or pupillary responses, and survival.

Biochemically, FHF is characterized by increased bilirubin, elevated transaminases, and prolonged prothrombin and partial thromboplastin times. If the onset of FHF was "hyperacute," initially the bilirubin may not be very elevated. In acute viral or toxic liver injury the transaminases are usually markedly elevated; in contrast it is unusual to find a serum aspartate amino transferase (AST) greater than 300 IU/liter in acute alcoholic hepatitis. Likewise, the AST is often not very high in fulminant Wilson's disease.

Table 32.3
Grades of Hepatic Coma

I.	Restless, euphoria, confused, asterixis
II.	Drowsy, inappropriate behavior, sphincter incompetence
III.	Stuporous, but rousable
IV.	Comatose, but may respond to pain

The best biochemical indicator of the severity of liver damage is the prothrombin time. Although a marked prolongation of prothrombin time, deep jaundice, and high transaminases are ominous findings at the time of presentation, they are of little prognostic significance once the patient has reached grade IV coma.

The white count is often elevated in the absence of infection. Profound hypoglycemia may occur due to failure of gluconeogenesis. Arterial ammonia is usually elevated, but is of limited clinical or prognostic use, although it may be helpful in assessing alcoholics with coma of undetermined etiology. Inappropriate fluid and electrolyte management may lead to abnormalities in sodium and potassium concentrations. Lactic acidosis is very common and may be the result of vasodilation and maldistribution of blood flow.

DIAGNOSIS

In the deeply jaundiced patient with high transaminases and markedly prolonged prothrombin time it is not difficult to make the diagnosis of FHF. As explained above, although plasma bilirubin and transaminase concentrations may not be alarmingly abnormal, usually the prothrombin time is significantly prolonged and will not correct with vitamin K. At the bedside, the combination of altered mental state, asterixis, and fetor hepaticus is virtually diagnostic. The etiologic diagnosis is usually made on historical and clinical features. Wilson's disease, a hereditary copper storage disorder, must be considered in all young patients. The absence of the greenish-brown corneal Kayser-Fleischer ring does not exclude the diagnosis. Urine and serum copper and ceruloplasmin must be measured in all young patients presenting with recurrent episodes of hepatic necrosis or hepatic necrosis associated with hemolytic anemia.

Acetaminophen poisoning is an extremely common cause of hepatic necrosis in Britain and Europe and is likely to become a major problem in North America. Acetaminophen may be measured in the blood and toxic levels identified by reference to Figure 33.2. The recommended treatment for acetaminophen poisoning is intravenous *N*-acetylcysteine (Parvolex).

Under special circumstances a liver biopsy may be helpful in the diagnosis of acute fatty liver of pregnancy, alcohol or halothane hepatotoxicity, and the acute Budd-Chiari syndrome. Because there is a risk of hemorrhage following biopsy it should only be performed in special centers and only under circumstances when the information to be gained is worth the risk taken.

TREATMENT

Although the mortality of FHF is high, the liver has a remarkable capacity for regeneration. If the patient survives he or she is likely to regain biochemically and histologically normal liver function. In an attempt to tide the patient over the acute phases of the illness a variety of heroic measures have been tried. These have included exchange transfusion, regular hemodialysis, total body washout, liver transplantation, pig liver perfusion, human cross-circulation, charcoal hemoperfusion, and polyacrylonitrile membrane hemodialysis. The majority of these techniques have not been subjected to controlled trials and remain of doubtful value. Those that have been properly studied did not significantly improve patient survival. Corticosteroids, L-dopa, and bromocriptine are also of no proven value.

Except in research centers, FHF is managed by conservative measures (Table 32.4). The frequency of clinical, biochemical, and bacteriologic monitoring will vary with the severity and rate of progression of the hepatic failure. Frequent clinical assessment is important, and blood glucose and gases are the most important treatable biochemical parameters. Care must be taken to protect the airway and to prevent accumulation of secretions. Ventilatory support may be needed as hypoxia will lead to lactic acidosis and CO_2 retention will aggravate cerebral edema. High concentrations of oxygen and positive end-expiratory pressure (PEEP) may be needed to achieve adequate oxygenation. Strict aseptic technique must be observed in all venipunctures and IV manipulations Daily cultures of sputum, urine, and blood should be obtained. If unexplained fever develops, IV sites should be relocated and cultured, and broad spectrum antibiotics should be considered on the basis of the patient's demonstrated flora and the particular nosocomial infections of the treatment unit.

Unless convulsions occur, sedatives must never be given. Because of the risk of hemorrhage, all medications must be given by the intravenous or subcutaneous route and never by intramuscular injection. Dietary protein is restricted (in research centers, special mixtures of amino acids are administered intravenously). At the beginning of therapy the colon should be cleaned with enemas and sufficient lactulose administered by mouth or nasogastric tube to ensure two to three loose bowel movements per day. If GI hemorrhage develops, more vigorous purgation may be necessary. Oral neomycin to "sterilize" the gut must only be used with caution, as significant amounts of this "nonabsorbable" antibiotic are absorbed and may result in nephrotoxicity or ototoxicity. The absorbed neomycin may also interfere with bacterial culture while not producing a cure in the infected patient.

Hypoglycemia must be avoided at all cost, but there are theoretical reasons for avoiding extreme hyperglycemia. Blood sugar should be checked at regular intervals by finger prick and dextrose stick or, if necessary, by venipuncture. Slow infusion of 10% glucose is usually sufficient to prevent hypoglycemia. Fluid and electrolyte balance must be carefully watched. Hyponatremia is common and is handled by restriction of free water.

Peripheral vasodilation, tachycardia, and hypotension are common, but sepsis, hypovolemia, and unrecognized blood loss must be considered in all cases of unexplained hypotension. Hemodynamic monitoring with a Swan-Ganz catheter may be necessary. Cerebral autoregulation may be lost, and pressor agents may be necessary to maintain adequate cerebral perfusion.

If the airway is protected or if the patient has a normal gag reflex and is nursed correctly, nasogastric intubation is not necessary, except possibly to administer oral medication. Nasogastric intubation in a supine patient may predispose to gastroesophageal reflux and, in a ventilated patient with large tidal excursions, a nasogastric tube may traumatize the lower esophageal mucosa as the gastroesophageal junction moves during respiration. Prophylactic cimetidine, 1.2–2.4 gm IV daily, may prevent bleeding from gastric or esophageal erosions, but it may not prevent their formation. Catastrophic GI hemorrhage is managed by infusion of fresh blood, fresh frozen plasma, and platelets. Prophylactic use of fresh frozen plasma or platelets is of no benefit.

Renal function is best monitored by serum creatinine because BUN may be elevated by GI hemorrhage or decreased by markedly impaired hepatic function. If volume overload, hyperkalemia, anuria, or marked elevation in creatinine occur, peritoneal or hemodialysis will be necessary. In the presence of renal impairment, aminoglycoside antibiotics must be used with caution.

If there is clinical evidence of cerebral edema it is best managed by judicious fluid restriction and hyperventilation. Corticosteroids are ineffective, and intracranial pressure monitoring is essential if mannitol therapy is to be used. However, these measures have not been proven to be of sustained benefit.

Fulminant hepatic Wilson's disease is universally fatal, and strong arguments have been made to proceed directly to liver transplantation. The role of transplantation in other forms of FHF is still uncertain.

The prognosis of FHF is grim. However, the liver has a great regenerative capacity and because the major neurologic defects are metabolic in origin, complete neurologic recovery can be expected if the patient survives. No supportive measures should be withheld, but the struggle may be considered lost when in the absence of seda-

Table 32.4
Management and Monitoring of Fulminant Hepatic Failure

General Management of FHF
Protection of airway, chest physiotherapy, aseptic technique, no sedatives, no intramuscular injections, protein restriction—20 gm daily for grades I and II, 0 gm for grades III and IV; enemas and laxatives; maintenance of H_2O, sodium, potassium balance
Specific Management of Complications
10% glucose IV; vitamin K_1, 5 mg, IV × 3; cimetidine, 1.2–2.4 gm, IV daily; ventilate if necessary; dialyze if indicated; antibiotics—infection documented or strongly suspected; anticerebral edema measures
Monitoring the Patient
Clinical: blood pressure, heart rate, respiration, temperature, level of consciousness, urine output, pupillary response, reflexes, oculocephalic, oculovestibular responses
Hemodynamic: by Swan-Ganz catheter
Biochemical: glucose, blood gases, electrolytes, prothrombin time, partial thromboplastin time, hemoglobin, WBC and platelets, creatinine and BUN
Bacteriology culture: sputum, urine, blood, IV sites when changed
Intracranial pressure: in selected cases

tives, hypothermia, and hypoglycemia, all brainstem reflexes are lost, and the EEG has been isoelectric on two occasions over a 48-hour period.

Suggested Readings

Bihari D: Acute liver failure. *Clin Anesthesiol* 3:973–997, 1985.

Bihari D, Gimson AES, Waterson M, Williams R: Tissue hypoxia during fulminant hepatic failure. *Crit Care Med* 13:1034–1039, 1985.

Canalese J, Gimson AES, Davis M, Mellon PJ, Williams R: A controlled clinical trial of mannitol and dexamethasone for the cerebral oedema of fulminant hepatic failure. *Gut* 23:625–629, 1982.

Crossley I, Wardle N, Williams R: Biochemical mechanisms of hepatic encephalopathy. *Clin Sci* 64:247–252, 1983.

Ede R, Gimson AES, Canalese J, Williams R: Cerebral oedema and monitoring of intracranial pressure in fulminant hepatic failure. *Gastroenterology* (Japan) 17:163–176, 1982.

Gazzard BG, Portmann D, Murray-Lyon IM, Williams R: Causes of death in fulminant hepatic failure and relationship to quantitative histological assessment of parenchymal damage. *Q J Med* 176:615–626, 1975.

Hanid MA, Silk DBA, Williams R: Prognostic value of the oculovestibular reflex in fulminant hepatic failure. *Br Med J* 1:1029, 1978.

MacDougall BRD, Bailey RJ, Williams R: H_2-receptor antagonists and antacids in the prevention of acute gastrointestinal hemorrhage in fulminant hepatic failure. *Lancet* 1:617–619, 1977.

Randomized trial of steroid therapy in acute liver failure. *Gut* 20:620–623, 1979.

Ring-Larsen H, Palazzo U: Renal failure in fulminant hepatic failure and terminal cirrhosis. *Gut* 22:585–591, 1981.

Trewby PN, Warren R, Contini S, et al.: Incidence and pathophysiology of pulmonary edema in fulminant hepatic failure. *Gastroenterology* 74:859–865, 1978.

Williams R, Gimson A: An assessment of orthotopic liver transplantation in acute liver failure. *Hepatology* 4 (suppl):225–245, 1984.

CHAPTER

33 Acute Poisonings

James E. Calvin, M.D.

Self-poisoning remains a major clinical problem, with over one million drug overdoses reported annually in the United States. The most common drugs used in overdose attempts are the benzodiazepines and aspirin. Barbiturates are not as prominent as they were in the 1960s. Recently, a major change in the pattern of drug overdose has been the overdose with multiple drugs (polypharmacy), a situation that understandably makes treatment more difficult.

PATHOPHYSIOLOGY

The most common serious systemic manifestations of a drug overdose are respiratory depression and hypotension. The respiratory depression is central in origin, resulting in systemic hypoxia and respiratory acidosis secondary to CO_2 retention. Hypotension is due to depressed cardiac output from either hypovolemia secondary to vasodilation and/or vascular injury with third-space fluid loss. A decrease in systemic resistance, and hence hypotension, may occur due to α-blocking properties of drugs, direct effects of vascular smooth muscle, or central vasomotor depression. In addition, the prolonged effects of hypoxia, acidosis, and hypotension may worsen myocardial depression, as described in Chapter 5 on shock.

Drug-induced arrhythmias are caused by general metabolic disturbances associated with drug overdose, hypotension, hypoxia, acidosis, and electrolyte imbalance. Also, drug-induced arrhythmogenesis may be a direct effect of sympathomimetic effects, anticholinergic effects, or changes in central nervous system (CNS) autonomic outflow.

Pulmonary edema may occasionally complicate serious drug overdose, especially with aspirin, narcotics, and lipid-soluble hypnotics. Although fluid overload may be a factor, primary changes in pulmonary capillary permeability (i.e., adult respiratory distress syndrome (ARDS)) are the most common causes of this type of edema (see Chapter 11). There are many theories about the precise mechanism of edema formation, including direct injury to the alveolar-capillary membrane and pulmonary venospasm secondary to either local hypoxia or increased CNS sympathetic outflow.

DIAGNOSIS (TABLE 33.1)

Every patient with an acute change in the level of consciousness must be considered potentially as a case of drug overdose. Overdose is frequently a diagnosis of exclusion, especially if there is no appropriate history from friends or police, and is considered only after a careful neurologic examination has ruled out other structural or metabolic causes for the depressed level of consciousness (see Chapter 18). The initial presentation may include confusion or restlessness, with a progression to drowsiness and coma. Respiratory depression with a slow respiratory rate is often noted. Deep tendon reflexes may be absent or decreased, and muscle tone is flaccid. In some cases of barbiturate poisoning, increased muscle tone and hyperreflexia may be noted. However, such signs may be secondary to tissue anoxia. Occasionally patients with a drug overdose may present with focal neurologic signs and not the typical picture of a global metabolic encephalopathy. Transient paresis or seizures require a complete neurologic workup (see Chapter 18) to exclude structural CNS lesions; this workup frequently includes an EEG, brain scan, or even computed tomography. Bowel sounds are often depressed in severe coma from whatever cause.

Proof of drug intoxication can be obtained by an analy-

Table 33.1
Monitoring of Poisoning Cases

System	Clinical examination	Diagnostic test
Respiratory	Respiratory rate	Blood gases, chest x-ray
CNS	Pupils, arousability, reflexes, response to command and stimuli	EEG (optional)
Cardiovascular	BP, pulse rate	ECG, CVP, PCWP, and CO (where applicable)
Renal	Urine output	BUN, creatinine, electrolytes

Table 33.2
Poisons Important to Identify and their Antidotes

Poison	Antidote	Dose
Carbon monoxide	Oxygen	100%; consider hyperbaric O_2 if available
Cyanide	Hydroxocobalamin sodium nitrate	25 mg/hr IV; 300 mg (10 ml of 3% solution at a rate of 2.5–5 ml/min IV)
	Sodium thiosulfate, amyl nitrate (inhaled)	12.5 gm IV 1 ampoule q 5 min × 4
Ethylene glycol methanol	Ethanol	1 ml of 100% ethanol per kg; maintain serum ethanol of 100 mg/dl
Organophosphate	Atropine	2 mg IV; repeat prn
Digoxin	FAB fragment of digoxin; specific IgG	IV FAB = total body load of digoxin in mg × 60
Acetaminophen	Acetylcysteine	IV—150 mg/kg over 15 min; then 50 mg/kg over 4 hours; then 100 mg/kg over 16 hours

sis of blood or urine. Barbiturate and salicylate levels can be done in most hospitals. Suspicion that drug overdose is secondary to another agent may be documented by specialized toxicologic analysis as provided by regional hospitals. Sending a sample of blood to a toxicology laboratory for documentation can prove to be life saving; sometimes the police can be called upon to transport the sample. In all cases the most helpful part of the investigation is the history, which involves contacting friends, relatives, or family doctors to determine what possible medication was potentially available to the patient, as well as documenting a history of previous drug ingestion and/or emotional illness.

Because some drugs have specific antidotes they are especially important to exclude. Table 33.2 provides a list of common poisonings or overdoses for which there are specific antidotes. These antidotes and their dosages are also described.

TREATMENT (FIG. 33.1)

The initial phase of treatment is primary resuscitation and respiratory/cardiovascular support. Formerly the major cause of early death was respiratory failure and pulmonary infection from prolonged supportive treatment. Now morbidity from drug overdose is low when the principles of resuscitation are initiated immediately. The airway must be protected by intubation if necessary. If the gag reflex is not depressed, the patient may be managed with an oropharyngeal airway to prevent the glottis from obstructing the upper airway. The need for assisted ventilation will depend on the respiratory rate, minute ventilation, and arterial blood gases as outlined in Chapter 4.

Hypotension accompanying drug overdose is most frequently due to vasodilation that causes a relative state of volume depletion. Fluid challenges should be initiated to maintain a central venous pressure (CVP) (or pulmonary capillary wedge pressure (PCWP)) of 10–12 mm Hg. Higher levels of preload (e.g., PCWP) may contribute

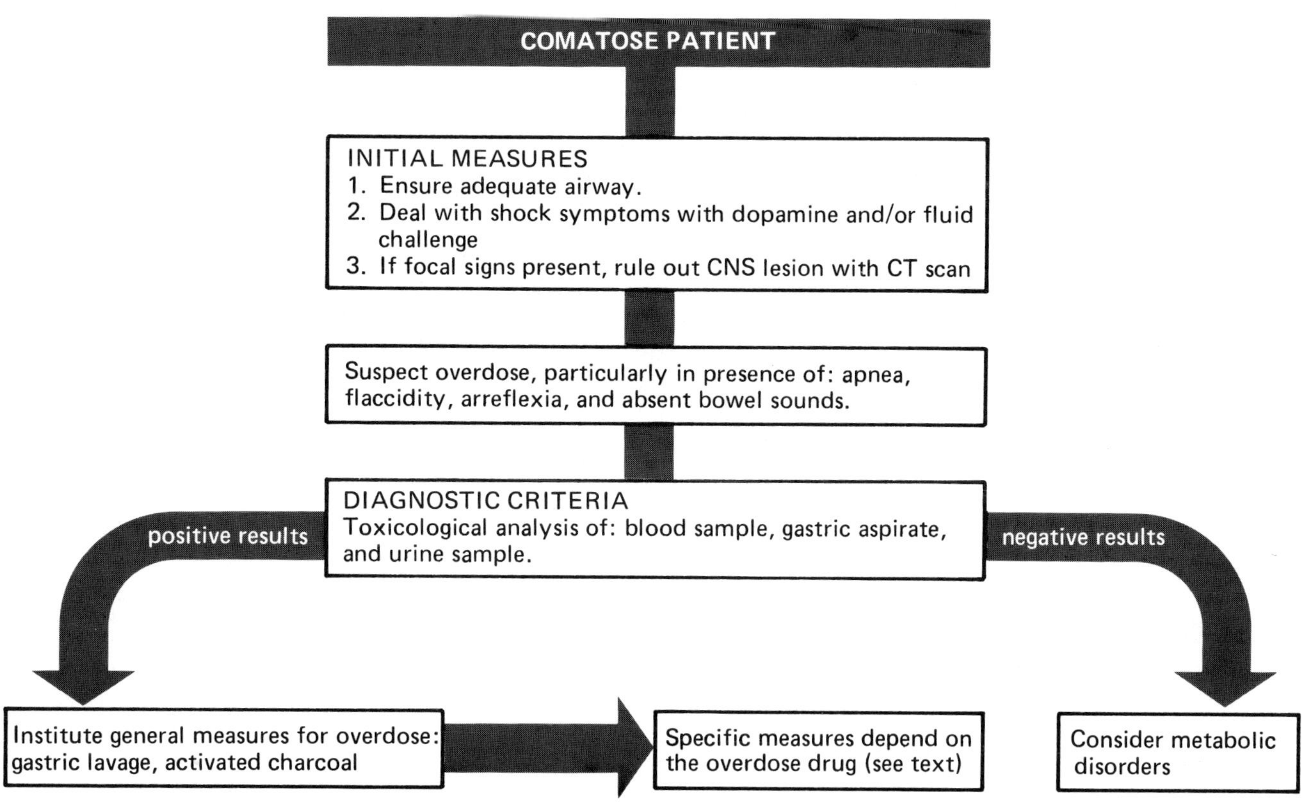

Figure 33.1. Management of the patient with a suspected overdose.

Table 33.3
Protocol for Forced Diuresis

Indications: Barbiturates, aspirin
Contraindications: Lipophilic hypnotics, tricyclic antidepressants
Method: 1st hour—IV 500 ml D5W with 50 mEq $NaHCO_2$
2nd hour—IV 500 ml D5W with 25 mEq KCl
3rd hour—IV 500 ml normal saline at 500 ml/hr
Add Lasix 20–40 mg IV to maintain urine output > 50 ml/hr

to pulmonary edema, especially with aspirin and narcotics ingestion. Inotropic drugs are instituted when fluid resuscitation does not quickly restore systemic perfusion. The inotrope of choice is dopamine, with the exception of overdose with tricylics and antipsychotic drugs when α-agonists are preferred.

Following initial resuscitation and stabilization of the cardiovascular and respiratory systems, the next priority is to enhance removal of the offending agent. The stomach must be emptied within 4 hours of ingestion of most agents, although in the case of enteric-coated tablets, remnants may still be found several hours later. In a patient who is fully conscious, syrup of ipecac may be helpful to induce emesis (10–15 ml) and can be repeated once within 15–30 minutes.

Gastric lavage is imperative if vomiting is not induced. In the unconscious patient, the airway should be protected with an endotracheal tube before a stomach tube is passed. The only contraindication to emptying the stomach is ingestion of strong corrosive agents, such as alkali, mineral acids, or petroleum distillates. In association with gastric lavage, nonspecific antidotes are administered. The most commonly used antidote is activated charcoal, an effective resin with virtually all chemicals (except cyanide), whether they be organic or inorganic, large or small compounds. It is important to give enough activated charcoal; the recommended dose is 1 gm/kg after lavage.

Enhanced drug elimination through forced diuresis, hemodialysis, and hemoperfusion is also a mainstay of treatment. Forced diuresis is used for both barbiturate and salicylic acid overdoses (Table 33.3). Significant complications include metabolic alkalosis, pulmonary edema, hypernatremia, and hypokalemia.

Hemodialysis effectively removes water-soluble drugs that are not protein bound. It can also be used to correct fluid and electrolyte disturbances. Theoretically, hemoperfusion may enhance the clearance of more lipid-soluble, protein-bound drugs with small volumes of distribution but is not frequently used except in specialized centers. It is associated with thrombocytopenia, hypocalcemia, and hypothermia and cannot correct fluid and electrolyte disturbances. Table 33.4 outlines drugs or poisons that can be removed by hemodialysis or hemoperfusion.

Table 33.4
Drugs Removable by Extracorporeal Techniques

Hemodialysis	Hemoperfusion
Barbiturates[a]	Barbiturates
Salicylates[a]	Salicylate
Methanol	Glutethimide
Ethylene glycol	Ethchlorvynol
Ethanol	Theophylline
	Tricyclics[b]
	Paraquat
	Methaqualone[b]

[a] Preferred extracorporeal method.
[b] May be of clinical benefit.

BARBITURATES

The pathophysiology of intoxication with barbiturates has been described above. The main cause of mortality is prolonged coma and its attendant sequelae, particularly hospital-acquired bronchopulmonary infection. The two principles of treatment are circulatory and ventilation stabilization as previously discussed and enhancing the rate of removal. There are two main types of barbiturates: (1) long-acting (phenobarbitones); and (2) intermediate-acting (butobarbitones). The first group are relatively little protein bound, whereas the intermediate-acting group are protein bound to a much greater extent. Serious poisoning occurs when the blood level of a long-acting barbiturate exceeds 20 mg/100 ml, or 4 mg/100 ml in the intermediate-acting group. The mortality rate of serious cases still exceeds 8%.

Measures to increase the rate of removal of barbiturates are primarily forced alkaline diuresis or dialysis. Studies have shown that the length of coma time is decreased by forced diuresis. Forced diuresis has been suggested as the treatment of choice after initial resuscitation in patients who have ingested long-acting drugs (for method, see Table 33.3). Careful attention must be paid to possible fluid overload, and therefore CVP monitoring is recommended. Hemodialysis is recommended in patients with renal failure, when barbiturate levels are greater than 20 mg/100 ml, when a demonstrable rise in serum barbiturate level occurred despite treatment, or when there is evidence of myocardial depression. Because of the relatively short coma time induced by the short-acting barbiturates, only supportive treatment and forced alkaline diuresis are recommended for their removal.

TRICYCLIC ANTIDEPRESSANTS AND ANTIPSYCHOTIC MEDICATION

These drugs include imipramine (Tofranil), amitriptyline (Elavil), doxepin (Sinequan), and chlorpromazine. Overdose may be manifested by coma, convulsions, and cardiac arrhythmias. Cardiovascular complications are more pronounced with tricyclics. Moderate overdose from both tricyclics and antipsychotics may be characterized by severe depression of consciousness, exaggerated limb reflexes, extensor plantar reflexes, gross muscle twitching, and, occasionally, fixed dilated pupils. Severe intoxication is characterized by hyperpyrexia, hypertension followed by hypotension, severe respiratory depression, cardiac arrhythmias, seizures, coma, and death. Electrocardiographic changes are common, including prolongation of the PR and QT intervals, U wave, and T wave abnormalities. Prolongation of QRS complex and atrioventricular block can occur. One recent study has demonstrated that prolongation of the QRS complex beyond 100 msec can predict patients who will develop neurologic complications and that prolongation beyond 160 msec can predict ventricular arrhythmia. Arrhythmias include atrial and nodal tachycardia, atrial fibrillation and flutter, ventricular premature beats, and ventricular tachycardia.

These drugs are rapidly absorbed, cleared from the serum, and concentrated in the fat stores of the body. Only 3% of tricyclics are excreted in the urine. Severe toxicity should be suspected when ingestion is in the range of 10–20 mg/kg. The half-life ranges from 25–81 hours.

Supportive care supplemented by gastric lavage is our current policy.The myocardial effects of tricyclics may be reduced by alkalinization to maintain the serum pH between 7.42 and 7.50. Alkalinization may also reduce the pharmacologically active free component. Management of hypotension is best accomplished through fluid infusion with close monitoring of the filling pressures, i.e., CVP, PCWP. If vasopressors are necessary, selective α-agonists may be used to offset the α-blockade of the ingestant. Patients should be monitored until they are arrhythmia-free for 24 hours. Sinus tachycardia does not need treatment unless myocardial ischemia is a problem; in that case, physostigmine may be effective. For ventricular tachyarrhythmias, Xylocaine and Dilantin are the drugs of choice. Quinidine, procainamide, and disopyramide (Norpace) should be avoided; Inderal may be used but is possibly dangerous with atrioventricular (AV) nodal conduction disturbances. Physostigmine may also be used for the treatment of supraventricular tachycardias because of its vagotonic effect. It is given by IV injection slowly over 30–60 seconds. Recommended doses are 0.5–2 mg repeated at 10- to 20-minute intervals until a maximum dose of 4 mg has been administered. Physostigmine may also reverse the mental obtundation associated with tricyclic overdose.

LIPOPHILIC HYPNOTICS

The drugs commonly seen in this category are ethchlorvynol (Placidyl), glutethimide (Doriden), methyprylon (Noludar), and methaqualone (Mequelon). These drugs are highly lipophilic or fat soluble and poorly water soluble. This binding to fat stores in the body, with subsequent slow release into the circulation, is responsible for the prolonged coma time and the poor response to dialysis. Overdose with glutethimide is characterized by profound coma that often fluctuates, fixed dilated pupils, papilledema, and periods of sudden apnea.

Forced diuresis is generally ineffective as only 20% of these drugs are excreted in the urine anyway. In fact, forced diuresis may increase pulmonary or cerebral edema. Dialysis does not reduce coma time, and its only role is in managing associated acute renal failure. Hemoperfusion does seem, however, to increase the clearance of ethchlorvynol and gluthethimide, although repeated perfusion may be necessary (Table 33.4). Because bowel sounds disappear in deep coma, it has been suggested that the unabsorbed drug may remain in the GI tract for a long time. It is therefore believed that castor oil may act as a ligand and prevent the unabsorbed drug from being absorbed. Certainly it has been shown in dogs that peak levels of ethchlorvynol can be reduced by concomitant administrations of castor oil.

A retrospective study at Victorial Hospital was done on two groups of patients who had ingested an overdose of lipophilic drugs. Both groups had been treated the same, except castor oil was added to the regime in one group. The castor oil group showed a 31% reduction in the half-life of the drug. The mainstay of lipophilic overdose treatment is supportive respiratory/cardiovascular support, with the addition of castor oil, 15 ml/kg every 12 hours (q12h).

SALICYLATE DRUG OVERDOSE

Salicylates are the most widely used medication in the world. A recent series of 73 cases showed that mortality with intoxication varies from 2–35%, with the highest mortality rate being observed in the older patient population who are taking the drug for medical problems and who become intoxicated slowly with a consequent delay in recognition.

Toxic levels result in tachypnea, respiratory alkalosis, metabolic acidosis, and hypokalemia. Pulmonary edema may also occur secondary to increased permeability of the lung microvessels (ARDS). Therapy should be aimed at fluid repletion with correction of hypokalemia and acidosis. Alkalinization of urine will enhance excretion. In severe cases, hemodialysis is effective.

STIMULANT DRUG OVERDOSE

Amphetamines, Cocaine, and Phencyclidine (PCP or Angel Dust)

The major cardiovascular effects of large doses of stimulant drugs are due to stimulation of the sympathetic nervous system: tachycardia, hypertension, arrhythmias, cardiovascular collapse, and respiratory arrest. Major causes of death include cerebral vascular accidents, arrhythmias, hyperpyrexia, and acute myocardial infarction.

The overstimulation of the sympathetic nervous system results from (1) displacement and release of stored catecholamines from nerve endings, (2) direct postsynaptic agonist activity, and (3) monoamine oxidase inhibition. Phencyclidine has been reported to have a direct vasoconstrictor effect.

Hypertension and tachycardia can be managed with α-(phentolamine) and β- (propranolol) blocking drugs. Hyperpyrexia responds to chlorpromazine. Fluid replacement is quite critical and may be large early on. Management remains supportive, with no role for hemodialysis or hemoperfusion.

ACETAMINOPHEN

The use of acetaminophen is increasing in Canada and the United States. Overdose is well known in Britain and is the main cause of fulminant hepatic failure in that country. Untreated ingestions of over 15 grams cause hepatotoxicity in 50–70% of patients, with the mortality rate from hepatotoxicity approximating 50%.

Acetaminophen is metabolized in the liver, and 90% is excreted in the kidney. In therapeutic amounts, it is metabolized to glucuronide and sulfate conjugates. At higher levels of ingestion, these enzyme systems are saturated, and a toxic alkylating intermediate, produced by "cytochrome P-450 mixed function oxidase," accumulates and causes hepatocellular necrosis.

Clinically the patients progress through three stages. The first stage, beginning within a few hours of ingestion, is characterized by anorexia, nausea, vomiting, and diaphoresis. In the second phase, about 24 hours after ingestion, these symptoms improve, but liver enzymes and the serum bilirubin increase. The third phase occurs between 3 and 5 days and is characterized by jaundice, a coagulopathy, and encephalopathy. The probability of hepatocellular injury can be predicted by half-life and serum levels. A level greater than 20 mg/100 ml at 4 hours postingestion or greater than 7.5 mg/100 ml at 12 hours (Fig. 33.2) is potentially associated with significant liver damage and should be aggressively treated.

Treatment is supportive, but if there is significant risk of hepatotoxicity as previously described, more active treatment is required. Amino acid precursors of glutathione or other sulfhydryl group donors have been used to prevent hepatotoxicity. Both cysteamine and methionine have been shown to be effective, but they have significant side effects and are not generally available. The current drug of choice is *N*-acetylcysteine (Mucomyst), which is effective if given within 10 hours of ingestion. It is given orally as a 40 mg/kg loading dose followed by 70 mg/kg every 4 hours for a total of 18 doses.

DIGOXIN

Intoxication with digoxin is a frequent cause of hospital admissions. Such side effects as yellow vision and nausea are distressing to the patient, but dangerous arrhythmias are the main concern. The therapeutic blood level for digoxin is 0.8–2.0 μg/100 ml. Treatment of ventricular irritability or tachyarrhythmias consists of intravenous KCl, Xylocaine, Inderal or Dilantin. Bradyarrhythmias or AV block is a contraindication for KCl or Inderal, and temporary ventricular pacing may be required for these disturbances.

The clearance of digoxin can be enhanced by the use of digoxin-specific antibodies. These antibodies produced by animal sera have been shown to reverse severe digoxin toxicity in animal models. Unfortunately these are not widely available yet. Hemodialysis does not enhance digoxin excretion, but may be useful for treating life-threatening hyperkalemia that is unresponsive to other treatment methods.

METHANOL

Methanol is the simplest of alcohols and is used as a solvent or antifreeze. Methanol ingestion is relatively rare. The toxic dose is quite variable; as little as 15 ml has caused blindness. Methanol is oxidized to formaldehyde and to formic acid. The rate of metabolism to the toxic metabolites is reduced by ethyl alcohol administration.

The symptoms of severe toxicity do not appear until 12–24 hours after ingestion. They consist of headache, dizziness, nausea, vomiting, severe abdominal pain, and back pain. In addition, CNS depression and respiratory failure may occur. Visual disturbance is universal and ranges from mild impairment to total blindness. Acidosis is frequent and may not be accompanied by respiratory compensation. Gastric lavage is useful in the first hour or two. Acidosis should be corrected with sodium bicarbonate. Peritoneal and hemodialysis are very effective and

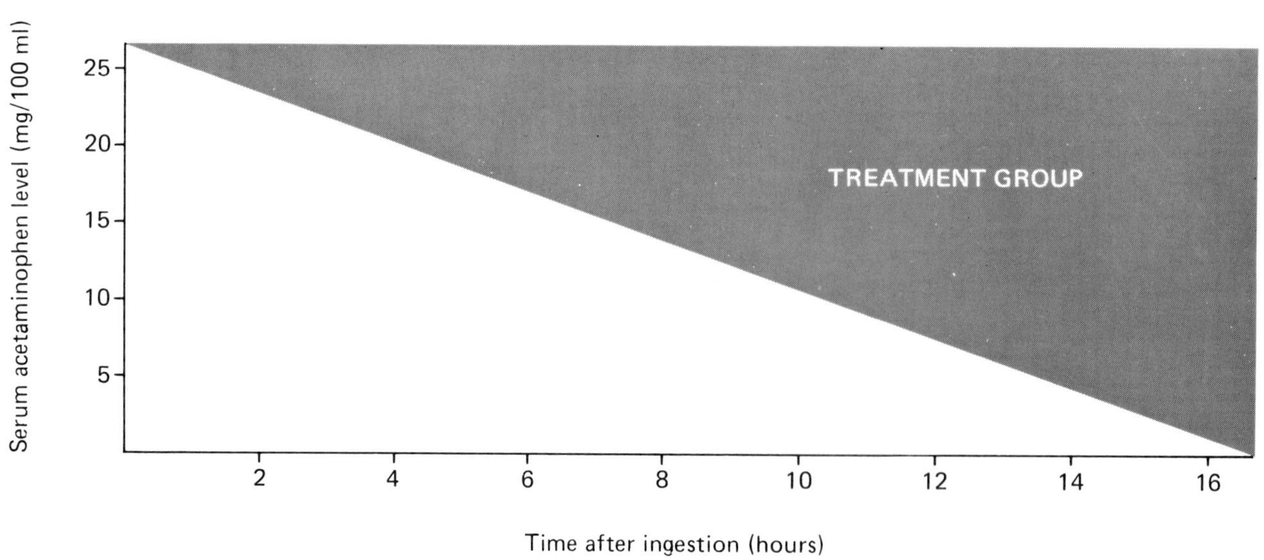

Figure 33.2. Estimation of serum acetaminophen levels.

Table 33.5
Brief Summary of the Management of Specific Drug Overdoses

Drug	Poisoning dose	Symptoms	Basic treatment
Barbiturates	Long-acting (phenobarbs): >20 mg/100 ml Intermediate-acting (butobarbs): >4 mg/100 ml	Stupor → coma, respiratory depression	Supportive measures Forced alkaline diuresis or dialysis
Tricyclic antidepressants	10–20 mg/kg body weight	Coma, convulsions, cardiac arrhythmias Moderate overdose: depression, exaggerated reflexes Severe overdose: hyperpyrexia, respiratory depression	Supportive care Drugs for tachycardia and hypotension Alkalinization
Lipophilic hypnotics	Plasma levels correlate poorly with clinical course	Deep coma, fixed dilated pupils, papilledema, sudden apnea	Supportive care Hemoperfusion for ethchlorynal and glutethimide
Acetaminophen	Hepatotoxicity: 15 gm Liver damage if 4 hours after ingestion >20 mg/100 ml, or 12 hours after ingestion >7.5 mg/100 ml	Initial reaction: anorexia, nausea vomiting, diaphoresis 24 hours after ingestion: liver enzymes and bilirubin increase 3–5 days after ingestion: jaundice, coagulopathy, encephalopathy	*N*-acetylcysteine (Mucomyst) (see Figure 33.2)
Digoxin	Serum levels >2.5 mg/ml	Yellow vision, nausea, arrhythmias	IV KCl, Xylocaine, Inderal, Dilantin Stop digoxin IV Fab
Methanol	Variable, but 15 ml can cause blindness	Headache, nausea, vomiting, abdominal and back pain, CNS depression, respiratory failure, acidosis	Gastric lavage Ethanol
Salicylates	Mild overdose >30 mg/100 ml Severe overdose >100 mg/100 ml	Tinnitus, respiratory alkalosis → metabolic acidosis. If severe, lactic acidosis due to mitochondrial dysfunction	Gastric lavage Forced alkaline diuresis If unresponsive to treatment, dialysis

can be life saving. In addition, 0.15 ml/kg ethyl alcohol q2h may inhibit the metabolism of methyl alcohol to its toxic metabolites.

For a summary of the management of specific drug overdoses, refer to Table 33.5.

Suggested Readings

Anderson RJ, Potts DE, Gabow PA et al: Unrecognized adult salicylate intoxication. *Ann Intern Med* 85:745, 1976.

Arena JM: Poisoning: treatment and prevention. *JAMA* 1975, part 1, 232:1272; part 2, 233:358; part 3, 233:900, 1975.

Benowitz N, Rosenberg J, Becker CE: Cardiopulmonary catastrophies in drug overdose patients. *Med Clin North Am* 63:267, 1981.

Boehnert MT, Lovejoy FH: Value of the QRS duration versus the serum drug level in predicting seizures and ventricular arrhythmias after an acute overdose of tricyclic antidepressants. *N Engl J Med* 313:474–479, 1985.

Corby DG, Decker WJ: Management of acute poisoning with activated charcoal. *Pediatrics* 54:324, 1974.

Crome P: Antidepressant overdosage. *Drugs* 23:431–461, 1982.

Diamond MJ, Brownstone VS, Erceg G, et al.: The reduction of coma time in lipophilic drug overdose using castor oil. *Can Anaesth Soc J* 1976, 23:170, 1976.

Ekins BR, Watanabe AS: Acute digoxin poisoning: review of therapy. *Am J Hosp Pharm* 35:268–277, 1978.

Goodman JM, Bischel MD, Wagers PW, Barbour BH: Barbiturate intoxication—morbidity and mortality. *West J Med* 124:179–186, 1976.

Hedley-White J, Burgess G, Feeley TW et al.: Management of poisoning. In Hedley-White J, et al.: *Applied Physiology of Respiratory Care*. Boston, Little, Brown and Co, 1976.

Hopewell PC, Murray JF: The adult respiratory distress syndrome. *Annu Rev Med* 27:343, 1976.

Marven GE, Lee HA: Value of forced diuresis in acute barbiturate poisoning. *Br Med J* 2:790, 1968.

Pond S, Rosenberg J, Benowitz NL, Takki S: Pharmocokinetics of haemoperfusion for drug overdose. *Clin Pharmocokin* 4:329–354, 1979.

Sitter JG, Maher JF, Schreiner GE: Barbiturate intoxication: evaluation of therapy including dialysis in a large series selectively referred because of severity. *Arch Intern Med* 117:224, 1966.

Shubin H, Weil MH: The mechanism of shock following suicidal doses of barbiturate, narcotic and tranquilizing drugs, with observations on the effects of treatment. *Am J Med* 38:853, 1965.

Thorstrand C: Cardiovascular effects of poisoning by hypnotic and tricyclic antidepressant drugs. *Acta Med Scand* 198 (suppl):583, 1975.

Walker S: Acetaminophen intoxication: mechanism and management. *Modern Med Can* 34:29, 1979.

Winchester JF, Gelfund MC, Knepshield JG et al.: Dialysis and hemoperfusion of poisoning drugs—update. *Trans Am Soc Artificial Internal Organs* 23:762, 1977.

CHAPTER 34

Management of the Bleeding Patient

John G. Kelton, M.D.

The optimal management of patients with life-threatening bleeding requires the rapid assessment of their status, prompt intervention to limit further blood loss, and institution of the appropriate replacement therapy. Often the bleeding is secondary to a local lesion, such as esophageal varices, or lacerations from trauma, and the patient does not have an underlying hemostatic defect. Other patients have an underlying hemostatic defect that must be recognized and treated appropriately.

PRINCIPLES OF HEMOSTASIS

The body's hemostatic system functions to prevent blood loss from intact vessels and to limit the amount of blood lost from transected vessels. The hemostatic system comprises three complementary components: (1) the platelets, (2) the coagulation factors, and (3) the vessels themselves. Mild-to-moderate defects in a single component usually do not lead to spontaneous bleeding, but do exacerbate trauma-induced bleeding. Relatively mild defects in two or more components of hemostasis can lead to spontaneous hemorrhage. Certain findings suggest defects in a particular hemostatic component (Table 34.1). The management of patients with bleeding disorders is presented according to the hemostatic defect responsible, and the general approach to each type of defect is described in Table 34.2.

MANAGEMENT OF THE PATIENT WITH BLEEDING CAUSED BY LOSS OF VASCULAR INTEGRITY

Loss of vascular integrity can be caused by trauma or by spontaneous vascular rupture, e.g., esophageal varices or a ruptured aneurysm. Management requires estimation of the blood loss, control of the bleeding, and blood and fluid replacement.

Management of the Patient in Shock Due to Blood Loss

Rapid Assessment of the Extent of the Blood Loss

The approximate amount of blood replacement needed by a particular patient depends upon the estimated blood

Table 34.1
History of Signs Suggestive of a Particular Hemostatic Defect

History	Potential Hemostatic Defect Contributing to Bleeding	Physical Finding
Trauma History suggestive of a ruptured aneurysm	→ BLOOD VESSELS ←	None except for massive bleeding
Anticoagulant therapy History of easy bruising—bleeding History of a bleeding disorder	→ COAGULATION FACTORS ←	Purpura Hemarthrosis Spontaneous bleeding into unusual locations (retroperitoneal hemorrhage)
Ingestion of certain drugs—(i.e. quinidine) Recent viral infection Uremia	→ PLATELETS ←	Petechiae, purpura, generalized ecchymoses
Comorbid conditions which predispose to DIC Infection Pregnancy Postsplenectomy Neoplasm	→ COMBINATION OF DEFECTS ← i.e. DIC ↑	Fever (sepsis), generalized bleeding, particularly from intravenous sites

Table 34.2
Hemostatic Defects That Cause Significant Bleeding

Defective hemostatic component	Usual cause of defect	Laboratory test useful to identify defect	Treatment
Vessel wall	Acquired (trauma)		1. Mechanical intervention to limit the blood loss 2. Replacement
Coagulation factors	Acquired or congenital	PTT, PT, TCT, plus specific factor assays if indicated	1. As above 2. As above 3. Specific factor replacement
Platelets	Acquired (consumptive)	Platelet count, bleeding time	1. As above 2. As above 3. Correct underlying cause if possible; treatment depends upon the cause
Coagulation factors and platelets	Acquired (DIC)	PTT, PT, TCT, platelet count	1. As above 2. As above 3. Treat initiating event 4. Coagulation factor and platelet replacement

loss (Table 34.3). Useful signs in assessing the extent of blood loss include (1) *an orthostatic drop in the blood pressure;* (2) *the capillary bed blood flow return time:* the nail bed capillaries are blanched by pressure and the time required for refilling is estimated (normal <2 seconds)—this physical sign becomes abnormal after an acute loss of 10–20% of blood volume; and (3) *the pulse-pressure:* the cardiac output is dependent upon venous return and the pulse pressure progressively narrows with increasing blood loss.

Measurement of the hematocrit or hemoglobin is of limited use in estimating the blood loss because of the time lag between hemorrhage and changes in these parameters.

Initiation of Treatment

The most important aspects of treatment are the control of bleeding and volume replacement.

Control of Bleeding

Bleeding from lacerated or transected vessels should initially be controlled by external pressure before more definitive treatment is instituted. Circumferential pneumatic compressive (CPC) devices are often used because they limit the blood loss through tamponade and acutely shift blood to the body core.

Volume Replacement

Adequate vascular access with at least two 16- to 18-gauge needles is important. Blood samples should be collected

Table 34.3
Assessment of the Extent of Blood Loss

Blood loss	Approximate amount of blood loss (ml)	Percent of total blood volume lost	Clinical signs	Replacement
Class I	750[a]	15	None	Crystalloid[b]
Class II	1200	20–25	1. Anxiety, tachycardia, tachypnea 2. Recumbent blood pressure may be normal, but there is usually orthostatic hypotension 3. Urine output normal	Crystalloid[b]
Class III	1500	30–35	1. Anxiety, tachycardia, tachypnea 2. Decrease in recumbent systolic blood pressure 3. Urine output decreased	Crystalloid[b] plus blood (component therapy)
Class IV	2000	40–50	1. Anxiety, tachycardia 2. Systolic blood pressure less than 100 mm Hg 3. Evidence of decreased blood flow to vital organs (confusion, oliguria)	Crystalloid[b] plus blood (component therapy)

[a] All blood loss estimates the acute losses in a 70-kg human.
[b] Replace approximately 3 ml of crystalloid/ml estimated blood loss, i.e., 2 liters for a class I hemorrhage and 3–4 liters for a class II hemorrhage.

for complete blood count (CBC), platelet count, coagulation screen (prothrombin time (PT), partial thromboplastin time (PTT), and thrombin clotting time (TCT)), glucose and electrolytes, and a sample of blood for cross-matching purposes.

If it is anticipated that large replacement volumes will be required, it is useful to insert a central line for monitoring the cardiac filling pressures.

Patients with a class 1 hemorrhage in whom bleeding is rapidly controlled can be managed with crystalloid solutions. Adequate replacement is usually considered to be three times the estimated loss, which allows crystalloid to be distributed throughout the extracellular compartment.

Class 2 hemorrhages (total blood loss estimated to be approximately 20–25% of blood volume or 1000–1500 ml) can be also managed using crystalloid solutions only. Patients with class 3 and 4 bleeding require blood replacement (see below).

Crystalloid Solutions

Infusion of iso-osmolar crystalloid solutions, such as 0.9% sodium chloride, or Ringer's lactate solution is the first line of treatment. These solutions are initially confined to the vascular compartment, but will distribute throughout all extracellular tissues. Preferences favoring Ringer's lactate or normal saline reflect personal bias and not carefully documented clinical evidence. Plasma expanders, such as dextran, should not be used because they interfere with platelet function.

Blood Replacement

Blood replacement is frequently life saving in these patients and should be administered without delay. Transfusion reactions may occur in the emergency situation and are often caused by "clerical errors" that occur when there is a break in routine procedure. The prompt administration of crystalloid solutions and the use of circumferential pneumatic compressive devices almost always allow sufficient time to be devoted to orderly patient-sample identification and processing of blood samples.

The use of "universal donor blood"—unmatched group O negative blood—is seldom justified, and there is almost always sufficient time to prepare group-specific blood. The blood group of the patient can be determined in minutes, and a "quick spin" emergency cross-match using donor cells and patient serum only requires an additional 1–2 minutes.

Choice of the Blood Component to Use

Blood is transfused to ensure adequate oxygen delivery to the tissues and can be given as fresh whole blood (not available in most centers), whole blood, or red cell concentrates (packed red cells) (Table 34.4). Some physicians favor the use of whole blood in emergency situations for two reasons: (1) it contains many coagulation factors; and (2) because it contains plasma, it is less viscous and can be infused at a faster rate than red cell concentrates. However, as shown in Table 34.4, whole blood does not contain all coagulation factors, and a dilutional coagulopathy can still occur with its use. Thus, the use of whole blood cannot be justified.

Table 34.4
Constituents of Various Blood Products

WHOLE BLOOD: 450 ml of blood plus approximately 60 ml of anticoagulant (CPD). Stored at 4 °C for 35 days. Contains erythrocytes plus coagulation factors, except very little factor VIII and decreased amounts of factor V. Whole blood does not contain viable platelets. Fresh whole blood is not available in most blood banks. Group-compatible blood is given only after a complete or "emergency" cross-match.

RED CELL CONCENTRATES: The red cells present in one unit of whole blood plus approximately 100 ml of plasma. Stored at 4 °C for 35 days. Group-compatible blood is given only after a complete or "emergency" cross-match.

FRESH FROZEN PLASMA: Approximately 200 ml of plasma separated from whole blood within 6 hours of collection. Stored for up to 12 months at −30 °C and therefore must be thawed before use (this takes 30 minutes). Contains all coagulation factors, but no viable platelets. Must be group compatible with the recipient's blood.

PLATELET CONCENTRATES: The platelets ($4–6 \times 10^{10}$) plus 50 ml of plasma separated from fresh whole blood and stored at 22 °C with constant agitation for up to 5 days. If possible, the platelets should be group specific, but ABO nonidentical platelets can be given.

CRYOPRECIPITATE: The concentrate of factor VIII and fibrinogen prepared by cold precipitation of fresh plasma. Cryoprecipitate contains approximately 80 units of factor VIII and up to 250 mg of fibrinogen in 5–10 ml of plasma. Can be stored frozen for up to 12 months and therefore must be thawed before use (this takes 10 minutes). It is preferable, but not essential, to give group-compatible cryoprecipitate blood.

A unit of whole blood or a unit of red cell concentrates has equal numbers of erythrocytes, but red cell concentrates (packed red cells) offer advantages to both the critical care physician and the blood bank. Most blood banks stock greater numbers of red cell concentrates because blood collection centers fractionate whole blood into its various components, an approach that allows the maximal utilization of a limited resource. A major disadvantage of packed cells is their slow infusion rate, but this is overcome by adding 100–200 ml of 0.9% sodium chloride to the cells and infusing them under pressure. Solutions containing calcium must never be added to a blood product because the calcium will initiate clotting. All blood should be infused through macropore (170-μm) filtration devices that should be changed after the infusion of every 4 units of red cells, or sooner if the rate of blood flow decreases.

A specific guide to replacement that is designed to avoid a dilutional coagulopathy is described in the section below.

Circumferential Pneumatic Compressive Devices

Large amounts of venous blood are present in the extremities. CPC devices may redistribute venous blood from the lower extremities and abdomen to organs above the diaphragm. These devices also increase extraluminal arterial pressure in the areas they cover, i.e., tamponade effect. The use of a CPC device in a hypovolemic patient usually results in an immediate rise in the blood pressure, which is maintained only while the garment is inflated. CPC devices only "buy time," and the actual amount of blood shifted is small.

CPC devices provide greatest benefit in the treatment of hypovolemic shock secondary to injuries below the diaphragm. A number of different devices are available, although the Military Anti-Shock Trousers (MAST suit) are most widely used. Inflation pressures of 20–25 mm Hg are usually adequate to induce the desired blood pressure response in the patient.

Congestive heart failure and pulmonary edema are contraindications to the use of the MAST suit because it could theoretically worsen these conditions. Other possible side effects include lactic acidosis secondary to decreased lower extremity perfusion, trophic skin changes, reduction in the vital capacity secondary to abdominal compression, and reduction of the glomerular filtration rate.

Only after the patient has received sufficient fluid replacement (see Table 34.3) and is no longer in shock should the CPC device be removed. The abdominal segment is slowly deflated until the patient's blood pressure decreases. If this occurs, deflation is stopped, and intravenous replacement is continued until the pressure again rises. If deflation of the abdominal cuffs does not cause a change in the blood pressure, the leg cuffs are slowly deflated while monitoring the blood pressure.

Development of a Dilutional Coagulopathy in the Massively Transfused Patient

Patients transfused with large volumes of crystalloid and red cell concentrates will develop a dilutional coagulopathy that is proportional to the severity of the initial hemorrhage and the type, volume, and rate of replacement. The blood volume is approximately 7% of the body weight, and after one blood volume replacement (5 liters in a 70-kg patient) only 25% of the original blood and coagulation factors remain in the circulation. Replacement with two blood volumes (10 liters) reduces the coagulation factors to 10%, and after three complete exchanges (15 liters), the factors are 4% of normal. A decline of all coagulation factors to 20–40% can contribute to bleeding, and therefore, factor replacement should begin during the first blood volume replacement.

The drop in the platelet count in the massively transfused patient is proportional to the number of complete exchanges that the patient has received, but is less dramatic than the drop in the coagulation factors. After two complete exchanges (10 liters), the platelet count is reduced by approximately 50%.

The rise of coagulation factors following replacement can be predicted, and one can prevent the dilutional coagulopathy. One unit of fresh frozen plasma (FFP) contains all coagulation factors and will result in a rise in each of approximately 2–5%. The maximal platelet rise per μl is approximately the number of units infused multiplied by 8,000, i.e., 8 units of platelets will result in a rise of in platelet count somewhat less than 64,000/μl. Two different approaches to blood replacement designed to avoid a dilutional coagulopathy are described below.

Approach 1. The patient is treated with red cell concentrates and crystalloid solutions (normal saline or Ringer's lactate). Colloid solutions, such as albumin, may also be used for volume expansion. After each blood volume exchange (5 liters), 6 units of plasma are given. After each two blood volume exchanges (10 liters) a further 6 units of plasma plus 5 units of platelet concentrates are given. Because plasma contains reduced amounts of factor VIII, 10 to 20 units of cryoprecipitate should be given after each two blood volume exchanges. A coagulation screen (PTT, PT, TCT) and platelet count should be performed after each blood volume exchange. This treatment should maintain coagulation factors above 20%.

Approach 2. The patient is treated with red cell concentrates and crystalloid solution (normal saline or Ringer's lactate). After each complete blood volume exchange (5 liters) the patient is given 10 units of cryoprecipitate to ensure adequate levels of factor VIII plus 6 units of plasma. After each two exchanges (10 liters), 5 units of platelet concentrates are given.

If the bleeding is relatively slow, and only one complete blood exchange is performed in 24 hours, a dilution coagulation defect will not develop, and "prophylactic" replacement is not necessary.

Fresh frozen plasma or platelet concentrates contain Rh-positive erythrocytes. If large quantities of these products are administered to an Rh-negative individual, particularly a young woman, the patient should receive Rhesus prophylaxis.

Other Adverse Effects of Massive Transfusions

Citrate Toxicity

Most blood components contain citrate to prevent clotting. Citrate binds calcium, and the infusion of citrate-containing blood products can cause hypocalcemia in the patient. However, this condition seldom is a problem unless (1) the patient is transfused at a rate of greater than 1 unit of blood every 5 minutes, (2) the patient has defective hepatic function and is unable to metabolize citrate, or (3) the patient is hypothermic or has severe hypotension. In these patients, hypocalcemia can occur with muscular and cardiac irritability and calcium supplementation is required.

Hyperkalemia

Each unit of 7-day-old red cell concentrate or whole blood contains 10–25 mEq of potassium/liter of supernatant plasma; however, hyperkalemia is rarely a problem during massive transfusion of adults, and its occurrence suggests the possibility of a transfusion reaction.

Hypothermia

The rapid infusion of blood that may be only slightly warmer than its 4 °C storage temperature can lead to hypothermia and clinical deterioration. Therefore, blood should be administered using a blood warmer, but care should be taken to ensure that the blood is not overheated because hemolysis will result.

Acid/Base Alterations

Stored blood contains up to 40 mEq/liter of acid that could exacerbate a patient's pre-existing acidosis. However, treatment with alkalinizing agents is usually not required. Freshly reconstituted blood less than 5 days old should be given to the neonate because acid/base imbalance can be a significant problem.

Altered Hemoglobin Function

The 2,3-diphosphoglycerate (2,3-DPG) content of hemoglobin declines dramatically in stored blood. This increases the affinity of hemoglobin for oxygen, which theoretically could contribute to tissue hypoxia; however, the adequacy of blood replacement is a more important determinant of oxygen delivery than its level of 2,3-DPG.

MANAGEMENT OF THE BLEEDING PATIENT WITH ISOLATED THROMBOCYTOPENIA

Platelet Function

Platelets are cytoplasmic fragments derived from the megakaryocytes of the bone marrow. Platelets contribute to hemostasis by forming the primary platelet plug and by interacting with certain components of the coagulation cascade. They adhere to the collagen exposed by breaks in the lining of vessels and bind together to form clumps (aggregation). They also provide a phospholipid surface (platelet factor III), on which many of the coagulation reactions occur.

The lower the platelet count, the more likely that the patient will develop spontaneous bleeding or have increased bleeding from transected vessels. Patients bleed excessively following trauma when the platelet count drops below 50–75,000/μl; when the platelet count is less than 10–20,000/μl, spontaneous bleeding can occur. Patients with a functional platelet defect (aspirin ingestion) have an increased risk of bleeding despite platelet counts that are only moderately decreased.

Treatment of the Thrombocytopenic Patient

Thrombocytopenic patients present with petechiae, purpura, and mucous membrane bleeding. Their bleeding time is prolonged, and laboratory studies demonstrate a low platelet count, but normal prothrombin, activated partial thromboplastin, and thrombin clotting times. Patients with severe thrombocytopenia seldom have massive bleeding, but a minor hemorrhage into a vital organ can be fatal. The usual cause of isolated thrombocytopenia is an increased rate of platelet destruction that is usually of immunologic origin. Rarely, bone marrow failure can present as isolated thrombocytopenia.

Life-threatening bleeding in a thrombocytopenic patient should be treated with high doses of intravenous IgG (1–2 gm/kg).

If the thrombocytopenia is caused by increased platelet destruction, all transfused platelets will have a shortened survival, but may have a hemostatic effect before being destroyed. The platelet count should be measured within hours of the platelet infusion for diagnostic and therapeutic reasons. Corticosteroids will usually cause the platelets to rise within several days if the patient has immune thrombocytopenia. IV IgG will raise the platelet count usually within 1 day of administration.

Some common disorders that present as isolated thrombocytopenia are described below.

Idiopathic Thrombocytopenic Purpura (ITP)

This common disorder of women is characterized by skin purpura, but otherwise the physical examination is normal. The majority of patients have a prompt rise in platelet count within 1 week of receiving 1 mg/kg of prednisone. Most patients relapse when the corticosteroids are discontinued and require splenectomy for disease control.

Drug-Induced Thrombocytopenia (DIT)

This disorder should be suspected in any patient who develops thrombocytopenia while receiving any type of medication. Treatment includes the immediate discontinuation of the offending agent and its replacement by another nonchemically related drug if indicated. Corticosteroids are administered, and severely thrombocytopenic individuals should be given platelet transfusions and intravenous IgG.

Septicemia

Bacterial septicemia is frequently associated with an isolated thrombocytopenia, which can vary from mild to profound. Control of the underlying infection leads to a rapid correction of the thrombocytopenia, and although corticosteroids are seldom indicated, prophylactic platelet transfusions may be indicated (see below).

Prophylactic Platelet Transfusions

Prophylactic platelet transfusions should be considered in patients who have septicemia or drug-induced thrombocytopenia and whose platelet count is lower than 20,000/μl because (1) these patients usually have a rapidly reversible thrombocytopenia that will not recur unless similar clinical circumstances occur, and (2) one cannot predict, particularly in the cases of patients with septicemic thrombocytopenia, that the platelet count will not continue to fall.

MANAGEMENT OF THE BLEEDING PATIENT WITH AN ISOLATED COAGULATION DEFECT

Coagulation Factors

The coagulation factors are plasma proteins, and except for fibrinogen, all are present in trace amounts (μg/ml). Von Willebrand factor is synthesized by endothelial cells, but other factors are primarily synthesized by the liver. Factors II, VII, IX, and X require postsynthetic modification by a vitamin K-dependent enzyme to become functional.

The process of coagulation involves a series of sequential enzymatic reactions that result in the conversion of soluble fibrinogen into insoluble fibrin (Fig. 34.1). Traditionally, the coagulation cascade can be considered to proceed through a "slower" intrinsic pathway or a "faster" extrinsic pathway. The intrinsic pathway is initiated by

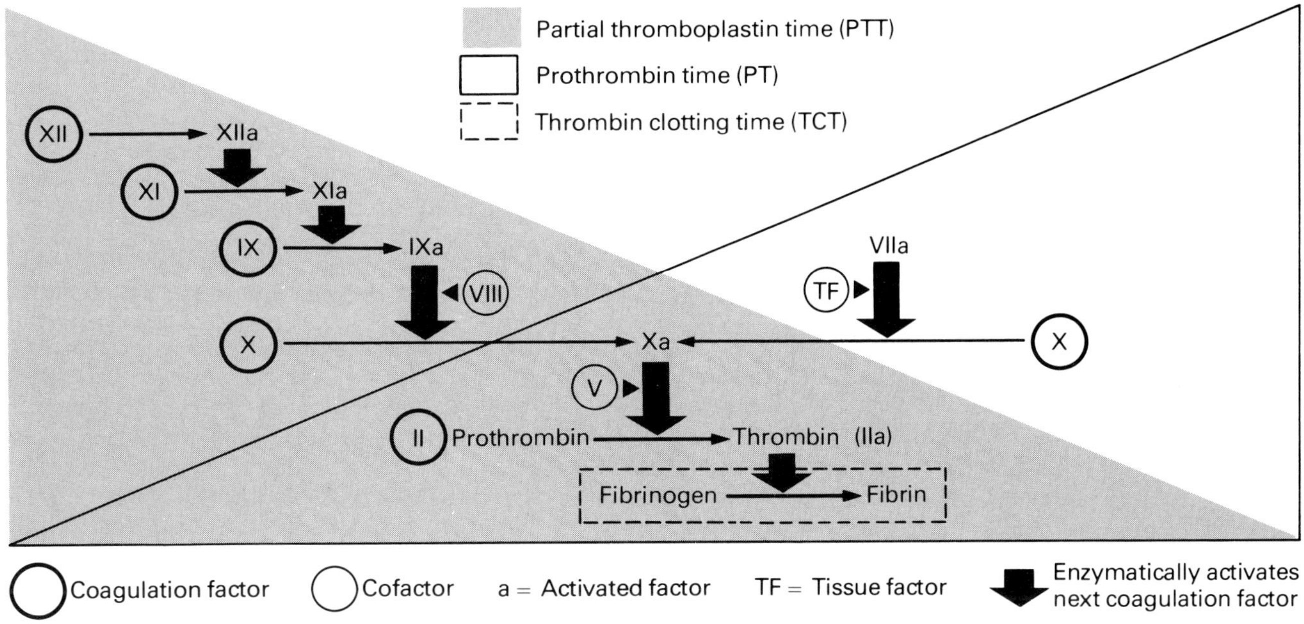

Figure 34.1. The clotting cascade.

the contact of factor XII with a nonendothelial surface, such as collagen, bacterial products, or immune complexes. Factor XII sequentially activates the other factors as shown in the figure. The integrity of the intrinsic pathway is assessed using the partial thromboplastin time (PTT). The PTT has a narrow normal range and is sensitive to a single coagulation factor deficiency of approximately 30% of normal or a global reduction of all factors to 40–50% of normal.

The extrinsic pathway is activated in vivo following tissue damage or by substances released from tumors, leukocytes, or leukemic cells. The integrity of this pathway is evaluated in vitro by the PT (Fig. 34.1). This test is sensitive to deficiencies of factor VII, V, and X and II, and fibrinogen, but the sensitivities vary among factors.

The thrombin clotting time (TCT) is prolonged if the level of fibrinogen is below 100–150 mg/dl or, depending upon the concentration of thrombin used, if there are inhibitors, such as a heparin or fibrin degradation products, in the patient's plasma.

These three tests enable one to diagnose the majority of clinically significant coagulation disorders. For example, a prolonged TCT but normal PT and PTT suggests a depletion of fibrinogen, defective fibrinogen function (dysfibrinogen), or the presence of inhibitor (heparin). Any patient receiving oral anticoagulants or with a vitamin K deficiency will have a prolonged PTT, a prolonged PT, but a normal TCT. Patients with the syndrome of disseminated intravascular coagulation (DIC) frequently have a prolongation of all three tests; however, if the PT and PTT are prolonged but the TCT is normal, DIC is unlikely. An isolated prolongation of the PTT occurs with deficiencies of factors XI, XII, IX, and VIII. Patients with hemophilia or Von Willebrand's disease (VWD) usually have a prolonged PTT.

Patients who bleed secondary to a coagulation factor deficiency may have either a congenital disorder or an acquired deficiency or defect. The common inherited disorders include Von Willebrand's disease and hemophilia A and B. The common acquired coagulation disorders include those caused by anticoagulant agents and disseminated intravascular coagulation.

Congenital Coagulation Disorders

Von Willebrand's Disease (VWD)

This is an autosomal inherited bleeding disorder that is caused by a deficiency or defect in the Von Willebrand factor, which is necessary for platelets to bind to transected vessels. The bleeding time is usually prolonged, and the PTT may or may not be prolonged.

Treatment of the bleeding patient with VWD involves correction of the deficiency of the coagulant component of factor VIII, if it is deficient in the patient. Factor VIII coagulant can usually be maintained at levels of greater than 50% in the adult by infusion of 15–20 units of cryoprecipitate once or twice daily. The deficiency of the Von Willebrand factor must also be corrected, which can be difficult because this factor cannot be directly measured. Sufficient amounts of cryoprecipitate are infused to return the bleeding time to normal. Large amounts (10–20 units) may need to be administered several times per day. The factor present in cryoprecipitate that shortens the bleeding time is not present in predictable amounts in concentrates of purified factor VIII, and these products should not be given unless cryoprecipitate is not available. One should always remember that blood products carry the risk of infection For this reason, increasing numbers of clinicians now use the synthetic vasopressin analogue DDAVP, rather than cryoprecipitate.

Women with VWD and menorrhagia are helped by oral contraceptive agents. Seldom is dilation and curettage of the uterus indicated unless there is a strong suspicion of underlying uterine pathology.

Hemophilia

Hemophilia is a sex-linked inherited coagulation disorder caused by deficient synthesis of the coagulant portion of the factor VIII molecule. The severity of hemophilia is proportional to the level of factor VIII in the plasma. The patient with no detectable factor VIII coagulant activity is usually severely affected and can bleed spontaneously into the joints, muscles, brain, or retroperitoneal space. Seldom is a patient with severe hemophilia not diagnosed at an early age; therefore, any patient first diagnosed as having severe hemophilia late in life should be investigated for an acquired inhibitor to factor VIII.

One unit of factor VIII is the amount of factor VIII in 1 ml of fresh, normal pooled plasma having 100% factor VIII activity. Ideally, 200 ml of FFP (the average volume of this product) should contain 200 units of factor VIII. However, for uncertain reasons, not all factor VIII can be recovered from the plasma. Furthermore, when the cryoprecipitate is prepared from the plasma, over 50% of the factor VIII is lost. When a bag of cryoprecipitate, which contains about 80 units, is infused into a patient with severe hemophilia (factor VIII level of 0%), the 80 units are distributed into a plasma volume of approximately 4% body weight or 2800 ml in a 70-kg human. This gives a final dilution of slightly less than 0.03 units per ml (or a level of 3% factor VIII). The actual rise in factor VIII per bag of cryoprecipitate infused into the average person is about 2%. The dose of factor VIII (in units) is usually calculated using the patient's weight: DOSE VIII (units) = body weight (kg) $\times$ 0.5 $\times$ desired rise in VIII.

The approximate amounts of factor VIII needed for certain situations are shown in Table 34.5.

Acquired Coagulation Disorders

Bleeding That Complicates Anticoagulant Therapy

Patients who are administered anticoagulant agents for the treatment or prevention of thrombosis are at particular risk for bleeding because these agents can cause bleeding if given in a sufficiently large dose.

Heparin Therapy

Increasing numbers of outpatients are receiving therapeutic doses of heparin administered by subcutaneous injection; therefore, some patients who bleed during heparin therapy are first seen in the emergency room. Bleeding can follow even minor surgical procedures, such as an arterial puncture, and these procedures should be avoided if possible.

The PTT, PT, and platelet count should be immediately assessed in any patient bleeding during heparin therapy. Therapeutic concentrations of heparin have minimal effects on the PT, and a significant prolongation of the PT suggests a concomitant vitamin K deficiency. The platelet count should be measured because heparin can cause thrombocytopenia.

If bleeding is serious, the anticoagulant effect of heparin can be reversed with protamine sulfate. Protamine sulfate is a strongly basic substance that combines with and inactivates heparin. If used within minutes of an intravenous injection of heparin injection, then a full neutralizing dose (1 mg of protamine/100 units of heparin) should be given. An occasional hypotensive response to rapid intravenous injection of protamine sulfate has been reported; therefore, it should be slowly injected over a 10–30 minutes. A bolus of 50 mg is usually sufficient to reverse the anticoagulant effect of 10,000 units of heparin administered 30 minutes previously. Because heparin clearance is rapid, only 50% of this dose of protamine sulfate needs to be given at 60 minutes after heparin in-

Table 34.5
Dose of Factor VIII Required for Hemophilia

Situation	Other management	Dose of Factor VIII
Mild to moderate hemarthrosis	1. Immobilization 2. Analgesics	10–15 units/kg, often a single dose is sufficient
Severe hemarthrosis	1. As above 2. As above 3. Ice Packs 4. Joint aspiration only if there is a very tense hemarthrosis and then only after VIII coverage	15–20 units/kg; given twice daily for several days
Muscle hematoma	1. Same as above 2. Monitor for nerve entrapment	15–20 units/kg; given twice daily for several days
Severe trauma, surgery, or cerebral hemorrhage	1. Supportive 2. Avoid extensive wound dressing and inspection	1. Raise level of VIII for 100% preoperatively or at presentation 2. Maintain level of VIII above 50% until wound healing is adequate (7–21 days)

jection and only 25% after 2 hours. Treatment with protamine sulfate may have to be repeated as protamine is cleared from the blood more quickly than heparin. The neutralizing effect is assessed by measuring the PTT or TCT immediately after a protamine injection.

After subcutaneous injection of heparin, protamine sulfate should be given in a dose equivalent to approximately 50% of the last heparin dose. This dose may have to be repeated because of delayed absorption of heparin from the subcutaneous depot.

It is possible to continue treatment at a lower dose of heparin in some patients who bleed during heparin therapy. If however, bleeding is potentially life threatening (e.g., gastrointestinal, retroperitoneal, cerebral, or into a deep abdominal wound), treatment with anticoagulants should be stopped, the effect of heparin reversed, and the thromboembolic event treated by other means, i.e., vena cava interruption.

Oral Anticoagulants

Bleeding due to oral anticoagulant therapy usually occurs at sites of recent surgery or trauma, from the gastrointestinal tract, or occasionally into the retroperitoneal space. Bleeding can also occur into unusual sites, including the adrenal gland, the ovary, the pancreas, and into the bowel wall.

Patients who bleed during therapy with oral anticoagulants but whose PT is within the therapeutic range often have a local lesion contributing to the bleeding. However, if the PT is markedly prolonged, it is usually not necessary to investigate the patient for possible underlying abnormalities. Treatment includes (1) cessation of anticoagulant therapy, (2) administration of vitamin K, (3) administration of plasma components that contain the vitamin K-dependent factors, and (4) volume replacement if indicated.

Life-threatening bleeding should be managed by infusion of prothrombin complex (II, VII, IX, and X concentrate) or, if not available, plasma. The large volume of plasma required to raise the coagulation factors to safe levels (50%) limits the usefulness of this approach.

If the PT is markedly prolonged but bleeding is not life threatening, then the anticoagulant effect can be reversed by intravenous or subcutaneous vitamin K. This treatment usually reverses the coagulation defect in 6–12 hours.

Hepatic Failure

Bleeding in patients with hepatic dysfunction can be caused by a variety of factors, including (1) decreased levels of all coagulation factors, except factor VIII, which is seldom decreased in liver failure; (2) defective coagulation factor function, such as dysfibrinogenemia; (3) excessive fibrinolytic activity; and (4) thrombocytopenia due to extrahepatic factors, such as hypersplenism. Bleeding in patients with hepatic dysfunction often originates in the gastrointestinal tract and can be due to gastric erosions or esophageal varices. Most patients who bleed as a direct or indirect consequence of hepatic dysfunction have a prolonged PTT and PT, but a normal TCT. Although fibrinogen is also made by the liver, deficient synthesis usually indicates severe acute failure or the end stage of chronic liver failure.

Management is difficult and often unsuccessful because of the global nature of the coagulation disorder. The bleeding patient should receive fresh frozen plasma and subcutaneous or intravenous vitamin K_1. Prothrombin concentrates can potentially correct the bleeding disorder, but can cause disseminated intravascular coagulation because activated factors in these preparations are not cleared by the liver.

MANAGEMENT OF THE PATIENT WHOSE BLEEDING IS CAUSED BY A COMBINATION OF HEMOSTATIC DEFECTS

A dramatic bleeding disorder characterized by thrombocytopenia plus a coagulopathy is the syndrome of disseminated intravascular coagulation (DIC). DIC is the pathophysiologic end point of a variety of initiating events that activate the coagulation cascade. Unlike physiologic thrombus formation, which is primarily extravascular, DIC is characterized by intravascular coagulation consumption and the deposition of fibrin within the microcirculation. The consumption of coagulation factors plus fibrin deposition can cause either bleeding or thrombus formation. The patient who survives the bleeding of the acute episode of DIC can die from ischemic damage to the lungs or kidneys.

There is a delicate balance between clot formation and clot lysis in the healthy individual. The same stimuli that cause the formation of the hemostatic plug also initiate the generation of the enzyme plasmin that will lyse the clot. DIC can result from (1) unopposed activation of the clotting cascade; (2) interference with the body's ability to clear activated clotting factors, a function of the reticuloendothelial system; or (3) defective fibrinolytic activity.

Most cases of DIC are caused by infection. Other causes include trauma, malignancy, surgery, and obstetrical emergencies (Fig. 34.2). The common malignancies associated with DIC are leukemia, lymphoma, and cancer of the lung, prostate, and breast.

The PTT, PT, and TCT are usually abnormal in patients with DIC, reflecting the global nature of the coagulation disturbance. In general, the more abnormal the test, the more severe the DIC. The TCT is a particularly useful test. Because fibrinogen is the final target for both the coagulation factors and plasmin, it is usually depleted in patients with DIC and the TCT is prolonged. Except under situations characterized by elevated fibrinogen levels, such as pregnancy, any patient with a normal TCT is unlikely to have clinically significant DIC.

The most important principles in the management of a patient with DIC are to correct the underlying cause and to maintain adequate tissue perfusion. If the patient is febrile, it is likely that the precipitating event is infection, and the patient should immediately be started on broad spectrum antibiotics.

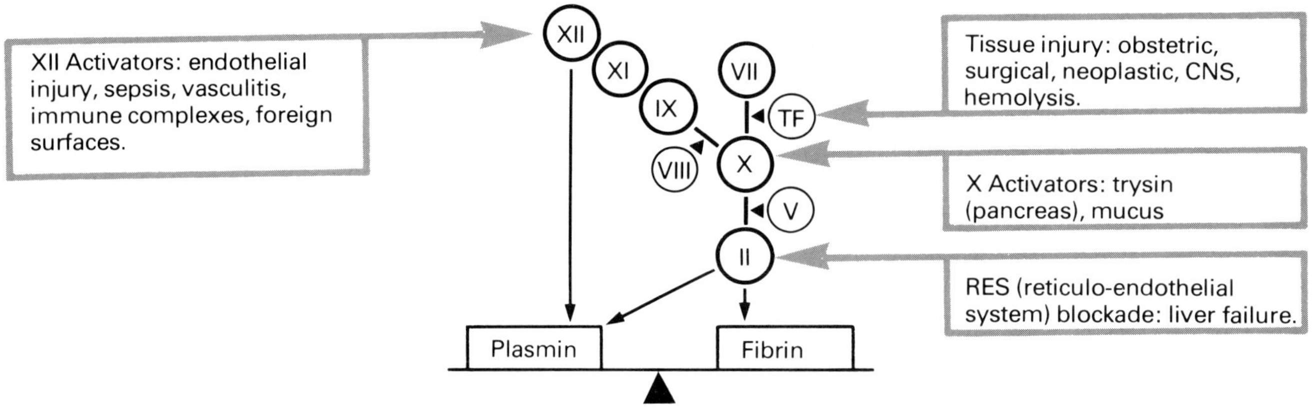

Figure 34.2. Initiation of disseminated intravascular coagulation (DIC). There normally is a balance between clot formation (fibrin deposition) and clot dissolution that is mediated by plasmin. Activation of the coagulation cascade results in the formation of fibrin, as well as plasmin. DIC can occur if there is excessive activation of the coagulation cascade. A number of entry points are illustrated in this figure. TF, tissue factor; CNS, central nervous system; and RES blockage, reticuloendothelial system blockade.

The levels of fibrinogen and factor VIII and V are often depressed in DIC, and the depleted factors should be replaced, particularly if the patient is bleeding or has a low fibrinogen level (a prolonged TCT). Replacement consists of cryoprecipitate, which contains both fibrinogen and factor VIII, and fresh-frozen plasma, which contains all the coagulation factors. Platelet transfusions may also be indicated. The replacement of the consumed coagulation factors in a patient with ongoing DIC was once considered analogous to "pouring gasoline on a fire" and was not done. However, there is no convincing evidence that DIC is worsened by factor replacement, and most clinicians now favor this approach in conjunction with adequate fluid replacement.

The use of heparin in patients with DIC is controversial. Heparin should be considered if the patient has evidence of end-organ dysfunction likely due to fibrin deposition, but it should be given only after coagulation factor replacement. A stronger case for immediate institution of full dose heparin therapy can be made for purpura fulminans, a disorder associated with certain bacterial septicemias.

Suggested Readings

Collins JA: Massive blood transfusion. *Clin Haematol* 5:201–222, 1976.

Hoffman JR: External counterpressure and the MAST suit: current and future roles. *Ann Emerg Med* 9:419–421, 1980.

Kelton G, Hirsh J: Bleeding associated with antithrombotic therapy. *Semin Hematol* 17:259–291, 1980.

CHAPTER 35

Nutritional Support of the Critically Ill Patient

Richard J. Finley, M.D.

Up to 40% of patients entering the hospital today demonstrate unequivocal signs of protein calorie malnutrition. The nutritional status and ongoing metabolic requirements of critically ill patients are small but crucial considerations in the broad spectrum of total patient care. However, failure to recognize their true importance can compound a patient's illness and lead to irreversible consequences.

DANGERS OF MALNUTRITION

The law of conservation of energy, as it applies to humans, states that any dietary calorie or protein deficit will result in consumption of structural body protein. This loss of protein, in the form of muscle or serum protein, is associated with increased morbidity and mortality in critically ill patients. In fact, patients who lose more than 30% of their total body protein have a mortality rate of 60% when they undergo an operation.

These increased complications in malnourished critically ill patients are due to two major problems: loss of skeletal muscle mass and hypoproteinemia. Wasting of the musculature involved with respiration compromises pulmonary function and results in inefficient ventilation, secretion retention, and pulmonary infection. In fact, pneumonia is the commonest cause of death in the malnourished patient. Hypoproteinemia is frequently observed in nutritionally depleted patients, but may also be seen in well-nourished individuals with sequestration of albumin at the site of extensive operative dissection, inflammation, or injury. This hypoproteinemia is associated with delayed wound healing, susceptibility to excessive salt and water retention, predisposition to hemorrhagic shock, delayed gastrointestinal transit time, poor tolerance of enteral feeds, and an impaired immune response to infection.

CAUSES OF MALNUTRITION

Malnutrition can be due to either a deficiency of the intake of protein (less than 0.7 gm/kg/day) or of calories (less than 30 calories/kg/day), or it may be due to increased consumption of protein or calories. Inadequate intake is usually due to withholding meals for diagnostic testing, a poor appetite, or a nonfunctioning gastrointestinal (GI) tract. Increased consumption of protein or calories can occur during any hypermetabolic state, such as in response to trauma, infection, burns, fever, cold ambient temperature, pain, and anxiety, and in certain endocrine disorders, such as hyperthyroidism. Every effort should be made to reverse the processes that increase protein and calorie consumption.

ASSESSMENT OF NUTRITIONAL STATUS

On admission to the hospital several objective criteria may be used to determine the nutritional status of the patient:

1. *Body weight and rate of weight loss:* A total weight loss of more than 10% or a recent rapid weight loss of up to 6% of the body weight indicates that appropriate nutritional therapy should be instituted.
2. *Anthropometric measurements:* Triceps skin-fold thickness and arm muscle circumference correlate reasonably well with body composition. Any loss of muscle mass or subcutaneous fat should be taken into account when evaluating the nutritional status of the patient.
3. *Evidence of disease:* cancer, infection, liver disease, or renal disease.
4. *Tests of immune function:* Total peripheral lymphocyte count (which can be done on a peripheral blood smear) and response to such skin tests as tuberculin or *Candida albicans* are reliable indicators of the immune competence of patients. These tests of immune function often show depressed values in malnourished patients and return to normal with nutritional repletion.
5. *Blood analysis:* Hemoglobin and red blood cell indices, serum albumin, and total protein concentration are valuable in the assessment of the nutritional status of critically ill patients. Serum albumin concentrations less than 2.8 gm/100 ml indicate severe malnourishment.

METABOLIC EFFECTS OF STARVATION

Body weight comprises water and minerals (65%), fat (25%), and protein (10%); the rest is carbohydrate stores. However, because of its anhydrous state, fat accounts for 90% of the calorie or energy stores in the body, whereas protein accounts for 9% and carbohydrates for 1% of the total body calorie stores. These carbohydrates in the form of glycogen are used for energy production in the first 24 hours of starvation. In the early stages of starvation there is an obligatory demand for glucose by the brain, red blood cells, bone marrow, and renal cortex. Carbohydrates in the form of glycogen meet these demands in the first 12 hours, after which the glucose is derived from protein breakdown. In order to preserve protein the demand for glucose diminishes as starvation progresses, so that, by the 17th day of fasting, fat accounts for more than 90% of the energy supply. The physiologic condition that produces this substrate mobilization in starvation consists of low serum insulin and high plasma glucagon concentrations. Therefore, during uncomplicated starvation, the body adapts to the loss of protein calorie intake by converting to a fat-consuming system, thus conserving the important total body protein stores.

In hypermetabolic states, such as sepsis and burns, this protein-conserving mechanism does not occur. In fact, infected patients may lose their protein stores up to six times faster than starving subjects with no complications. Therefore, it is imperative to support these patients with protein and calories at a very early stage.

INDICATIONS FOR NUTRITIONAL SUPPORT

Nutritional supplementation is indicated in the following disease states:

1. Abnormalities of the GI tract leading to subacute or chronic malnutrition: inflammatory bowel disease; GI fistula; prolonged paralytic ileus; short bowel syndrome; malabsorption syndrome; carcinoma of the pharynx, esophagus, or stomach; chronic pancreatitis; hepatic failure, GI complications from radiotherapy or chemotherapy;
2. Hypermetabolic states: burns, multiple trauma, infection, pancreatitis;
3. Those patients in whom oral feeding is hazardous: cerebral vascular accident, laryngeal incompetence, reversible coma, tetanus;
4. Severe preoperative malnutrition;
5. Anticipated protein calorie deficiency of greater than 5 days, e.g., esophagectomy or colectomy.

BASIC NUTRITIONAL REQUIREMENTS

When designing feeding solutions it is best to calculate the nutritional requirements in terms of kilograms of *ideal* body weight. The fluid, electrolyte, calorie, protein, vitamin, and trace mineral requirements needed to keep the patient in an anabolic state are described below.

Fluids

The basic fluid requirements are 30–40 ml/kg of ideal body weight/day. Additional losses from the GI tract, etc., must be tabulated on a daily basis and replaced, volume for volume. Electrolytes in these losses must also be analyzed and replaced.

Electrolyte Replacement

Sodium: 2 mEq/kg/day, plus losses or 0.5 mEq/kg/day plus losses in cardiac patients. Potassium: 1.25 mEq/kg/day plus losses. Magnesium: 0.15 mEq/kg/day.

Calorie Requirements

Basal calorie needs are 35 kcal/kg of ideal body weight/ day. The calorie requirements increase as the metabolic rate of the patient increases. Patients with intestinal fistulas require 40 kcal/kg/day. Patients with infections require 50 kcal/kg/day. Patients with severe burns require around 70 kcal/kg/day. These calories can be supplied as dextrose (3.4 kcal/gm), protein ((4 kcal/gm) and fat (9 kcal/ gm).

Protein

The protein requirements of most patients are 0.7–1 gm/ kg/day. These may increase in patients with hypermetabolic diseases, such as sepsis; these patients require up to a level of 3 gm/kg/day with a calorie:nitrogen ratio of 100:1.

Trace Elements and Vitamins

Mineral and trace element requirements are outlined in Table 35.1; Table 35.2 describes vitamin requirements.

Table 35.1
Essential Minerals and Trace Elements in Diets for the Critically Ill Patient

Sodium chloride	Administration based on usual fluid and electrolyte therapy.
Potassium	Moves into the cell with glucose and amino acids. Is retained in a ratio of 3 mEq for each 1 gm nitrogen, unless previous intracellular deficiencies existed. Inadequate administration may limit nitrogen accumulation.
Phosphorus	The importance of inorganic phosphate for synthesis of high-energy organic bonds demands an adequate supply of this ion. Deficiencies are reported with parenteral diets free of phosphorus; symptoms include weakness, malaise, anorexia, bone pain, muscle weakness, hyperventilation, and mental depression. Serum concentrations are markedly reduced, and red cell ATP and 2,3 DPG levels fall, causing shifts in the oxyhemoglobin-dissociation curve. Phosphorus may be administered as a potassium salt (KH_2PO_4), but is present in some hydrolysates and in soybean oil emulsion. Because phosphorus moves into the cell with nitrogen, this effect is dependent on the quantity of calories. The quantity of phosphate necessary is related to the calorie intake; 20 mEq potassium dihydrogen phosphate is necessary per 1000 IV calories.
Magnesium	Deficiencies observed after 3–4 weeks of deprivation in nutritionally intact individuals. Losses increase with diarrhea or fistula output. Deficiency frequently observed in alcoholic patients. Acute deficiency associated with hypocalcemia and hypokalemia, accompanied by anorexia, nausea, and vomiting.
Zinc	The body contains 1–2 gm zinc, which is an essential co-factor in a variety of enzyme systems. Increased catabolism results in the

Table 35.1 (continued)

	rapid mobilization of zinc from its intracellular stores and excretion. If zinc is omitted from the diet, particularly during repletion in adults or in the growing infant, deficiency will occur; it is characterized by diarrhea and mental depression, perioral and perinasal dermatitis, and alopecia. Intravenous infusion of 40–80 mg of zinc sulphate per day will reverse the zinc deficiency state.
Iron	The requirements for iron are well known. However, the lack of response of the bone marrow to iron during critical illness and the normal fall in blood levels that occur during infection suggest that iron should not be administered during the acute phase of most catabolic disease processes, particularly when associated with infection.
Calcium	Large calcium deposits are present in the body, and normal endocrine mechanisms should function to maintain normal serum levels. In addition, patients who remain in bed increase their urinary and fecal calcium losses, and the added effect of calcium infusion in adults must be undertaken with caution. Infusion of phosphate in large doses will lower serum calcium, and it has been suggested that calcium be induced in the nutritional mixture when phosphate is given to prevent signs of hypocalcemia. Low-dose phosphate infusion in patients with normal serum calcium levels does not cause a fall in serum calcium. Calcium is essential to the growing infant.
Copper	Deficiency state in long-term maintenance parenteral nutrition is manifested by pancytopenia and cerebellar degeneration. May accumulate with hepatic disease.
Chromium	Impaired glucose tolerance, ataxia, and peripheral neuropathy seen in deficiency state.
Manganese	Nausea and vomiting seen in deficiency state.

TYPES OF NUTRITIONAL FOODS

After calculating the nutritional requirements of the patient, one can choose from a number of enteral and intravenous fluids the solution that best suits the patient's needs.

Enteral Diets

If a patient has a functioning GI tract with no evidence of obstruction or malabsorption, then enteral feeding techniques are the most efficient and cheapest way to meet the patient's nutritional needs.

Regular Hospital Diets

Dietary composition can be altered by the dietitian to satisfy individual patient requirements. Some of the usual diets provided in the hospital include (1) mechanically soft diets for patients who have difficulty chewing; (2) bland diets from which caffeine, spices, and alcohol have been excluded to prevent irritation of the GI tract; (3) residue-restricted or residue-added diets for patients with inflammatory disease of the intestinal tract; (4) modification of carbohydrate and fat content in the diet for patients with abnormalities in lipid metabolism; (5) lactose-restricted or lactose-free diets for patients with known lactose intolerance; and (6) low-sodium or low-caloric diets.

Blended Tube Feedings

This is a cheap balanced diet of protein, fat, and carbohydrates that is ideal for a patient with complete GI function, e.g., patient in coma. It must be given into the stomach as it needs pancreatic and bile secretion for proper absorption.

Liquid Diet

Liquid diets can be given down nasogastric tubes much like blended tube feeding diets. Liquid diets available on the market are outlined in part A of Table 35.3.

Elemental Diet

These solutions comprise hydrolized fat, protein, and carbohydrate that are easily absorbed from the GI tract. This

Table 35.2
Vitamin Requirements in Normal and Critically Ill Individuals

Vitamin	Biochemical action	Signs of deficiency or toxicity	Clinical history, predisposing deficiency	Normal	Moderate injury	Severe injury
A (Retinol)	Maintains epithelial integrity and retinal pigments	Night blindness, xerosis. Toxicity usually associated with food faddism; manifested by malaise, dermatitis, peripheral edema, and yellow tint to skin	Protein deficiency, fat malabsorption	5000 IU	5000 IU	5000 IU
D	Metabolism of calcium and phosphorus	Rickets, hypocalcemia. Toxicity manifested by elevation of serum calcium and phosphorus, soft tissue calcification, and renal calculi	Malnutrition, fat malabsorption	400 IU	400 IU	400 IU

Table 35.2 (continued)

Vitamin	Biochemical action	Signs of deficiency or toxicity	Clinical history, predisposing deficiency	Normal	Moderate injury	Severe injury
E (Tocopherol)	Antioxidant preventing oxidation of polyunsaturated fatty acids	Hemolytic anemia in children, impaired red cell survival in adults	Fat malabsorption	15 IU	—	—
K (Phylloquinone)	Catalyzes prothrombin synthesis in the liver	Decreased prothrombin time	Prolonged antibiotic therapy; bile fistula, obstructive jaundice	0.4 mg	2 mg	20 mg
C (Ascorbic acid)	Maintains intracellular matrices of cartilage and bone, important in collagen synthesis	Poor wound healing, hemorrhage, infection	Malnutrition	45 mg	75 mg	300 mg
Thiamine (B_1)	Decarboxylation of alphaketo acids; requirement proportional to carbohydrate in diet	Beri-beri, decreased appetite, cardiomyopathy, neurologic symptoms	Alcoholism, sepsis, trauma	1.5 mg	2 mg	10 mg
Riboflavin (B_2)	Contributes to flavo-proteins involved in oxidative process	Cheilosis, bleeding gums, seborrheic dermatitis, magenta-colored tongue	Kwashiorkor, severe malnutrition	1.8 mg	2 mg	10 mg
Niacin	Coenzyme in carbohydate metabolism	Pellagra, dermatitis, dementia. Toxicity manifested by flushing and burning sensations	High-corn diets, diets low or lacking in tryptophan	20 mg	20 mg	20 mg
Pyroxidine (B_6)	Participates in a variety of enzyme systems associated with amino acid metabolism	Mental depression, dermatitis, increased excretion of tryptophan metabolites	Malnutrition, pyroxidase antagonists (isoniazid used in treatment of tuberculosis)	2 mg	2 mg	40 mg
Pantothenic acid	Converted to coenzyme A, which participates in biologic acetylation reactions	Decreased antibody production in humans, fatigue, nausea	Severe malnutrition	5–10 mg	18 mg	40 mg
Folic acid	DNA synthesis, transfer of one-carbon units	Megaloblastic anemia	Malnutrition, malabsorption, folic acid antagonist	0.4 mg	1.5 mg	2.5 mg
Vitamin B_{12}	Maintains normal folic acid metabolism, myelin synthesis, reducing agent; participates in metabolism of fat, carbohydrate, and protein	Pernicious anemia, neurologic symptoms	Malnutrition malabsorption, ileal resection; HCl and intrinsic factor also necessary for absorption	3 mcg	2 mcg	4 mcg

Table 35.3
Nutritional Content of Liquid, Elementary, and Supplementary Diets

	Volume *(ml)*	Calories *(kcal)*	Carbo-hydrate *(gm)*	Fat *(gm)*	Protein or protein equivalent *(gm, source)*	Nitrogen: calorie ratio	Osmo-lality *(mOsm)*	Na *(mEq)*	K *(mEq)*
				LIQUID DIETS					
Complete B	1000	1000	120	40	40	1:156	517	60	37
Ensure	944	1000	137	35	35	1:179	460[d]	30	31
Nutri-1000	944	1000	100	52	32	1:195	400	22	36
Isocal	960	1000	125[b]	42	32	1:192	350	22	32
				ELEMENTAL DIETS					
Vivonex	1000	1000	226	0.1	20 (amino acids)	1:306	500[c]	37	30
Vivonex HN	1000	1000	210	0.4	42 (amino acids)	1:150	844	34	18
Flexical	1000	1000	154	34.0	22 (casein hydrolysate)	1:286	724	15	38
Precision LR[a]	926	1000	226	0.7	22 (egg albumin)	1:283	600	27	20
Precision HN[a]	1000	1000	207	0.5	42 (egg albumin)	1:150	580	41	22
				DIETARY SUPPLEMENTS					
Meritene powder with 8 oz whole milk	240	275	31	9	18	1:95	690	11	20
Meritene liquid	240	240	28	8	14	1:107	560[c]	10	10
Sustacal vanilla powder with 8 oz whole milk	240	318	43	8	19	1:106	—	12	21
Sustacal liquid	240	240	33	5	14	1:104	756	10	13
Sustagen powder in water	240	390	66	4	24	1:104	1170	11	20
Nutramigen	240	160	20	6	6	1:167	—	3	4
Carnation Instant Breakfast	240	267	33	8	14	1:116	—	11	18

[a] Similar to defined formula diets but contains egg albumin as protein source.
[b] Lactose free.
[c] Increases with flavoring.
[d] More concentrated formula provided in Ensure.

type of diet does not require pancreatic and biliary secretion for its absorption so it may be given into the jejunum. It is low in residue and is ideal for the short gut syndrome, low GI fistulas, and inflammatory bowel disease, and as a bowel preparation for colonic surgery. The available low residue diets are outlined in part B of Table 35.3.

Dietary Supplements

Studies of critically ill hypermetabolic patients demonstrate that food intake from meals is approximately 15% less than before the injury, although energy requirements may be twice as great. If the patient is able to eat, the hospital diet can be supplemented by interval liquid feedings. Available dietary supplements are outlined in part C of Table 35.3.

Intravenous Alimentation

If a patient is unable to take enough nutrients by the GI tract, then calories and/or protein must be given intravenously.

Glucose Alone

The daily infusion of 2000 ml of 5% dextrose in water (D5W) will reduce the glucose demand of a starving patient by 50% and thus decrease the muscle protein breakdown by 50%. This is called the protein-sparing effect of glucose. Glucose is the most readily utilized caloric source, and there are no known toxic side effects to its infusion. A solution of D5W is an ideal nutritional regimen for a patient who will be able to take proteins and calories by mouth in less than 5 days. When using concentrations of glucose greater than 10%, it must be given through central veins to avoid the problems with venous thrombosis and phlebitis.

Amino Acids Alone

Nonobese Patients

Infusion of 3% amino acids into postoperative patients has been shown to conserve total body protein better than 5% glucose solutions. This system is expensive and has not been shown to be superior to 5% glucose in routine postoperative patients, however.

Obese Patients

Infusion of amino acids (0.7 gm/kg/day) into fasting obese patients spares protein, yet allows the burning of fat for energy needs. This system is ideal in fat patients who want to lose fat but keep protein mass. Amino acids alone may be given through a peripheral vein because the amino acid solution is iso-osmolar. Essential amino acids are those amino acids that the body cannot synthesize and that must be provided in the diet. Isoleucine, leucine, lysine, methionine, phenylalanine, threonine, tryptophan, and valine are essential amino acids. Nonessential amino acids are those that the body can synthesize from dietary proteins in other nitrogenous food stuffs. The nonessential amino acids include alanine, arginine, cysteine, glutamate, glycine, histidine, proline, serine, and tyrosine. The optimal mixture of amino acids is 45% essential amino acids, 55% nonessential amino acids.

For optimal utilization it is important that all the essential amino acids be given simultaneously and that they be combined with a nonprotein energy source, such as carbohydrate or fat. The optimal pattern for nonessential amino acids is not yet known, but excess ingestion of any single amino acid may create toxicity. The optimal utilization of amino acid mixtures occurs when the ratio of total nonprotein calories to grams of nitrogen is between 150:1 and 200:1 in noncatabolic patients and approximately 100:1 to 80:1 in hypercatabolic septic patients. One gram of nitrogen is equivalent to 6.25 gm of protein. Also required for optimal utilization of intravenous amino acids is simultaneous administration of electrolytes, vitamins, and trace elements. In the past, the amino acids were given in the form of protein hydrolysate, but this has now been replaced by pure synthetic amino acid mixtures. These mixtures are advantageous because they contain all the L-isomer amino acids, they contain no peptides, and are associated with a decreased incidence of sensitivity reactions. The pure amino acid solutions are also preferred because the risk of sepsis is less. Physical activity improves the retention of amino acid nitrogen better than increasing the supply of protein and calories.

Amino Acids Plus Nonprotein Calories

In any state in which protein anabolism is desired, the use of amino acids plus nonprotein calories is mandatory. Therefore, the infusion of 1000 ml of 5% amino acids (0.7 gm/kg/day) when combined with at least 40 kcal/kg/day results in weight gain (0.5 kg/day) and retention of nitrogen as protein. The nonprotein calories can be supplied by hypertonic 25% glucose and lipid. Hypertonic 25% glucose (1500 ml of 50% glucose daily will give 3000 calories or about 45 nonprotein calories/kg/day) is hyperosmolar (1200 mOsm/liters) and must be given into a central vein through a subclavian catheter. In order to avoid fatty acid deficiencies with this regimen, 500 ml of 10% lipid must be given three times weekly. Fat emulsions (10% and 20% lipid) are desirable in parenteral nutrition because they are concentrated sources of calories (kcal/gm), they supply essential fatty acids in the form of linoleic acid, they are isotonic and may be given peripherally, and they are a valuable source of phosphate. Lipids should not be given to patients with type 1 or type 5 hyperlipoproteinemias. They are contraindicated in all patients with pancreatitis until serum triglyceride levels are known. The daily infusion of 1500 ml of 10% lipid and 1000 ml of 12.5% glucose provides about 2500 nonprotein calories/day. Although more expensive than glucose, this solution may be given through a peripheral IV because it is iso-osmolar with blood. It is the solution of choice for short-term alimentation or for patients with diabetes mellitus.

INSERTION OF CENTRAL VENOUS FEEDING CATHETERS

Extensive experience has shown that infusion of hypertonic nutrient solutions can be accomplished via indwelling polyvinyl, Silastic, or Teflon catheters directed into the superior vena cava following percutaneous or cut-down insertion into the external or internal jugular vein or the cephalic, basilic, or saphenous vein. However, infraclavicular percutaneous subclavian vein puncture is the safest and most effective technique for long-term catheterization of the superior vena cava in adults and in infants weighing more than 10 pounds. Either subclavian vein may be used safely for this technique, unless a specific contraindication exists, such as the presence of ipsilateral giant emphysematous bullae, other apical disease, previous radical neck dissection, clavicular fracture, or radical mastectomy. Despite the theoretical possibility of thoracic duct injury, especially on the left side, this complication has rarely been observed. It is the responsibility of the physician to be thoroughly familiar with the anatomy of the lower neck and upper chest region both in the operating room and at the autopsy table.

Before attempting percutaneous central venous catheterization, it is essential to position the patient head down at 15° (Trendelenburg position) to allow hydrostatic dilation of the subclavian vein. Doing so provides a larger target for the needle and increases central venous pressure, thus minimizing the risk of air embolization during the procedure. To gain the easiest access to the subclavian vein the patient's shoulders should be hyperextended over a rolled sheet that is placed longitudinally between the scapulae under the thoracic spine. With the hyperextended shoulders depressed caudally and the head turned to the opposite side, the subclavian vein becomes most accessible for percutaneous catheterization. However, after successful puncture of the vein has been accomplished, it is often helpful to have the patient rotate the head back to the neutral position in order to reduce the chances of the catheter passing up into the jugular vein.

The skin over the neck, shoulder, and upper chest should be carefully shaved; cleansed with ether, acetone, or some other organic solvent to remove skin oil; and then prepared with either a 2% tincture of iodine or thimerosal or povidone-iodine in a manner identical to preoperative skin preparation. Using strict aseptic techniques with sterile gloves and instruments, the operator drapes the area with three or four sterile towels and infiltrates a local anesthetic agent (1% lidocaine or procaine) into the skin, subcutaneous tissue, and periosteum at the inferior border of the midpoint of the clavicle. Five to ten minutes later, a 2-inch, 14-gauge needle is attached to a 2- or 3-ml syringe that is inserted, bevel down, through the skin wheal. It is advanced beneath the inferior margin of the clavicle in a horizontal (coronal) plane, with the needle tip aimed at the anterior margin of the trachea at the level of the suprasternal notch (Fig. 35.1A). With the needle and syringe parallel to the surface of the patient's bed and adjacent to the anterior deltoid prominence, the needle should enter the anterior wall of the subclavian vein in the direction of its long axis. As the needle is advanced beneath the clavicle, a slight negative pressure achieved by withdrawing the syringe piston 1 cm will indicate the accuracy of the venipuncture by a flashback of blood. The needle should always be advanced a few millimeters beyond the point at which the blood first appears in the syringe to ensure the placement of the entire beveled tip of the needle inside the vein. The patient is asked to perform a Valsalva maneuver or to hold his or her breath in full inspiration to minimize the risk of inadvertent air embolism. The syringe is then removed carefully while the needle is held firmly in place with a hemostat. If the patient is unable to cooperate at this step in the procedure, pressure can be placed on the abdomen by an assistant in order to prevent the patient from inspiring while the centrally placed needle is open to atmospheric pressure.

A 16-gauge, 8-inch radiopaque catheter is introduced immediately through the needle and threaded its full length into the venous system (Fig. 35.1B). The catheter should advance easily if the needle tip is entirely within the lumen of the vein and if the original direction of the needle has been maintained. If any difficulty is encountered during the advancement of the catheter through the needle, the needle and catheter must be withdrawn carefully as a unit and another attempt at venipuncture made. The catheter must never be withdrawn through the needle after having been passed beyond the tip of the needle because transection and embolization of the catheter can result.

When the catheter has been advanced its full length, it is attached to the solution container by sterile intravenous administration tubing and immediately flushed with isotonic fluid to minimize intraluminal clotting. At this point, the needle is withdrawn, and the catheter is secured by a 3-0 silk suture placed lateral to the skin puncture site. The solution bottle or bag is momentarily lowered below bed level to ensure free back flow; it is then raised rapidly several feet above the patient's head to ensure free forward flow, an indication that the catheter tip is properly placed within the central vein.

A broad spectrum antimicrobial ointment or povidone-iodine antiseptic ointment is applied to the puncture site (Fig. 35.1C), and covered with polyurethane dressing. To prevent accidental disengagement of the administration tubing from the catheter hub and possible subsequent air embolism, the tubing-catheter connection is carefully reinforced with adhesive tape (Fig. 35.1D). The administration tubing is looped and secured again with tape to the dressing or skin to guard against accidental traction on the catheter (Fig. 35.1D).

Before infusion of the hypertonic nutrient solution is started, an anteroposterior chest x-ray must be obtained to verify the position of the catheter tip in the midportion of the superior vena cava. Failure to verify the location of the catheter tip in the superior vena cava has resulted in unjustifiable venous thrombosis. When the catheter is found to be malpositioned it must be removed and a new catheter inserted. Manipulation of a catheter back and forth to achieve a more favorable position is condemned.

The same basic techniques can be used with commercially available 6-inch internal needle and external catheter combinations. The longer needle in this apparatus may be helpful in reaching the subclavian vein in large-framed or obese individuals. However, the longer needle is more difficult to control, can inadvertently reach a greater number of vital structures, and can present significant difficulties when attempts are made to advance the catheter over it. It is advisable to make a small skin incision before inserting such needles in order to minimize the friction of the skin on the external wall of the catheter as it is advanced.

Indwelling parenteral feeding catheters may also be placed percutaneously into the superior vena cava via an external or internal jugular vein, or by the supraclavicular approach to the subclavian vein. Because of the mobility of the neck and proximity of hair-growing areas, these puncture sites are less comfortable to the patient and are more difficult to keep sterile than is the infraclavicular access to the subclavian vein.

In infants weighing less than 10 pounds, the small subclavian vein and high apex of the lung can make percutaneous subclavian puncture difficult and very dangerous. Long-term intravenous catheterization in such patients is achieved more safely by inserting the catheter via an external or internal jugular vein cut-down, using a 1-cm incision either at the base of the neck or at the angle of the jaw (Fig. 35.2). Advancement of the catheter tip into the superior vena cava through the venotomy can be facilitated by gentle traction on the vein, thereby straightening out many of the angulations along the course of the vein. After proper placement of its tip into the superior vena cava, the catheter is secured to the vein

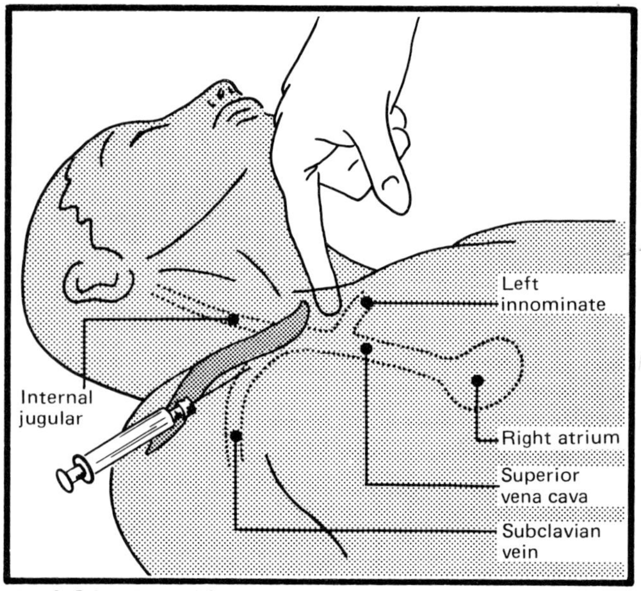

A. A 2 in. long 14 gauge needle is inserted at the inferior border of the middle of the clavicle and directed towards a fingertip which is pressed firmly into suprasternal notch.

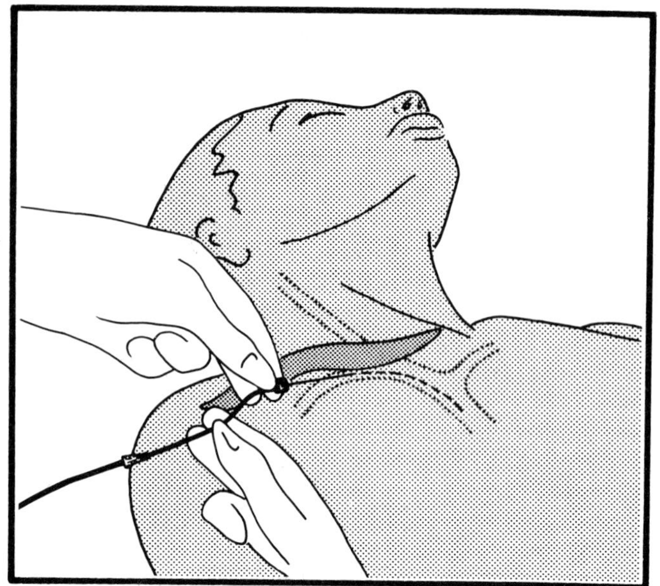

B. With the bevel of the needle directed caudally in the direction of venous flow, the 16 gauge catheter is advanced into the superior vena cava.

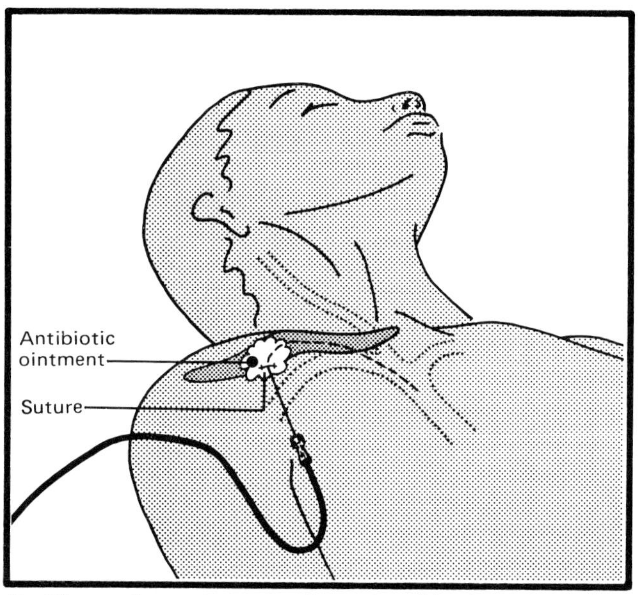

C. The catheter is sutured to the skin lateral to the puncture site to prevent motion in either direction, and antimicrobial ointment is applied to maintain antisepsis.

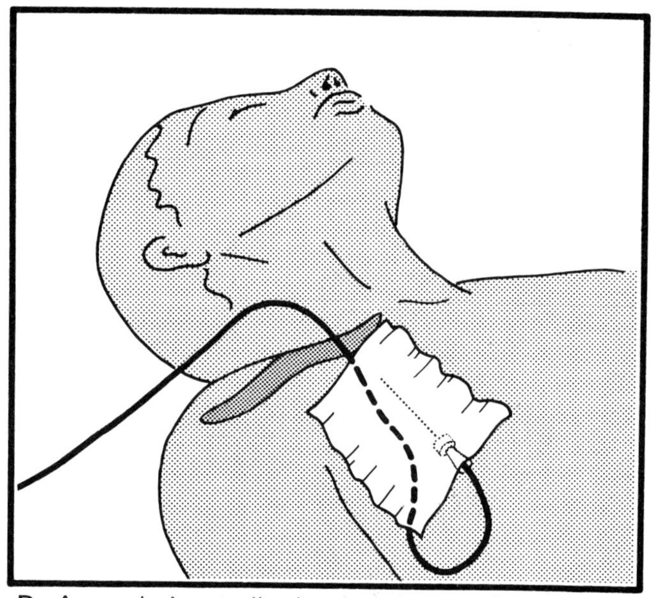

D. An occlusive sterile dressing protects the catheterization site and secures the infusion tubing without interfering with neck or shoulder motion.

Figure 35.1. Percutaneous insertion of the subclavian catheter.

by two or three sutures, and the proximal end is brought out through a subcutaneous tunnel in the postauricular area to a tiny stab wound in the parietal scalp. The skin exit site is thus removed to a point distant from the phlebotomy site, thereby reducing the risk of infection and mechanical kinking and facilitating aseptic catheter maintenance. The neck wound is closed, and the catheter is sutured at the scalp exit site with 4-0 silk. An antiseptic ointment is applied, and the scalp is dressed in a manner similar to that used in the infraclavicular subclavian catheterization technique.

To achieve safe, long-term central venous catheterization, meticulous and compulsive care and maintenance of the catheter are just as important as proper insertion. Every 2 or 3 days, the dressing over the puncture site should be removed and the administration tubing changed. Using aseptic techniques and sterile gloves, the nurse or physician again removes oil from the skin around the exit site with acetone, ether, or an organic solvent and prepares the skin with tincture of iodine or thimerosal or povidone-iodine. Antiseptic ointment is again applied around the catheter, and the sterile occlusive dressing is

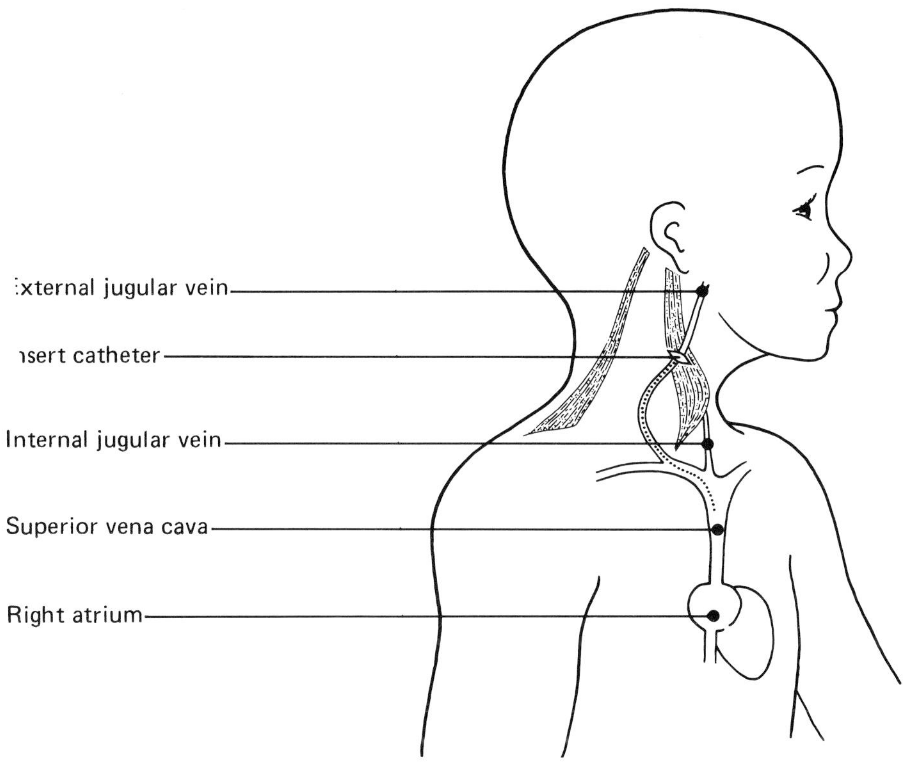

Figure 35.2. Insertion of the jugular catheter in children. The fine catheter is inserted via a cut-down in the neck into the external jugular vein, as illustrated, or into the internal jugular vein directly or via a common facial branch.

replaced. Administration or withdrawal of blood through the nutrient catheter should be avoided, because these practices significantly increase the possibility of contamination or clotting of the catheter. Neither antibiotics nor steroids are added routinely to the nutrient solutions, but these or other medications may be administered through a Y-tubing attached to the central venous catheter, if indicated or desired. The use of multilumen catheters is advocated because drug administration, as well as measurement of central venous pressure, may be carried out safely without contamination of the nutrient solutions.

COMPLICATIONS OF ALIMENTATION

Enteral

Aspiration

In order to avoid aspiration of tube feedings in critically ill patients the following precautions should be taken: (1) color tube feedings so that aspiration can be recognized; (2) use a small no. 8 feeding tube and check the position by x-ray before starting tube feedings; (3) feed with the head up; (4) use continuous feedings; and (5) avoid nighttime feedings.

Dehydration and Hyperosmolarity

It is imperative to start any enteral feedings using one-quarter strength solutions at 50 ml/hour. The volume of fluid should be increased daily until 40 ml/kg/day plus losses are reached. Only at this time should the concentration of the feedings be increased. If this technique is not used, the patient is faced with a high osmotic load leading to diarrhea and an osmotic diuresis, resulting in dehydration, hyperglycemia, hyperosmolarity, coma, and possible death.

Intravenous

Complications of the Subclavian Catheter

It is essential to know that the catheter is properly placed before the infusion is started. The catheter should lie in the superior vena cava on chest x-ray, and blood should be drawn back easily. Complications of the catheter include misplacement, pneumothorax, hemothorax, infection, and thrombophlebitis. If the infusion of hyperalimentation fluid is associated with a new fever, the solution should be stopped and replaced with 10% glucose to avoid hypoglycemia. If the fever persists, the catheter should be removed and cultured.

Metabolic Complications

Potential metabolic complications are shown in Table 35.4.

MONITORING THERAPY

Standing orders regarding TPN monitoring are an integral part of any feeding program, both to monitor ther-

Table 35.4
Potential Metabolic Complications of Intravenous Hyperalimentation

Problems	Possible causes
Glucose metabolism	
Hyperglycemia, glycosuria, osmotic diuresis, hyperosmolar nonketotic dehydration, and coma	Excessive total dose or rate of infusion of glucose, inadequate endogenous insulin and glucocorticoids, sepsis
Ketoacidosis in diabetes mellitus	Inadequate endogenous insulin response, inadequate exogenous insulin therapy
Postinfusion (rebound) hypoglycemia	Persistence of endogenous insulin production secondary to prolonged stimulation of Islet cells by high-carbohydrate infusion
Amino acid metabolism	
Hyperchloremic metabolic acidosis	Excessive chloride and monohydrochloride content of crystalline amino acid solutions
Serum amino acid imbalance	Unphysiologic amino acid profile of the nutrient solution; differential amino acid consumption with various disorders
Hyperammonemia	Excessive ammonia in protein hydrolysate solutions; arginine, ornithine, aspartic acid, and/or glutamic acid deficiency in amino acid solutions; primary hepatic disorder
Prerenal azotemia	Excessive protein hydrolysate or amino acid infusion
Calcium and phosphorus metabolism	
Hypophosphatemia: decreased erythrocyte 2, 3-diphosphoglycerate, increased affinity of hemoglobin for oxygen, aberrations of erythrocyte-intermediary metabolites	Inadequate phosphorus administration. Redistribution of serum phosphorus into cells and/or bone
Hypocalcemia	Inadequate calcium administration; reciprocal response to phosphorus repletion without simultaneous calcium infusion; hypoalbuminemia
Hypercalcemia	Excessive calcium administration with or without high doses of albumin; excessive vitamin D administration
Vitamin D deficiency; hypervitaminosis D	Inadequate or excessive vitamin D administration
Essential fatty acid metabolism	
Serum deficiencies of phospholipid, linoleic, and/or arachidonic acids; serum elevations of α-5,8,11-eicosatrienoic acid	Inadequate essential fatty acid administration; inadequate vitamin E administration
Miscellaneous	
Hypokalemia	Inadequate potassium intake relative to increased requirements for protein anabolism; diuresis
Hyperkalemia	Excessive potassium administration especially in metabolic acidosis; renal decompensation
Hypomagnesemia	Inadequate magnesium administration relative to increased requirements for protein anabolism and glucose metabolism
Hypermagnesemia	Excessive magnesium administration; renal decompensation
Anemia	Iron deficiency; folic acid deficiency; vitamin B_{12} deficiency; copper deficiency; other deficiencies
Bleeding	Vitamin K deficiency
Hypervitaminosis A	Excessive vitamin A administration
Elevations in SGOT, SGPT, and serum alkaline phosphatase	Enzyme induction secondary to amino acid imbalance; excessive glycogen and/or fat deposition in the liver
Cholestatic hepatitis	Decreased water content of bile
Serum triglycerides and cholesterol	Lipid emulsion in excess of tolerance

apy and avoid complications. As therapy is established and measured parameters remain within acceptable limits, the frequency of monitoring may be decreased on the attending physician's order. Recommended monitoring frequencies are given in Table 35.5.

DESIGNING NUTRITIONAL THERAPY

A simple approach to designing nutritional therapy is essential in order to cut costs, avoid complications, and ensure fulfillment of the patient's dietary requirements.

The standardized form used by the pharmacy at Victoria Hospital, which includes an ideal weight-for-height table and a chart for calculating additional stress requirements, is shown in Figure 35.3.

Table 35.5
Recommended Monitoring Frequencies

Test	Frequency
Clinical assessment	Daily
Temperature, pulse, and respiratory rate	q8h
Body weight	Three times/weekly
Blood: Hb, Hct, WBC, electrolytes, SMA12	Twice weekly
Triglycerides, cholesterol, PT, serum osmolality	Once weekly
Creatinine clearance, blood culture, blood gases	As necessary
Urine: sugar and ketones, electrolytes	q6h, with diabetic protocol as necessary

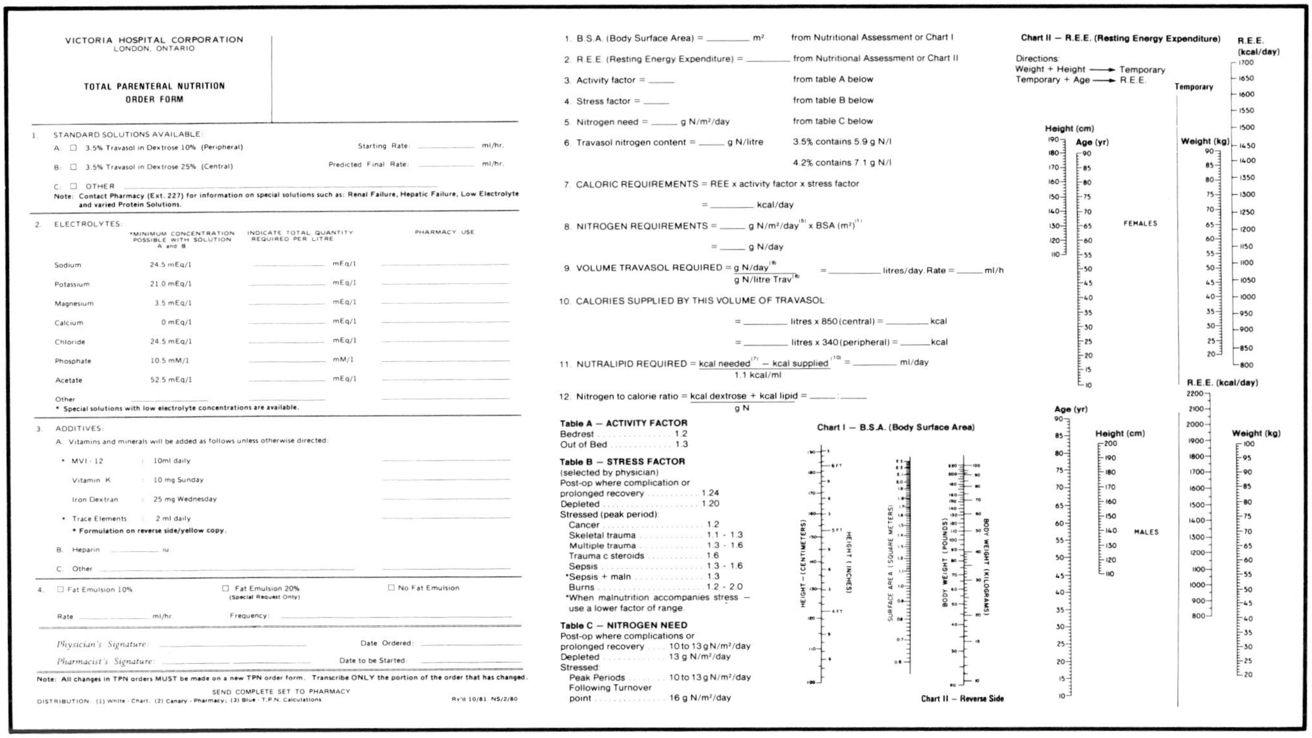

VICTORIA HOSPITAL CORPORATION
LONDON, ONTARIO

TOTAL PARENTERAL NUTRITION
ORDER FORM

1. STANDARD SOLUTIONS AVAILABLE:
A: ☐ 3.5% Travasol in Dextrose 10% (Peripheral) Starting Rate: ______ ml/hr.
B: ☐ 3.5% Travasol in Dextrose 25% (Central) Predicted Final Rate: ______ ml/hr.
C: ☐ OTHER ______
Note: Contact Pharmacy (Ext. 227) for information on special solutions such as: Renal Failure, Hepatic Failure, Low Electrolyte and varied Protein Solutions.

2. ELECTROLYTES:

	*MINIMUM CONCENTRATION POSSIBLE WITH SOLUTION A and B	INDICATE TOTAL QUANTITY REQUIRED PER LITRE	PHARMACY USE
Sodium	24.5 mEq/1	______ mEq/1	______
Potassium	21.0 mEq/1	______ mEq/1	______
Magnesium	3.5 mEq/1	______ mEq/1	______
Calcium	0 mEq/1	______ mEq/1	______
Chloride	24.5 mEq/1	______ mEq/1	______
Phosphate	10.5 mM/1	______ mM/1	______
Acetate	52.5 mEq/1	______ mEq/1	______
Other ______		______	______

* Special solutions with low electrolyte concentrations are available.

3. ADDITIVES:
A. Vitamins and minerals will be added as follows unless otherwise directed:
* MVI - 12 : 10ml daily
Vitamin K : 10 mg Sunday
Iron Dextran : 25 mg Wednesday
* Trace Elements : 2 ml daily
* Formulation on reverse side/yellow copy.
B. Heparin ______ iu
C. Other ______

4. ☐ Fat Emulsion 10% ☐ Fat Emulsion 20% (Special Request Only) ☐ No Fat Emulsion
Rate ______ ml/hr. Frequency: ______

Physician's Signature: ______ Date Ordered: ______
Pharmacist's Signature: ______ Date to be Started: ______

Note: All changes in TPN orders MUST be made on a new TPN order form. Transcribe ONLY the portion of the order that has changed.
SEND COMPLETE SET TO PHARMACY
DISTRIBUTION: (1) White - Chart; (2) Canary - Pharmacy; (3) Blue - T.P.N. Calculations Rv'd 10/81 NS/2/80

1. B.S.A. (Body Surface Area) = ______ m^2 from Nutritional Assessment or Chart I
2. R.E.E. (Resting Energy Expenditure) = ______ from Nutritional Assessment or Chart II
3. Activity factor = ______ from table A below
4. Stress factor = ______ from table B below
5. Nitrogen need = ______ g N/m²/day from table C below
6. Travasol nitrogen content = ______ g N/litre 3.5% contains 5.9 g N/l; 4.2% contains 7.1 g N/l
7. CALORIC REQUIREMENTS = REE x activity factor x stress factor = ______ kcal/day
8. NITROGEN REQUIREMENTS = ______ g N/m²/day[5] x BSA (m²)[1] = ______ g N/day
9. VOLUME TRAVASOL REQUIRED = $\frac{\text{g N/day}^{(8)}}{\text{g N/litre Trav}^{(6)}}$ = ______ litres/day. Rate = ______ ml/h
10. CALORIES SUPPLIED BY THIS VOLUME OF TRAVASOL:
= ______ litres x 850 (central) = ______ kcal
= ______ litres x 340 (peripheral) = ______ kcal
11. NUTRALIPID REQUIRED = $\frac{\text{kcal needed}^{(7)} - \text{kcal supplied}^{(10)}}{1.1\ \text{kcal/ml}}$ = ______ ml/day
12. Nitrogen to calorie ratio = $\frac{\text{kcal dextrose + kcal lipid}}{\text{g N}}$ = ______ : ______

Table A — ACTIVITY FACTOR
Bedrest 1.2
Out of Bed 1.3

Table B — STRESS FACTOR
(selected by physician)
Post-op where complication or prolonged recovery 1.24
Depleted 1.20
Stressed (peak period):
Cancer 1.2
Skeletal trauma .... 1.1 - 1.3
Multiple trauma .... 1.3 - 1.6
Trauma c steroids 1.6
Sepsis .... 1.3 - 1.6
*Sepsis + maln 1.3
Burns .... 1.2 - 2.0
*When malnutrition accompanies stress — use a lower factor of range.

Table C — NITROGEN NEED
Post-op where complications or prolonged recovery .... 10 to 13 g N/m²/day
Depleted .... 13 g N/m²/day
Stressed:
Peak Periods .... 10 to 13 g N/m²/day
Following Turnover point .... 16 g N/m²/day

Figure 35.3. Order form for nutritional therapy.

Two examples of different patients requiring nutritional therapy are given, using the following method for calculating dietary requirements:

1. Patient's ideal weight: . . . kg (from table supplied on order form).
2. Nonprotein calories required (maintenance level) = 36 × no. kg = . . . kcal. Additional stress requirements calculated from chart on order form. Optimal calorie:nitrogen ratio = 150–200:1, therefore:
3. Nitrogen required = $\frac{\text{Total cal}}{180}$ = . . . gm.
4. Protein required = Gram nitrogen × 6.25 (Travasol) = . . . gm.
   Note: 3.5% Travasol = 35 gm protein/liter = 5.6 gm nitrogen/liter. 10% dextrose = 100 gm/liter × 3.4 =

EXAMPLE 1

1. 70 kg man ideal weight; basal state.
2. # cal = 70 x 36 = 2520 Kcal/day.
3. Nitrogen required = $\frac{2520}{180}$ = 14 g.
4. Protein required (ie Vamin - N) = 14 x 7.45 = 104.3 g.
5. # Litres Vamin - N = $\frac{104.3}{35}$ = 2.98.
6. Calories:
   Central = 2.98 x 850 = 2533 Kcal.
   Peripheral = 2.98 x 340 = 1013 Kcal.
7. Nutralipid = $\frac{\#2 - \#6}{1.1}$
   Central: not necessary; use 2-3 500 ml bottles/wk for essential fatty acids.
   Peripheral = $\frac{2520 - 1013}{1.1}$
   = 1370 ml Nutralipid = 55 ml/hr.

EXAMPLE 2

1. 60 kg female; 20% body burn, therefore ↑ BMR by 50% (see chart on order form).
2. Basal cals = 60 x 36 = 2160 Kcal.
   20% burn = ↑ BMR x 50%.
   Total cal = 2160 x 1.5 = 3240 Kcal.
3. Gram nitrogen = $\frac{3240}{180}$ = 18 g.
4. Gram protein (Vamin - N) = 18 x 7.45 = 134 g.
5. # Litre amino acids = $\frac{134}{35\ \text{g/l}}$ = 3.8 litres.
6. Cals Provided (central recommended) = 3.8 x 850 = 3256 Kcal.

This would sustain calculated metabolic requirements. Regular monitoring is even more important in a case such as this.

340 kcal. 25% dextrose = 250 gm/liter × 3.4 = 850 kcal. 10% fat emulsion, 500 ml = 550 kcal.

5. Liters amino acid solution required =
$$\frac{\text{Gram protein required}}{\text{Gram protein per liter}} = \ldots \text{l.}$$
6. Calories provided. Central: 850 × no. 5 = . . . kcal; peripheral: 340 × no. 5 = . . . kcal.
7. No. ml of 10% fat emulsion required =
$$\frac{\text{No. 2–No. 6}}{\text{1.1 cal/ml}} = \text{ml/24 hr.}$$

Suggested Readings

Abel RM, Beck CH, Abbott WM, et al.: Improved survival from acute renal failure after treatment with intravenous essential L-amino acids and glucose. *N Engl J Med* 288:695–702, 1973.

Hausman D, Mosebach KD, Caspar R: Combined enteral-parenteral nutrition versus total parenteral nutrition in brain-injured patients. A comparative study. *Intens Care Med* 11:80–84, 1985.

Hinton P, Allison SP, Littlejohn S, et al.: Insulin and glucose to reduce catabolic response to injury in burned patients. *Lancet* 1:767–769, 1971.

Jeejeebhoy KN, Langer B, Tsallas G, et al.: Total parenteral nutrition at home: studies in patients surviving 4 months to 5 years. *Gastroenterology* 71:943–953, 1976.

Lemoyne M, Jeejeebhoy KN: Total parenteral nutrition in the critically ill patient. *Chest* 89:568–75, 1986.

Long JM III, Wilmore DW, Mason AD Jr, et al.: The effect of carbohydrate and fat intake on nitrogen excretion during total intravenous feedings. *Ann Surg* 185:417–422, 1977.

Ryan JA Jr, Abel RM, Abbott WM, et al.: Complications of total parenteral nutrition: a prospective study of two hundred consecutive patients. *N Engl J Med* 290:757, 1974.

Sax HE, Talamini MA, Fischer JE: Clinical use of branched-chain amino acids in liver disease, sepsis, trauma and burns. *Arch Surg* 121:358–66, 1986.

Wilmore DW: *The Metabolic Management of the Critically Ill.* New York, Plenum Publishing, 1977.

Wolfe BM, Culebras JM, Sim AJW, et al.: Substrate interaction in intravenous feeding: comparative effects of carbohydrate and fat on amino acid utilization in fasting man. *Ann Surg* 186:108, 1977.

CHAPTER 36 Disorders of Body Temperature

Gerald Bristow, M.D. and Bryan W. Kirk, M.D.

Most patients, like the one illustrated in Figure 36.1, maintain a remarkably constant core temperature of 37 ± 0.5°C. In order to understand the pathophysiology and treatment of disordered temperature regulation, one must first examine the mechanism by which normal temperature is maintained.

Body temperature is constant when heat production and heat loss are equal. Heat is lost by three processes: radiation, mainly as infrared photons from the warm skin to surrounding cooler surfaces; convection, from warm skin to moving air that has a specific heat of 0.22 cal/liter; and by evaporation, in which each liter of vaporized water removes 580 kcal from the skin surface. In the example shown in Figure 36.1, a skin temperature of 33°C provides thermal balance between resting body heat production and environmental temperature. Note that the heat in this patient is lost almost equally by radiation and convection, both of which are dependent on skin temperature.

CONTROL OF SURFACE TEMPERATURE

Skin temperature is controlled as illustrated in Figure 36.2 by regulating cutaneous blood flow. To warm the skin and lose body heat, cutaneous vasodilation directs blood flow to the surface. To cool the skin, sympatheti-

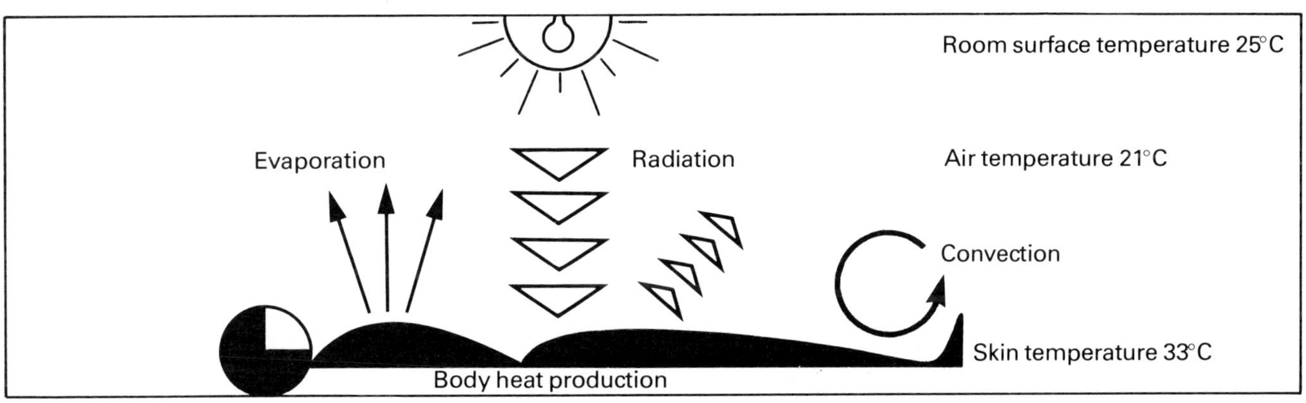

Body heat production

$$2064\ \text{kcal/day} = \underline{86}\ \text{kcal/hour}$$

Radiant heat loss

$$1\ \text{m}^2 \times (T_{skin}\ 33° - T_{surf}\ 25°) \times K_{rad} = -\underline{42}\ \text{kcal/hour}$$

Convection heat loss

$$1\ \text{m}^2 \times (T_{skin}\ 33° - T_{air}\ 21°) \times K_{conv.} = -\underline{36}\ \text{kcal/hour}$$

Evaporative heat loss

$$R_{sweating}\ 0.013\ 2/\text{hour} \times 580\ \text{Kcal} = -\underline{8}\ \text{kcal/hour}$$

Total heat loss $= 86$ kcal/hour

Thermal balance at 37° core $= \underline{0}$

Figure 36.1. Mechanisms of normal body temperature. Balance between heat production (thermogenesis) and heat loss for a patient lying exposed in bed, assuming 1 m^2 skin exposed and environmental temperatures illustrated. K_{rad} is 7.0 kcal/hour/m^2/°C temperature difference. K_{conv} is 6 kcal/m^2/hour/°C and assumes an air velocity of 9 cm/second.

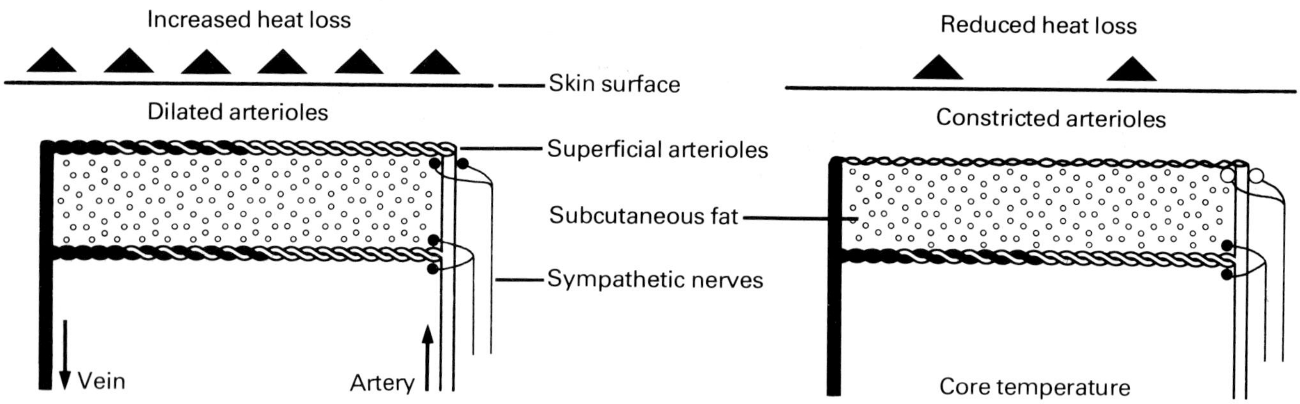

Figure 36.2 Thermal regulation by skin. Skin temperature controls body heat loss at rest. Dilation of superficial arterioles brings heat to surface, warming the skin. Constriction interposes insulating fat and skin cools. The insulating property of skin can be varied by a factor of 10.

cally mediated dermal vasoconstriction interposes the insulating subcutaneous fat between the environment and the core, conserving body heat. Shifting cutaneous blood flow in this way can alter the insulating properties of the skin by a factor of 10, resulting in a range of mean skin temperature from about 27°–36°C.

In a very hot environment, vasodilation, with radiant and convection heat loss, can remove only modest amounts of heat, becoming less effective as environmental temperature approaches body temperature. Sweating, on the other hand, can remove up to 2000 kcal/hr from the body surface, making it the major adaptive mechanism to heat stress. Humans are thus much better adapted to heat than to cold. For the unclothed person, the zone of comfort is about 28–31°C, a temperature that could be uncomfortably hot to personnel working in an intensive care unit.

Pathophysiology of Surface Temperature Control

Severe damage to the brainstem or spinal cord often results in cutaneous vasodilation and loss of muscle tone, and it is therefore common to see hypothermia in these injuries. Drugs may produce cutaneous vasodilation by a direct action on blood vessels and/or a blockade of sympathetically mediated vasoconstriction. Alcohol and opiates act directly on vessels to produce cutaneous vasodilation and will hasten the development of hypothermia during cold exposure. Chlorpromazine, a phenothiazine, produces vasoplegia by both direct dilation and α-adrenergic blockade mechanisms and has been widely used to induce hypothermia in anesthesia. In contrast, loss of control of both vasomotion and sweating in quadriplegia may result in hyperthermia when environmental temperature is high. In midbrain injury, cutaneous vasoconstriction plus increased muscle tone can lead to severe hyperthermia.

THERMOGENESIS

The ancients viewed the body as a furnace that produced heat if it was adequately stoked with food. The oxidation of 180 gm of glucose, for example, produces 686 kcal of energy as follows:

$$C_6H_{12}O_6 + 6H_2O + 134.4 \text{ liter } O_2 = 134.4 \text{ liters } CO_2 + 108 \text{ ml } H_2O + 686 \text{ kcal/180 gm}$$

Thus, we normally estimate metabolic rate by measuring either oxygen consumption or CO_2 production. One liter of oxygen consumed in an average diet results in the production of 4.83 kcal and 1 liter of CO_2, if the respiratory quotient (RQ) is one.

All organs produce heat as a by-product of their metabolic activity, but only muscle and brown fat seem to be capable of substantial increases in body heat production in response to cold stress. In response to a fall in environmental temperature, shivering and muscle tone are the most important sources of heat production. Nevertheless, shivering is not very efficient from a thermoregulatory viewpoint, because roughly half the heat produced is lost through increased superficial blood flow.

Pathophysiology

Malignant hyperthermia, discussed in more detail later, is a major problem resulting from "runaway" thermogenesis in muscle during anesthesia. Uniformly fatal until recently, it can now be prevented in most susceptible individuals.

Curare, succinylcholine, and other muscle relaxants abolish muscle heat production. They are very useful in the management of hyperpyrexia secondary to prolonged seizure activity or as an adjunct to surface cooling in central hyperpyrexia. However, hypothermia is a common complication of muscle relaxant administration in the critically ill patient, and body temperature must be monitored when muscle relaxants are used.

Nonshivering thermogenesis produces heat by mechanisms other than muscle contraction. It seems to be based on a calorigenic response to norepinephrine. Whether it is important in adult humans is not known. However, it is possible that nonshivering thermogenesis could account for the high caloric requirements observed in the early period following traumatic quadriplegia.

CENTRAL REGULATION

Body core temperature is normally regulated about set point by coordination of thermogenesis and skin temperature. It is likely that most, if not all, of normal central thermosensitivity in humans occurs in the hypothalamus. However, spinal centers of thermosensitivity, as demonstrated in animals, may account for the later return of thermoregulation following high spinal section in humans.

Pathophysiology

Central hyperthermia can result when the set point is increased by infection or midbrain injury. In both situations, the body responds as it normally would to a fall in core temperature with cutaneous vasoconstriction and shivering thermogenesis. As is discussed later, attempts at surface cooling in this situation result in a vigorous defense of the elevated temperature.

Central hypothermia usually occurs ominously following severe midbrain damage. Cutaneous vasodilation and flaccid muscle lead to a fall in core temperature that must be countered by surface heating.

DISORDERS OF TEMPERATURE REGULATION

Hypothermia

Hypothermia exists when the body's core temperature falls below 35°C. From the previous discussion on the regulation of core body temperature, it can be seen that hypothermia may occur due to decreased heat production, increased heat loss, or disordered central thermal regulation. Often, however, hypothermia occurs as a consequence of an abnormality in two or all three of the aforementioned areas. Whether hypothermia occurs depends as much on the body's ability to mount thermogenesis and constrict cutaneous vessels as it does on environmental temperature. For instance, hypothermia may occur at relatively mild ambient temperatures in the quadriplegic and those patients suffering from vasoplegic drug intoxication, including alcohol. Thermoregulation is poor in the newborn due to a combination of factors, such as restricted energy supplies, absence of shivering, poor vasoconstrictive activity, and a large body surface area to mass ratio. In addition, thermoregulation may be defective in the elderly, the drug and alcohol intoxicated, and the critically ill patient.

Hypothermia can complicate hypothyroidism, contributing to myxedema coma. We have seen one such patient in whom surface warming was necessary for 3 weeks.

For an unclothed, healthy person an air temperature under 15°C constitutes severe thermal stress. Wet exposure under 15°C, whether an individual is dressed or not, increases that stress 20 to 30 times because of the much greater thermal conductivity of water than of air. The most profound cases of accidental hypothermia in the northern hemisphere usually occur as a result of alcohol and drug abuse in the winter in urban settings, immersion in cold water, or in mountainous areas where air temperature may fall rapidly and winter rainfall occurs.

In order to simplify the approach to the hypothermic victim from the standpoint of prognosis and treatment, it is convenient to divide hypothermia into three types: mild, where the core temperature is between 30–35°C; moderate, where the core temperature is between 25–30°C; and severe, where the core temperature is less than 25°C.

Diagnosis

Most clinical mercury thermometers do not register below 34°C. In our experience, this has been a major source of failure to diagnose hypothermia. For this reason, most emergency departments now use either a glass laboratory thermometer, which must be held in place while read, or, more commonly, an electronic thermistor probe inserted into the esophagus at the level of the heart or into the rectum. When dealing with the hypothermic victim a simple diagnosis of hypothermia is insufficient, except in the case of pure exposure hypothermia, because drug or alcohol toxicity or physical illness may well be present as the predisposing factor. These conditions should be looked for assiduously.

Physiologic Response to Hypothermia

When subjected to cooling, awake, normal subjects develop tachypnea, tachycardia, hypertension, and shivering that begin almost immediately upon skin cooling and before the core temperature has reached 35°C. Oxygen consumption and heat production increase up to 500%. Physical performance, as measured by muscle strength, agility, and speed of movement, diminishes rapidly and profoundly even at temperatures as high as 35°C. Defects in cognition, memory, confusion, and disorientation begin to be manifested at temperatures under 32°C. Shivering ceases and consciousness is lost at temperatures below 30°C. One practical implication of the loss of consciousness is that, in individuals with core temperatures greater than 30°C who are suffering from hypothermia and who are unconscious, another cause for the disordered level of consciousness must always be sought. Generally, at core temperatures between 25–30°C tachypnea, tachycardia, hypertension, and muscle rigidity give way to deep coma, slow or absent respiration, bradycardias, and hypotension, which together may simulate clinical death.

Clinical death occurs usually with the onset of ventricular fibrillation. In the healthy individual, ventricular fibrillation is rarely seen at temperatures greater than 30°C, occasionally at temperatures between 25–30°C, and commonly at temperatures less than 25°C; however, individuals may not fibrillate in the accidental hypothermic state with core temperatures as low as 16°C. The cause of the wide variation in the fibrillation temperature of apparently healthy individuals is unknown, although alcohol seems to lower the temperature at which ventricular fibrillation occurs. The antiarrhythmic bretylium has also been noted to have this effect in animals.

An interesting and clinically very important fact when dealing with the hypothermic victim of cardiac arrest is that the biologic survival time, or that time during which the brain can tolerate a no blood flow state, is considerably lengthened in the hypothermic individual. It is lengthened because all tissue, particularly the brain, has a diminished need for oxygen. The relationship is such that for every 10°C fall in core body temperature, the safe circulatory arrest time without CPR is more than doubled.

In practical terms, then, an individual arresting at a core body temperature between 20–25°C (not an unlikely scenario) may well be able to sustain that absent circulation without cerebral damage for at least 15 to 20 minutes before the onset of CPR.

Treatment

Treatment depends on the severity of hypothermia, the presence of cardiac arrest, and the facilities at hand. Over the years, we have developed a protocol based on the experience in our emergency department that is suitable for most community hospitals. Table 36.1 summarizes the treatment of hypothermia.

Warming

If the core temperature is 30°C or greater, use surface or "shell" rewarming by applying dry warm blankets to the body surface, circulating warm water blankets to front and back, and immersing the patient in water at 40–45°C or a heat cradle. Warmed intravenous crystalloid may also be administered initially at the rate of 2–3 liters per hour, and the inspired gases may be warmed. Rectal temperature and cardiac rhythm should be monitored continuously.

If the core temperature is less than 30°C, surface rewarming is contraindicated. Because the shell is colder than the core, the vasodilation of surface warming can induce a fall in core temperature—the so-called afterfall—with a subsequent risk of intractable ventricular fibrillation. Therefore, below 30°C, we recommend peritoneal lavage. Peritoneal dialysis fluid with potassium supplemented to 4 mEq/liter warmed to 45°C is run in and out as rapidly as possible, 1–2 liters at a time depending on body size. If peritoneal dialysis fluid is not available, 0.9% sodium chloride with added potassium may be used and warmed before peritoneal installation by running through a blood warmer. Treatment may be stopped when the core temperature reaches 35°C.

Table 36.1
Management of Hypothermia

Immediate
• Airway and CPR if necessary
• Attach to ECG monitor
• Insert esophageal or rectal probe
• Send blood gas, electrolytes, and glucose
• Insert central line, Foley catheter
Warming
Above 30°C core temperature
• Use surface rewarming with circulating hot water blankets or heat cradle
Below 30°C core temperature
• Use peritoneal dialysis with 45° fluid
• CPR may be required until core temperature restored
Support
• Increase FiO_2
• Use warm saline and colloid for hypotension
• Administer bicarbonate 0.4 mEq/kg × corrected base deficit
• Antiarrhythmic drugs—avoid if possible

Cardiac Arrest

When cardiac arrest accompanies hypothermia, CPR must be carried out together with peritoneal lavage. We and others have seen periods of cardiac arrest in hypothermia where CPR exceeded 3 hours and the patient recovered with no neurologic sequela. Where an experienced pump team is available, cardiopulmonary bypass has also been used successfully to treat hypothermia with cardiac arrest. In profound hypothermia, the diagnosis of clinical death is impossible and must await rewarming. An old adage states that, when dealing with the hypothermic victim of cardiac arrest, death is not pronounced until the victim is "warm and dead." Remember there may be considerable discrepancy between clinical and biologic death in the hypothermic victim!

Supportive Care

Abnormalities of blood gases and acid/base balance are common. The interpretation of these values is confused by the difference between the body temperature and the measurement temperature, i.e., the hypothermic core body temperature and the electrode temperature of 37°C. Although there is some controversy in this area, the current wisdom is that PaO_2 should be temperature corrected, whereas the $PaCO_2$ and pH should not be corrected. Lactic acidosis during rewarming is a real problem that results from low cardiac output. Sodium bicarbonate may be required. Hypoxia, if present, should be corrected by a high FiO_2.

Dysrhythmias are the rule in severe hypothermia. An initial and persistent sinus tachycardia occurs until approximately a core temperature of 30°C is reached; ventricular tachycardia and ventricular fibrillation are seen usually at core temperatures less than 25°C. A host of other supraventricular and ventricular dysrhythmias, such as sinus bradycardia, junctional bradycardia, atrial fibrillation with slow ventricular response, frequent premature atrial contractions, and frequent premature ventricular contractions, may also occur. Unless these latter rhythms are hemodynamically significant, they should not be treated until rewarming is complete. Ventricular fibrillation often occurs after arrival in the hospital and once established is remarkably resistant to defibrillation and drugs. Most dysrhythmias respond simply to rewarming the heart. There is some evidence that bretylium in doses of 5–10 mg/kg may actually prevent or convert ventricular fibrillation in the hypothermic individual.

Hypotension during rewarming is usually secondary to cutaneous vasodilation in the presence of a low cardiac output. Administration of warmed saline or colloid is usually necessary. Theoretically at least, inotropic agents may produce cardiac dysrhythmias, and they should not be used routinely.

Increased Body Temperature

Fever

In the critical care unit, fever is most commonly the result of infection. In bacterial infections the mechanism is currently believed to be as follows. Bacteria release exogenous pyrogens. The ingestion of "exogenous pyrogen" (i.e., endotoxin) by leukocytes and other phagocytes results in the synthesis of an endogenous pyrogen, a lipoprotein peptide. Endogenous pyrogen in the blood seems to act in the central thermoregulatory center by increasing the core set point, an effect probably mediated by prostaglandins of the E series. An upward movement of the set point brings about a graded response of vasoconstriction and thermogenesis.

Fever, with its greater metabolism, results in an increase in calorie requirements, oxygen consumption, and cardiac output. An increase in body temperature of 1°C increases metabolic rate by about 10%. Thus, a patient with a temperature of 40°C has a 34% increase in both oxygen consumption and in cardiac output.

Treatment

There is still controversy over whether the fever of infection has any benefit as a host defense. Reviews of the available evidence suggest that an increase of 1–2°C in core temperature is neither detrimental nor beneficial. Thermal damage to tissue does not appear to occur below 42°C; thus, aside from discomfort, there is little reason to treat a fever under 40°C with urgency. On the other hand, calorie requirements increase one-third from 37° to 40°C, and over days or weeks, calorie depletion would result where the hypermetabolism of fever outstripped calorie intake.

Surface cooling in fever usually results in cutaneous vasoconstriction and shivering thermogenesis, increasing caloric requirements and requiring increased cardiac output. Thus, centrally acting antipyretics are the method of choice when the central set point is elevated by infection. Table 36.2 lists a number of antipyretic agents that, despite diverse chemical structure, all seem to act by prostaglandin synthetase inhibition. Acetylsalicylic acid and acetaminophen seem to be the most available and least toxic preparations in the critically ill patient.

The antipyretic dose of aspirin is 10–20 mg/kg q6h.

Table 36.2
Antipyretic Agents

Salicylates	Acetylsalicylic acid (aspirin)
***p*-Aminophenol**	Phenacetin
	Acetaminophen (Paracetamol)
Pyrazolon	Phenylbutazone
	Oxyphenbutazone
	Aminopyrine
Indomethacin	Indomethacin
	Sulindac (Clinoril)
Tolmetin	Tolmetin
Fenamate	Mefenamic acid
	Flufenamic acid
Propionic acid	Ibuprofen
	Naproxen

Aspirin tablets readily dissolve in water and can be administered down a nasogastric tube. Aspirin suppositories (300 mg) result in irregular, slower absorption, but are usually adequate for fever. Aspirin should not be used in patients with ongoing bleeding or thrombocytopenia because acetylation of the platelet cyclo-oxegenase markedly inhibits platelet aggregation. Gastric bleeding is increased by salicylates.

Acetaminophen (Tylenol) in a dose of 5–10 mg/kg is also antipyretic. Unlike most of the agents in Table 36.2, it does not affect platelet function or cause bleeding. However, because acetaminophen is metabolized in the liver repeated doses should be avoided in patients with liver impairment as the drug itself is hepatotoxic at levels above 100–125 μ/ml.

We prefer to use aspirin when a rectal suppository is required and acetaminophen liquid when the GI tract is functioning. Neither aspirin nor acetaminophen is ideal for use in the ICU. Unfortunately, a parenteral antipyretic is not available in either Canada or in the United States at this time.

Heat Stress Illness

Up to five abnormalities are recognized as a result of the human's attempt to cope with a heat load. These are muscle cramps, heat edema, heat syncope, heat exhaustion, and heat stroke. However, only the latter two actually represent a disorder of temperature regulation and are discussed here.

Heat exhaustion represents a failure of cardiovascular adaptation to high external temperature with attendant sodium and water loss. This sodium and water loss is a result of the body's attempt to maintain normal temperature; it usually occurs in unacclimatized individuals, most frequently in elderly persons receiving diuretics. Although symptoms may occur suddenly, they often develop over a day or two. Symptoms and signs are related to the CNS, GI tract, and cardiovascular system and include dizziness and lethargy; anorexia, nausea, vomiting, and diarrhea; and tachycardia and hypotension, particularly of the postural variety. The victim is usually pallid, cool, and clammy, although the temperature may be mildly elevated to the range of 38–39°C. When the temperature is raised in heat exhaustion, it represents a failure of the body to maintain a normal core temperature through the sweating process. Such patients may go on to develop heat stroke. Recovery from heat exhaustion is usually rapid when the patient is placed supine in a cool area and is given oral, or preferably parenteral, crystalloid.

Heat stroke or heat stress hyperpyrexia is a disease of rapid onset and high morbidity and mortality. Following head and cervical spine injuries, it is the third most common cause of death in athletes in North America. Occurring usually in the unacclimatized individual, it is the result of excessive heat production from exercise, febrile illness, or certain drug effects combined with a poor dissipation of heat because of such factors as a high ambient temperature and humidity, wearing heavy clothing, or anticholinergic drug usage. These factors may be combined with an absolute gain of heat from the surrounding atmosphere and objects. Sweating, which may be the only practical method of heat loss in these situations, soon becomes exhausted, at which point heat production and/or gain from the atmosphere will be greater than dissipation. Body temperature then begins to rise. This rise is usually dramatic over the course of several hours.

The clinical symptoms and signs of heat stroke stem usually from the cardiovascular and CNS systems; they include tachycardia, hypotension related to hypovolemia, weakness, disorientation, frank psychosis, seizures, or coma. The diagnosis of heat stroke is usually associated with core temperatures greater than 42°C. At temperatures above 42°C the pathophysiology of heat stroke includes, in addition to hypovolemia and hypoxia, denaturation of cellular proteins and cell membrane disruption. Survival is rare when the temperature exceeds 44°C, although recently a patient has survived from heat stroke with a presenting temperature of 47°C.

With any associated seizure activity, muscle temperature may greatly exceed core temperature. With heat stroke there is disruption of muscle cells (rhabdomyolysis), and myoglobin reaches the circulation through damaged capillaries. Cell damage also increases the levels of serum potassium and phosphate. Loss of plasma into the damaged muscle results in hypovolemia, which compounds the hypovolemia that is usually present as a result of prior sweat loss. The combination of reduced renal blood flow and filtered myoglobin seems to be a potent cause of acute renal failure. Liver cell necrosis is a common occurrence; the severity seems to parallel the maximum core temperature, and thus severe hepatic dysfunction should be anticipated when the core temperature exceeds 42°C. Finally, widespread tissue and capillary damage activates the clotting mechanism and intravascular coagulation leading to, at a minimum, thrombocytopenia and, at maximum, a consumption coagulopathy with bleeding.

Treatment

Treatment must be directed at multiple problems in a prioritized fashion. Table 36.3 summarizes the early management of severe hyperpyrexia. The first priority is to establish an airway, followed by an intravenous line through which colloid and inotropic agents can be administered. Cooling should, however, not be delayed. The most effective method is curarization (pancuronium, 0.1 mg/kg), tracheal intubation, and ventilation followed by immersion in ice water. Most centers, however, pack plastic bags filled with ice over the trunk, axillae, and groin. This method, although somewhat less effective, allows better access and monitoring during cooling. Esophageal temperature should be monitored and cooling discontinued when the core temperature reaches 38°C. Rectal temperature is not as reliable an indicator of core temperature in this situation as esophageal temperature. Hypovolemia must be treated with an infusion of colloid. Dopamine, up to 20 μg/kg min, may be required for severe hypotension until the temperature is reduced, acidosis is corrected, and volume is restored. Dopamine dosage should be rapidly tapered as the blood pressure returns to normal because the combination of dopamine in the α-adrenergic range above 10 μg/kg/min plus circulating myglobin could jeopardize renal function. Mannitol should be given initially 200 mg/kg (50–100 ml of 20% solution) over 5 minutes followed by bolus doses of 0.5–2.0 gm to keep the urine output over 100 ml/hour and to prevent precipitation of myoglobin in the renal tubules. Acidosis must be treated with hyperventilation and then sodium bicarbonate 0.4 mEq/kg x base deficit. Usually, the consumption coagulopathy and later hepatic insufficiency can be treated expectantly.

Table 36.3
Early Management of Severe Hyperpyrexia

In Operating Room
- Discontinue anesthetic, and hyperventilate with 100% O_2.
- Give dantrolene, 1 mg/kg, and repeat 5–10 minutes up to 10 mg/kg.
- Pack body cavities with iced saline if open.

In Emergency Room
- Intubate.
- Paralyze with pancuronium 0.1 mg/kg.
- Hyperventilate with 100% O_2.
- Pack body, axillae, and groin with bags of ice.

General Management
- Do ECG, central arterial line, Foley catheter.
- Monitor frequently blood gas, sodium, potassium, platelets.
- Administer bicarbonate 0.4 mEq/kg × base deficit.
- Administer mannitol 200 mg/kg.
- Treat hypovolemia with colloid.
- Early dialysis for potassium and phosphate may be required.

Malignant Hyperthermia

This anesthetic emergency results from runaway thermogenesis due to a striated muscle abnormality in genetically susceptible persons (Fig. 36.3). The muscle contracture seems to be due to a failure of endoplasmic reticulum to bind calcium following exposure to depolarizing muscle relaxants and/or hydrocarbon anesthetics.

In the typical case, relaxation of the jaw fails to occur following succinylcholine, a tachycardia appears, and skeletal muscles are firm. Temperature rises rapidly to as high as 46°C. Hypercarbia results from hypermetabolism, and lactic acidosis occurs because of anaerobic muscle metabolism. Muscle myoglobin and potassium are released. Secondary damage occurs in surviving patients in the form of hepatic cell damage (probably temperature induced), renal failure secondary to rhabdomyolysis and hypotension, and coagulation disorder due to cell damage; these conditions are hardly surprising when tissue temperatures may have exceeded 48°C!

Treatment

A history of anesthetic misadventure in family members, muscle hypertrophy, or elevated creatinine phosphokinase may provide some warning of this disastrous event. Suspect patients should be investigated, and premedication with large doses of dantrolene is necessary. Atro-

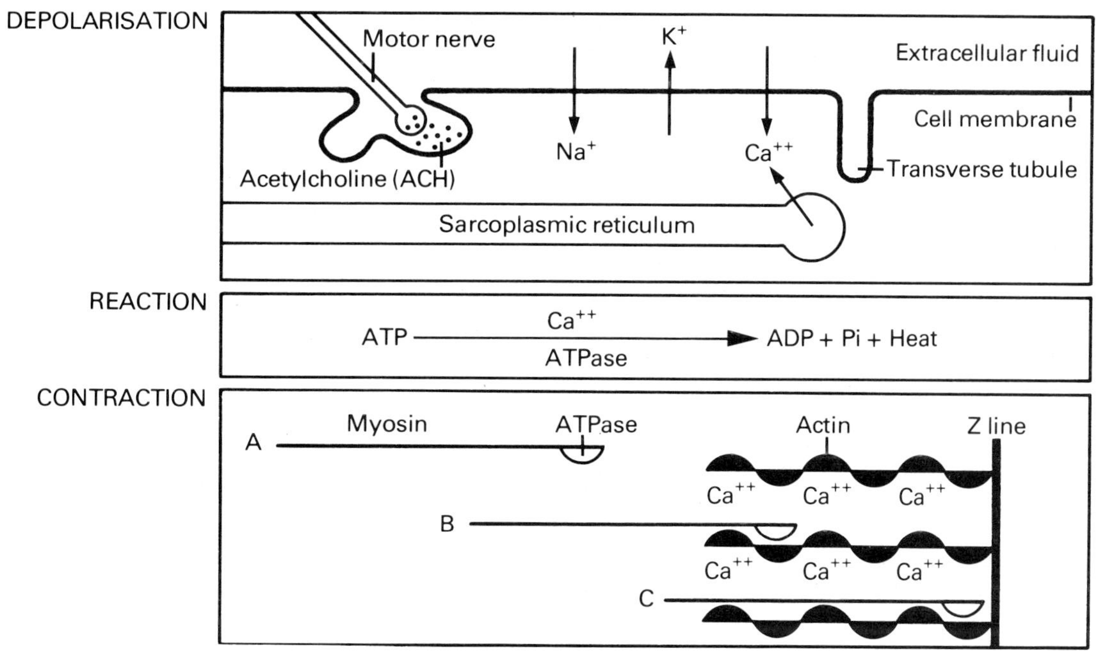

Figure 36.3. Muscle heat production. Acetylcholine release at the motor endplate triggers entry of calcium (Ca^{++}) from the extracellular fluid, which, in turn, triggers the entry of Ca^{++} from the extracellular fluid, which, in turn, triggers the entry of Ca^{+-} from the sarcoplasmic reticulum. The increase in calcium concentration activates contraction. At the end of contraction, Ca^{++} is pumped back into storage sites in the sarcoplasmic reticulum, sarcolemma, and extracellular fluid. Malignant hyperthermia appears to result from interference with the calcium pump in endoplasmic reticulum by muscle relaxants and volatile anesthetics resulting in sustained contraction. Core temperature may rise above 44°C.

pine, succinylcholine, and hydrocarbon anesthetics should be avoided.

Dantrolene, which interferes with the release of calcium from muscle sarcoplasmic reticulum, is the drug of choice for specific treatment of malignant hyperthermia. The starting dose of 1 mg/kg and up to 10 mg/kg has been used. Oral dantrolene 1–2 mg/kg q6h has been used to prevent recurrence or as prophylaxis. In the operating room, the body should be packed with ice and the body cavities with iced saline until esophageal temperature reaches 38°C. Extremely vigorous ventilation with 100% oxygen will be required to reduce arterial PCO_2.

The rest of the course of treatment of malignant hyperthermia is very similar to that outlined for heat stroke. Generally, however, cell damage is much more severe. Thus, fasciotomy may be required in the lower legs to prevent secondary ischemia induced by swelling muscle. Early hemodialysis may be required to reduce levels of potassium, phosphate, and other products of cell damage that may rapidly accumulate in the extracellular fluid. Bleeding is more likely to occur and may require the administration of fresh frozen plasma and platelets.

Neuroleptic Malignant Syndrome (NMS)

Typically, this hyperpyrexic syndrome develops over 24–72 hours in patients who are administered neuroleptic agents or following the withdrawal of levadopa. Drugs implicated in this syndrome are shown in Table 36.4. Predisposing factors seem to be exhaustion, dehydration, and organic brain damage. There is no relation to duration of neuroleptic administration. The major features are hyperpyrexia (up to 41°C), skeletal muscle rigidity, fluctuating level of consciousness, and autonomic instability. NMS, as do other hyperpyrexic syndromes, results in large increases in serum levels of muscle creatinine kinase and may increase liver enzymes. Rhabdomyolysis can result in renal failure.

Treatment

Obviously neuroleptics should be stopped, but where depot neuroleptics are involved symptoms can return for up to 3 weeks. The postulated mechanism is central; thus both central and peripherally active drugs could be effective. Dantrolene in doses of 0.8–10 mg/kg/day has been used with reported success, as has bromocryptine mesylate in doses of 2.5–10 mg orally q8h and amantidine hydrochloride in doses of 100 mg orally twice daily. Both of these drugs are central dopamine agonists. Dantrolene and bromocryptine have been used successfully in combination.

Table 36.4
Drugs Associated with Neuroleptic Malignant Syndrome

Phenothiazines
Butyrophenones (Haloperidol)
Thioxanthenes
Other antipsychotic drugs
Withdrawal of Levodopa
Amantadine

Suggested Readings

Abbot R, Loizou L: Neuroleptic malignant syndrome. *Br J Psychiatr* 148:47–51, 1986.

Bristow G: Clinical aspects of accidental hypothermia in living in the cold, physical and biochemical adaptations. Heller HG, Musachia XQ, Wang LC (eds): Elsivier Science Publishing Co, 1986.

Bristow G, Smith R, Lee J, et al: Resuscitation from cardiopulmonary arrest during accidental hypothermia due to exhaustion and exposure. *J Can Med Assoc* 117:247–249, 1977.

Guze B, Baxter L: Current concepts, neuroleptic malignant syndrome. *N Eng J Med,* 313:163–166, 1985.

Hirvonen J: Accidental hypothermia. In Lomax P, Schonbaum E (eds): *Body Temperature.* New York, Marcel Dekker, 1979, pp 561–585.

Kugelberg J, Schuller H, Breg, B, et al: Treatment of accidental hypothermia. *Scand J Thorac Cardiovasc Surg* 1:142–146, 1967.

Leithead CS, Lind AR: *Heat Stress and Heat Disorders.* Philadelphia, FA Davis, 1964.

McElroy E, Auerbach PS: Heat illness. In: *Current Perspectives in Management of Wilderness and Environmental Emergencies.* New York, MacMillan Publishing Co., 1983.

Pickering RG, Bristow, GK, Craig DB: Core rewarming by peritoneal irrigation in accidental hypothermia with cardiac arrest. *Anesth Analg* 56:574–577, 1977.

Stine RJ: Heat illness. *JACEP* 8:154–160, 1979.

CHAPTER 37

Multiorgan Failure in Critically Ill or Injured Patients

John H. Duff, M.D.

In the past, death of the critically ill or injured patient usually occurred quite suddenly from shock. Blood pressure could not be maintained by available methods of treatment, and death occurred from cardiac or respiratory arrest. Today, the mode of death in critically ill patients is different. Although a fall in blood pressure still is the terminal event, often the patient has been resuscitated from shock only to develop multiorgan failure that then leads directly to death. The downhill course, which often is prolonged, is characterized by muscle wasting, rapid weight loss, and impaired function of lungs, kidneys, liver, brain, heart, and GI tract.

The postmortem diagnoses that used to be made in patients dying from shock are now diagnosed before death as multiorgan failure. Many patients survive a prolonged critical illness. The concept of multiorgan failure has been described only since modern intensive care has prolonged the lives of patients seriously ill from trauma, sepsis, hemorrhage, and complicated major surgical procedures.

Because proper functioning of the body's organs and systems is based on great interdependence among them, single organ failure is exceptional as a cause of death in seriously ill patients. Rather, organ failure follows a sequential pattern, with the first organ to fail usually being the kidney or lung (Fig. 37.1). Unless recovery occurs, there is further failure of heart, brain, liver, and gut.

FACTORS PRECIPITATING MULTIORGAN FAILURE

Sepsis

Focal or diffuse abdominal sepsis is the most frequent cause of multiorgan failure. Intestinal anastomotic leak, peritonitis, pancreatitis, and postoperative abscess are some of the prominent septic problems. A hyperdynamic circulation is often an initial finding and is characterized by high cardiac output, low systemic resistance, and narrow arteriovenous oxygen difference. Protein catabolism is marked, with increased nitrogen excretion in urine, and eventually, skeletal muscle wasting is obvious. For a time, septic patients can be adequately supported with intravenous fluids, nutritional solutions, and antibiotics. However, if the infection cannot be drained or resolved by antibiotics, organ failure supervenes. The onset usually occurs days after sepsis is diagnosed and the catabolic deficits of body protein are well established. In such patients, there is indirect evidence that visceral protein lysis follows a long period of skeletal muscle protein lysis.

In contrast, multiorgan failure may occur quickly within 48 hours of the onset of sepsis. The following case illustrates this sequence of events.

Mr. Q, 28, had a motorcycle accident from which he sustained blunt chest, abdominal, and head trauma; face and scalp lacerations; crush and laceration injuries of the abdominal wall; and fractures of pelvis, tibia, fibula, and radius. Initially, he was conscious and stable. But 24 hours after admission, his condition had deteriorated, and celiotomy was performed. The abdominal wall injury was debrided of crushed muscle and fascia, and two tears of proximal jejunum were repaired. Apart from minor mesenteric tears and hematomas, there were no other intra-abdominal injuries. Operation appeared to have little influence on his clinical course. He was febrile. His mental status gradually deteriorated, and he became unresponsive. By the second postoperative day, renal failure was established with a creatinine of 6 mg/dl, and there were signs and x-ray evidence of respiratory failure. He required mechanical ventilation. His course was stormy for the next 8 days, with progressive deterioration in the function of his lungs, kidneys, brain, and liver. Blood cultures grew a non-spore-forming anaerobe not identified further. Numerous Gram negative oganisms were grown from swabs of the abdominal wound, tracheal aspirate, and urine. No distinct focus of infection or pus could be diagnosed. Repeat celiotomy was performed 9 days after the first because of progressive multiorgan failure. No infection was found. A tracheostomy was performed. Renal hemodialysis was required. The liver enzymes peaked at 5 times the normal values, and the serum bilirubin rose to 8 mg/dl. Other manifestations of organ failure were low blood platelets (<75,000) and prolonged paralytic ileus.

The progressive multiorgan failure stopped 15 days after the injury, and by the 20th day, recovery was well underway. He left the ICU and was fit for discharge from hospital 55 days after his injury.

Trauma

Like sepsis, trauma from an accident or major surgery is often the first event that is followed by multiorgan failure. Sepsis may be suspected, but is never proven.

Mr. W, aged 75, was admitted to the hospital with anemia and rectal bleeding. Investigation revealed carcinoma of cecum and a mass within the bone of the sacrum that was benign on needle biopsy. At operation, cancer of the cecum without lymph node metastases was removed by right hemicolectomy. There was no other intra-abdominal disease. The

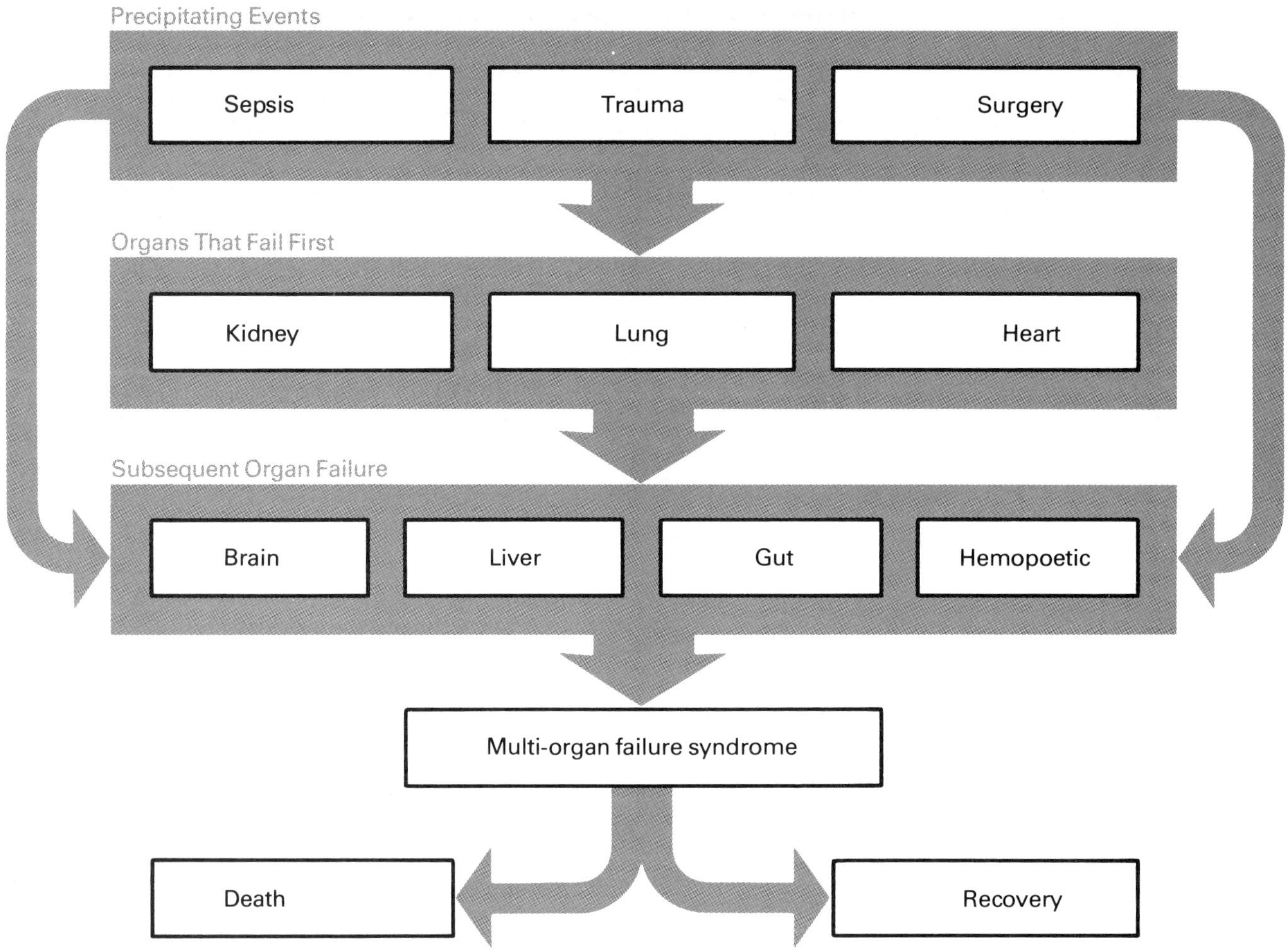

Figure 37.1. Development of multiorgan failure syndrome.

sacral tumor could not be felt. Blood transfusion was not required. No intraoperative hypotension was recorded. On the first postoperative day, breathing was labored, and the patient became confused. He was transferred to the ICU for closer observation. On the second postoperative day, respiratory failure was obvious. Intubation and mechanical ventilation were established. His mental condition became worse, and he responded only to painful stimuli. On the third postoperative day, both feet became ischemic, despite adequate popliteal and foot pulses. Venous thrombosis and gangrene were suspected, but could not be proven by venography. Renal failure occurred with elevated blood urea nitrogen and serum creatinine. He was febrile and mildly hypotensive. Cultures of blood, urine, and sputum were negative. Although there were no signs of intra-abdominal infection, his deteriorating condition suggested a septic focus. The two possible locations were the abdominal cavity and the gangrenous foot, which by this time had demarcated. A celiotomy was performed, and no intra-abdominal infection was found. A left below-knee amputation was done at the same time. There was no dramatic improvement in his multiorgan failure, and a tracheostomy was required. With continued supportive therapy, improvement began. One month later on the medical ward, he was alert and able to conduct some of his personal affairs. The tracheostomy was closed. His other foot forepart had fully demarcated dry gangrene.

ORGANS THAT FAIL IN THE CRITICALLY ILL PATIENT

Heart

Cardiovascular failure may be defined as a cardiac index of less than 2.5 liters/min/m^2 with normal or elevated filling pressures, or a dependence on inotropic drugs to maintain adequate tissue perfusion as assessed by clinical criteria.

Failure of the heart may be due directly to coronary artery occlusion, valvular disease, or myopathy, but such distinct lesions are not often seen in the heart failure of sepsis. If one accepts the definition of heart failure as inability of the heart to maintain adequate blood flow despite adequate preload, then heart failure in septic patients is relatively common. By contrast, many septic patients have increased cardiac output with normal or elevated filling pressure. They do not have cardiac failure, but usually show evidence of failure in other organs or systems.

There is seldom a correlation between the clinical and postmortem findings in septic patients judged to have cardiac failure by hemodynamic criteria. In patients dying following shock due to trauma, fatty degeneration of the myocardium has been observed. In experimental hemorrhagic shock, microscopic changes in the form of muscle necrosis, loss of striations, and fatty change have been observed within 24 hours of the onset of shock. In humans, gross changes in the heart are rare, and microscopic abnormalities are mild and nonspecific. Nonetheless, these histologic changes may be indications of quite significant metabolic and functional changes in the myocardium.

Lung

Pulmonary failure may be defined by either a fall in arterial PO_2 to less than 50 mm Hg on room air, the need for mechanical ventilation for longer than 48 hours because of hypoxemia or hypoventilation, or pulmonary edema on chest x-ray with a pulmonary capillary wedge pressure of less than 18 mm Hg.

Adult respiratory distress syndrome (ARDS), "shock lung," "Vietnam lung," and "lung lesion of sepsis" all describe a type of respiratory failure that is often the first manifestation of multiorgan failure in the critically ill or injured patient. The various names incorporate the three most prominent initiating events: shock, trauma, and sepsis.

The first clinical sign is dyspnea, and the earliest laboratory abnormality a fall in PO_2. As respiratory failure increases, there is pulmonary edema on chest x-ray, and the PCO_2 may rise. By this time, most patients require intubation and mechanical ventilation to prevent death from respiratory arrest. The lesion must be distinguished from other conditions that give a similar x-ray picture of pulmonary edema, such as crystalloid fluid overload, left heart failure, neurogenic pulmonary edema, aspiration pneumonia, fat embolism, and overwhelming bacterial pneumonia. X-ray changes may be absent during the first 12 hours of the syndrome when the only findings are hyperventilation and a fall in arterial PO_2. The earliest x-ray change is interstitial edema. As the condition worsens, patchy densities develop and progress to a diffuse symmetrical alveolar pattern in both lungs with an air bronchogram.

The pulmonary edema of ARDS does not respond to diuretics and digitalis, as would be expected of the pulmonary edema of heart failure or pure fluid overload. The complications of ARDS include secondary bacterial infection and pneumothorax. When resolution of the lung lesion occurs, it is characterized radiologically by cystic-like shadows that are due to localized interstitial emphysema and fibrosis.

The pathophysiology of lung failure is obscure, but there is evidence from clinical and experimental studies that the edema is due to increased permeability of the pulmonary capillaries. A few seriously ill patients would be expected to have edema on the basis of the hydrostatic and oncotic pressures alone, but in the majority, the edema cannot be explained by a simple subtraction of the hydrostatic from the oncotic pressure, as calculated from the pulmonary capillary wedge pressure (PCWP) and the serum albumin.

When death occurs, the postmortem examination reveals heavy lungs with congestion and edema on sectioning. Pleural effusions are present. Microscopically, the alveoli are fluid filled, and there is interstitial edema. The alveolar septa are thickened. There is focal hemorrhage. Microthromboemboli are often observed in pulmonary capillaries. In some cases hyaline membranes are seen covering alveolar walls and terminal bronchioles. Although none of these changes is specific for the pulmonary edema of the multiorgan failure syndrome, together they suggest that the lung is reacting to circulating factors that are highly toxic to capillary endothelium (see Chapter 11).

Brain

Central nervous system failure may be defined as a decreased level of consciousness ranging from confusion to coma in the absence of CNS infection or structural abnormalities. A more precise assessment may be determined by using the Glasgow Coma Scale (see Chapter 19).

In the multiorgan failure syndrome, there is often a noticeable degree of brain impairment. Initially, there is loss of interest in surroundings. Patients stop reading or watching television; they do not know their nurses or doctors. With worsening, drowsiness, confusion, and, eventually, coma occur. On examination, it is difficult to elicit responses to questioning, and patients will not carry out simple commands. Muscle stiffness and meningism are common signs suggesting that a neurologic complication has occurred. However, localizing signs are absent, and lumbar puncture is negative. The EEG is abnormal but nonspecific and, along with the neurologic examination, prompts the neurologic consultant to diagnose a "metabolic" or "anoxic" encephalopathy. But these diagnoses do not correlate with the laboratory studies, which show no significant electrolyte or glucose abnormality, and there has usually not been an episode of hypoxia. Of all the organs that fail in this syndrome, there is least understanding or knowledge of why or how brain failure occurs.

There is also a lack of correlation between the profound clinical changes and the pathology of the brain at postmortem examination.

Liver

Liver failure may be defined by a rise in serum bilirubin greater than 4 mg/dl or a serum glutamic oxaloacetate transaminase (SGOT) greater than twice normal in the absence of duct obstruction, hemolysis, or hepatitis of viral or toxic etiology.

When liver failure is part of the multiorgan failure syndrome, jaundice is usually the first sign. Liver tests are abnormal. They show a rising serum bilirubin and alkaline phosphatase with elevation of the liver enzymes—SGOT, serum glutamic phosphotransferase (SGPT), and lactic dehydrogenase (LDH). These changes suggest cholestatic jaundice, but the causative factor is unknown.

Changes in blood amino acids related to liver function also occur. There is consistent elevation of phenylalanine, an amino acid metabolized only in liver. Blood phenylalanine is known to be elevated in liver failure from other causes. The sulfur-containing amino acids—taurine, cysteine and methionine—also metabolized in the liver, have been shown to be elevated. Liver failure is not usually fulminant when part of multiorgan failure, but may be followed by renal failure in a pattern much like the hepatorenal syndrome seen in other types of liver disease.

At postmortem, the morphologic changes include focal necrosis, fatty change, congestion, and enlargement of sinusoids and cholestasis. The multitude of liver functions make assessment of liver failure a complex problem. As well as metabolic function, the liver functions as a barrier between the splanchnic and systemic circulations. Impaired function may allow toxic factors from the gut, such as bacteria and endotoxin, to have serious, if not fatal, extrahepatic effects.

Kidney

Renal failure is indicated by a serum creatinine of greater than 2.0 mg/dl or double the previous level if pre-existing renal impairment was present, creatinine clearance less than 30 ml/min, or urine output of less than 30 ml/hr over a 24-hour period despite adequate hydration.

Renal failure is almost always part of the multiorgan failure syndrome. Prerenal failure is excluded by a high urine sodium concentration. Renal failure is reversible, but usually persists 10 days or more and is associated with mortality of 50%.

The pathophysiology of renal failure is not fully known. Acute tubular necrosis may or may not be present, and this change has been observed in the kidneys of patients who did not have renal failure. Decreased renal blood flow, endotoxin, and vasoconstriction of renal arteries have been postulated as mechanisms of renal failure.

Fortunately, renal failure can be treated by hemodialysis until recovery of function occurs. However, if there is no recovery of the other organs that have failed, particularly the liver, return of renal function is not likely.

Gastrointestinal Tract

Gastrointestinal failure may be defined by the inability of patients to tolerate enteral feeding in the absence of mechanical obstruction and after an initial postoperative period of 5 days following abdominal surgery; acalculous cholecystitis; pancreatitis in the absence of gallstones, trauma, or alcohol abuse; or gastrointestinal bleeding requiring transfusion of greater than 2 units of packed cells in 24 hours.

Ulceration, loss of barrier function, and malabsorption are the mechanisms of failure for the gastrointestinal (GI) system. Ulceration most frequently occurs in the stomach and duodenum, but may be found in virtually any part of the GI tract. Hemorrhage is the obvious manifestation, although many ulcers do not bleed. The etiology of GI ulceration as part of the multiorgan failure syndrome is not known. Gastric acid secretion tends to be increased in critically ill patients, and duodenogastric reflux of bile has also been observed. Further support for gastric acid as a prominent cause of ulceration is the observation that antacids given according to gastric pH monitoring sharply decrease the incidence of bleeding.

Lower GI bleeding is uncommon and difficult to localize. Recently, acute bleeding rectal ulcers within reach of the examining finger have been reported in ICU patients with multiorgan failure.

Acute acalculous cholecystitis has been observed in patients who are critically ill from trauma or sepsis. Conscious patients may complain of right upper quadrant pain several days after their accident or the onset of illness. Examination reveals upper abdominal tenderness and sometimes a mass in the right upper quadrant. In confused or comatose patients, there may be minimal abdominal findings. These patients have fever and may appear to be deteriorating without an evident cause. Gangrenous acalculous cholecystitis is at times a surprising finding when laparotomy is performed in a deteriorating patient to rule out intra-abdominal sepsis. The pathologic findings range from a perforated gangrenous cholecystitis to an enlarged, tense gallbladder with patchy areas of gangrene, walled off by an inflamed, edematous greater omentum. The cystic artery is usually patent. Histologically, there is focal or diffuse necrosis with denuded hemorrhagic mucosa. The etiology of this GI manifestation of multiorgan failure is unknown. Most patients are receiving parenteral nutrition and, having no stimulus for gallbladder contraction, would tend to have bile stasis in a distended gallbladder. Many have had periods of hypotension and presumably decreased splanchnic blood flow. Ischemic gallbladder mucosa may lose its barrier function and allow concentrated bile to damage the stretched gallbladder wall.

Although difficult to measure, it is likely that in some critically ill patients the GI tract fails in its barrier function, allowing abnormal absorption of bacteria and toxins. Failure of this function should not be surprising in view of the massive denudation of GI tract mucosa observed frequently at postmortem in patients dying from multiorgan failure. In experimental hemorrhagic or traumatic shock, there is increased absorption of endotoxin. Indeed, some believe that loss of the gut barrier function in hypovolemic shock is the reason for irreversibility, i.e., death despite adequate volume replacement. Direct evidence for loss of gut barrier function comes from experiments that showed that, whereas curare given by mouth to normal dogs is harmless, when given to dogs in hemorrhagic shock it causes paralysis.

Finally, it is not surprising, in view of the above evidence, that there is failure of the digestive and absorptive function of the gut in seriously ill patients. Attempts to feed critically ill patients by nasogastric tube are often met by vomiting, diarrhea, and continued weight loss.

Morphologic changes in the gut in patients dying in multiorgan failure and GI tract involvement are well described. They are similar to those seen after death from hemorrhagic shock. Erosions are widely distributed in segmental fashion from esophagus to anus. The bowel mucosa is hemorrhagic. Histologically, there are dilated capillaries and veins, scant inflammatory reaction, and relative sparing of the muscular and serosal layers.

Hemopoietic System

The criteria for failure of the hemopoietic system are a platelet count of less than 50,000 in the absence of previously documented autoimmune thrombocytopenia; disseminated intravascular coagulation documented by fibrinogen levels of less than 200 mg/dl, fibrin-fibrinogen degradation products greater than 10 ug/ml, or a positive protamine sulfate test; or clinical bleeding diathesis as indicated by spontaneous bleeding from mucous membranes or bleeding from puncture sites.

MANAGEMENT AND PROGNOSIS

With an incidence of approximately 8% in medical surgical intensive care units, multiorgan failure is commonly encountered by those managing critical illness. No specific therapy exists because the precise etiology of multiorgan failure is obscure. Supportive therapy, which has allowed the syndrome to be observed in the first place, is the mainstay of present-day management. The lung and kidneys can be supported by mechanical devices for a long time, but no such support exists for the heart, liver, and brain. Parenteral nutrition supports one aspect of the failing GI system, but no procedure as yet is available to maintain the barrier function and to prevent mucosal ulceration and hemorrhage. Although a few patients show spectacular recovery from timely drainage of an intra-abdominal abscess, most patients with intra-abdominal sepsis and multiorgan failure succumb whether or not the abscess is drained. Blind laparotomy has been suggested for patients with multiorgan failure and presumed intra-abdominal sepsis without localizing findings on investigation. Studies in the literature of this problem suggest that pus will be found in a significant number of such patients, but survival remains poor. Few patients over age 50 with multiorgan failure recover following laparotomy whether or not a drainable pus is found.

MULTIPLE ORGAN FAILURE: A COMMON THEME

Although most would agree that the syndrome of multiorgan failure exists, there is only speculation about a common thread that binds the various parts of the syndrome together.

Hypoxia is not likely the cause because most patients have normal or increased oxygen uptake. Their arterial blood lactate levels, a metabolic index of tissue hypoxia, tend to be only slightly elevated, and their arteriovenous blood oxygen differences, if anything, are narrowed.

Metabolic abnormalities are obviously present in each of the organs that fail, but there is no evidence from the commonly measured parameters, such as pH, blood glucose, cortisol, thyroxine, and catecholamines, of a metabolic abnormality profound enough to cause such a widespread derangement of organ function.

A more plausible hypothesis is that organs fail because of a metabolic fuel deficit. Of the body's fuel stores, liver glycogen is depleted 48 hours after fasting, and fat, the major fuel reserve, is poorly metabolized during critical illness due to sepsis or trauma. Body protein becomes a source of fuel, with skeletal muscle being the initial site of protein lysis. Because all of the body's protein has a metabolic function, it follows that depletion of protein will immediately and progressively impair the function of the tissue or organ from which it is lost. This hypothesis fits the patient in whom multiorgan failure develops during a relatively prolonged catabolic illness. However, it does not explain the sometimes rapid development of organ failure long before a significant protein deficit could be reasonably expected.

Finally, it has been suggested that multiorgan failure is based on the toxic action of free radicals (O_2^-, OH^-, H_2O_2). In multiple trauma, following major operation, or in sepsis, complement is activated with the release of factor C5a. This factor causes margination and aggregation of granulocytes that then release free radicals in an amount sufficient to cause cellular damage, dysfunction, and possibly organ failure. Accumulation of granulocytes has been observed in lung, liver, and kidneys in experimental sepsis. Anoxia and drugs have been shown to cause release of free radicals. The free radical theory is attractive because it offers an explanation of how predisposing factors other than sepsis and trauma may cause multiorgan failure.

Suggested Readings

Bell RC, Colson JJ, Smith JD, Johanson WG: Multiorgan system failure and infection in adult respiratory distress syndrome. *Ann Intern Med* 99:293, 1983.

Bounous G, McArdle AH, Hodges DM, et al: Biosynthesis of intestinal mucin in shock: relationship to tryptic hemorrhagic enteritis and permeability to curare. *Ann Surg* 164:13, 1966.

Brigham KL, Bowers RE, Haynes J: Increased sheep lung vascular permeability caused by *Escherichia coli* endotoxin. *Circ Res* 45:292, 1979.

Duff JH, Wright FF: Acute and chronic benign ulcers of the rectum. *Surg Gynecol Obstet* 153:398–400, 1981.

Eisenman B, Beart R, Norton L: Multiple organ failure. *Surg Gynecol Obstet* 144:323–326, 1977.

Faist E, Baue AE, Dittmer H, Heberer G: Multiorgan failure in polytrauma patients. *J Trauma* 23:775, 1983.

Ferraris VA: Exploratory laparotomy for potential abdominal sepsis in patients with multiorgan failure. *Arch Surg* 118:1130, 1983.

Freiman DG: Hemorrhagic necrosis of the gastrointestinal tract. *Circulation* 32:329, 1965.

Fry DE, Pearlstein L, Fulton RL, Polk HC: Multisystem organ failure. *Arch Surg* 115:136, 1980.

Hackel DB, et al: The heart in shock. *Circ Res* 35:805, 1974.

Hinsdale JG, Jaffe BM: Reoperation for intra-abdominal sepsis. *Ann Surg* 199:31, 1984.

Lucas CE; Stress ulceration: the clinical problem. *World J Surg* 5:139–151, 1981.

Machiedo GW, LoVerme PJ, McGovern PJ, Blackwood JN: Patterns of mortality in a surgical intensive care unit. *Surg Gynecol Obstet* 152:757, 1981.

Nolan JP: The role of endotoxin in liver injury. *Gastroenterology* 69:1346–1356, 1975.

Norton LW: Does drainage of an intra-abdominal pus reverse multiorgan failure? *Am J Surg* 149:347, 1985.

Pine RW, Wertz MJ, Lennard SE, Dellinger EP, Carrico CJ, Minshew BH: Determinants of organ malfunction or death in patients with intra-abdominal sepsis. *Arch Surg* 111:242, 1983.

Sibbald WJ, Anderson RR, Holliday RL: Pathogenesis of pulmonary edema associated with the adult respiratory distress syndrome. *Can Med Assoc J* 120:445, 1979.

Teasdale G, Jennet B: Assessment of coma and impaired consciousness: a practical scale. *Lancet* II:81, 1974.

CHAPTER 38 Host Defense Mechanisms in Critically Ill Patients

John A. McCredie, M.B.

Primary alterations in host defense mechanisms are important elements in the establishment of infections and the subsequent prognosis of survival or death of critically ill patients. In this chapter, host defense is considered to be synonymous with the immune response, i.e., it includes humoral and cellular defense mechanisms that are and are not dependent on previous exposure to foreign antigens. Diseases that are associated frequently with a decrease in host resistance are burns, multiple trauma, intestinal fistula, advanced cancer, and local and systemic sepsis. Treatment of disease also can be immunosuppressive, such as operation, radiotherapy, chemotherapy, and the administration of immunosuppressive drugs, i.e., prednisone, Pentothal. The extremes of age are also accompanied by a decrease in immunity.

Acute or chronic malnutrition also seems to play a major role in producing immunosuppression seen in most of these patients. Protein-calorie malnutrition is present in most critically ill surgical patients; it leads to a loss of structural body proteins and hypoproteinemia. This decrease in plasma proteins may be due to inadequate intake or to a hypermetabolic state, as in the stressed patient, especially with burns and infections.

Formerly, the history, body weight, physical examination, and serum albumin were the only means of assessing host resistance. Now it is possible to quantitate a greater number of aspects of host resistance, and such tests have provided additional help in timing elective surgical procedures and determining the need for surgical intervention or change in treatment in critically ill patients. Because of the close relation between host resistance and nutrition, tests of the nutritional status are most frequently clinically employed in assessing a patient's host resistance.

PHYSIOLOGY

Natural Immunity

Natural humoral agents that help in combatting infections are lysozymes, opsonins, the properdin system, and complement (Table 38.1). Examples of the natural cellular resistance are phagocytosis of particles by granulocytes and macrophages. The number of polymorphonuclear (PMN) cells is important as is their function, such as their ability to adhere to membranes, chemotaxis (i.e., their attraction to the site of an infection), and their ability to mediate intracellular killing of organisms. The presence of opsonins that enhance phagocytosis are essential for normal PMN cell function.

Table 38.1
Host Defense Mechanisms

NATURAL	HUMORAL:	Lysozymes, opsonins, the properdin system, complement
	CELLULAR:	PMN cells Lymphocytes—NK cells Large mononuclear cells
ACQUIRED	HUMORAL:	B cells → plasma cells → cytotoxic or blocking antibodies
	CELLULAR:	Lymphocytes—T cells and K cells Large mononuclear cells

Recently, a family of lymphocytes has been discovered that recognizes and attacks a foreign cell in the absence of prior exposure to the cell or the presence of antibody or complement. It is known as the natural killer (NK) cell lymphocyte.

Acquired Immunity

In contrast to natural immunity, acquired humoral and cellular immune responses require previous sensitization to the foreign organism or antigen. The cells responsible for acquired immunity are the lymphocytes, plasma cells, and macrophages (Table 38.1).

Bursal-derived lymphocytes, B cells, play an important role in the reaction of the host to a foreign antigen (Fig. 38.1). On specific sensitization, either B cells become plasmablasts, which then divide producing plasma cells, or B cells change directly into plasma cells. Plasma cells synthesize cytotoxic or blocking antibodies that interact with the foreign antigen, either destroying it or enhancing its presence. Antibodies are immunoglobulins in the γ-globulin fraction of the serum proteins and are subdivided into the classes IgG, IgA, IgM, IgD, and IgE. IgG activates complement and plays an important part in conferring immunity to bacterial infections. IgM also activates complement and is important in resistance to infections, especially those caused by Gram negative organisms. IgA is found in respiratory and gut secretions and counteracts infections in these systems. IgD is found on the surface of immunocompetent cells where it serves as a specific antigen receptor. IgE is responsible for allergic reactions, as in asthma and hay fever, and for the

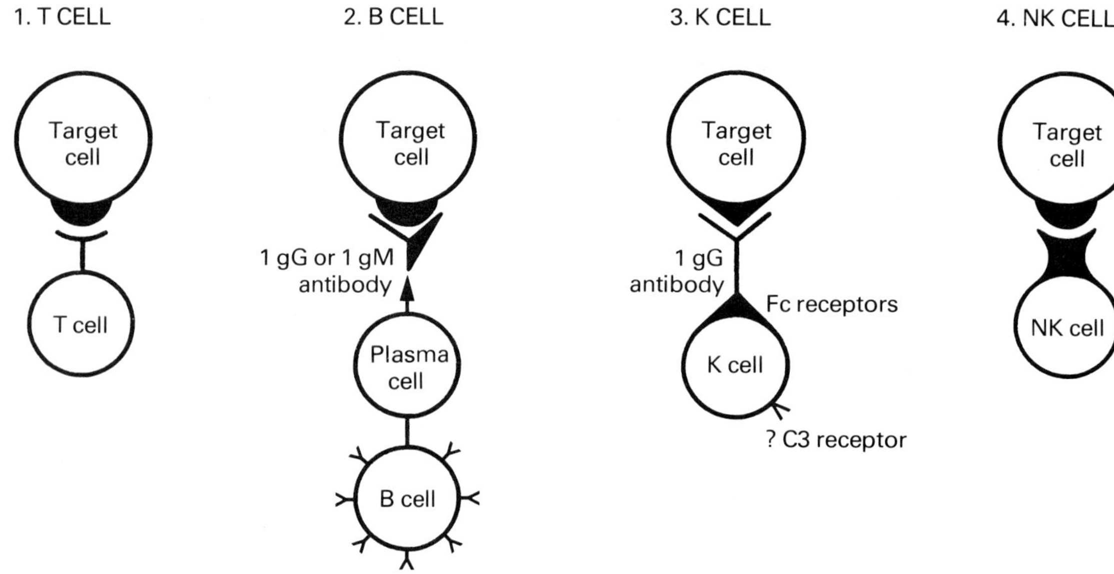

Figure 38.1. Effector functions of lymphocytes. Thymic-dependent lymphocytes, T cells, interact with a specific target cell. B cells on sensitization become plasma cells that produce immunoglobulins that react specifically with the target cells in the presence of complement. Killer cell lymphocytes, K cells, are not specifically programmed for the target cell, but react with it if antitarget cell IgG antibody is present. The cells were initially called "null" cells, in that they were thought to have no markers on their surface, but they do have Fc receptors and possible also C3 receptors. Natural killer lymphocytes, NK cells, are the simplest to understand; they recognize the target cell as foreign and react with it without the presence of complement or antibody.

rapid vascular changes seen in the inflammatory response.

Thymic-dependent lymphocytes, T cells, play a major role in defense against specific fungal and viral infections. There are many clones of T cell lymphocytes, with each programmed for one or a small number of antigens. A clone is a family of cells derived from one cell. When the specific lymphocyte—a "memory" T cell—interacts with its specific antigen, the cell is triggered and becomes a larger mononuclear cell that divides, giving rise to more T cells. The T cells then either interact with the antigen, causing its destruction by "effector" T cells, or promote its continuance by "suppressor" T cells. "Helper" T cell lymphocytes also act in cooperation with B cells to amplify the antibody response against bacterial infections.

Another family of lymphocytes has been recognized that attacks a foreign cell only if the cell is coated with specific antitarget cell IgG antibody. This lymphocyte is known as a "killer" (K) cell or antibody-dependent cellular cystotoxicity (ADCC) lymphocyte. The K cell does not require prior exposure to the target cell and so could be described as a natural immunity cell. However, because specific antitarget cell antibody must be present, it is generally included in acquired cellular immunity.

Macrophages of the lymphoreticular system are important in mediating the protective effects in acquired humoral and cell-mediated immunity. When memory T cells recognize their special antigen, large mononuclear cells take up the foreign antigen, process it, and pass on the information to a specific helper T cell. The helper T cell then helps in the sensitization of B cells. Therefore, a complicated series of events including large mononuclear cells, helper T cells, and B cells is involved in the triggering of acquired humoral immunity. The uptake of antigen by the large mononuclear cells and passing on the information as a specific RNA or RNA-antigen complex are important in the sensitization of T cells that give rise to effector and suppressor T cells. The large mononuclear cell thus plays a role in acquired cellular immunity.

DIAGNOSTIC TESTS OF HOST RESISTANCE

Body Weight

In view of the close relation between nutrition and the immune response, quantitation of the nutritional status of the host is a useful indicator of cellular and humoral immunity (Tables 38.2 and 38.3). A decrease in body weight was the first recognized sign to be associated with an increase in infection and in mortality. In patients operated on for peptic ulcer, mortality was 33% in those

Table 38.2
Tests for Host Resistance

Nutritional
Body weight, anthropometric measurements, serum albumin, serum transferrin
Natural immunity
Cellular—PMN cells, number and function
· Lymphocytes—NK cells
· Large mononuclear cells—number and function
Acquired immunity
Humoral—B cells, plasma cells, and immunoglobulins; cellular—delayed hypersensitivity skin reactions, T cells, K cells, and large mononuclear cells

Table 38.3
Host Resistance: Normal Values

	Normal values	Immuno-depressed patient
Serum albumin (gm/100 ml)	4.25 ± 0.06[a]	<2.8
Serum transferrin (m/100 ml)	260 ± 12	<160
Lymphomononuclear cell count (cells/mm^3)	2200 ± 72	<1100

[a] Mean ± SEM.

who had a marked decrease in body weight and only 4% in those who had no change. The weight/height ratio is a more accurate index than body weight.

Anthropometric and Biochemical Measurements

A number of anthropometric and biochemical tests have been used to assess the nutritional status of patients. The weight/height ratio and midarm circumference are used to quantitate protein-calorie malnutrition. Creatinine is a catabolic product of muscle breakdown and is therefore a good indicator of breakdown of body proteins. The ratio of the amount of creatinine in a 24-hour urine collection to body height is related to total cell mass. Some have found that anthropometric measurements are useful, although others have found that they are of little value in assessing an individual patient's nutritional status.

Serum Albumin

Albumin is synthesized exclusively in the liver, and the amount in the serum is a good indicator of the nutritional status of the host. In 70 critically ill patients, we found that the serum albumin was decreased by 25% in those who had lived and by 40% in those who died, thus apparently predicting survival or death.

Serum Transferrin

The serum β-globulin, transferrin, is also a good indicator of the nutritional status of the host. Iron is transported in the serum in conjunction with transferrin. The level is increased in iron deficiency and in those on oral contraceptives. It is decreased in acute and chronic sepsis and in the presence of tissue necrosis. The normal serum value is 250 mg/dl.

Polymorphonuclear Cells

The number of PMN cells is of no value in predicting prognosis in critically ill surgical patients. Views differ on the prognostic value of tests of PMN cell function. In septic patients, Meakins et al. found that chemotaxis was decreased, whereas we found that only immune adherence was decreased. The function of PMN cells is also dependent on the presence of opsonic factors, such as fibroneatin or cold-insoluble globulin that can be measured in the serum. Severe systemic sepsis is characterized by depressed opsonic (fibronectin) activity, which may be responsible for poor lymphoreticular clearance of bloodborne debris.

Lymphomononuclear Cells

The simple observation of the number of lymphomononuclear (LMN) cells in the peripheral blood seems to be useful in predicting the outcome of a critically ill patient and in monitoring the course of the illness. We found that LMN cell count was decreased by 55% in survivors and was lower in those who died than in those who lived. Values continued to decrease in those who died and rapidly returned to normal in survivors. In absolute numbers, an initial count of 1100/mm^3 indicated that the patient was extremely ill and had a high likelihood of death unless treatment caused a reversal, such as drainage of an occult abscess. With the approach of death, the value decreased to 800/mm^3.

Skin Tests

Delayed hypersensitivity skin tests, using recall or neoantigens, have proven to be useful indicators of host resistance. The delayed hypersensitivity skin reaction is complicated, including T cells, B cells, and large mononuclear cells, and is therefore not a simple test of T cell function. A recall antigen is one to which the patient has previously been exposed. There is therefore a cutaneous response following intracutaneous injection of the antigen that can be measured after 48 hours. A neoantigen is one to which the patient has not previously been exposed. The antigen is injected subcutaneously, the patient becomes sensitized after 10 days, and a response develops 48 hours after the second challenge with the antigen. Recall antigens are therefore more clinically useful because results can be obtained after 48 hours, whereas neoantigens require prior sensitization and results cannot be obtained until after 10 days. The commonly used antigens are purified protein derivative (PPD), histoplasmin, *Trichophyton, Candida,* mumps, and tetpolio. Patients who do not respond to any of the antigens are described as anergic and as relatively anergic if they respond to only one antigen.

Meakins et al. found that in normal reactors the incidence of postoperative sepsis was 7% and mortality was 2%, whereas in those who did not respond to any of the antigens the incidence of sepsis was 52% and the mortality was 36%. Schackert et al. studied 302 surgical patients of whom 42 had complications, mostly from sepsis. In anergic patients, the complication rate was 10.6% compared with 7.5% in normergic patients. They found serum albumin and white blood count were of no value in predicting the complication rate.

T Cells and B Cells

In vitro tests for cell number and function have proven to be of little value in monitoring surgical patients. Changes in B cells are variable and may be normal, increased, or decreased prior to death. Views differ on the value of in vitro tests for T cells. Uptake of tritiated thymedine after stimulation of peripheral blood lymphocytes with the mitogen phytohemaglutinin (PHA) has been used as a measure of T cell function. O'Gorman et al. found that in 30 patients with gunshot wounds, lymphocyte stimulation was decreased when compared with healthy controls and that recovery of lymphocyte function was associated with improvement in the patient's condition. It is interesting that these authors found that skin tests, white blood cell count, anthropometric measurements, and albumin level were of no value in predicting the clinical outcome.

K Cells

K cell function is one of the most sensitive indicators of the immune state of the patient. We found that K cell activity was decreased in critically ill surgical patients at the time of admission compared with healthy individuals, patients with benign diseases, and patients with early cancer. In survivors, there was no significant changes in K cell level, but in those who died there had been a decrease of 58%. In nonsurvivors, the values continued to decrease and were 64% lower than the initial values. K cell function is therefore a sensitive indicator of the immune status and can be repeated daily.

TREATMENT OF THE PATIENT WITH IMPAIRED HOST DEFENSE

Sepsis Control

The possibility of therapeutic reversal of immunodepression is important. From the foregoing discussion, it is apparent that drainage of an abscess or specific treatment of an infection will result in a marked improvement in host resistance and improved likelihood of survival.

Correction of Malnutrition

The close relation between acute and chronic weight loss and immune deficiency suggests that correction of malnutrition by the oral, peripheral, or central venous routes might result in a decrease of sepsis and increased survival. Admittedly, there are few studies that have prospectively proven this suggestion, although it seems common sense to provide aggressive alimentation to the critically ill patient manifesting increased catabolic activity and subsequent ongoing depression of host defense if left in the "starved" state.

Immune Stimulation

Pharmacologic attempts to improve host immunity have included administration of thymosin, interferon, levamisole, dinitrochlorobenzene zinc, *Corynebacterium parvum,* large doses of vitamin A, C, and E, immune ribonucleic acid, and bacille bilié de Calmette-Guérin and its methyl extraction residue. The possibility of immunizing patients at high risk of developing infections with antibacterial vaccines (i.e., *Pseudomonas* vaccine in the burned patient) has also been considered. This is currently an exciting field of investigation. None of these treatments, however, has been shown to be effective in a controlled clinical trial.

SPECIAL SITUATIONS

Splenectomy

Splenectomy is frequently necessary as an emergency procedure in the critically ill surgical patient with multiple trauma or as a result of injury during operation. It is also sometimes performed in a patient with Hodgkin's disease and hematologic diseases, such as idiopathic thrombocytopenic purpura and hemolytic anemias. Initially it was thought that only in infants did splenectomy decrease resistance to infections by encapsulated organisms, such as the pneumococcus and hemophilus influenza. Now it is recognized that splenectomy increases the propensity for serious infection at all ages. Efforts are therefore being made to maintain splenic function by treating splenic injuries without operation, by repairing a tear, by performing partial splenectomy, or by transplanting splenic tissue into the greater omentum. Pneumococcal vaccine, 0.5 ml subcutaneously every third year, is given to enhance host resistance against the pneumococcus in splenectomized patients. In those patients who have had the spleen removed, prophylactic antibiotics are also indicated when the patient develops even a minor infection.

The Critically Ill Cancer Patient

In the patient with early cancer, most of the tests of the immune status are normal. In those with advanced disease, the values are markedly decreased. The decrease is therefore the result of the presence of a large amount of cancer. Cancer tissue produces an increase in metabolism and a decrease in appetite. The cachexia may be the result of a decrease in the taste and smell of food and impairment of hypothalamic food control. The resulting weight loss may be the major factor in decreasing host resistance. Preoperative nutritional supplementation by the oral, peripheral venous, or central venous routes can lead to an increase in weight, an improvement in host resistance, and a decrease in postoperative complications, such as the development of infections and intestinal fistulas following gut resection.

The Burn Patient

The burn patient rapidly develops impaired host resistance. The hypermetabolic state results in malnutrition from the increased autoconsumption of proteins and other caloric sources. The exposed burn surfaces readily become infected and contribute to a further decrease in host resistance. A patient with a 50% burn that is infected may require 3500–5000 calories/day to maintain body weight. During simple starvation, the metabolism of fats yields the main source of energy, with subsequent conservation of tissue protein. However, in the septic burn patient there is initial metabolism of glycogen, followed closely by body protein. The marked third-space loss of proteins from the surface and into burned tissues results in further hypoproteinemia. It is therefore essential to supply adequate calories and amino acids by the oral, peripheral, or central venous routes at an early stage in the illness. All devitalized tissues must be excised and skin coverage obtained as rapidly as possible. This will minimize loss of fluids and proteins, maintain host resistance, and decrease infection.

SUMMARY

A number of objective measurements of host resistance can be made that are of value in monitoring the course of an illness. Body weight, anthropometric measurements, serum albumin, and transferrin reflect the severity of malnutrition. The number of PMN cells is of no value, although certain aspects of their function, such as adherence and chemotaxis, may be. The number of LMN cells in the peripheral blood is decreased by one-half in critically ill patients who are likely to die. Delayed hypersensitivity skin tests, using recall antigens, are useful in defining those who are anergic, who subsequently have had a high incidence of postoperative sepsis and death. K cell activity is a sensitive indicator of cell-mediated immune status.

The possibility of therapeutic reversal of immunodepression is vital to survival. Correct treatment of sepsis can cause a dramatic reversal and is probably the most important therapeutic procedure. Correction of malnutrition likely improves host resistance. Immune stimulants have also been used, but none has been shown to be effective in a controlled clinical trial.

Suggested Readings

Alexander JS, Stinnett JD, et al: A comparison of immunologic profiles and their influence on bacteremia in surgical patients with a high risk of infection. *Surgery* 79:94–104, 1979.

Brennan MF: Total parenteral nutrition in the cancer patient. *N Engl J Med* 305:375–382, 1981.

Forse RA, Shizgal HM: The assessment of malnutrition. *Surgery* 88:17–24, 1980.

Lewis RY; Albumin: role and discriminative use in surgery. *Can J Surg* 23:322–328, 1980.

McCredie JA: Antibody-dependent cellular cytotoxicity in critically ill surgical patients. *Surgery* 88:544–550, 1980.

McCredie JA, MacDonald HR: Antibody-dependent cellular cytotoxicity in cancer patients: lack of prognostic value. *Br J Cancer* 41:880–885, 1980.

McCredie JA, Austin TW, Holiday RL, et al: Predictive value for survival of lymphocytes and polymorphonuclear leukocytes in patients with sepsis. *Can J Surg* 22:447–451, 1979.

Sinclair NR St C, McCredie JA: Immune response in tissue transplantation and critically ill surgical patients. In *Basic Surgery,* ed 2. New York, Macmillan Publishing, 1986, pp 65–79.

Meakins JL, Pietsch JB, Bubenick O, et al: Delayed hypersensitivity: indicator of acquired failure of host defenses in sepsis and trauma. *Ann Surg* 186:241, 1977.

Meakins JS, Wicklund B, Armour-Frose R, et al: The surgical intensive care unit: current concepts in infection (Symposium on surgical infections, Alexander, J.W. geust ed). *Surg Clin North Am* 60:117–132, 1980.

O'Gorman RB, Feliciano DV, Matthews KS, et al: Correlation of immunologic and nutritional status with infectious complications after major abdominal trauma. *Surgery* 549–555, 1986.

Ota DM, Copeland EM, Corriere JN, et al: The effects of nutrition and treatment of cancer on host immunocompetence. *Surg Gynecol Obstet* 148:104–111, 1979.

Schackert HK, Betzler M, Timmermann GF, et al: The predictive role of delayed cutaneous hypersensitivity testing in postoperative complications. *Surg Gynecol Obstet* 162:563–568, 1986.

Seigel HH, Cerra FB, Coleman B, et al: Physiological and metabolic correlations in human sepsis. *Surgery* 86:163–193, 1979.

Studley HO: Percentage of weight loss (a basic indicator or surgical risk in patients with chronic peptic ulcer). *JAMA* 106:458–460, 1936.

CHAPTER 39

Severe Acute Pancreatitis: Current Diagnosis and Management

Alain Gilbert, M.D., David Leasa, M.D., and Brian Taylor, M.D.

In 5–15% of patients with acute pancreatitis the disease takes a fulminant course. Of these patients 20–60% will either die or face life-threatening complications. It is this lethal form of the disease that requires vigorous supportive therapy in the critical care environment and judicious surgical intervention. This chapter describes the general aspects of acute pancreatitis, particularly the critical care management of the complicated, high-risk patient.

ETIOLOGY

Alcohol and biliary disease (gallstones) are the most frequent causes of acute pancreatitis. Trauma (penetrating or blunt), infection (mycoplasma), drugs (azathioprine, thiazides), metabolic factors (hyperlipidemia, hyperparathyroidism), ischemia, and neoplasms are the other common etiologic agents. More recently, pancreatitis has been observed to follow endoscopy, pancreatography, and cardiopulmonary bypass. Pancreatitis in the postoperative setting usually follows surgery on the pancreas, biliary tract, stomach, or duodenum.

PATHOPHYSIOLOGY

The pancreatic proteolytic enzymes—trypsin, chymotrypsin, and elastase—are normally secreted as inactive proenzymes and activated only after contact with duodenal enterokinase. The key event in acute pancreatitis seems to be an abnormal activation of these and other enzymes that destroy tissue in and around the pancreas. A cascade of other enzymes, such as phospholipase A, is also involved. In addition to the local effects on the pancreas, a fluid rich in activated enzymes, histamine-releasing factors, vasoactive amines, and some other unidentified substances exudes into the surrounding tissue and peritoneal cavity. Once released from the pancreas, these substances are absorbed into the bloodstream from the peritoneal cavity. They then have profound effects on myocardial function, vascular tone, endothelial integrity, and complement activation.

CLINICAL PRESENTATION

The typical clinical presentation of acute pancreatitis is that of upper abdominal pain with radiation through the back that is associated with nausea, vomiting, and low-grade fever. Symptoms usually remain very nonspecific, and other intra-abdominal (and intrathoracic) problems can cause the same symptoms. Sometimes a patient has no pain, but presents with distension, ileus, fever, and tachycardia; this form of presentation is particularly prevalent following pancreatitis secondary to open heart surgery.

Mild pancreatitis is usually limited to local abdominal manifestations and will subside within a few days. In more severe cases, the cardiovascular system is always involved. Tachycardia and hypotension are the characteristic changes. These alterations are caused by the combined effects of increased capillary endothelial permeability, relative myocardial depression despite increased cardiac output, and decreased peripheral vascular resistance. The shock state is the major cause of death in the first week of acute pancreatitis.

Impaired respiratory function (e.g., hypoxemia, reduced functional residual capacity, decreased pulmonary compliance, and pleural effusions) is also a frequent feature of the initial phase of acute pancreatitis. An increase in pulmonary microvascular permeability to proteins and an increase in lung water (ARDS) may complicate acute pancreatitis. The specific agent of the alveolocapillary membrane injury is unknown, although liberated pancreatic enzymes, vasoactive substances, platelet microemboli, and endotoxins have been implicated. A particularly attractive hypothesis holds that phospholipase A, a lecithinase released in acute pancreatitis, destroys the phospholipid components of the pulmonary membranes, including surfactant.

Renal failure, generally secondary to hypotension, may also be seen. However, renal function may deteriorate without any period of hypotension and could be associated with circulating vasoactive substances that cause intrarenal vasoconstriction and increased renal vascular resistance with reduced glomerular filtration. Histologic studies have shown deposits of fibrin in the glomeruli, possibly secondary to activation of the coagulation cascade by trypsin.

DIAGNOSIS

The total serum amylase level has always been the classical laboratory test for acute pancreatitis. Its value is based on its high sensitivity of over 90%. However, amylase is nonspecific for pancreatic disease. The enzyme can be produced by many tissues other than pancreas, such as salivary glands, prostate, breast, and lungs. A simple way to improve the specificity of serum amylase may be to increase its cut-off number to twice the upper limit of normal, i.e., specificity increases from 82% to 98% while keeping the sensitivity over 90%. A normal serum amylase is rare in cases of acute pancreatits; however, the peak amylase level may be missed if the patient presents a few days after the onset of symptoms.

Caution is advised when interpreting elevated serum amylase levels as hyperamylasemia is frequently due to elevations in the nonpancreatic isoamylase fractions. A recent study in an ICU population demonstrated that 26% of patients with an increased serum amylase had pancreatic isoenzyme elevation solely, 17% had both pancreatic and extrapancreatic isoamylase elevation, and 57% had nonpancreatic fraction alone.

Pancreatic isoenzyme, even if specific for pancreas, can be elevated in many other intra-abdominal problems, including cholecystitis, perforated gastroduodenal ulcer, intestinal obstruction, and ischemic bowel. For this reason, determination of serum amylase isoenzymes is not of much help in acute abdominal situations. However, serum amylase isoenzymes may still be beneficial in distinguishing between pancreatic (or intra-abdominal) and extra-abdominal disease.

Serum lipase is mainly produced in the pancreas and has the advantage of remaining elevated in the blood for many days. However, it too is nonspecific and may be elevated with intestinal obstruction, perforation, or infarction.

At one time, amylase-creatinine clearance ratio had been proposed to improve the specificity of increased serum amylase in the diagnosis of acute pancreatitis, but at present it does not seem to be sufficiently reliable in distinguishing acute pancreatitis from other illnesses. New sophisticated tests, such as measuring serum elastase, pancreatic polypeptide, and trypsin, have been proposed, but have no great advantage over amylase and lipase, considering their time delay and costs.

Radiographic Tests

The plain film of the abdomen is most useful in excluding other abdominal conditions, usually free air or bowel obstruction. In acute pancreatitis, an ileus may be seen involving the small bowel (sentinel loop) or sometimes the transverse colon (the classical "colonic cut-off"). GI contrast studies are not sensitive tests for acute pancreatitis; however, widening of the duodenal C-loop, anterior displacement of the stomach, and narrowing or downward displacement of the transverse colon may be seen secondary to pancreatic edema or pseudocyst formation.

Chest x-ray may reveal pleural effusion(s), an elevated immobile diaphragm, patchy atelectasis, or diffuse parenchymal infiltrates (ARDS). Approximately 15% of patients with acute pancreatitis have an associated pleural effusion that is usually left-sided, as anatomically the tail of the pancreas is in direct contact with this diaphragm.

Ultrasonography and computed abdominal tomography have largely superseded the plain film or GI contrast series in pancreatic investigation. Ultrasonography is a simple, safe, and readily available test that can reveal diffuse pancreatic enlargement, pseudocyst, or abscess formation. Its other major use is evaluation of the biliary tree to rule out biliary obstruction. The major problem with ultrasonography is the interference caused by intestinal gas, a feature frequently observed with pancreatitis-induced ileus. For this reason, 40% of patients with acute pancreatitis will not have a good evaluation of their pancreas, and consequently no ultrasonographic diagnosis can be made.

In contrast to ultrasonography, computed abdominal tomography is not affected by air interference and will visualize the pancreas in almost every patient. Only those with complete absence of retroperitoneal fat will have inadequate visualization of the pancreas. Nevertheless, one-third of patients with acute pancreatitis may show no abnormality on CT scans, despite excellent visualization of their pancreas.

Radionuclide biliary excretion scans (e.g., HIDA scan) have been used to try to differentiate intraluminal obstruction of the bile duct by a stone from extrinsic compression by a swollen pancreas; that is, to distinguish between biliary and alcoholic pancreatitis. Evidence to date suggests that these tests are inadequate for the task.

PROGNOSIS

Ranson has described a multifactoral assessment of 11 signs to predict prognosis early in the course of pancreatitis. Five are determined at the time of admission, and the remaining six within the first 48 hours of hospitalization (Table 39.1). Ranson indicated that the mortality was 0.9% in patients with two or less prognostic signs, 16% in patients with three and four signs, 40% with five and six signs, and 100% with seven or more signs.

Even though these signs may not be very useful when a particular patient presents with abdominal pain, they can predict a reasonable prognosis after 48 hours. For example, a patient with five or six prognostic signs who looks clinically well after 2 days should probably be watched closely, maybe in an ICU, because his or her course may abruptly change. The other use of these prognostic signs is to stratify groups of patients for a more accurate comparison of the effects of different treatments for acute pancreatitis.

TREATMENT: MEDICAL

Unfortunately the medical treatment of acute pancreatitis is mainly supportive. Many specific treatments have been tried in the past to decrease the inflammatory reaction or block the enzymatic damage, but without success.

Resting the Pancreas

The first principle of therapy has been to "put the pancreas to rest" by reducing stimulation from gastric distension and acid-induced secretion of secretin. Nasogastric suction, cimetidine, glucagon, and atropine have all good theoretical application, but none has been proven

Table 39.1
Prognostic Signs Early in Acute Pancreatitis[a]

Admission	First 48 hours
Age > 55 years	Hematocrit fall > 10 percentage points
Blood glucose > 11 mmol/liter (200 mg/dl)	Serum calcium < 2.0 mmol/liter (8 mg/dl)
WBC > 16,000	Arterial PaO2 < 60 mm Hg
AST > 250 U/liter	BUN increase > 1.8 mmol/liter (5 mg/dl)
LDH > 350 U/liter	Base deficit greater than 4 mEq/liter
	Fluid replacement greater than 6 liters

[a]Adapted from Ranson JHC: Etiological and prognostic factors in human acute pancreatitis: a review. *Am J Gastroenterol* 77:633–638, 1982.

effective in improving the survival. Nonetheless, nasogastric suction is useful in decreasing the patient's discomfort secondary to ileus, nausea, or vomiting. Prevention of stress ulceration with antacids or H_2 receptor antagonists is also important.

The other aspect of specific medical treatment is the inhibition of pancreatic enzymes. The most popular drug for this use is aprotinin (Trasylol), which was shown by Trapnell in 1974 to be effective in this regard. However, many subsequent randomized, double-blind clinical studies have shown no benefit. Until studies show any beneficial specific treatment for acute pancreatitis, supportive therapy will be the only approach to the disease.

Cardiovascular Support

Aggressive fluid resuscitation is essential considering the large third-space volume losses and the associated vasodilation. Significant fluid and electrolyte losses may occur secondary to vomiting and nasogastric suctioning. There is no advantage in colloid over crystalloid resuscitation. In severe acute pancreatitis a pulmonary artery catheter may be necessary for adequate fluid resuscitation, especially if hypotension and hypoperfusion persist despite restoration of intravascular volume. Vasopressors (dopamine, levarterenol) may be required if hypotension and marked peripheral vasodilation persist despite apparent restoration of the intravascular volume (PCWP>15 mm Hg). A urinary catheter is essential for hourly urine output.

Respiratory Support

Respiratory problems are common, and arterial blood gases should be monitored frequently. Hypoxemia is initially corrected with oxygen supplementation; however, endotracheal intubation with mechanical ventilation and positive end-expiratory pressure (PEEP) may be necessary if respiratory failure occurs; i.e., if there is (1) failure to maintain adequate arterial oxygenation secondary to ARDS or atelectasis or (2) ventilatory insufficiency attributable to increased abdominal pressure, reduced diaphragmatic excursion, and reduced functional residual capacity as third-space losses increase.

Electrolyte and Acid/Base Balance

Hyperglycemia, hypomagnesemia, hypocalcemia, hypophosphatemia, and metabolic acidosis may occur. Insulin may be required to control hyperglycemia. Although hypoalbuminemia accounts for a large fraction of the drop in total calcium seen, a true decrease in ionized calcium does occur. When ionized calcium is significantly reduced, treatment with parenteral calcium is indicated. Metabolic acidosis may be secondary to alcoholic ketoacidosis, lactic acidosis, diabetic ketoacidosis, or renal failure.

Pain Relief

Because the pain associated with acute pancreatitis may be very severe, effective analgesia is important. Meperidine is preferred to morphine because it may cause less spasm of the ampulla of Vater. Epidural anesthesia may be beneficial because it avoids ampullary spasm and increases pancreatic blood flow; however, it is contraindicated in severe acute pancreatitis with hemodynamic instability. It may also mask abdominal findings.

Nutrition

Nutritional support should be instituted in any patient anticipated to be fasting for a long time. We generally consider total parenteral nutrition (TPN) as a supportive rather than a therapeutic measure. Enteral feeding offers more physiologic nutritional support with less complication and should be used when possible. Feeding jejunostomy can be performed if any intra-abdominal surgery has to be done during the disease. The nutritional regimen (total daily calorie and protein requirements) must be modified according to the patient's level of stress.

Antibiotics

Antibiotics have been proposed by many authors to decrease the risk of abscess formation, but no clinical study has indicated any benefit. However, all the studies have been done in mild to moderate pancreatitis, and the value of prophylactic antibiotics in severe necrotizing pancreatitis is unknown. We generally reserve antibiotics for pancreatitis associated with biliary tract infection, pancreatic abscess, or suspected sepsis.

Peritoneal Lavage

The value of peritoneal lavage, a compromise between medical and surgical treatment, has been debated in the last 10 years. The rationale is simple: it facilitates the clearance of the toxic factors liberated in the abdominal cavity by pancreatic inflammation. These toxins are those associated with the hemodynamic and respiratory instability in the acute phase of pancreatitis.

Ranson and Spencer demonstrated that patients with three or more prognostic signs did better in the first week with peritoneal lavage. However, overall hospital mortality was not changed. Apparently, lavage did not prevent the septic complications of acute pancreatitis.

Recently a prospective, randomized, controlled study was conducted in 91 patients who had objective evidence of severe acute pancreatitis. This multicenter study concluded that the outcome was not influenced by peritoneal lavage (2 liters/hr for 3 days). However, although the role of peritoneal lavage has been seriously challenged, lingering suspicion remains of its benefit for a few selective patients, i.e., those with severe hemodynamic and respiratory instability and massive pancreatic ascites.

TREATMENT: SURGICAL

Except for biliary pancreatitis, there is no specific surgical treatment for acute pancreatitis. There are three major indications for surgery in acute pancreatitis: (1) to rule out another surgically correctable disease when the diagnosis of pancreatitis is in doubt, (2) to operate on the biliary tree in gallstone pancreatitis, and (3) to remove necrotic or infected foci during the septic phase of hemorrhagic or necrotizing pancreatitis.

Ruling out Surgically Correctable Disease

As mentioned earlier, several acute abdominal situations can have the same clinical presentation as acute pancreatitis, i.e., leaking abdominal aneurysm, perforated gastroduodenal ulcer, acute cholecystitis, and mesenteric thrombosis. Consequently, surgery may be performed for an acute abdominal problem, without a specific diagnosis, in the hopes of finding a correctable lesion. If acute pancreatitis is found without any sign of pathology in the biliary system, local drainage with or without lavage is the accepted treatment.

Biliary Pancreatitis

This constitutes the only specific treatment of acute pancreatitis; that is, the only procedure directed to its cause. The treatment is clear—cholecystectomy/cholecystostomy with exploration of the common bile duct. However, the timing of surgery is controversial.

The most debated issue is whether early operative intervention, within 24 to 36 hours of the onset of symptoms, will reduce the incidence of hemorrhagic pancreatitis, presumably by stopping the progression of the inflammatory process. Studies of early surgery (first 48–72 hours) found impacted stones in over 60% of patients. Other investigators claim that the mortality is increased by performing the surgery in the acute phase of the disease. They recommend delaying the surgical treatment until the physiologic parameters return to normal and the patient is clinically well. More recently, endoscopic sphincterotomy has been proposed for the acute phase. The studies are so far small, but results are encouraging. Endoscopic sphincterotomy in experienced hands allows prompt decompression of the biliary tree without the need for a technically difficult laparotomy in a very ill patient.

Excision and Drainage of Necrotic or Infected Foci

This third indication for surgery in acute pancreatitis is the most challenging one. The main problem is to find some objective evidence of necrosis or infection. No specific test presently exists for either of these complications. A patient who rapidly deteriorates in the first few days after the onset of symptoms should make the physician suspect pancreatic necrosis. Computed abdominal tomography scan is the best diagnostic test, but may not distinguish between severe inflammation and necrosis, especially if no fluid collection is seen; therefore, clinical judgment becomes all important.

Surgical treatment of pancreatic necrosis consists of debridement of all nonviable tissue and adequate drainage. Some surgeons advocate pancreatic resection in order to try to stop the inflammatory process, but this is a formidable procedure once the disease process has progressed over several days. At the time of laparotomy, we usually place gastrostomy and feeding jejunostomy tubes, in addition to the biliary and pancreatic drains. If there is extensive necrosis, plans are made to return the patient to the operating room every 48 hours for debridement until the necrotic tissue has been completely removed. In most cases, the abdomen is best left open for drainage, with the bowel packed off until adhesions develop to prevent evisceration.

Pancreatic infection or abscess will usually appear after 7 to 15 days. Here again, clinical signs of sepsis are usually the main factors in the diagnosis. A computed abdominal tomography scan may show a collection of fluid but will not indicate whether it is infected. Percutaneous aspiration under computed abdominal tomography guidance can be done for diagnosis. Evolution toward multiple organ failure may be the only sign of infection and should be considered an indication for surgical exploration if no other obvious reason can explain the deterioration, even in the absence of radiologic findings. The mortality of pancreatic abscesses without drainage is virtually 100%. Percutaneous drainage under computed abdominal tomography guidance has a success rate of approximately 60%; however, multiple abscesses may be present and very thick material may be difficult to drain. Therefore, surgical exploration with adequate drainage, using soft sump drains, is usually the preferred approach to pancreatic abscesses.

Pancreatic necrosis and infection also cause local complications, i.e., hemorrhage from erosion of major blood vessels and intestinal fistulas, usually involving the transverse colon. Considering that hemostasis is difficult to accomplish in necrotic and friable tissue, angiographic embolization is the best initial management of severe local bleeding, but surgical exploration may well be necessary. Colonic fistulas require a transverse colostomy, proximal to the area of fistulization, and drainage of the pancreatic abscess.

Suggested Readings

Geokas MC, Baltaxe HA, Banks PA, Silva J, Frey CF: Acute pancreatitis. *Ann Intern Med* 103:86–100, 1985.

Mayer AD, McMahon MJ, Corfield AP, Cooper AP, Williamson RCN, Chir M, Dickson AP, Shearer MG, Clement WI: Controlled clinical trial of peritoneal lavage for the treatment of severe acute pancreatitis. *N Engl J Med* 312:399–404, 1985.

Moossa AR: Diagnostic tests and procedures in acute pancreatitis. *N Engl J Med* 311:639–643, 1984.

Pellegrini CA: The treatment of acute pancreatitis: a continuing challenge. *N Engl J Med* 312:436–438, 1985.

Ranson JHC: Etiological and prognostic factors in human acute pancreatitis: a review. *Am J Gastroenterol* 77:633–638, 1982.

Weaver DW, Busuito MJ, Bouwman DL, Wilson RF: Interpretation of serum amylase levels in the critically ill patient. *Crit Care Med* 13:532–533, 1985.

CHAPTER

40 Emotional Concerns and Ethical Issues in Critical Care

Irene Tiegs, M.S.W.

Physicians and health care professionals working in a critical care environment should be cognizant of possible emotional responses of the critically ill patients and their families so that they will be prepared to respond appropriately to them or request intervention from support services as needed. Patients who experience a trauma may suffer from posttraumatic stress disorders, and physicians should be aware of early interventions that may be productive in reducing the possible long-term negative psychological effects. In addition to discussing emotional responses to a critical illness or a trauma, this chapter also addresses ethical concerns that may arise in the decision-making process regarding diverting efforts from aggressive to compassionate care.

POSSIBLE PSYCHOLOGICAL RESPONSES

Anxiety

A critically ill patient may become very anxious when he or she awakes in an uncomfortable position, in an unfamiliar environment, and surrounded by an array of overwhelming equipment. Fear of the unknown is a common cause of anxiety. Patients may also perceive the illness as a threat to their body image and integrity. They may fear death, disability, or disfigurement. Patients may also become anxious about peripheral concerns, such as financial loss, assumption of their responsibilities, or care of their children during the hospitalization.

To reduce anxiety, the lucid patient should be oriented to the critical care setting; this orientation should include information about the surrounding equipment, as well as any planned procedures or treatments. When it is known that an individual will be admitted to the unit, such as a patient who is scheduled for coronary artery bypass surgery, information about what to expect should be prospectively given or ideally the patient may be offered a tour preoperatively.

An effort should be made to establish the source of the individual's anxiety. However, isolating the source may be particularly difficult with intubated patients. If they are capable of writing, writing tools should be provided. With individuals who are unable to write, family members may be helpful in suggesting what issues may be concerning the patient. Family members are generally better at lip reading than are staff.

Depression

Depression occurs in approximately 30% of all admissions and is particularly common in the critical care setting. Lucid patients who are in critical care for lengthy periods of time are particularly vulnerable to depression. With restricted mobility, they may experience a loss of control over their environment, body, and activities. Their total dependence on others may result in a feeling of helplessness and, often, hopelessness.

Depressive symptoms in the critical care setting include a loss of interest in visitors, suicidal ideation, crying, difficulty making decisions, withdrawal or failure to respond to stimuli in the environment, feelings of being punished, a sense of failure, and failure to communicate needs to staff.

To combat depression, patients should be encouraged to engage in self-care when feasible, even if it only entails washing their own face or hands. They may be encouraged to engage in decision making, including the timing of their bathing or in which direction they would like to be turned first. Within reason, control of visitors should be the lucid patient's decision. Demand analgesic offers the patient some control over pain management. The overall goal should be to encourage the patient to maintain a sense of autonomy that will not substantially interfere with prescribed treatment plans.

Another factor contributing to depression is a lack of external stimulation. A "Walkman" or a battery-operated radio with earphones may be helpful in providing the patient with music; the radio may also provide contact with the outside world through the current events of news broadcasts. Patients with young children or grandchildren who are unable to visit may benefit from hearing tapes of the children's voices. Pictures of family or close friends may be taped on intravenous poles in the unfamiliar environment. Visitation from family members is also important in reducing depressive symptoms.

Crisis intervention in the form of psychotherapy may be productive in reducing depressive symptoms. However, if the depression persists and sleep is disrupted, an antidepressant may be required.

Anger

Anger may be associated with feelings of humiliation, guilt, frustration, or unfocused rage. The patients in the critical care setting may feel alienated by the healthy staff all around them, or they may experience feelings of withdrawal. The patients may feel that no one appreciates what they may be experiencing. Anger may also be expressed by victims of accidents or injury caused by others.

Patients who attempted suicide may feel angry that they did not succeed. Their anger may be, however, derived from guilt when they realize the distress they have created for their family members. Guilt-produced anger may also be expressed by patients who failed to seek medical attention and ignored early symptoms of their disease process. Individuals who survive a trauma may experience unwarranted guilt over their survival as they come to realize that others were killed. Some critically injured patients may experience guilt because they feel that they deserved the injury for previous "wrongdoings." These emotions may be particularly prevalent in religious patients who feel that they must bear the burden for previous sins that they committed. Patients experiencing guilt may overtly express their anger or they may withdraw. These individuals may require professional intervention to enable them to reframe their thinking by placing the events into perspective. Understanding guilt is the initial stage in resolution.

Because some individuals may be humiliated by the loss of dignity in their naked state, all patients should be discretely covered and curtains should be drawn during bathing or periods of necessary exposure.

Most patients experience frustration with the loss of mobility and discomfort associated with intubation. Angry patients may attempt to extubate themselves, and such staff responses as "you must," "you should," or "you have to" may elicit defensive responses. Empathy, with an emphasis on responding to the feelings as opposed to the content of the patient's message, is generally more productive in eliciting a more cooperative response in the lucid patient. Staff members should attempt to convey to the patients that they understand what they may be experiencing and, if indicated, offer reassurance that they will be extubated when their condition improves.

A patient's anger should be validated, and the expression of their anger should be encouraged. To improve communication with the intubated patient, the staff should establish nonverbal codes, such as blinking or squeezing hands with individuals who are unable to write and who cannot be understood by lip reading.

ICU Syndrome

The critical care unit with its high-technology equipment, continuous lighting, medical jargon, and absence of meaningful stimuli creates an environment that may cause confusion, hallucinations, and paranoia in the alert patient. The unit may be compared to a "spy camp" in which patients are exposed to intermittent pain stimuli, varying levels of lighting and noises, a lack of differentiation between night and day, a loss of autonomy, and deprivation of oral consumption.

The brain needs to be continuously stimulated by changes in sensation and to experience meaningful contact with the outside world. With an absence of stimuli, patients become easily distracted and bored and consequently experience disruptions in perceptions. Dream-like states and hallucinations may prevail as the cortex arranges available stimuli to find meaning in the environment or to maintain arousal. In the critical care unit, the patient is socially isolated and hence experiences perceptual and sensory deprivation. Prolonged deprivation and alienation, compounded by delusional thoughts, may develop into psychosis. Uncertainty and confusion may lead to paranoia.

Immobility

Patients in the critical care unit experience restricted mobility as they are attached to such machines as ventilators and have nasogastric tubes, intravenous lines, and chest tubes in place. Immobilized healthy individuals may develop disturbing symptoms, such as changes in body image, depersonalization, aches and pains, and impairment in intellect, cognitive, and psychomotor functioning.

Patients should be encouraged to mobilize their limbs if feasible. Patients who are immobile may benefit from passive range of motion exercises that may be done in conjunction with their bathing.

Sensory Deprivation

There is minimal visual stimulation in the critical care environment. The unadorned walls are usually sterile white, beige, or a muted tone that blends in with the drab color scheme of much of the ancillary apparatus. There are generally no clocks or calenders to stimulate the disoriented patient. Most units lack windows, which makes it more difficult for the socially isolated patient to differentiate between day and night in a unit that remains lit all the time. Taste and smell are affected by nasogastric tubes. Familiar sounds and voices are generally absent.

Some patients who appear withdrawn or lethargic with staff may respond to familiar voices of family and friends. Radios and television are also useful means of providing stimulation and contact with the outside world. If eyeglasses and hearing aids are generally worn, they should be used so that the patient may benefit from what limited stimuli are available.

Medical jargon is the most common language of a critical care unit and is perceived by the patient as a foreign language. A study conducted to assess postoperative psychosis found that a language barrier may contribute to the psychosis. Of the non-English-speaking individuals in the study, 29.4% suffered from postoperative psychosis in comparison to 3.9% of the English-speaking group.

Sensory Overload

A critical care unit is illuminated 24 hours a day, and the noise level of the monitoring equipment can become intolerable. One author compared an ICU to a busy typing office with phones ringing continuously. In a study conducted to establish the focal point of hallucinations of patients in a unit, the source seemed to be unexplained environmental noises. The most annoying noise identified by the patients was the voices of staff discussing personal affairs with other staff and the voices of staff talking with other patients in the room.

In an effort to reduce the noise level, staff should eliminate unnecessary alarms at night, and they should position the ventilators so that the bellows are not next to the ears of the patients. The staff should attempt to minimize unnecessary conversation.

Sleep Deprivation

The major disturbing factor for patients in the critical care unit is sleep deprivation, which is of particular concern because sleep is essential to the healing process. The cells of the body are continuously being degraded and renewed. Wounds heal through the same process of cell division and protein synthesis. Activities of wakefulness enhance catabolism (degradation), whereas sleep shifts the balance to anabolism (renewal). Sleep positively inhibits the secretion of cortisol, a catabolic hormone, and deep sleep is the normal stimulus for the release of the growth hormone, as well as the anabolic hormone that increases the synthesis of protein and mobilizes free fatty acids to provide energy.

Because sleep is an essential element of the healing process, it is imperative that staff make conscious efforts to minimize sleep deprivation for the critically ill patient. Staff should organize activities to allow for long periods of uninterrupted sleep. The lights should be dimmed, and staff should refrain from talking near the bedside.

"CABG Syndrome"

Following coronary artery bypass graft (CABG) surgery, patients may experience changes in intellectual functioning. These changes are usually temporary, but can concern the patients, and hence they should be addressed to help reduce the patients' anxiety and frustration. The following residual problems have been noted: impaired concentration, diminished judgment of distance, increased visual disturbances, difficulty with arithmetic, and impaired handwriting. They generally disappear after 6–8 weeks.

POSTTRAUMATIC STRESS DISORDERS

Critically ill patients are susceptible to posttraumatic stress disorders, and hence it is beneficial to have an appreciation of possible long-term psychological difficulties that the patient may experience. Staff may be helpful in reducing the negative effects of these disorders.

Anxiety Attacks

Individuals who suffer emotionally from a traumatic experience and are unable to ventilate their fears may suffer from anxiety attacks. Victims of motor vehicle accidents, shootings, stabbings, and physical abuse and witnesses of trauma are particularly susceptible to anxiety attacks. These attacks have also been observed in some patients following major surgery who may have failed to express their preoperative fears. Postoperatively, when they are relieved and less defensive, their repressed fears may surface in the form of anxiety attacks. The onset is generally sudden, and patients usually experience difficulty comprehending these intense emotions. Critical care patients who are lucid may repress anxiety that results from a loss of control and feelings of being victimized as a dependent patient.

Anxiety attacks may occur when individuals are in a secure environment and they consciously or subconsciously recall the trauma. These attacks mimic cardiac difficulties, with respiratory distress, rapid palpitations, profuse sweating, nausea, trembling, and/or tightness in the chest. Often individuals may not appreciate the source of the anxiety because it generally has a sudden onset and may occur during periods of relaxation. Ventilation of their fears and discussing the incident and their emotional responses at the time of the trauma will generally reduce the frequency of these attacks.

Sleep Disorders

Individuals who are traumatized may also have sleep disorders. They may have difficulty falling asleep because they are preoccupied with their negative experience. Others may be emotionally exhausted and fall asleep initially; however, they may awaken after only a few hours of sleep and experience difficulty falling asleep again. Some patients may experience hypersomnia, which involves sleeping excessively during the night and often during the day. Sleeping may be an escape or a diversion from their depressing thoughts.

Some trauma victims may experience disturbing dreams or nightmares. Their dreams may be depressing or involve violence. When analyzed, these dreams are often reflective of their fears and negative feelings associated with their trauma. Individuals who experience sleep disorders readily become emotionally and physically fatigued and hence are unable to cope effectively with daily activities. Psychotherapy may be productive in assisting these individuals to deal with their repressed negative feelings that may be the source of their sleep disturbances.

Difficulty with Memory and/or Concentration

Traumatized individuals may experience difficulty concentrating because they may be preoccupied with their trauma. This deficit may affect their short-term memory. These individuals may read a page and not be able to recall immediately what they have read. They may have difficulty retaining information heard verbally or memories of events that lack an emotional component.

Individuals who experience difficulty with memory or concentration may become frustrated and withdraw socially. Frustrated students may need to be reassured that this deficit may be only temporary. Intervention may be productive in assisting the individual to grieve overtly or express repressed concerns that may be the source of the difficulties.

These deficits may be the result of a head injury or an organic brain disorder. However, these individuals may also suffer impairment of orientation, intellect, and judgment and lability of affect. Formal psychological testing may be helpful in diagnosing the source of the impairment.

Psychological Flashbacks

Individuals who are unable to express negative feelings when experiencing a trauma that has a visual component may be distressed by psychological flashbacks of the incident at a later time. These visual hallucinations are most likely to occur when the individual is fatigued or when efforts are made to relax.

Family members who view a critically injured patient may also experience psychological flashbacks. To prevent this stress disorder for family members, an attempt should be made to prepare them for what they may expect when they view the patient. When visiting, they should be encouraged to ventilate their negative feelings.

Loss of Interest in Premorbid Activities

A loss of emotional investment in people and activities may occur after a trauma. The individual may be so preoccupied with his or her negative feelings that loss of libido or sexual drive may be experienced. The traumatized victim may suffer from anhedonia, which is the inability to experience pleasure from any source, as well as the loss of the pleasure-seeking drive. He or she may experience difficulty accepting or demonstrating affection without a concentrated effort. In a broad sense, the traumatized patient loses interest in most things in the world outside of self.

Individuals who have experienced a trauma may express feelings of estrangement or detachment from their family and friends because they feel no one understands what they have experienced. Family and friends may become very frustrated with these individuals as time passes and they remain obsessed with their trauma. Research has shown that traumatized victims may experience residual emotional concerns for as long as 2 years.

This estrangement may be particularly difficult for family members to comprehend and may consequently lead to family discord. It may be especially stressful on the marital relationship; a separation may result if intervention is not provided to help the spouse appreciate what the victim is experiencing. Both victims and their families may require intervention in coping with these symptoms.

Phobias

A traumatic event that poses a threat to his or her security may create a phobia in an individual with a premorbid personality of anxiety proneness, emotional dependence, and/or psychosexual immaturity. Traumatized individuals suffering with agoraphobia have anxiety or panic attacks when they venture outside their homes. They may experience associated fears of losing control, going beserk, becoming insane, fainting, or collapsing. These patients may be able to venture out into social situations only when accompanied by a supportive individual.

Depression

An individual who is traumatized or suffers from a critical illness may be susceptible to residual depression. Symptoms may include loss of appetite, apathy, loss of self-esteem, insomnia, irritability, feelings of bodily malaise, loss of confidence, loss of insight, impaired memory, and loss of interest in work or recreational activities. Some may experience feelings of total personal inadequacy combined with feelings of hopelessness and helplessness. Suicidal thoughts may also prevail in some individuals.

Individuals suffering a loss are prone to experiencing depressive symptoms. Losses include not only death of a loved one but also loss of limbs, body parts, or ability. Studies have also indicated a higher incidence of depression in individuals who have suffered a myocardial infarction or a life-threatening illness.

Traumatized individuals suffering with depression may benefit from psychotherapy; however, when the condition persists, sleeping medication may be required. A minor tranquilizer or an antidepressant may be indicated in certain situations.

GRIEF RESPONSES OF RELATIVES

The family members and significant others of patients in critical care may experience similar emotional responses to those of patients. Patients' loved ones may express feelings of anger, guilt, fear, helplessness, frustration, and/or relief.

Relatives of critically ill patients may share angry feelings toward patients who may have failed to seek medical attention. Family members of a traumatized patient may express anger toward the individual who may have inflicted the injury or toward their loved one who was careless. Relatives of industrial accident victims may ventilate anger toward the employer for hazardous working conditions or toward their loved one for performing an unsafe act or failing to take safety precautions. Frequently, family members feel anger directed to their family physician or physicians in smaller centers whom, they feel, failed to make an accurate diagnosis or waited too long to initiate treatment or transfer to a better-equipped facility. Staff members must be cautious not to pass judgment upon another physician's actions. It is, however, ethical to suggest to the family that they address their concerns with the responsible physician.

Occasionally, feelings of anger with the patient may be misdirected toward staff. It is therapeutically beneficial if staff members refrain from responding defensively. If family members express complaints regarding the patient's care, the concerns should be addressed both at a "content" level and "feeling" level.

Family members may also ventilate warranted and unwarranted guilt if they failed to act on or encourage the patient to seek medical attention when initial symptoms were observed. These feelings are particularly prevalent if the critically ill patient is a child whose condition deteriorated over a period of days as opposed to a sudden onset. Family members may also experience guilt over anger or negative feelings expressed toward the traumatized victim before the trauma occurred. Loved ones who have had minimal recent contact with the patient, due to other commitments or priorities, may have a need to share their guilt. Staff should also be cognizant that personal guilt may be misdirected in the form of anger toward other family members or staff. The medical team should be cautious not to become enmeshed in the struggles of feuding family members. Encouraging the family to select a spokesperson may alleviate this problem.

Relatives may benefit from ventilating their fears of losing the patient. They may need to express their anxiety about the prognosis, treatment, or surgical interventions. Some family members may appear to be unconcerned; however, some individuals fail to ask questions because they are fearful of the answers. Others are intimidated by health professionals and are afraid to demonstrate their ignorance by asking inappropriate questions. It is important that physicians establish a comfortable rapport with the family spokesperson so that any misconceptions may be corrected.

Family members may also express feelings of helplessness when visiting because they sense the patient's distress and are unable to offer any relief. Parents and spouses are particularly susceptible to feelings of helplessness as they were accustomed to addressing the individual's premorbid needs.

Feelings of frustration may occur when the critically ill patient's progress is slow or if recovery is delayed by complications, such as sepsis. Although there may be little change in the patient's condition, it is important that physicians maintain regular contacts with the discouraged family member who may otherwise misinterpret that physicians have "given up."

Loved ones may experience feelings of relief when life supports are withdrawn or when treatment is diverted from aggressive to compassionate care. They may view it as an end either to the patient's or their own emotional suffering. Family members may have difficulty accepting these feelings of relief, and they may need to be reassured that individuals grieve on two levels. At a cognitive level, they may resign themselves to the inevitable or realize that the condition is irreversible and nothing is to be gained from further intervention. However, on the emotional level it is difficult to "let go" because they appreciate the permanency of death. Although family members may request that life support machines be discontinued, at the same time they may experience difficulty coping with their loss.

Family members need to be reassured that these feelings are a normal response to a loss. They should be encouraged to grieve overtly as crying is a positive release of tension and frustration. They should also be encouraged to utilize past experiences and strengths as coping mechanisms. Reminiscing is also a constructive technique in the grieving process.

Relatives often suffer a loss of appetite, and thus they should be encouraged to maintain their own health by eating a balanced diet and obtaining enough sleep. Individuals should be alerted to the fact that stress depletes their energy resources. If they suffer from insomnia, they may benefit from sleeping medication because it is difficult to cope if one is fatigued. However, they should be discouraged from taking tranquilizers or antidepressants during the day as these drugs may only block the grieving process.

Family members frequently need "permission to leave" because many feel that they should remain in the waiting room 24 hours a day. They fear the patient may awaken or deteriorate in their absence, and they will then have to cope with their guilt of missing that event. If rooms are available in close proximity to the hospital, family members may be convinced to go to them to sleep for short periods of time. Staff should reassure the relatives that they will be contacted if the patient awakens or if their condition deteriorates. Family members should also be advised that they may call if they awaken during the night and are concerned about the patient's condition. This may be helpful in reducing any unnecessary anxiety.

In a study conducted by Molter in 1979 family members of critically ill patients identified their most important visiting needs as the need to visit their relatives frequently and to be able to visit whenever they wanted. A study conducted by Stillwell in 1984 confirmed these findings. Thus, critical care staff members need to examine existing visitation policies that conflict with the needs of the patient and family. Although visitation policies may be necessary to ensure that patients receive adequate rest that is important in the healing process, staff need to be flexible and assess each situation individually, rather than adhere to rigid policies.

Intervention provided by social workers and/or chaplains should be available to grieving relatives. Social workers may act as liaisons between medical staff and families and, as such, may be helpful in setting up information sessions between relatives and physicians. Supportive intervention should be provided for the family of suspected brain-dead patients before requesting organs for purposes of transplantation. Supportive intervention involves creating privacy, clarifying any misconceptions, keeping the family well informed of the patient's deteriorating condition in efforts to lessen "the blow," encouraging ventilation, and validating feelings and concerns. Although it is not helpful to destroy the hope maintained by relatives, it is not constructive to offer false reassurance. Staff should be honest with relatives because it is difficult to cope effectively if they have no appreciation of the situation with which they are confronted.

VISITATION BY CHILDREN

Children should be spared the trauma of visiting a critical care unit if staff are convinced that the patient will eventually be transferred out of the unit. However, if the patient is suspected to be brain dead or unlikely to survive and his or her appearance is not grossly disfigured, it is not unreasonable to permit a child to visit. It is less devastating for a child to say goodbye to a person who is warm to the touch and appears to be sleeping than to a cold body in a funeral home.

It is important that children be adequately prepared for the visit. It may be helpful for a social worker or a nurse to explain to the child what he or she may expect to observe when visiting. During the visit, the child should be encouraged to ask questions, and time should be made available after the visit to address any negative feelings that may arise. Staff may also reduce the negative aspects of the experience by drawing curtains around patients in close proximity to the parent or grandparent whom the child is visiting so that the child only views the loved one. The child's parent or caregiver should alert staff to any emotional difficulties that may be observed after the visit. Changes in appetite, sleep disturbances, and changes in play may be indicators of such difficulties.

Children suffer from sleep disorders and other emotional disturbances if they are not adequately prepared for the visit, if they repress their negative feelings, or if they are forced to do something that they are uncomfortable doing. Thus, adequate preparation, encouragement of ventilation of any negative feelings that may arise, and refraining from encouraging the child to visit or do something that he or she is opposed to should prevent any residual difficulties.

ETHICAL DILEMMAS IN CRITICAL CARE

Because of recent technological advances, the line between life and death has become finer and at times blurred. Intensivists are challenged daily with decisions either to implement their knowledge of medicine and advanced technology aggressively or to withhold or withdraw life-sustaining machines, drugs, interventions, and nourishment. This decision-making process in the critical care unit has ethical, legal, and economic implications. Factors influencing this decision include patient autonomy, quality of life, prognosis, and treatment options. These factors need to be considered for both patient groups: the competent critically ill patient and the incompetent patient with an irreversible illness.

Competent Patient

Traditionally, physicians have adopted a paternalistic approach to decision making; however, paternalism runs counter to the patient's autonomy. The competency of critically ill patients may be difficult to assess when they are intubated, and competency is a prerequisite to autonomy. A physician may find it difficult to respect the wishes of critically ill patients who may be hypotensive or receiving analgesics and who experience fluctuations in their medical status. However, it is the ethical and legal right of patients to be informed of their diagnosis, available treatment options, risks involved, probable benefits, possible side effects, and likely costs. This objective information should be made available to the competent patient who then has the right and the liberty either to accept or reject treatment. The competent patient has the ultimate option to die with dignity.

There exist, however, certain situations where physicians may choose to take a paternalistic approach. The patient may have expressed a desire not to know, or the physician may perceive that informing the patient may generate emotional responses that may negatively affect the patient's condition. It is the general consensus, however, that patients cope more effectively if they express their fears and concerns, rather than suppressing or denying their feelings that may arise. Often, patients are already aware or suspicious of their prognosis, and they readily adopt mechanisms to cope with distressing news.

Competent patients must be involved in the decision-making process because they alone can define the quality of their lives. Studies have revealed that individuals fear abandonment, loneliness, and the process of dying more than death itself. Although most individuals do not want to die, few actually fear death, and given the choice some would choose death as opposed to existing in a dependent state that may involve emotional and/or physical suffering.

Cassel defines suffering as "the state of severe distress associated with events that threaten the intactness or wholeness of the person"; thus, suffering can only be defined by the patient. It may occur in the absence of symptoms and may be experienced by the family member who must view a loved one suffering.

According to Cassell, patients can tolerate severe physical pain for short periods if they anticipate or if they are reassured that the pain will be short lived. However, patients may become intolerant of minor pain or other symptoms that may cause suffering if they view it as chronic or never ending or if they feel their condition is considered hopeless.

To respond to the patient's suffering, Cassell suggests that diagnostic and therapeutic goals must be set (1) in terms of the patient and not the disease, (2) to maximize the patient's function and not the length of life, and (3) to minimize the patient's and the family's suffering actively. Hence, relief of suffering is a goal, and adequate pain relief is a hallmark of good care. Intensivists require special skills in providing compassionate care: effective communication skills so that a positive rapport may be established with the competent patient and a familiarity with the pharmacology of relieving symptoms. Treatment enhancing the support mechanisms of the patient's family and other health professionals can generally best be provided outside the critical care setting if feasible. Hence, a treatment goal in providing compassionate care may be to stabilize the patients so that they may be discharged to private rooms on medical floors where their families may visit for indefinite periods. If the prognosis is considered to be grave and the patient and the physicians are in agreement, nursing staff should be informed and a do not resuscitate (DNR) order should be written on the chart to prevent an unwarranted readmission to critical care.

If the patient and the physician disagree on the mode

of treatment, the physician should make an attempt to entertain the patient's concerns. Frequently, the patient has misinterpreted the information and the physician may need to utilize supportive and educative skills to alleviate any of the patient's misconceptions. If the patient and the physician still disagree, a second opinion should be obtained. If the patient still refuses treatment, the patient's wishes should be respected. However, a physician should not feel compelled to continue working with the patient. It is the physician's prerogative to withdraw from the case if he or she is uncomfortable either with continuing or withdrawing treatment contrary to the patient's request. The patient's care should be transferred to another physician.

Incompetent Patient

Caring for the incompetent patient presents more troubling ethical dilemmas for intensivists. With the exception of the patients who are brain dead, the neurologic recovery of many of the critically ill patients is difficult to predict. Physicians are compelled to exhaust all resources before practicing passive euthanasia, which allows the patient to die comfortably and naturally by withholding extraordinary procedures and medications that seem to be prolonging only misery.

Although incompetent patients are not capable of participating in the decision-making process, the physician may gain direction from other resources. These patients may have previously shared their wishes with their physician, a family member, or with a lawyer. Although the "living will" is legally recognized in only some states in the United States, it is a helpful guide for physicians because it reflects the patient's premorbid wishes.

Physicians should request that one family member be designated as the family spokesperson. This individual will take on the responsibility as the liaison with medical staff. The physician should meet with the spokesperson on a regular basis so that the eventual decision evolves as a process or consensus and not as an isolated event.

Family members or a patient's surrogate may offer valuable information about the patient's premorbid values and appreciation of an acceptable quality of life. However, occasionally, family members are unable to separate their feelings from those of the patient, and a health professional skilled in crisis intervention may be productive in assisting the family to ventilate their emotional concerns and view the decision more objectively. This objective opinion may be referred to as "substituted judgment."

The quality of a patient's life is difficult for a physician to assess unless he or she had previously received directive information from the patient. In a study conducted by Pearlman and Jonsen, the vagueness of the criterion of quality of life was shown when 205 physicians were asked to decide whether or not to intubate an elderly gentleman with chronic obstructive pulmonary disease. Eighty-seven percent of the physicians who chose not to intubate the patient indicated that the consideration of the patient's quality of life supported their decision. Of the physicians who chose to intubate the patient, eighty-two percent stated that the patient's quality of life positively supported their decision. The authors concluded, "It is noteworthy that these divergent evaluations of an individual's quality of life were used to justify polar treatment decisions of clinical significance."

There is, however, a point where the quality of life falls below a minimum standard, and continued treatment merely maintains organic life. Civetta suggests that the goal of preserving life should be replaced by the goal of alleviating suffering when a patient reaches his or her "x-point," which he defines as the point beyond which life cannot be extended with value, dignity, or meaning.

Because it is difficult to predict the prognosis of some critically ill patients, there is unfortunately no list of symptoms that can be devised based on diagnoses. Some authors suggest that extraordinary measures should be discontinued when the disease is irreversible and the patient receives no pleasure or satisfaction from continued existence, whereas others for whom a better prognosis exists could benefit from scarce life-support resources. In addition to a poor prognosis, the emotional costs to the family and staff of prolonging life should be considered.

Dyck offers three criteria for the decision-making process: factual knowledge, a vivid understanding of how everyone is affected by such actions and policies, and impartiality.

Although family members should be included in the decision-making process, they should not be approached to make the decision to change from aggressive to compassionate care. Family members may later feel guilty if they make this decision. They should be informed of the final decision, which should be made by physicians and their medical teams on the basis of their medical knowledge, technological background, experience, research, advice of colleagues, and in many facilities, an ethics committee for consultation in difficult cases.

The physician and the medical team may employ the "best interest" test or the "reasonable man" test, which is the treatment option that is in the best interest of the individual patient. Diverting from aggressive to compassionate care does not necessarily imply extubating the patient. Physicians may choose not to resuscitate or add any additional treatment, or they may choose to discontinue antibiotics, feedings, medications for supportive cardiac function, blood transfusions, and/or fluids.

In some circumstances, the family may require a period of time to accept the medical team's decision. However, this period should not exceed 24 hours. If after that period, the family is not prepared to accept the physician's decision, a second opinion should be obtained, followed by a submission to the ethics committee. In a complex situation where the family is still opposed to the treatment proposed, a concerned party may utilize the courts as a final resort. Physicians should be cognizant that the fear of litigation or the contemplation of potential litigation occurs more often than the reality. Physicians should not utilize the law as an excuse not to exercise good critical care decision making.

Suggested Readings

Cassell E: The relief of suffering. *Arch Intern Med* 143:522–523, 1983.

Civetta JM: Beyond technology: intensive care in the 1980's. *Crit Care Med* 9:763–767, 1981.

Dyck AJ: Ethical aspects of care for the dying incompetent. *J Am Geriatr Soc* 32:665–669, 1984.

Graham NK: Psycho-traumatology: crisis therapy in the trauma room. *Design Emerg Med* 1:1–3, 1981.

Meisel A, Grenvik A, Pinkus RL, Snyder JV: Hospital guidelines for deciding about life-sustaining treatment: dealing with health "limbo." *Crit Care Med* 14: 1986.

Pearlman RA, Jonsen A: The use of quality-of-life considerations in medical decision-making. *J Am Geriatr Soc* 33:342–52, 1985.

Rhodes J (ed): Psychology crises in the critical care unit. *Crit Care Q* 6:1–80, 1984.

Sherlock R, Dingus M: Families and the gravely ill: roles, rules and rights. *J Am Geriatr Soc* 33:121–124, 1985.

Wallace-Barnhill GL, Roth MD, Armstrong CJ, Hixon SE: Health care law update: legal protection for critical care physicians; state of the art determination of life support and living will legislation. *Crit Care Med* 12:56–61, 1984.

APPENDICES

CHAPTER

41 Appendix 1: Monitoring Techniques and Normal Values

William C. Ballantyne

The modern critical care unit provides many important facilities integral to the total care of the critically ill patient. One of the most important features is the capacity to monitor a wide variety of physiologic parameters and organ functions. This capacity allows the definition of existing abnormalities and the individual tailoring of therapy to meet the needs of each patient. The ideal monitoring system would be simple to institute and maintain, inexpensive, and of minimal risk to the patient. Unfortunately such a system is not available, so the benefits as well as the potential complications of each invasive monitoring technique must be well understood.

The purpose of this appendix is to outline important basic and advanced monitoring techniques and parameters presently available to the practicing physician, with their formulas, units of measure, and expected normal ranges. It is important to realize that "normal" values of commonly monitored physiologic variables may not be appropriate for the critically ill patient and may at times be misleading. The body responds to stress with physiologic compensations that attempt to preserve homeostasis, and these compensations may depart from physiologic norms. Appropriate care demands the proper understanding of these mechanisms and the reason for their deviation from expected values before any attempts to normalize these values are made.

All parameters should be viewed in the light of the clinical situation and only after a thorough physical examination of the patient. When measured indices and laboratory results conflict with clinical judgment, beware of technical error.

Collected data are most useful when they are efficiently displayed using a flow chart format. The charting system employed in the Critical Care/Trauma Centre at Victoria Hospital, London, Ontario, is reproduced in Figure 41.1.

Adequate monitoring of a critically ill patient begins with routine laboratory and hemodynamic parameters and is followed by more intensive investigation of basic organ systems. These are analyzed as follows: (1) cardiovascular, (2) pulmonary, (3) renal, (4) central nervous system, and (5) nutrition.

CARDIOVASCULAR SYSTEM

Most crucial to the welfare of critically ill patients is the maintenance of adequate cardiovascular function. The traditional approach to cardiovascular monitoring has included such parameters as heart rate, systemic blood pressure, urine output, central venous pressure, and the electrocardiogram. Although more sophisticated present-day monitoring techniques may overshadow these simple measurements, they should not be dismissed from consideration. For example, pulse rate is a more sensitive early indicator of hypovolemic shock than systemic blood pressure, and urinary output is likely one of the best and most readily available indicators of adequate tissue perfusion.

Simplified invasive cardiovascular techniques using balloon flotation catheters (Swan-Ganz catheter*), can now produce data at the bedside that reflect fundamental aspects of cardiovascular function. These techniques can simplify therapeutic decision making and lead to improved patient management. As invasive cardiac monitoring becomes more practical and more accessible, a larger number of physicians will feel comfortable with, and be able to interpret accurately, standard hemodynamic indices.

Noninvasive techniques have also become more sophisticated. Radionuclide angiography, using a mobile gamma camera, has led to a knowledge of ventricular volumes, varying myocardial contractile states, and dimensional ventricular geometry, all of which facilitate selection of therapies most likely to be successful.

Orderly monitoring of the cardiovascular system first requires the definition of its basic hemodynamic components. The following statements are derived from physiologic principles:

1. Blood pressure = cardiac output × systemic vascular resistance;
2. Cardiac output = heart rate × stroke volume;
3. Stroke volume is determined by (1) cardiac contractility; (2) preload (filling pressures), and (3) afterload (impedance to ejection or ventricular wall tension).

All cardiovascular derangements may be explained by an alteration in one or more of the components found in the preceding equations. As a result of modern technology, each variable can either be measured directly or derived from collected data. (Table 41.1)

*Edwards Laboratories, Santa Ana, California.

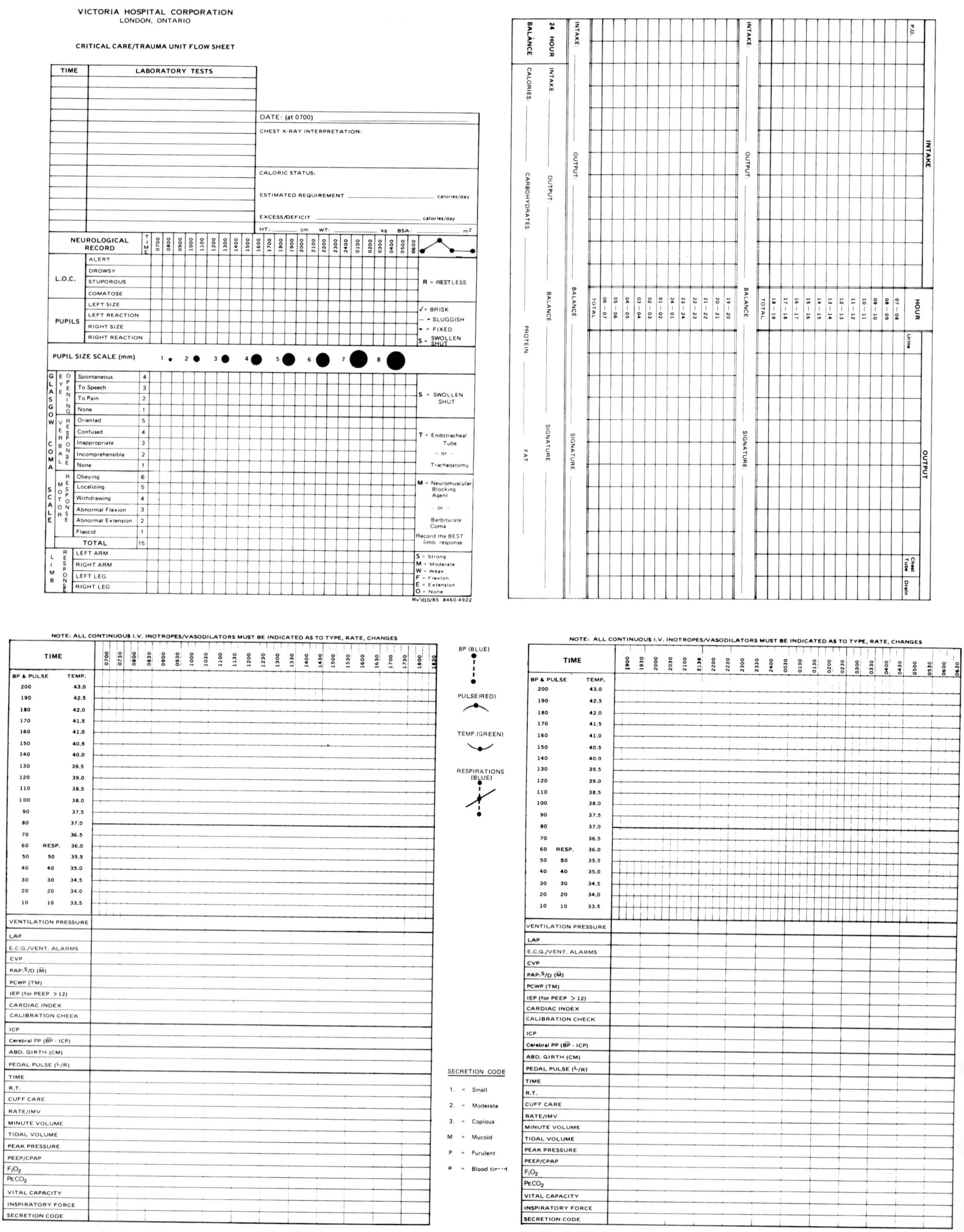

VICTORIA HOSPITAL CORPORATION
LONDON, ONTARIO

CRITICAL CARE/TRAUMA UNIT FLOW SHEET

TIME	LABORATORY TESTS

DATE: (at 0700)

CHEST X-RAY INTERPRETATION:

CALORIC STATUS:

ESTIMATED REQUIREMENT ______ calories/day

EXCESS/DEFICIT ______ calories/day

HT: ____ cm WT: ____ kg BSA: ____ m^2

NEUROLOGICAL RECORD		TIME	0700	0800	0900	1000	1100	1200	1300	1400	1500	1600	1700	1800	1900	2000	2100	2200	2300	2400	0100	0200	0300	0400	0500	0600	
L.O.C.	ALERT																										R = RESTLESS
	DROWSY																										
	STUPOROUS																										
	COMATOSE																										
PUPILS	LEFT SIZE																										✓= BRISK
	LEFT REACTION																										— = SLUGGISH
	RIGHT SIZE																										= = FIXED
	RIGHT REACTION																										S = SWOLLEN SHUT

PUPIL SIZE SCALE (mm) 1 2 3 4 5 6 7 8

GLASGOW COMA SCALE			
EYE OPENING	Spontaneous	4	S = SWOLLEN SHUT
	To Speech	3	
	To Pain	2	
	None	1	
VERBAL RESPONSE	Oriented	5	T = Endotracheal Tube — or — Tracheostomy
	Confused	4	
	Inappropriate	3	
	Incomprehensible	2	
	None	1	
MOTOR RESPONSE	Obeying	6	M = Neuromuscular Blocking Agent — or — Barbiturate Coma
	Localizing	5	
	Withdrawing	4	
	Abnormal Flexion	3	
	Abnormal Extension	2	
	Flaccid	1	Record the BEST limb response
	TOTAL	15	

LIMB RESPONSE		
	LEFT ARM	S = Strong
	RIGHT ARM	M = Moderate, W = Weak
	LEFT LEG	F = Flexion, E = Extension
	RIGHT LEG	O = None

Rv'd10/85 8460-4922

INTAKE — P.O. — HOUR: 07–08, 08–09, 09–10, 10–11, 11–12, 12–13, 13–14, 14–15, 15–16, 16–17, 17–18, 18–19, TOTAL — INTAKE: OUTPUT: BALANCE: SIGNATURE:

OUTPUT — Urine — Chest Tube — Drain

HOUR: 19–20, 20–21, 21–22, 22–23, 23–24, 24–01, 01–02, 02–03, 03–04, 04–05, 05–06, 06–07, TOTAL — INTAKE: OUTPUT: BALANCE: SIGNATURE:

24 HOUR BALANCE — INTAKE ____ OUTPUT ____ BALANCE ____ SIGNATURE ____

CALORIES: ____ CARBOHYDRATES ____ PROTEIN ____ FAT ____

NOTE: ALL CONTINUOUS I.V. INOTROPES/VASODILATORS MUST BE INDICATED AS TO TYPE, RATE, CHANGES

TIME: 0700 0730 0800 0830 0900 0930 1000 1030 1100 1130 1200 1230 1300 1330 1400 1430 1500 1530 1600 1630 1700 1730 1800 1830

BP & PULSE	RESP.	TEMP.
200		43.0
190		42.5
180		42.0
170		41.5
160		41.0
150		40.5
140		40.0
130		39.5
120		39.0
110		38.5
100		38.0
90		37.5
80		37.0
70		36.5
60		36.0
50	50	35.5
40	40	35.0
30	30	34.5
20	20	34.0
10	10	33.5

VENTILATION PRESSURE
LAP
E.C.G./VENT. ALARMS
CVP
PAP: S/D (M̄)
PCWP (TM)
IEP (for PEEP >12)
CARDIAC INDEX
CALIBRATION CHECK
ICP
Cerebral PP (B̄P - ICP)
ABD. GIRTH (CM)
PEDAL PULSE (L/R)
TIME
R.T.
CUFF CARE
RATE/IMV
MINUTE VOLUME
TIDAL VOLUME
PEAK PRESSURE
PEEP/CPAP
F_iO_2
P_ECO_2
VITAL CAPACITY
INSPIRATORY FORCE
SECRETION CODE

BP (BLUE)
PULSE (RED)
TEMP. (GREEN)
RESPIRATIONS (BLUE)

SECRETION CODE
1. = Small
2. = Moderate
3. = Copious
M = Mucoid
P = Purulent
P = Blood tinged

NOTE: ALL CONTINUOUS I.V. INOTROPES/VASODILATORS MUST BE INDICATED AS TO TYPE, RATE, CHANGES

TIME: 1900 1930 2000 2030 2100 2130 2200 2230 2300 2330 2400 0030 0100 0130 0200 0230 0300 0330 0400 0430 0500 0530 0600 0630

(Same BP & PULSE / RESP. / TEMP. scale and row labels as above.)

Figure 41.1. Critical care flow sheet.

Table 41.1
Cardiovascular Indices

Formula	Normal value
Stroke volume (Sv) (ml/beat) = $\frac{\text{CO (ml)}}{\text{Heart rate}}$	60–70 ml/min
Stroke index (SI) (ml/min/m^2) = $\frac{\text{Stroke volume}}{\text{Body surface area}}$	35–45 ml/min/m^2
Mean arterial pressure (MAP) = $\frac{\text{Pulse pressure}}{3}$ + diastolic pressure	85–95 mm Hg
Mean pulmonary artery pressure ($\overline{\text{PA}}$) may be directly measured from digital display or calculated as in MAP.	10–17 mm Hg
Right ventricular stroke work (RVSW) (gm/M/m^2) = SI × $\overline{\text{PAP}}$ (mm Hg) × 0.0136	8–12 gm/M/m^2
Left ventricular stroke work (LVSW) (gm/M/m^2) = SI × MAP × 0.0136	51–61 gm/M/m^2
Pulmonary vascular resistance (PVR) (dynes/sec/cm^{-5}) = $\frac{\overline{\text{PA}}\text{ (mm Hg)} - \overline{\text{PWP}}\text{ (mm Hg)} \times 79.9}{\text{CO (liter/min)}}$	150–250 dynes/sec/cm^{-5}
Systemic vascular resistance (SVR) or total peripheral resistance (TPR) = $\frac{\text{MAP (mm Hg)} - \text{CVP (mm Hg)} \times 79.9}{\text{CO (liter/min)}}$	900–1200 dynes/sec/cm^{-5}

Systemic Blood Pressure

Systemic blood pressure can be measured by both invasive and noninvasive techniques. The traditional cuff method is acceptable in many cases, but an inlying arterial cannula provides the continuous oscilloscopic and digital displays necessary for the management of an unstable cardiovascular system. The arterial line also provides a convenient access site for blood gas determinations.

Radial artery cannulation by either percutaneous or cutdown techniques should be done only after the performance of an Allen test to ensure adequate ulnar collateral arterial flow to the hand. Other peripheral arterial sites are equally acceptable, including dorsalis pedis and superficial temporal arteries. More central sites, such as femoral and brachial arteries, should be used when fewer options exist, due to the inherent complications of more centrally placed arterial lines.

A disparity routinely exists between indirect and direct blood pressure measurements. The majority of these discrepancies are minor and can be attributed to the anatomy of the human arm. The inlying radial pressures should always be higher than cuff-occluded brachial pressures. Discrepancies of over 20 mm Hg in the absence of peripheral vasoconstriction or shock are usually due to less than ideal technique and/or equipment problems.

In the shock state, sympathoadrenal discharges are responsible for the preferential shunting of blood to vital structures and away from nonessential areas, such as extremities and skin. For this reason the technically correct reading obtained from a peripheral artery may be far below actual core blood pressures.

Cardiac Output

Cardiac output (CO) determinations have been simplified with the use of thermodilution Swan-Ganz pulmonary artery catheters. A thermodilution computer measures the time interval required for a 10-ml bolus of iced saline to travel from the central venous pressure (CVP) port to the catheter tip and from this computes cardiac output. Normal CO = 5–6 liters/min.

Cardiac Index

Cardiac index (CI) is cardiac output that has been corrected for the patient's body surface area (BSA), thus allowing a standardized index for comparative purposes. CI = CO (liters/min)/BSA (m^2). Normal CI = 2.5–3.5 liters/min/m^2; values of less than 2.0 liters/min/m^2 indicate severe cardiac dysfunction.

Preload

Preload refers to the end-diastolic volume present in the ventricle just before its contraction. It is routinely measured as the end-diastolic pressure. From the work of Otto Frank and Ernest Starling we know that the pumping action of the ventricle is dependent on the volume of blood delivered to it in diastole. Preload = ventricular end-diastolic volume (Normal = 70 ml/m^2). Measured pressures (i.e., pulmonary capillary wedge pressure (PCWP) do not accurately reflect ventricular compliance relationships discussed below.

Central Venous Pressure and Pulmonary Wedge Pressure

Central venous pressure (CVP) reflects right-sided venous pressure and end-diastolic volume. Pulmonary wedge pressure (PCWP) accurately reflects left-sided filling pressures by measuring the pressure in a static-free column of blood extending from the catheter tip to the left atrium. CVP will only secondarily reflect altered left-sided function and may be unreliable when rapidly changing cardiac status is present or in the presence of pre-existing pulmonary vascular disease. In general, hemodynamic trends are more valuable than isolated readings when an unstable circulatory system exists. Normal CVP = 5–12 cm H_2O. Normal PCWP = 5–12 cm H_2O.

Ventricular Compliance

Ventricular compliance refers to ventricular distensibility. It is commonly decreased after episodes of myocardial ischemia and infarction; therefore, higher preloads (end-diastolic pressures) represent a constant volume necessary to maintain cardiac output. Patients with reduced compliance respond less efficiently to altered filling pressures caused by blood loss or fluid challenge (Fig. 41.2).

Afterload

Afterload describes the impedance or resistance against which the ventricle must contract after the semilunar valves are open. It also represents ventricular wall tension developed for ejection purposes. Afterload is primarily a function of peripheral resistance, and these resistances may be calculated for both pulmonary and systemic circulations. As mentioned previously, blood pressure is intimately associated with peripheral resistance (afterload). Decreased afterload may lead to increased cardiac output and vice versa. This is the key consideration in afterload reduction therapy (see Chapter 5). Measured pressures (i.e., pulmonary capillary wedge pressure (PCWP)) do not accurately reflect ventricular preload because of the ventricular compliance relationships discussed below (Figure 41.2).

Myocardial Oxygen Consumption

The determinants of myocardial oxygen consumption MVO_2 include (1) heart rate, (2) contractility, (3) afterload, and (4) myocardial wall tension. Clinically, MVO_2 = HR × systolic BP product (see Chapter 5).

PULMONARY

The monitoring of pulmonary function can be divided into three areas of consideration: (1) oxygenation, (2) ventilation, and (3) lung-thorax mechanics.

Oxygenation

The arterial partial pressure of oxygen (PaO_2) is the best index of oxygenation, but it is of minimal clinical importance without knowledge of the inspired oxygen concentration (FiO_2). A simple means of relating these two measurements is the PaO_2/FiO_2, which reflects the efficiency of oxygen uptake by the lungs, but does not identify the cause of hypoxia. Normal $PaO_2/FiO_2 = 400–500$. Severe dysfunction = <300.

Alveolar-Arterial Oxygen Gradient

Alveolar-arterial oxygen gradient (A-a O_2) helps define the cause of hypoxemia. In the normal person a minimal barrier exists to the diffusion of oxygen across the alveolocapillary membrane, and the small differential that normally exists from the alveolus to mixed arterial blood can be explained by several factors:

1. Venous blood entering the left heart, i.e., bronchial blood flow and Thebesian veins;
2. Anatomic shunts present in the lung; normally 2–5% accounting for 50% of the A-a O_2;
3. Regional disparities of ventilation to perfusion ($\dot{V}a/\dot{Q}t$)—physiologic shunts.

An increased A-a O_2 can be due to (1) diffusion block at the alveolocapillary membrane (e.g., pulmonary edema) and (2) pathologic right-to-left shunts, e.g., arteriovenous malformation, atrial septal defect with reverse flow, and $\dot{V}a/\dot{Q}t$ abnormalities. Administration of 100% oxygen will improve the A-a O_2 due to diffusion block, but will not improve that due to shunting.

The alveolar oxygen tension on 100% oxygen can be calculated by subtracting the water vapor pressure (PH_2O) and the $PaCO_2$ from the barometric pressure (P_B). $P_AO_2 = P_B - (PH_2O + PaCO_2)$. Therefore A-a $O_2 = P_A - PaO_2$. The trend is more important than the ab-

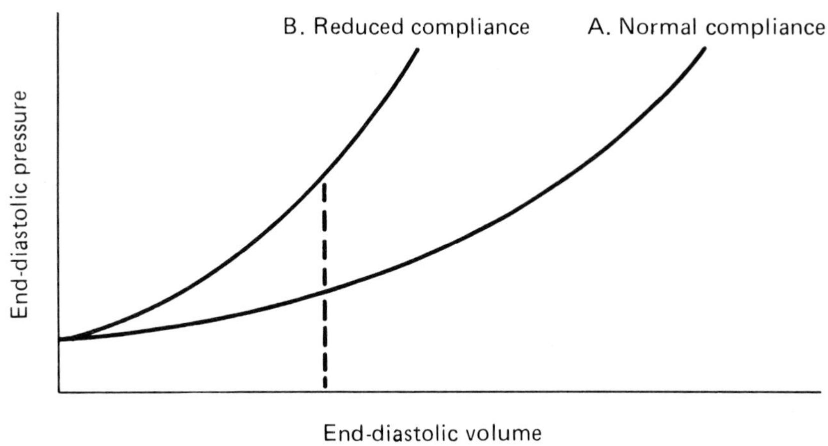

Reduced compliance (B) leads to a larger increase in end-diastolic pressure for any given volume increase, compared to normal compliance (A). This increases the chances of pulmonary edema formation with small increases in EDV in a noncompliant ventricle.

Figure 41.2. Effect of altered ventricular compliance.

solute value, and although a normal gradient of A-a O_2 is 10–20 mm Hg, a value of less than 200 may be acceptable in postinjury patients.

Pulmonary Shunt

Pulmonary shunt ($\dot{Q}s/\dot{Q}t$) can be measured following ventilation on 100% oxygen for 20 minutes using the modified Berggren's formula. Mixed venous and arterial blood must be analyzed for blood gases and oxygen saturation.

$$\frac{Qs}{Qt}=\frac{(P_AO_2-PaO_2)\times 0.0031}{(CaO_2-CvO_2)+(P_AO_2-PaO_2)\times 0.0031}$$

where $CaO_2=1.39\times Hb\times SaO_2+(PaO_2\times 0.0031)$ and $CvO_2=1.39\times Hb\times SvO_2+(PvO_2\times 0.0031)$. This calculation describes how many alveoli are perfused but not ventilated. Normally a shunt of 5–8% exists.

Ventilation

Ventilation refers to the movement of gases from the atmosphere to the alveolar sites of gas exchange. Arterial CO_2 tension ($PaCO_2$) is the best index of alveolar ventilation due to its rapid capillary-alveolar diffusability. Under normal circumstances ventilation will excrete all CO_2 produced by the tissues and hence maintain a normal $PaCO_2$.

Adequate ventilation is the end result of several factors that can be manipulated in the critically ill patient.

1. Tidal volume (V_T): normal = 500 ml;
2. Respiratory rate (RR): normal = 18–20/min;
3. Minute volume (MV) ($V_T\times$ rate): normal = 8–10 liters/min;
4. Dead space (V_D): normal = 150 ml.

Clinical experience with ventilated patients has shown that tidal volumes of 10–15 ml/kg are required to avoid small airway closure. With these high volumes, a slower rate of 10–15 respirations/min is necessary to avoid hypocarbia. If the MV is greater than expected to maintain normal $PaCO_2$, this may indicate increased CO_2 production, often seen in sepsis or with hyperalimentation.

The relationship of total dead space—the sum of "anatomic" plus "alveolar" dead space (i.e., alveoli ventilated but not perfused)—to tidal volume is also useful when the $PaCO_2$ of expired air ($PeCO_2$) can be measured.

$$\frac{V_D}{V_T}=\frac{PaCO_2-PeCO_2}{PaCO_2}\qquad \text{Normal} < 0.3.$$

Lung-Thorax Mechanics

All mechanical disorders of the lungs and chest increase the work of breathing. A few simple measurements exist that adequately describe lung mechanics.

Vital Capacity

Vital capacity (VC) is defined as the largest volume of gas expired after maximal inspiration. It is a simple measurement of ventilatory reserve, which is a valuable monitoring index. In patients with neuromuscular disorders or other restrictive disease of lung and chest wall, vital capacity often correlates well with dyspnea; marked decreases can occur before blood gas abnormalities become evident. If the vital capacity is more than three times the patient's normal tidal volume, hypoventilation should not occur while at rest. Mechanical abnormalities most commonly causing dyspnea are increased airway resistance and decreased lung and chest wall compliance. Normal VC = 65–75 ml/kg.

Flow Rate

Flow rate measurements during a maximum effort expiratory maneuver have a useful relationship to airway resistance. The most common, simple measure of airway resistance is the forced expiratory volume over a 1-second interval (FEV_1). Normal values for a variety of populations are available, as well as correlation with the degree of clinical disability and long- and short-term prognoses for impairment due to a variety of disorders.

Compliance

Compliance refers to the ability of the lung to expand. Most lung disorders associated with critical illness cause a reduction in compliance, thereby increasing the work of breathing. A simple measure of effective compliance in ventilated patients is volume change per unit of pressure applied:

Effective compliance

$$=\frac{\text{Tidal volume } (V_T)}{\text{Peak inspiratory pressure (PIP)}}$$

(Normal = 30–35 ml/cm of H_2O)

RENAL MONITORING

Renal dysfunction is a serious and all too common complication of critical illness. Certain key principles are useful in avoiding acute renal failure in the critically ill patient. These include avoidance of sustained hypotension, careful regulation of potentially nephrotoxic agents, and the prevention of sepsis.

The monitoring of renal function requires an assessment of the adequacy of plasma volume, specific renal function tests, and the exclusion of obstruction. Improved methods of fluid resuscitation and estimating effective circulating plasma volume have decreased the incidence of prerenal oliguria.

Clearance

Clearance refers to removal of a substance from the blood by the kidney. Clearance = UV/P, where U = concentration of substance in urine (mg/ml), V = volume of urine per minute, P = concentration of substance in plasma (mg/ml).

With certain substances (e.g., insulin, mannitol), clearance is equal to the glomerular filtration rate (GFR). Clinically, creatinine clearance is used as a measure of GFR. Tissue trauma and altered muscle metabolism after trauma may lead to increased loads of creatinine being presented to the kidney. Therefore an apparently normal creatinine clearance may be misleading; the GFR may in fact be decreased by a factor of two or three.

Urinary Sodium

Urinary sodium is important in the evaluation of acute oliguria and may help in differentiating acute tubular necrosis from prerenal azotemia. Urinary sodium concentration should be low (10–20 mEq/liter) in patients with intravascular volume depletion without intrinsic renal damage. In oliguric acute renal failure (ARF), urinary sodium is usually greater than 30–40 mEq/liter. These values are unreliable in the face of recent diuretic administration.

Simultaneous measurements of urine and plasma concentrations of solutes can be helpful as a simple spot check of renal function. A valuable measure is the urine to plasma osmolar ratio (U/P osm). This represents the work of the kidney done to concentrate urine. The maximum value seen is 4, and a U/P osm above 1.7 indicates good concentrating ability. Several other tests based on simultaneous measurements are helpful, including U/P urea nitrogen and U/P creatinine ratios. Two calculated indices that may be more specific in separating prerenal from oliguric acute renal failure are (Table 41.2):

1. Renal failure index $= \dfrac{\text{U Na}}{\text{U/P creatinine}}$
2. Fractional excretion of filtered sodium (FeNa) $= \dfrac{\text{U/P Na}}{\text{U/P creatinine} \times 100}$

Renal monitoring can be separated into general and specific considerations. The general considerations include arterial BP, intake/output, ECG, CVP and PCWP, and serum electrolytes, BUN, creatinine. Specific urinary indices include urine osmolality, urine Na (mEq/liter), U/P urea nitrogen, U/P creatinine, renal failure index, and fractional excretion of filtered sodium.

It is important to emphasize that a small but significant percentage of patients with either prerenal oliguria or oliguric ARF may have intermediate values, making a sharp distinction between groups impossible. Also, patients with nonoliguric ARF may have intermediate values, suggesting that the urinary diagnostic indices listed in Table 41.2 are predominantly of value in the oliguric patient. Both the renal failure index and the fractional excretion of sodium (FeNa) minimize the overlap between prerenal and oliguric ARF groups and are therefore the most reliable indices for differentiating between these two forms of oliguria.

Acute glomerulonephritis may present with urinary diagnostic indices similar to prerenal oliguria (i.e., high U/P osmolar ratios), thereby suggesting that renal tubular function is intact early in the course of acute glomerular lesions. In this situation the clinical history and urinalysis can usually distinguish between these entities. In the majority of cases, these few simple tests, combined with general monitoring parameters, will specify the etiology of oliguric renal dysfunction.

Table 41.2
Valves for Specific Urinary Indices in Oliguric Renal Failure

Index	Prerenal	Oliguric ARF
Urine osmolality	>500	<350
Urine Na (mEq/liter)	< 20	> 40
U/P urea nitrogen	> 8	< 3
U/P creatinine	> 40	< 20
Renal failure index	< 1	> 1
Fractional excretion of filtered sodium	< 1	> 1

CENTRAL NERVOUS SYSTEM

Frequent clinical examination to assess responsiveness, both level of consciousness and neurologic status, remains the most valuable monitor of cerebral function. Skilled observation is by far the most discriminating method of cerebral monitoring. A standardized method of recording pertinent findings for therapy and prognosis is found in the Glasgow Coma Scale (see Chapter 19 and Table 41.3).

However, clinical examination often lacks objectivity and quantification and may therefore have some disadvantages. Also, the peripheral neurologic manifestations of illness may not reflect minute-to-minute changes that are occurring centrally. Certain clinical situations obscure physical findings and necessitate other means of cerebral monitoring, e.g., Pentothal coma or pharmacologically induced paralysis. Objective monitoring methods are therefore necessary.

Electroencephalogram

The electrical activity arising from cortical neurons may be recorded at the skin surface as an electroencephalogram (EEG). Frequency and amplitude of electrical wave patterns can indicate depth of coma, as well as region and extent of injury. Conventional EEG recording has not been widely accepted as a means of continuous monitoring, but it has been useful in supporting a diagnosis of brain death.

Intracranial Pressure

Increased intracranial pressure (ICP) is an important factor governing cerebral demise in critically ill neuro-

Table 41.3
Glasgow Coma Scale

	Response category[a]		
Score	Motor	Verbal	Eye opening
6	Obeys		
5	Localizes	Oriented	
4	Normal flexor (good withdrawal)	Confused	Spontaneously
3	Abnormal flexor (purposeless, random)	Inappropriate, but says words	To sound
2	Extensor (decerebrate)	Incomprehensible, but utters sounds	To pain
1	Nil	Nil	Nil

[a]Note: record best response, from best side. Any falloff in numerical score is a danger sign.

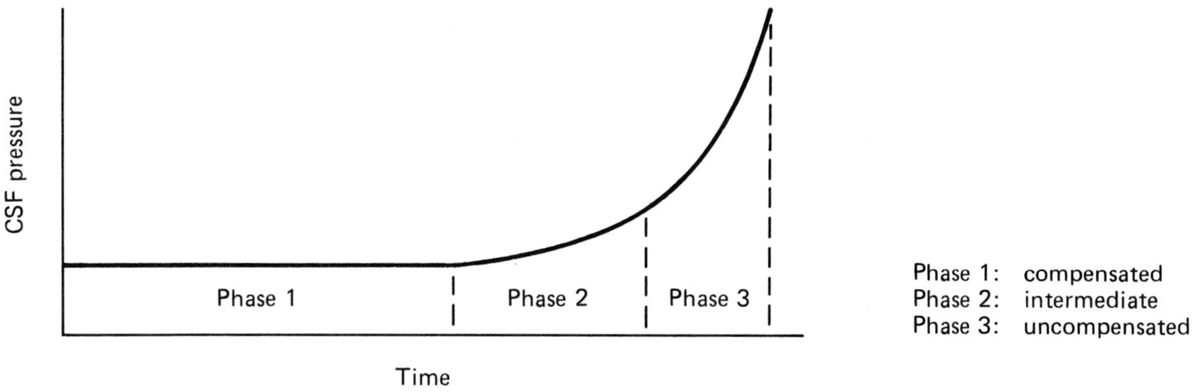

Figure 41.3. Intracranial pressure-volume curve.

surgical patients. The intracranial contents are brain, blood, and cerebrospinal fluid (CSF). The closed-box theory of intracranial pressure states that any space-occupying lesion expands at the expense of one or more of the three basic contents. An intracranial pressure line gives information about the state of intracranial compression produced by space-occupying disease states, whether hemorrhage, tumor, or edema.

The intracranial pressure-volume curve (Fig. 41.3) has three phases. *Phase 1* is the compensated phase during which intracranial pressure rises little with expansion of the space-occupying lesion. *Phase 2* is the intermediate stage. *Phase 3* is the uncompensated terminal phase during which ICP rises rapidly with minimal increases in volume of the lesion.

There are several approaches to ICP monitoring: intraventricular and subarachnoid, which are both direct, and subdural and extradural, which are indirect. Intraventricular lines allow direct access to CSF for drainage purposes to lower ICP, for acid/base measurements, and for the assessment of intracranial compliance. Subarachnoid bolts provide access to CSF as well, but in our experience the pressure readings are less reliable than those from intraventricular lines. Subdural and extradural transducers provide indirect measurements, but are not used in our critical care/trauma unit.

Cerebral Perfusing Pressure

Cerebral perfusing pressure is defined as mean arterial pressure (MAP)-ICP. ICP monitoring is of value in the management of the acute stage of severe head injury, providing early warning of intracranial bleeding or cerebral edema. It is also of value in the monitoring of cerebral edema therapy by such techniques as hyperventilation, dehydration, or steroids. Normal cerebral perfusing pressure = 60–80 mm Hg.

NUTRITION

The past decade has witnessed a growing awareness of nutritional problems in hospitalized patients, stimulated by the knowledge that malnutrition will interact with all disease processes to impair significantly host responses to stressful illness. The basic factors determining metabolic energy requirements are

1. Nutritional state of the patient before the illness;
2. Extent of catabolism associated with the disease process;
3. Time elapsed from the onset of the disease process.

The nutritional problems of hospitalized patients may be separated into two major groups. Group 1 patients have standard nutritional requirements, but because of illness they are unable to maintain an adequate oral intake. These patients are starvation adapted, for they efficiently utilize body stores of fat and protein to maintain basal metabolic requirements while at the same time attempting to spare protein reserves. Supplemental carbohydrate, protein, and fat are well accepted by these patients.

Group 2 patients have dramatically increased nutritional requirements as a result of the metabolic stress associated with their illness (Fig. 41.4). This problem is also complicated by the less efficient management of existing body energy stores. These catabolic patients characteristically utilize protein stores as their primary endogenous energy source, leading to a rapid depletion of both visceral and somatic protein reserves. A delay in the recognition of group 2 patients or in the institution of adequate nutritional support can contribute to their early demise.

Unfortunately, no individual parameter exists that will provide a completely accurate assessment of nutritional status and ongoing nutritional requirements. For this reason a battery of tests must be employed in a serial fashion to determine nutritional status and the response to nutritional therapy.

Nutritional support during illness is directed primarily toward the preservation of each patient's lean body mass, which is the metabolically active, oxygen-consuming, and work-performing tissue of the body. The most important components of this lean body mass are the somatic and visceral protein stores; namely, skeletal muscle and the body organs. For this reason, an accurate nutritional assessment should reflect the body's protein reserves.

In the healthy individual, body weight provides a simple monitor of general nutritional status. It may also be helpful in uncomplicated starvation adaptation, but be-

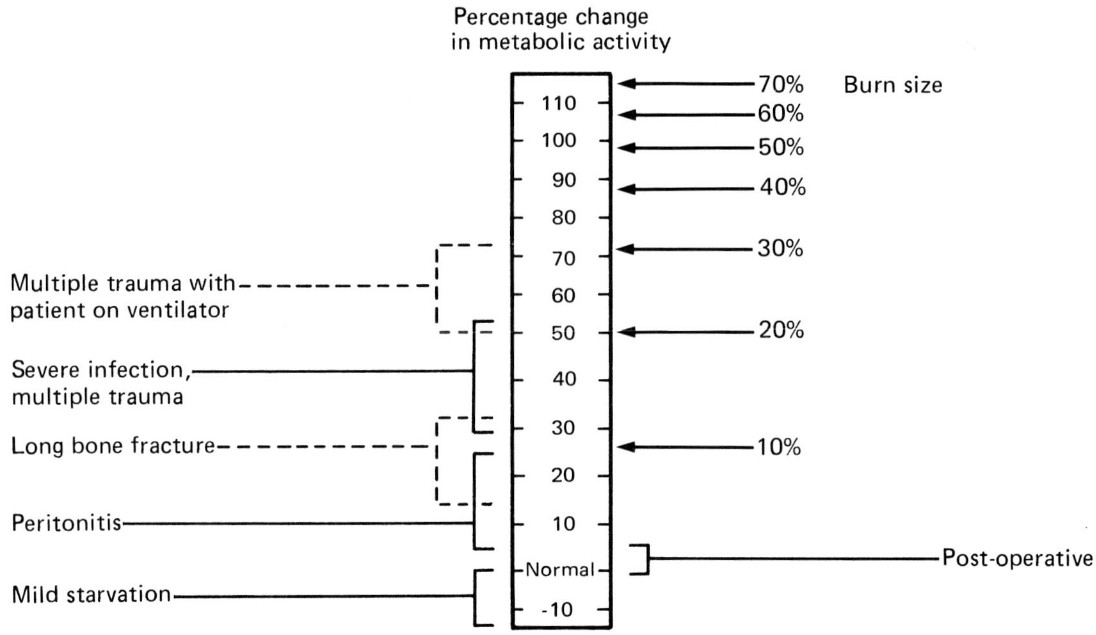

Figure 41.4. Estimation of energy requirements for the critically ill patient.

cause catabolic illness is often characterized by large swings in fluid volume status, body weight is of little use in assessing nutritional status. *Anthropometric measurements,* such as midarm circumference and triceps skin fold, are an attempt to characterize skeletal muscle and fat stores.

The *creatinine-height index* is based on the knowledge that creatinine is elaborated from muscle at a constant rate that is proportional to the patient's muscle stores. Tables of ideal urinary creatinine for height are employed to calculate this index.

$$\text{Creatinine height index} = \frac{\text{Actual urinary creatine}}{\text{Ideal urinary creatinine}} \times 100$$

The result is expressed as a percentage of normal. Again this test is more reliable in starvation adaptation than during catabolic illness, and it relies heavily on normal renal function.

Many attempts have been made to correlate the levels of circulating substances, including albumin, transferrin, and total proteins, with nutritional status. Albumin and transferrin concentrations often fall as a reflection of chronic malnutrition, but are of questionable value during an acute illness.

Probably the most important function of the visceral protein compartment is immune competence, and logically, immune competence may be altered by malnutrition. Many other factors can be responsible for altered immune function, but during the last decade a clear correlation between nutrition and immune competence has been established. Delayed hypersensitivity skin testing to a series of antigens provides information on the cellular component of immune function and therefore can provide a useful index of nutritional status.

The somatic protein compartment has formerly been examined with nitrogen balance studies, but these can be both expensive and cumbersome. Wilmore has described a simple method of calculating clinical nitrogen balance from the equation:

$$\text{Nitrogen balance} = \text{Nitrogen in} - \text{Nitrogen out}$$

Dietary nitrogen represents nitrogen intake, and nitrogen excretion is calculated using a simple formula that allows for unmeasured losses in sweat and feces.

$$\begin{aligned}&\text{Nitrogen loss (gm/day)}\\&= \text{Urinary urea nitrogen (mg/100 ml)}\\&\quad \times \text{urinary volume (1/day)} \div 100\\&\quad + 20\%\ \text{urinary urea loss} + 2\ \text{gm.}\end{aligned}$$

Example: Urinary urea nitrogen = 500 mg/100 ml, urine volume—2 liters.

$$\begin{aligned}\text{Nitrogen loss} &= 500 \times 2 \times \frac{1}{100} \times 120\% + 2\\ &= 10 \times \frac{120}{100} + 2 = 12 + 2 = 14\ \text{gm}\end{aligned}$$

Sophisticated experimental techniques exist that will more accurately define the lean body mass, but their principles and applications are beyond the scope of this text.

Early recognition of patients with increased metabolic requirements and early institution of alimentation by the most readily available route are the keys to nutritional monitoring and support. The GI tract should be the preferred route because of the expense and potential complications associated with intravenous alimentation.

Suggested Readings

Carrico CJ, Horonitz JH: Monitoring the critically ill surgical patient. *Adv Surg* 11:101–127, 1977.

Gorlin R: Practical cardiac hemodynamics, current concepts in cardiology. *N Engl J Med* 296:203, 1977.

Guenter CA, Welch MH, Hogg JC: *Clinical Aspects of Respiratory Physiology*. Philadelphia, JB Lippincott, 1978.
McDowall DG: Monitoring the brain. *Anaesthesiology* 45:117–134, 1976.
Miller TR, Anderson RJ: Urinary diagnostic indices in acute renal failure. *Ann Intern Med* 89:47–50, 1978.
Pietsch JB, Meakins JL: Predicting infection in surgical patients. *Surg Clin North Am* 59:185–197, 1979.
Swan HJC: The role of hemodynamic monitoring in the management of the critically ill. *Crit Care Med* 3:83–89, 1975.
Wilmore DW: *The Metabolic Management of the Critically Ill*. New York, Plenum Medical Book Co, 1977.

CHAPTER

42 Appendix 2: Drugs Used in the Treatment of the Critically Ill Patient

Sandra G. Campbell, B.Sc. Phm.

The management of the critically ill patient has become a highly specialized and sophisticated field in which pharmacologic intervention plays a major role. The use of newly developed antimicrobial, antihypertensive, and inotropic agents and improved understanding of older agents have enhanced the practitioner's ability to modify the underlying disease process and thus care for his or her patients.

Unfortunately, the use of these new drugs does not in itself promote better health care or guarantee benefit to the patient. For with all the advantages of availability, potency, and selectivity come the risk and dilemmas of toxicity, adverse effects, and drug interactions in an already severely compromised patient. No longer is it sufficient or wise to administer the "usual" or "standard" dose of a drug without consideration of concomitant therapy, alterations in homeostasis, and the implications of alternate therapeutic modalities. To be able to weigh all the factors affecting therapy and thereby achieve rational drug usage, the practitioner must keep abreast of the current explosion of pharmaceutical literature. The purpose of this chapter is to fulfill, in part, that need and to provide the various members of the health team dealing with the critically ill patient a working manual of pharmaceutical knowledge. It is not intended to be an all-inclusive reference text, but it is meant to highlight important aspects of drug therapy seen in critical care situations and supplement other readily available information sources. Many of the recommendations made are based on experience gained in the Critical Care Trauma Centre at Victoria Hospital.

FORMAT

This chapter contains a list of drugs that are used frequently in the ICU setting. Information is contained under several different headings enabling the user to find the desired information quickly. Drugs are listed alphabetically by generic name, and proprietary names are given in parenthesis. The abbreviations used are *po,* by mouth; *SC,* subcutaneous, *q6h,* every 6 hours; *D5W,* 5% dextrose and water; *NS,* normal saline; and *RL,* Ringer's lactate. References, coded by superior number in the text, are listed at the end of the chapter. The description of each drug starts with a statement of the drug's pharmacology and major effects and is subdivided as follows:

Dosage

The adult dosage and dosage ranges used in the ICU are listed in this section; among these the reader will find several nonapproved routes of administration. Our positive experiences, in combination with extensive monitoring, have validated the safety and efficacy of drugs administered via these routes in our unit. Pediatric doses are not included. The user is encouraged to read the rest of the description, paying particular attention to the section, "Dosage Adjustments and Precautions," before prescribing the drug.

Pharmacokinetics and Biopharmaceutics

Pharmacokinetics is defined as the study of the movement of drugs within biologic systems as affected by absorption, distribution, metabolism, and elimination; it can be applied clinically to improve usage of specific agents. This study can show the effects of physiology and pathology on drug distribution and elimination, dosage adjustment in disease states, and the evaluation of drug interactions. In its most sophisticated form, pharmacokinetics can be used to develop therapeutic models and thus individualize dosage regimens with the aid of monitoring blood levels of the agent.

This section provides information on currently known pharmacokinetic parameters of the drugs used in the treatment of the critically ill patient. Terms such as bioavailability, half-life (T½), apparent volume distribution (Vd), and the metabolic fate of the agents are given, as well as information concerning the time required to achieve the peak effect and the duration of the therapeutic effect. Where applicable, this section equates responses elicited by the various routes of administration and dosage equivalents.

Bioavailability is a term that describes the extent of a drug's absorption from various dosage forms. Factors affecting bioavailability include the formulation of the dosage form and the first-pass effect. Certain agents, although readily absorbed from the GI tract, undergo extensive metabolism before reaching the systemic circulation. This results in the large dose disparities between oral and intravenous dosage forms.

The *half-life* of a drug is one of the most useful pharmacokinetic parameters in clinical practice. It is defined as the time required for one-half of the drug in the body to be eliminated. This variable is important in determining the dosing interval and the time required to excrete the drug. The half-life of an agent is also the sole determinant of the time needed to reach steady state plasma concentrations.

The *apparent volume of distribution* (Vd) reflects the extent of a drug's distribution. It must be remembered that the numerical value is "apparent" and does not necessarily refer to a real volume, but is instead a mathematical parameter that estimates the exposure of the body to a given drug. The Vd has been defined as the relationship of the plasma concentration achieved to the dose administered. Apparent distribution volumes that are very large and thus have no tangible physiologic meaning indicate that the particular agent is distributed throughout tissues or binds selectively to specific areas. Conversely, if the drug is restricted to a certain segment of the body water, the Vd will be equivalent to that of the compartment.

The Vd is a measure of the total amount of drug in the body and is thus used to estimate loading doses necessary to attain desired plasma concentrations.

Adverse Effects

Adverse effects listed are generally the short-term effects, i.e., effects that would occur in the ICU. If a more extensive list is required, the user is referred to other texts.

Dosing Adjustments and Precautions

In this section particular emphasis is placed on the pathologic states that alter drug effects or therapy. Included are such conditions as renal, hepatic disease, congestive heart failure (CHF), and hypoalbuminemia. Contraindications are not found within these descriptions, but it is under this subheading that precautions may be found that, depending on the situation, may represent relative or absolute contraindications.

Nursing Implications and Methods of Administration

This is a very broad section containing compatibility data, methods of administration, monitoring parameters, infusion guidelines, and dilutions commonly used.

Interactions

This section deals with drug/drug and drug/laboratory test interactions. This list is not exhaustive; however, it covers the drug combinations that may be used in the intensive care setting. The concomitant administration of two potential interactants may not necessarily produce a clinically significant effect.

AMRINONE (INOCOR)

Amrinone is a nonglycosidic, nonadrenergic inotropic agent. The exact mechanism of action is unknown; however, part of its activity could be related to its ability to inhibit myocardial phosphodiesterase. Amrinone acts as a vasodilator and reduces left ventricular filling pressures.[16,61]

Dosage

A loading dose of 0.75 mg/kg; IV below drip chamber (BDC) over 2–3 minutes. This dose may be repeated 30 minutes after therapy has begun. The initial loading dose is followed by a maintenance infusion of 5–10 μg/kg/min (maximum 20 μg/kg/min). Dosing adjustments should be made at a minimum of 1-hour intervals. The total daily dose should not exceed 10 mg/kg/day.[31,32]

Pharmacokinetics and Biopharmaceutics

IV duration: 60–90 minutes. Vd: 1.2 liter/kg; increased in congestive heart failure to 1.3–1.6 liter/kg. Protein binding reported range: 10–49%. Elimination T½: 3.6 hours; metabolized hepatically and 10–40% excreted unchanged by the kidney.[12,104]

Adverse Effects

Thrombocytopenia (dose-dependent), ventricular and supraventricular arrhythmias, hypotension, hepatotoxicity, fever, burning at the injection site.[31,100]

Dosage Adjustments and Precautions

The distribution and elimination of amrinone may be altered in congestive heart failure and renal and hepatic disease. Dosage reductions may be required; however, these have not yet been defined. Cautious use is advised in patients with aortic or pulmonic valvular disease, thrombocytopenia, or those receiving other drugs known to produce thrombocytopenia.[31]

Nursing Implications and Method of Administration

Amrinone may be given IV BDC and as a continuous infusion. The concentration recommended is 1–3 mg/ml, and amrinone must be mixed in a saline-containing solution (NS, 0.45 sodium chloride). It is not compatible with dextrose because a chemical interaction occurs resulting in a loss of potency. The prepared amrinone infusion may be piggy-backed into a running dextrose solution, if necessary. The undiluted solution must be protected from light for storage purposes. Start the dose of amrinone low and increase at hourly intervals according to cardiac indices. Monitor platelet count, hepatic function, HR, PCWP, MAP, CO, and ECG.[31,101]

Interactions

Amrinone + dopamine/dobutamine → improvement of cardiac function, probably secondary to amrinone's vasodilating properties; amrinone + disopyramide → decreased BP.[16,31]

ATROPINE

Atropine is a naturally occurring alkaloid of belladonna with parasympatholytic activity. Effects seen with increasing doses are *initial bradycardia* with atrioventricular (AV) dissociation followed by tachycardia, reduction of secretions and airway resistance, pupillary dilation, ciliary paralysis, and reduced GI motility and urinary bladder contractility.[61]

Dosage

0.6 to 1.0 mg IV repeated every 3 minutes until a total dose of 2.0 mg has been given. This dose may be repeated every 3–4 hours. Endotracheally: 1–2 mg in 10 ml water produces rapid and effective reversal of bradycardia.[66,78]

Pharmacokinetics and Biopharmaceutics

Onset (IV): rapid; Vd: 2–4 liters/kg. Fate: 30–50% eliminated unchanged in urine, the rest as metabolites. Primarily metabolized by enzymatic hydrolysis in the liver. $T\frac{1}{2} = 2–3$ hours.[61]

Adverse Effects

Dose dependent, from low to high doses: dryness of nose and mouth, bradycardia, fever, accelerated heart rate and mydriasis, flushed skin, tachycardia, palpitations, blurred vision, increased CNS involvement.[61]

Dosing Adjustments and Precautions

Caution in patients with glaucoma, obstruction of GI tract, paralytic ileus, unstable cardiovascular status.[26]

Nursing Implications and Methods of Administration

IV usual route of administration but may be given IM or SC; monitor vital signs; observe for changes in quality and rate of pulse and respiration; incompatible with alkalies, such as sodium bicarbonate.[26,61,101]

Interactions

Atropine + propranolol → reversal of propranolol-induced bradycardia; atropine + quinidine → additive vagolytic effects. Atropine + cimetidine → enhanced effect on depression of H ion secretion.[39,61]

BRETYLIUM

Bretylium is a class III antiarrhythmic agent that has antifibrillatory activity. It is useful in the management of serious ventricular arrhythmias, such as ventricular fibrillation and tachycardia that are refractory to conventional forms of treatment. Bretylium increases the action potential duration and prolongs the effective refractory period. It does not adversely affect myocardial contractility, although bretylium is a sympatholytic that results in vasodilation.[23,61]

Dosage

Ventricular fibrillation: 5 mg/kg, then 5–10 mg/kg at 15–30 minute intervals prn (maximum cumulative dose 30 mg/kg). Ventricular tachycardia: 5 mg/kg initially, 5 mg/kg may be repeated in 1–2 hours; maintenance therapy: 5–10 mg/kg q6–8h or continuous infusion of 1–2 mg/min. There is little experience with doses exceeding 40 mg/kg/day.[31,61]

Pharmacokinetics and Biopharmaceutics

Onset (IV): antifibrillatory activity begins within minutes; suppression of ventricular tachycardia or premature ventricular contractions may not occur for 20 minutes–6 hours. Duration: 6–24 hours. Vd: 3.4–9.5 liters/kg; plasma protein binding is negligible, extensive distribution appears to be secondary to uptake by adrenergic nerves, the myocardium, and the spleen. Excretion: bretylium undergoes extensive renal clearance, approximately 90%; $T\frac{1}{2}$: 13.5 hour (4–17 hour). Plasma concentrations of bretylium were not related to either myocardial concentrations or antiarrhythmic actions of the drug.[3,61,81]

Adverse Effects

Transient hypertension, hypotension, bradycardia, tachycardia, arrhythmias (ventricular tachycardia and fibrillation) nausea, and vomiting with rapid IV administration.[31,61]

Dosing Adjustments and Precautions

Dosage should be reduced in renal failure; exact guidelines are not available. It has been suggested that with a GFR less than 10–50 ml/min, give 25–50% of the usual dose and do not use bretylium when GFR is less than 10 ml/min.

Bretylium initially causes a catecholamine release, and a transient hypertension may be observed. This phenomenon may aggravate digoxin-induced arrhythmias, and for this reason, digitalis toxicity is a contraindication to bretylium administration. Bretylium should be used cautiously in fixed cardiac output states.[11,31]

Nursing Implications and Method of Administration

In the treatment of ventricular fibrillation administer bretylium undiluted BDC rapidly, over approximately 1 minute. With other life-threatening diseases, dilute the dose to a concentration of 10 mg/ml with D5W or NS and give over 8–10 minutes. A continuous infusion may be mixed in a concentration of 2 gm/500 ml of D5W or NS. Bretylium is compatible with dopamine, lidocaine, nitroglycerin, and procainamide. Monitor BP, ECG.[61,101]

Interactions

Bretylium + sympathomimetics → enhanced sympathomimetic effect; bretylium + β-blockers → significant bradyarrhythmias; bretylium + tricyclic antidepressants → decreased bretylium effect; bretylium + other antiarrhythmics → increased toxicity; bretylium + quinidine → decreased bretylium effect.[23,31,61]

β-BLOCKING AGENTS—PROPRANOLOL

Propranolol is the prototype β-blocking agent. It produces bradycardia and diminished cardiac output, and blood pressure. Proposed mechanisms of its antihypertensive action include central effects on blood pressure control, reduction of plasma renin, and a decrease in heart rate and contractility. Propranolol also reduces automaticity conduction velocity and rate of rise of the action potential. Prolongation of the effective refractory period is also observed.

Other β-blockers with various degrees of cardioselectivity include metroprolol, atenolol, timolol, and pindolol.[61]

Dosage

po: initiate therapy at low doses and increase according to effect and patient tolerance. General doses for angina pectoris, 160–240 mg/day; hypertension, 80–320 mg/day; arrhythmias, 40–320 mg/day. IV: 0.53–3.0 mg slowly IV BDC (rate 1 mg/min), which may be repeated after 2 minutes. Maximum dose is 0.15 mg/kg. Continuous infusion: 3–5 mg/hr (adjusted to clinical parameters).

EQUIVALENT DOSES (MG/DAY)

Propranolol	Metoprolol	Atenolol
<80	50	50
80–120	100	50
120–160	150	50
>160	200	100[31,44]

Pharmacokinetics and Biopharmaceutics

Absorption: variable bioavailability, 16–60%. Onset (po): 1–2 hours: (IV): 2–4 minutes. Duration: variable, dependent upon dose, route, and duration of therapy; following single IV dose, reversal of, β-blockade occurs in 10–15 minutes. Vd: 6 liters/kg. Protein binding: 90–95% to alpha, acid glycoprotein. T½ (IV)—2, 4 hours; (po)—3.3 hours. Fate: complex metabolic pathway involved; major metabolite, 4-hydroxypropranolol, is active, and is formed after po but not IV administration. Considerable first pass effect occurs (up to 80% initially).[15,31,61]

Adverse Effects

Seen in approximately 10% of patients. These include fatigue, weakness, dizziness, nausea, vomiting, impaired AV conduction, CNS symptoms (depression, insomnia, hallucinations, acute brain syndrome), bradycardia, bronchospasm, hypotension, heart failure, and acute pulmonary edema and are not necessarily dose related.[31,61]

Dosing Adjustments and Precautions

Use of these agents is contraindicated in several disease states, including sinus bradycardia, cardiogenic shock, and ventricular failure. Large interpatient variability occurs, and dosing adjustments may be required in liver disease, renal failure, young smokers, and elderly patients. May mask signs of hypoglycemia. If the drug is to be discontinued after prolonged administration, this should be accomplished gradually over a 2-week period.

Nursing Implications and Methods of Administration

IV (push): at maximum rate of 1 mg/min. IV (infusion): 10 mg/100 ml. Monitor blood pressure, ECG, (↑ PR interval), and heart rate (should be maintained at minimum of 60/min unless otherwise indicated). Requires careful monitoring and administration via infusion pump, preferably into a central vein.

Interactions

Propranolol + β-sympathomimetics (e.g., salbutamol) → antagonizes bronchodilation; propranolol + amiodarone → bradycardia, sinus arrest; propranolol + epinephrine → increased BP, decreased HR → fatal; propranolol + lidocaine → lidocaine toxicity; propranolol + procainamide → increased procainamide levels; propranolol + theophylline → mutual antagonism of therapeutic effect, decreased theophylline metabolism; propranolol + verapamil → hypotension, changes V block; propranolol + methyldopa → reduction of antihypertensive effect; propranolol + neuromuscular blockers → enhanced neuromuscular block; propanolol + cimetidine → enhanced bradycardia.[27,33,36,42,43]

CIMETIDINE (TAGAMET)

Cimetidine is a competitive inhibitor of histamine at H_2 receptor sites of gastric parietal cells; it inhibits gastric acid secretion and reduces the total pepsin output as a result of a decrease in volume of gastric juices. It is efficacious in the treatment of duodenal ulcer, gastric ulcer, and stress ulcer phophylaxis. It has also been used for metabolic alkalosis and aspiration pneumonia. Ranitidine is similarly effective and less toxic.[26,31]

Dosage

300 mg po/IV q6h or by continuous infusion at 2–4 mg/kg/hr.[26]

Pharmacokinetics and Biopharmaceutics

Onset (IV): rapid. Peak (po): 60–90 minutes. Vd = 1.5–3.4 kg. T½: 2 hours, reduced in burns. Fate: 70–80% unchanged in the urine; also metabolized in liver and excreted via kidney; trace amounts in feces.[26,31,60]

Adverse Effects

Usually mild (headache, fatigue, diarrhea, skin rash, dizziness) but gynecomastia, bradycardia, confusion, delusion, depression, hallucination, pancreatitis, renal dysfunction, hepatotoxicity, fever, and bacterial colonization have also been reported. The drug has been implicated in neutropenia, agranulocytosis, aplastic anemia, pancytopenia, and eosinophilia. Cimetidine also suppresses response to immediate skin test.[18,34,35,48,72,86,87,98,107]

Dosing Adjustments and Precautions

Renal failure (if creatinine clearance is 10 ml/min or less, reduce dose to 300 mg q12h); hemodialysis removes 80%. Patients with renal and multiple organ failure are more susceptible to adverse effects. Burn patients may require higher doses (0.8 mg/kg/hr).[11,60]

Nursing Implications and Methods of Administration

IV use: minimum volume for dilution of 300 mg is 20 ml. Rapid IV infusion results in hypotension, sinus arrest, or cardiac arrest. Recommended dilution is 300 mg in 50 or 100 ml D5W or NS. Cimetidine is compatible with a large number of drugs and IV solutions, including amino acids and nitroprusside.[31,101]

Interactions

Cimetidine + warfarin → increased anticoagulant effect; cimetidine + diazepam → enhanced sedation; cimetidine + ketoconazole → decreased oral absorption of ketoconazole; cimetidine + lidocaine → enhanced lidocaine toxicity; cimetidine + phenytoin → enhanced phenytoin toxicity; cimetidine + propranolol, labetalol, metoprolol → increased β-blocker levels; cimetidine + propranolol → enhanced bradycardia; cimetidine + theophyline → increased theophylline effect. Cimetidine may increase serum creatinine and serum transaminases.[10,18,26,43,46,52,55,56,73,91,106]

DIAZOXIDE (HYPERSTAT)

Diazoxide is a nondiuretic thiazide that reduces systemic vascular resistance and blood pressure by peripheral vasodilation. This profound hypotension is accompanied by a reflex tachycardia and an increased cardiac output with resultant increased organ perfusion.

Dosage

300 mg push is no longer recommended; *"mini-bolus"* 1–3 mg/kg to a maximum of 150 mg repeated at 5–15 minute intervals dosing appears safer and equally effective. Some authors report the use of even smaller doses i.e., 25 mg every 20 minutes.[31,79]

Pharmacokinetics and Biopharmaceutics

Onset (IV): 1–2 minutes. Peak: 3–4 minutes. Duration: 4–12 hours. Protein binding: 90–95% (reduced in renal failure). Vd: 0.2 liter/kg. T½: 20–40 hours (does not correlate with hypotensive effect). Fate: 60% metabolized to nonactive metabolite and eliminated via glomerular filtration; there is a significant degree of tubular reabsorption.[2,31,61]

Adverse Effects

Hyperglycemia (usually transient), edema, tachycardia, pronounced hypotension, cardiac and cerebral ischemia.[26,31]

Dosing Adjustments and Precautions

Caution—in patients with hyperglycemia, coronary artery disease, dissecting aortic aneurysm, cerebrovascular disease; titrate dose to individual; approximately 15% of patients are refractory.[61]

Nursing Implications and Methods of Administration

Preparation for IV use only; given by IV bolus injection; slow administration is reported to diminish the antihypertensive effect in acute hypertension; slow infusions will produce some effect. Slow infusion may be helpful to avoid precipitous drops in blood pressure. Monitor blood pressure (arterial line) frequently—as often as every 5 minutes for the first 15–30 minutes, then on an hourly basis; monitor blood sugar.[38,64,101]

Very alkaline pH; avoid extravasation. If it occurs, treat the area with warm compresses.

Interactions

Diazoxide + furosemide (and other thiazides) → reduced edema and sodium retention, increased hyperglycemia; diazoxide + warfarin → increased hypoprothrombinemia effect; diazoxide + phenytoin → decreased levels of phenytoin; diazoxide may increase plasma uric acid.[43,61]

DIGOXIN (LANOXIN)

Digoxin is a cardiac glycoside that produces a positive inotropic effect by a direct action on the myocardium, increasing force and velocity of myocardial contraction. In the failing heart, cardiac output increases, systolic emptying is more complete, and diastolic heart size decreases; in the nonfailing heart cardiac output is unchanged and peripheral vascular resistance increases. Digoxin shortens atrial refractory period and increases atrioventricular (AV) and ventricular refractory periods. In patients without CHF heart rate is slowed due to sympatholytic and vagal effects on sinoatrial (SA) node. Toxicity is due to direct depression of SA node and increased automaticity everywhere else in the heart.

Dosage

Digitalization. *Loading dose (LD):* for *congestive heart failure,* 8–10 μg/kg; for *atrial fibrillation,* 13–15 μg/kg based on lean body weight. The total dose is given in three divided doses every 6 hours. *Maintenance dose* (MD): MD = LD × fraction lost daily = LD × (14 + CrCl/5)% where CrCl is creatinine clearance in ml/min. (Example: 70 kg male in atrial fibrillation with CrCl 55 ml/min. LD = 1.0 mg (15 μg/kg × 70 kg). MD = LD (14 + CrCl/5)% = 1 (14 + 55/5)% = 0.25 mg daily.[90]

Pharmacokinetics and Biopharmaceutics

Onset (IV): 15–30 minutes. Peak: 1.5–5 hours. T½: 33–51 hours. Vd: 6–10 liters/kg, reduced in renal failure. Plasma levels (therapeutic): 0.6–2.6 mg. Bioavailability: large variation—50–93%, assumed to be 80% for conversion purposes. Fate: eliminated primarily by kidney, 14% of drug metabolized.[1,61]

Adverse Effects

Nausea, vomiting, slow pulse rate, headache, fatigue, cardiac arrhythmias, and visual disturbances are associated with toxicity but all have low specificity as indicators; also gynecomastia, rash may occur.[1,95]

Dosing Adjustments and Precautions

Low therapeutic index, reduce dose in the elderly, in renal failure, and in myxedema; hyperthyroid patients and those with high creatine clearances may require larger doses. Hypokalemia, hypoxemia, hypercalcemia, and hypomagnesemia may predispose to toxicity. Many patients in normal sinus rhythm may not require continued therapy with digoxin.[1,26,49,61]

Nursing Implications and Methods of Administration

IV or po; do not give SC or IM. Rapid IV administration may cause vasoconstriction and decrease in cardiac output. Dilute in normal saline and run in over 15–50 minutes; monitor rate and quality of pulse, ECG, electrolytes, plasma levels. May be given below the drip chamber (BDC), but infusion is preferred method.[1,26]

Interactions

Digoxin + aluminum hydroxide, magnesium hydroxide, kaolin-pectin → decreased po absorption of digoxin; digoxin + cholestyramine → decreased po absorption of digoxin; digoxin + diuretics (thiazides/furosemide) → predispose to toxicity via electrolyte disturbance; digoxin + other potassium depleters (corticosteroids, laxatives, amphotericin B) predispose to toxicity; digoxin + calcium (IV) → increased risk of toxicity; digoxin + quinidine or spironolactone → increased digoxin effect; digoxin + sympathomimetic amines → increased risk of arrhythmias; digoxin + verapamil → increased serum digoxin levels.[1,4,21,53,93]

DOBUTAMINE (DOBUTREX)

Dobutamine is a synthetic analogue of isoproterenol for use in the treatment of cardiac decompensation due to refractory heart failure or cardiac surgery. It produces increased myocardial contractility and increased cardiac output by direct stimulation of β-1-adrenergic receptors and has little effect upon heart rate at lower dosages.[17]

Dosage

Initiate treatment at 2.5 μg/kg/min and adjust according to cardiac outputs up to maximum of 10μg/kg/min. Maximum dosage is 40 μg/kg/min.[25]

Pharmacokinetics and Biopharmaceutics

IV infusion only. Onset: 1–2 minutes. Peak: minutes. T½: 2 minutes. Fate: metabolized to conjugates of dobutamine and 3–0 methyl dobutamine.

Adverse Effects

Nausea, vomiting, headache, chest pain, increased heart rate. Increased systolic pressure (7.5% have 50 mm Hg or greater increase at low doses). Arrhythmias in 5% of patients—usually manifested as PVCs. Pronounced hypotension at higher doses.[5]

Dosing Adjustments and Precautions

Correct hypovolemia before initiating therapy. Caution in patients with hypertension, coronary artery disease (CAD), presence of arrhythmias, with or after general anesthetics. *Doses of 20 μg/kg/min or greater* may cause tachycardia, arrhythmias, and hypotension.

Nursing Implications and Methods of Administration

IV infusion only. Dilute 500 mg in 500 ml of D5W, NS or LR. The solution is stable for 24 hours; incompatible with alkali solutions, such as sodium bicarbonate. A pink discoloration of the solution may occur; this does not represent a significant loss of potency. Dobutamine has minimal direct pressor activity other than by increasing cardiac output (at higher doses blood pressure will decrease). Monitor ECG, blood pressure, pulmonary capillary wedge pressure (PCWP), cardiac output, and cardiac index. Weaning should be accomplished slowly. Infuse via central vein if possible.

Interactions

Dobutamine + other sympathomimetics → increased risk of toxicity; dobutamine + theophylline → increased risk of toxicity; dobutamine + general anesthetics (with or shortly after) → increased risk of toxicity; dobutamine + propranolol → blockade of inotropic effect; dobutamine + nitroprusside (and other vasodilators) → more favorable hemodynamic effects than when either agent administered alone.[5,77]

DOPAMINE (INTROPIN)

Dopamine is a naturally occurring catecholamine that exerts a positive inotropic effect by a direct action on β-adrenergic receptors and by releasing norepinephrine; it also has a unique dopaminergic effect on the kidney with resultant increase in renal blood flow and urine output at low doses. Dopamine also stimulates α-adrenergic receptors and may be used as a pressor agent.[25]

Dosage

IV (infusion only): Effect is dose-dependent with three dosage levels identified. Note that considerable difference in opinion exists as to the dose associated with various levels. The dosage ranges listed below are only guidelines, and practitioners should be aware that the values for the different levels are by no means absolute.

Dopaminergic effect (0.5–2 μg/kg/min): increase in renal blood flow and urine output, may raise cardiac output slightly; *beta effect* (5–10 μg/kg/min): increase in cardiac output with little effect on arterial blood pressure or heart rate; *alpha effect* (above 10 μg/kg/min): increase in systemic peripheral vascular resistance; doses in excess of 20 μg/kg/min may reverse dopaminergic effect.[25,26]

Pharmacokinetics and Biopharmaceutics

IV infusion only. Onset: rapid. Peak: 5 minutes. Duration: 10 minutes. T½: 1.75 minutes. Fate: 75% metabolized in liver, kidneys, and plasma; 25% is converted to noradrenaline.[31,61]

Adverse Effects

Nausea, vomiting, tachycardia, ectopic beats, angina pectoris, vasoconstriction, palpitations, hypertension, extravasation.[25,74]

Dosing Adjustments and Precautions

Correct hypovolemia and arrhythmias before administration; caution in sensitive patient, e.g., vascular disease; cirrhotics may require increased doses. Dopaminergic doses may impair hypoxic ventilatory drive.[26,68,74]

Nursing Implications and Methods of Administration

IV infusion only. Usual concentrations are 1600 μg/ml (400 mg in 250 ml). Stable for 24 hours in D5W, NS (D5/NS), D5/RL, and RL. Yellowish color indicative of decomposition; unstable in alkaline solutions, such as sodium bicarbonate. Also reported incompatible with amphotericin B. Monitor for changes in skin color or temperature, blood pressure, urine output, and heart rate. If hypotension occurs, increase rate of infusion; if it persists, a change in therapy is indicated. If diastolic BP or heart rate increases, reduce infusion rate if possible; wean slowly, i.e., 5 ml/30 min. Infuse via central vein whenever possible using pump.[36,74,101]

Interactions

Dopamine + α-blockers (e.g., phentolamine) → blockade of high dose alpha effects of dopamine; dopamine + phenytoin (*IV*) → profound hypotension. Refer to dobutamine section for other interactions.[14,40]

FUROSEMIDE (LASIX)

Furosemide is a potent diuretic that inhibits sodium reabsorption in ascending limb of Henle's loop, as well as both proximal and distal tubules. A decrease in peripheral vascular resistance and left ventricular filling pressure occurs prior to diuresis. It also reduces renal vascular resistance.[26,61]

Dosage

IV: 20–120 mg over 1 minute, or slower po: 40–120 mg/day in 1 or 2 doses. Initiate regimen with small dose and titrate upward to meet needs of individual.[26]

Pharmacokinetics and Biopharmaceutics

Onset: (po)—30–60 minutes; (IV)—5 minutes. Peak: (po)—1–2 hours; (IV)—20–60 minutes. Duration: (po)—6–8 hours; (IV)—2 hours. T½: 30–70 minutes (increased in renal failure). Vd: 0.1 liter/kg. Protein binding: 90–95% (decreased by 9–14% in acute renal failure). Bioavailability: although the bioavailability of oral is 50% that of parenteral, a similar response is obtained with equal doses of po and IV. Fate: 60–80% eliminated unchanged, remainder is excreted in feces, and some eliminated in urine as metabolites.[29]

Adverse Effects

Fluid and electrolyte disturbances, hypochloremic alkalosis, hyperglycemia, hyperuricemia. Reduces serum calcium. Ototoxicity is usually reversible and occurs especially with rapid IV administration in renally impaired patients.[26,31,61]

Dosing Adjustments and Precautions

Although it is a sulfonamide derivative, little cross-sensitivity to other sulfas is seen (ethacrynic acid may be used as alternative). Higher doses of up to 1 gm/day may be required in renal failure. When using furosemide for its calciuretic effect, replace sodium, potassium, and magnesium losses. Elderly and very young are prone to volume depletion. In septic patients start with small dose (i.e., 10 mg) and titrate upward slowly.[61]

Nursing Implications and Methods of Administration

Monitoring of electrolytes is essential. Divided doses produce greater overall effect. Also monitor serum glucose, uric acid. Suggested vehicles for administration are NS and RL. Acidic solutions, such as multiple vitamin infusion, dopamine, dobutamine, and commercial dextrose solutions with pH <5.5, will cause precipitation. Suggested rate for direct IV administration: 20 mg/min.[26,101]

Interactions

Furosemide + cephalosporin → possible additive nephrotoxicity; furosemide + corticosteroids/amphotericin B/laxatives → increased potassium loss; furosemide + digitalis → increased risk of digitalis toxicity; furosemide + aminoglycosides → additive ototoxicity; furosemide + phenytoin → decreased diuresis with furosemide; furosemide may increase blood ammonia, amylase, blood glucose, and uric acid levels.[43]

HEPARIN

Heparin is an anticoagulant that enhances antithrombin III activity, resulting in a rapid inhibition of thrombin. It also neutralizes activated forms of factors XII, IX, X, XI, and perhaps VII.

Dosage

Titrate individually. Adjust to partial thromboplastin time (PTT) (1½–2½ times control value). IV for thrombophlebitis/pulmonary embolus; bolus of 5000–10,000 units followed by continuous infusion of 1000 units/hr. (Note that patients with pulmonary embolus may require larger doses initially). SC for prophylaxis of postoperative deep venous thrombosis: 3000–5000 units SC q8–12h until ambulatory.[61]

Pharmacokinetics and Biopharmaceutics

Onset: rapid. Duration: short (see below); effect may continue for 4 hours after drug stopped. T½ anticoagulant effect: 1.5 hours; pharmacologic T½: dose dependent—of little clinical relevance. Vd: 0.05–0.2 liter/kg. Protein binding: 95%. Therapeutic level is 1½–2½ × control value of activated partial thromboplastin time (PTT). Fate: Primarily metabolized by liver but with doses larger than 5000 units increasing amounts are eliminated unchanged.[31]

Adverse Effects

Hemorrhage, thrombocytopenia, osteoporosis.[24,26]

Dosing Adjustments and Precautions

Elderly females and patients with hepatic failure are particularly at risk of bleeding. Overdose treated by discontinuing infusion, administering blood products, and, when needed, administering protamine sulphate.[70]

Nursing Implications and Methods of Administration

IV continuous infusion methods superior to intermittent method; use infusion pump. Avoid IM use both for heparin and other drugs while receiving heparin. SC heparin to be administered into abdomen using ½- or ⅝-inch needle. Watch for signs of bleeding—hematuria, hemapositive stools, etc. Thrombocytopenia may occur early in therapy, so platelet counts should be obtained on a regular basis. Incompatible with aminoglycosides, meperidine, hydroxyzine, and promethazine.[61,101]

Interactions

Heparin + anticoagulants/antiplatelet drugs → prolonged bleeding time; heparin may increase free thyroxine levels and increase T_3 and uptake.[43]

HYDRALAZINE (APRESOLINE)

Hydralazine is an antihypertensive agent that reduces arteriolar blood pressure by direct smooth muscle relaxation. In heart failure, hydralazine exerts its principal effects on resistance vessels and reduces afterload. Reflex tachycardia is frequently seen.[7,61]

Dosage

po: 10 mg four times a day, increasing to a maximum of 200–300 mg/day. IM/IV: 10–50 mg q4–6h. IV (infusion): 50 mg/500 ml at initial rate of 0.5 mg (5 ml)/hr increased gradually every 40–60 minutes while maintaining a heart rate of less than 120 beats/min.[61]

Pharmacokinetics and Biopharmaceutics

Onset: (po)—within 1 hour; (IV)—10–20 minutes. Peak: (po)—1–2 hours; (IV)—20–40 minutes; Duration: 3–8 hours. Vd: 0.3–0.7 liter/kg. Protein binding: 87%; T½: 1.5–8 hours (varies with acetylator type; clear distinction between fast and slow acetylators has not been found). Fate: acetylation is relatively unimportant after first pass effect; extensive hydroxylation in the liver, small amounts eliminated unchanged.[31,61]

Adverse Effects

Tachycardia, headache, palpitations, flushing, systemic lupus erythematus (SLE), angina pectoris, arrhythmias, dizziness, hypersensitivity, drug fever, fluid retention, peripheral neuropathy, hypotension, hepatotoxicity.[61]

Dosing Adjustment and Precautions

Caution in patients with congestive heart failure, angina pectoris, mitral valve, and abdominal aortic aneurysm. May require reduced dose in renal failure. Slow acetylators more prone to peripheral neuropathy, SLE.[1,26,30]

Nursing Implications and Methods of Administration

IM and IV slowly (rate of 5 mg/min) or as infusion solution (50 mg/500 ml) in either NS or LR, but not dextrose solutions as there are conflicting compatibility data. Avoid mixing with barbiturate and aminophylline solutions. Monitor BP (arterial line), heart rate, and antinuclear antibody (ANA) periodically. Generally heart rate should not exceed 120 beats/min. Infuse with pump preferably through central vein.[26,101]

Interactions

Hydralazine + β-blockers → reduction of hydralazine-induced tachycardia; hydralazine + thiazides → reduction of hydralazine-induced sodium retention and enhancement of hypotensive effect; hydralazine may produce a positive direct Coombs test.[61]

ISOPROTERENOL (ISUPREL)

Isoproterenol is a direct acting β-adrenergic receptor stimulator that causes bronchodilation, cardiac stimulation, and peripheral vasodilation. Myocardial oxygen consumption increases and cardiac efficiency decreases. Conduction time is shortened and the refractory period of the atrioventricular (AV) node is reduced.[26,61]

Dosage

IV (bolus): 0.5–1.0 mg IV push diluted in 10 ml NS; IV (infusion for cardiac use): 1–4 μg/ml adjusted according to heart rate, systemic blood pressure, and urine output.[31,61]

Pharmacokinetics and Biopharmaceutics

Onset: rapid. Duration: short, approximately 15 minutes. Fate: 50% excreted unchanged, 25–35% metabolized by COMT (catecholamine-*o*-methyltransferase); termination of drug effect is due to uptake into adrenergic neuron, not metabolism.[31,61]

Adverse Effects

Flushing, sweating, mild tremors, nervousness, headache, tachycardia, anginal pain, arrhythmias.[26,61]

Dosing Adjustments and Precautions

Correct hypovolemia. Caution in patients with ischemic heart disease, hypertension, and hyperthyroidism.[61]

Nursing Implications and Methods of Administration

Solution becomes pink-to-brown color on exposure to air, metal, alkali, or increased temperature and should not be used. Solution contains 2 mg/500 ml D5W (4μg/ml) and is incompatible with sodium bicarbonate and aminophylline. If heart rate increases over 110 beats/min or there are premature beats, a reduction in dosage may be required. Monitor heart rate, blood pressure, urine output. Administer via an infusion pump.[26,101]

Interactions

Isoproterenol + epinephrine (and other catecholamines) → increased cardiac stimulation; isoproterenol + propranolol → blocks beta effects.[43]

LIDOCAINE (XYLOCAINE)

Lidocaine is an antiarrhythmic agent similar in cardiac actions to phenytoin. It suppresses automaticity in the His-Purkinje system and spontaneous depolarization of ventricles during diastole. It is used primarily for treatment of ventricular arrhythmias.[41]

Dosage

Loading dose: 100 mg given over 2 minutes and repeated once in 10 minutes, or 50 mg over 1 minute repeated every 5 minutes for 3 doses. Maintenance dose: 1–4 mg/min; in circulatory failure 10 μg/kg/hr.[61,108]

Pharmacokinetics and Biopharmaceutics

IV use only, IM use to be avoided. Onset: 45–90 seconds (bolus). Duration: 10–20 minutes (bolus). T½ (alpha): 7–30 minutes. T½ (beta): 1.5–2 hours. Vd: 1.7 liters/kg, decreased by 50% in patients with left ventricular failure. Fate: metabolized (approximately 90%) in liver to active metabolite, less than 10% eliminated unchanged by kidney. Therapeutic serum levels: 6–21 μm/liter.[61,108]

Adverse Effects

CNS effects (drowsiness, seizures, agitation) are due to both lidocaine and a metabolite that has a longer T½ than parent drug and therefore may occur after the infusion has been stopped. Cardiac arrhythmias, cardiac depression, decreased blood pressure may also occur.[61]

Dosing Adjustments and Precautions

Reduce dose in CHF and liver disease. Note that loading dose in cardiac failure should also be reduced due to decrease in Vd. Infusing beyond 36 hours may necessitate decreasing dose.[37,61]

Nursing Implications and Methods of Administration

Infusions are administered as a 2 gm/500 ml solution. Lidocaine may be given as a direct injection, rate not to exceed 50 mg/min. During infusion, monitor ECG (lidocaine shortens QT interval), blood pressure, and heart rate. Incompatible with amphotericin B, sulfas, and perhaps ampicillin. Lidocaine may be piggybacked with sympathomimetics, but direct admixture is not recommended.[8,101]

Interactions

Lidocaine + neuromuscular blocking agents → increased blockade; lidocaine + propranolol → prolonged lidocaine T½.[61,66]

MANNITOL

Mannitol is an osmotic diuretic that is filtered by the glomeruli and excreted unchanged in urine, with only minimal reabsorption occurring in tubules. Reabsorption of water and sodium is inhibited in the proximal tubule, and excretion of these substances, as well as potassium, calcium, and phosphate, is increased. Mannitol has been used therapeutically in the treatment of patients with intractable edema states, to increase urine flow, to flush out debris from renal tubules in patients with acute tubular necrosis (ATN), to increase toxin excretion in patients with drug intoxication, and to decrease cerebral edema. Diagnostically, it is useful in evaluating an acutely oliguric patient.[26,65]

Dosage

(1) *Diagnostically in an acutely oliguric patient:* Test dose of 12.5–25.0 gm mannitol (20–25%) given IV push over 3–5 minutes. Urine volume and specific gravity should be measured hourly. A positive response is a urine output of >50 ml urine/hr. If <50 ml urine/hr is excreted after first hour, the same dose should be repeated. If still no response, no further mannitol should be given and therapy should be instituted for treatment of ATN. (2) *Prevention of acute renal failure:* Test dose as above followed by a priming dose of sufficiently concentrated mannitol, over an hour, to bring the dose to 50 gm. Thereafter, maintain urine output at 50 ml/hour with IV infusion of 5% mannitol. Addition of sodium chloride 20 mEq/liter and calcium gluconate 1 gm/liter has been recommended due to electrolyte loss. (3) *Adjunctive therapy for intoxications:* Test dose and priming dose as above. Maintain urine output at 150–500 ml/hr with infusion of 5% solution. Repletion of electrolytes may be accomplished by administering 45 mEq NaCl, 24 mEq sodium acetate, 1 gm calcium gluconate, 1 gm magnesium sulfate, and 20 mEq potassium acetate. (4) *Treatment of elevated intracranial or intraocular pressure:* Administer 1.5–2.0 gm/kg (15–20%) over 30–60 minutes and repeat as necessary to control pressure.[61,65]

Pharmacokinetics and Biopharmaceutics

IV only. Onset: 1–3 hours for diuresis; 30 minutes for reduction of intracranial pressure (ICP). Duration: 3–8 hours. T½: 15 minutes in patients with normal renal function. Fate: Primarily eliminated unchanged in urine.[61,65]

Adverse Effects

Fluid and electrolyte imbalances, hypo-/hypernatremia, hyperosmolality, cellular dehydration, pulmonary edema, congestive heart failure especially in patients with poor renal function.[26,61,65]

Dosing Adjustments and Precautions

Patients with poor renal function may be at greater risk of adverse effects. Drug should not be used in very severe renal disease. A positive fluid balance of 1–2 liters should be maintained.[65]

Nursing Implications and Methods of Administration

May crystallize out in concentrations of greater than 15%. These crystals may be redissolved by heating and shaking. Drug should be administered through an inline filter. *Electrolytes should not be added to solution of 20% or more.* Urine and serum sodium, urine and serum osmolality, and urine output should be monitored.[61,65,101]

METHYLDOPA (ALDOMET)

Methyldopa is an antihypertensive agent that exerts its effect primarily through a central action, although a false neurotransmitter mechanism may also be involved. Hypotension produced is slow in onset and does not affect cardiac output or renal blood flow.[61]

Dosage

IV: 250–500 mg q6h (maximum, 1 gm q6h); po: 250 mg, 2 or 3 times a day and increase to 2–3 gm/day.[26,61]

Pharmacokinetics and Biopharmaceutics:

Onset (IV): 4–6 hours. Duration (IV): 10–16 hours. Vd: 0.5 liters/kg. T½: 2 hours. Fate: orally, 50% is absorbed, with most of oral drug being metabolized in the gut wall. Cleared by glomerular filtration with up to 90% of IV dose in urine. Major metabolite of methyldopa has some antihypertensive activity.[65]

Adverse Effects

Drowsiness (initially), depression, impotence, postural hypotension, drug fever (1–3%), diarrhea, constipation, skin rash, sodium retention, and hypertension (with IV formulation). Methyldopa may cause hemolytic anemia and hepatitis. The hepatitis that occurs is indistinguishable from that of viral origin and seems to occur more often in females.[1,26]

Dosing Adjustments and Precautions

Reduction of dose may be necessary in renal failure.

Nursing Implications and Methods of Administration

Desired dose to be added to 100 ml of solution and administered over 30–60 minutes; incompatible with sulfas, barbiturates, and amphotericin B. Do not give IM/SC. Blood pressure must be monitored, and patient's urine may darken on standing. Hemodialysis removes 60% over 6 hours.[101]

Interactions

Methyldopa + phenothiazines → increased blood pressure; methyldopa + propranolol → loss of blood pressure control. Methyldopa may cause a positive Coombs test.[43]

MORPHINE

Morphine is a narcotic alkaloid of opium that produces analgesia, CNS depression, respiratory depression, emesis by direct stimulation of chemoreceptor trigger zones, constipation, hypotension, and a reduction of pulmonary vascular resistance.[65]

Dosage:

Parenterally: 0.1–0.15 mg/kg; doses of 2 mg IV may produce analgesia; continuous IV infusion 1–10 mg/hr, titrated to effect; epidural: 4–5 mg. Hypotensive use may require higher doses, i.e., up to 10 mg.[65]

Pharmacokinetics and Biopharmaceutics

Onset: IV—1–2 minutes; epidural—6–30 minutes. Peak: (IV)—20 minutes. Duration: IV—4–7 hours; epidural—4–36 hours. Vd: 3–4 liter/kg. T½: 2–2.5 hours. Fate: extensively metabolized, 3–10% excreted unchanged by kidneys.[65]

Adverse Effects

Nausea, vomiting, respiratory depression, biliary colic.[26]

Dosing Adjustments and Precautions

Caution is advised when treating patients with liver disease, hypoalbuminemia, and obstructive lung disease.[65]

Nursing Implications and Methods of Administration

Preferred route of administration is IV below the drip chamber (BDC). Monitor vital signs and alertness of patient. May also be given po, SC, IM, epidural.[26,101]

Interactions

Morphine + CNS depressants → additive CNS depression; morphine + phenothiazines → additive CNS depression; morphine + neuromuscular blockade → increased blockade. Morphine may increase serum amylase.[43]

NITROGLYCERIN

Nitroglycerin's vasodilating action causes venous pooling of blood, thereby reducing preload. It also enhances flow in collateral coronary arteries and ischemic areas. The drug produces only minor effects on afterload and cardiac output.[6,7,57]

Dosage

Sublingual: should be used only in stable angina patients due to unpredictability of effects. Ointment: 2.5–5 cm lightly to skin, adjusted to patients' needs q4h. IV (infusion): the dosage range is varied; start at 5 μg/min; increase by 5 μg/min until desired response is seen. Doses are titrated to effect. Note that upper dosage limit has not yet been determined.[26,75]

Pharmacokinetics and Biopharmaceutics

Ointment: onset—30 minutes; duration—at least 3 hours. IV (infusion): onset—immediate; duration—short: T½: 30 minutes. Fate: extensively metabolized by liver and other peripheral sites.[65]

Adverse Effects

Headache, dizziness, flushing, postural hypotension, tachycardia, alcohol intoxication with IV preparation, methemoglobinemia.[26,60,61,92]

Dosing Adjustments and Methods of Administration

Correct hypovolemia prior to administration. Because major effects are on preload (pulmonary wedge pressure (PWP)), it should be normal to elevated. Nitroglycerin should be used cautiously in patients with elevated intracranial pressure.[6,61,78]

Nursing Implications and Methods of Administration

Ointment: prescribed amount measured according to manufacturer's guide and applied in a thin layer to the skin. Covering the skin with plastic improves absorption. Gloves should be used and the old ointment removed prior to the next application. The chest area provides psychological benefits; however, other surfaces may be used. IV infusion: 50 mg/250 ml (200 μg/ml) D5W/NS in glass bottles. Nitroglycerine adsorbs to polyvinyl chloride of IV bags and administration sets. It is incompatible with hydralazine and phenytoin. Doses required may vary when nonabsorbable administration sets are used; monitor BP, PWP, and heart rate.[61,101]

Interactions

Nitroglycerin + vasodilators → enhanced hypotension; nitroglycerin and pancuronium bromide → enhanced neuromuscular blockade. Nitroglycerin may increase urinary catecholamine and vanillylmandelic acid (VMA) excretion.[31,43]

NOREPINEPHRINE BITARTRATE (LEVOPHED)

This is an agent that causes marked vasoconstriction with resultant increase in total peripheral resistance and elevation of blood pressure. Renal artery constriction may occur with resultant decrease in urine output. Although primarily an α-adrenergic receptor stimulant, it does have beta effects and produces a positive inotropic effect.[26,41,96]

Dosage

IV infusion only. Run infusion at 2–12 μg/min initially and adjust to maintain systolic blood pressure of 80–100 mm Hg or no less than 40 mm Hg below pre-existing pressure.[26,31,96]

Pharmacokinetics and Biopharmaceutics

IV only. Onset: rapid. Duration: 1–2 minutes. Fate: Primarily metabolized by catecholamine-*O*-methyltransferase (COMT) and monoamine oxidase (MAO). Effect is terminated by uptake into adrenergic neurons.[31,61]

Adverse Effects

Hypertension, bradycardia, decreased urine output, and arrhythmias.[26,61]

Dosing Adjustments and Precautions

Before administration correct hypovolemia. Also pre-existing arrythmias, hypoxia, and acidosis should be corrected. Elderly are at high risk of developing toxicity.[36,96]

Nursing Implications and Methods of Administration

Solution used is 4 mg (1 amp) NE 250 ml NS/D5W. Color change from clear-to-brown indicates a loss of potency. Extravasation should occur; monitor for coldness, pain, pallor, and discomfort at the site and infiltrate the area as soon as possible with 5–10 mg phentolamine. Dosages are expressed in terms of norepinephrine base (4-ml amp contains 8 mg norepinephrine as bitartrate, which is equivalent to 4-mg base). Monitor blood pressure, heart rate, ECG, urine output. Dopamine at low doses may be used to maintain urine output while NE is being infused. When discontinuing, gradually reduce infusion rate. Incompatible with sodium bicarbonate, lidocaine, aminophylline, and barbiturate solutions. Use infusion pump or some other precision device to administer, and administer by central vein.[26,96]

Interactions

Norepinephrine + anesthetics → increased risk of cardiac arrhythmias; norepinephrine + atropine → blockade of levarterenol-induced reflex bradycardia.[43,61]

PANCURONIUM BROMIDE (PAVULON)

This drug is a nondepolarizing neuromuscular blocker used to induce skeletal muscle relaxation during anesthesia and to facilitate the management of patients undergoing mechanical ventilation.

Dosage

Variable individual response. IV (bolus): 0.06–0.1 mg/kg initially and 0.015 mg/kg every 25–60 minutes. IV (infusion): 1.5–2 mg/hr.[26,61,83]

Pharmacokinetics and Biopharmaceutics

IV use only. Dose-dependent response. (1) 0.04 mg/kg: Onset: 45 seconds. Peak: 4.5 minutes. Duration: <1 hour. (2) 0.08 mg/kg: Onset: 30 seconds. Peak: 3 minutes. Duration: <1 hour. Vd: 0.08–1.9 liter/kg. $T_{1/2}$: dose-dependent, prolonged in renal/hepatic impairment. Fate: 60% primarily eliminated unchanged, although some (40%) may be metabolized.[31,83]

Adverse Effects

Anxiety, prolonged respiratory depression, increased heart rate and blood pressure, local reactions.[26,83]

Dosing Adjustments and Precautions

Precaution should be taken in patients with myasthenia gravis, renal failure, hepatic insufficiency. *Caution in patients with tachycardia.* Electrolyte imbalances should be corrected.

Nursing Implications and Methods of Administration

Patients if possible should be made aware of paralysis, and alarm systems should be operational at all times. Standard dosage 50 mg/500 ml is usually run at 15–20 ml/hr, but may also be given by direct injection. Refrigerate ampules for long-term storage; for short-term storage, drug is stable at room temperature for 6 months. Do not store solution in plastic syringes. Eyes should be kept moist (if not closed). The solution is stable for 24 hours; discard if color change is noted. Pancuronium is incompatible with barbiturates.[83,101]

Interactions

Pancuronium bromide + antagonists (acetylcholine, anticholinesterases, potassium, and calcium) → reduction of blocking effect; pancuronium bromide + agonists (halothane, quinidine, magnesium, aminoglycosides, polymyxin B, clindamycin, tricyclic antidepressants) and drugs that cause hypokalemia, such as diuretics → potentiation of neuromuscular block.[43,61]

PHENTOLAMINE (REGITINE)

Phentolamine is an α-adrenergic blocking agent that causes a marked arteriolar dilation and significant venodilation with a corresponding reduction in afterload and preload. It produces an increase in cardiac index, stroke volume, and heart rate. The only approved indications are for the control and diagnosis of pheochromocytoma and to prevent necrosis and sloughing of tissues following extravasation of sympathomimetic amines. Phentolamine is expensive.[61]

Dosage

As a vasodilator, 0.1–2 mg/min. Treatment of sympathomimetic extravasation: 5–10 mg infiltrated into the affected area.[2,61]

Pharmacokinetics and Biopharmaceutics

IV infusion. Onset: immediate. Duration: 3–10 minutes. Fate: 10% of drug is excreted unchanged in urine; the fate of remainder is unknown.[31]

Adverse Effects

Hypotension, tachycardia, cardiac arrhythmias, weakness, dizziness, flushing, anginal pain, nasal stuffiness, abdominal discomfort, sedation.[26,61]

Dosing Adjustments and Precautions

Correct hypovolemia prior to administration. Cautious use in patients with recent myocardial infarction. *Tachyphylaxis* may occur.

Nursing Implications and Methods of Administration

Concentration of infusion solution is 300 mg/500 ml NS/D5W. In refrigerated vials drug is stable for 7 days. Compatible with dobutamine and verapamil. Each vial contains 5 mg phentolamine, 25 mg mannitol. Monitor heart rate, ECG, and pulmonary capillary wedge pressure (PCWP). Administer via infusion.[26,61,80,101]

Interactions

Phentolamine + α-adrenergic agents → decreased alpha effect.

PHENYTOIN (DILANTIN)

Phenytoin is an anticonvulsant that is effective against most types of epileptic seizures with the exception of petit mal. Phenytoin produces a stabilizing effect on the convulsive threshold and protects against hyperexcitability caused by excessive stimulation. It is also effective in treatment of ventricular arrhythmias caused by digitalis toxicity.[41]

Dosage

Loading dose: 14 mg/kg (maximum IV rate is 50 mg/min). Maintenance dose: 100 mg po/IV q6–8h.[19]

Pharmacokinetics and Biopharmaceutics

Onset: with loading dose—20 minutes (time required to administer dose at maximum rate 50 mg/min); without loading dose—steady state not reached for 5–15 days. Vd: 0.6 liter/kg. T½: 8–60 hours (mean 24 hours), reduced to 8 hours in uremia. Oral bioavailability: 90%. Protein binding: 90%, which is reduced in renal failure. A 1% increase in free drug occurs with every 0.1-gm reduction in plasma albumin below 3 gm/dl. Therapeutic range: 40–80 μm/liter. Fate: primarily metabolized by liver with 60–75% excreted in urine as nonactive metabolite.[61]

Adverse Effects

Nystagmus, ataxia, drowsiness, slurred speech, gingival hyperplasia, pain from injection, megoblastic anemia, folic acid deficiency, rash, hirsutism, reduced automaticity of ventricles. Abrupt withdrawal may precipitate seizures.[26,61]

Dosing Adjustments and Precautions

Dosage adjustment may be required in patients with liver disease (theoretical), renal disease, and hypoalbuminemia. Phenytoin reverts from first order to zero order kinetics in range of 27–40 μm/liter, and small increments in dose may produce pronounced effects. Patients with cardiovascular instability may require a slower rate of administration.[19,61]

Nursing Implications and Methods of Administration

Administered IV below the drip chamber (BDC) at a maximum rate of *50 mg/min* (rapid administration may cause hypotension, cardiovascular collapse, and CNS depression). Do not administer IM. Although not recommended, if necessary phenytoin may be admixed with NS or RL, if the solution is used immediately, not piggybacked to another IV line and is no more concentrated than 18 mg phenytoin/ml.[19]

Interaction

Phenytoin + warfarin → variable effect on warfarin metabolism; phenytoin + chloramphenicol → increased phenytoin effect through reduced metabolism; phenytoin + dexamethasone → increased dexamethasone metabolism; phenytoin + sulfonamides → possible increased phenytoin effect; phenytoin + dopamine (IV phenytoin only) → profound hypotension; phenytoin + quinidine → decreased effect of quinidine; phenytoin + isoniazid (INH) → increased phenytoin effect; phenytoin + theophylline decreased theophylline effect.[14,19,43,59] Phenytoin may produce alterations in thyroid tests.

PROCAINAMIDE (PRONESTYL)

This drug is classically described as a type 1 antiarrhythmic used for the treatment of ventricular arrhythmias. Procainamide acts by decreasing membrane sodium conductance to produce a concentration-dependent decrease in automaticity and also decreases excitability and conduction velocity.[41,61]

Dosage

po/IM: 15 mg/kg as a loading dose and then 5–6 mg/kg q3h. IV: loading dose of 17 mg/kg over 1 hour (not more than 20–50 mg/min); maintenance dose of 2.8 mg/kg/hr, 1.4 mg/kg/hr in patients with renal failure (i.e., greater than 130 μM/liter serum creatinine (SCr). Alternative method is to administer 100 mg IV q10 minutes, until 1 gm dose achieved. Therapeutic serum levels: procainamide—17–68 μm/liter; procainamide + NAPA—43–128 μm/liter.[26,58]

Pharmacokinetics and Biopharmaceutics

Onset: po—unknown; IM—10 minutes; IV—immediate. Peak: IM—15–60 minutes. T½: 2.5–4.5 hours. Vd: 1.7–2.2 liters/kg. Fate: 50–60% eliminated unchanged by kidneys; 40% metabolized by liver to active metabolite *N*-acetylprocainamide (NAPA), which is then eliminated by kidneys; T½ of NAPA is 6 hours.[61]

Adverse Effects

GI effects, weakness, hypotension, heart block, confusion, arrhythmias (prolongation of PR, QRS, QT intervals), positive antinuclear antibody (ANA) with and without systemic lupus erythematosus (SLE), and thrombocytopenia.[61]

Dosing Adjustments and Precautions

A reduction in dose in renal failure may be necessary (as above). In patients with severely impaired cardiac function, a loading dose of 12 mg/kg and maintenance dose of 1.4 mg/kg/hr have been used. Reduce dose in liver disease. Variations in oral bioavailability occur. Most patients experience decrease in systolic and diastolic blood pressure of approximately 10% from IV administration; if greater than this, decrease infusion rate. If QRS interval is prolonged by 30–50%, dose is probably excessive.[8,58]

Nursing Implications and Methods of Administration

Procainamide may be given IV or IM. IV rate, BDC should not exceed 50 mg/min. IV infusion is 2 gm/500 ml. Solution may change from a clear solution to yellowish color upon standing; if darker than light amber solution, the solution should be discarded. Compatible with bretylium, lidocaine, dobutamine. Monitor ECG, heart rate, blood pressure, and periodically ANA, serum levels.[26,101]

Interactions

Procainamide + antihypertensives → increased hypotensive effect; procainamide + neuromuscular blockers → increased neuromuscular block; procainamide + cimetidine → enhanced procainamide effect. Procainamide may produce a positive Coombs test.

QUINIDINE

Quinidine is an alkaloid of cinchona species that produces its antiarrhythmic effects by decreasing excitability and conduction velocity. Direct depressant effects upon cardiac tissue are complicated by indirect vagolytic effects. It prolongs QRS and QT interval.[8,41,62]

Dosage

Oral, (premature atrial and ventricular tachycardia): 0.2–0.3 gm, 3 or 4 times a day. Maximum dose 2400 mg/day. IM (treatment of acute tachycardia): 600 mg followed by 400 mg q2h; evaluate after each dose. IV: 800 mg/50 ml D5W at not greater than 1 ml/min.[26] There are no good dosing guidelines for IV quinidine, however.

Pharmacokinetics and Biopharmaceutics

po bioavailability: well absorbed, it approximates parenteral. Quinidine sulfate contains 87.4% quinidine. Quinidine gluconate contains 62.3% quinidine. po (peak): 1.3 hours. Therapeutic range: 4.6–12 μm/liter. Protein binding: 60–80% to alpha, -acid glycoprotein. T½: 6–7 hours. Vd: 3 liters/kg. Fate: hydroxylated by liver and excreted by kidney both in unchanged form and as metabolites.[8,26]

Adverse Effects

Diarrhea, from po forms, which is not dose related and may be treated with Amphojel; hypotension (usually from parenteral forms), cinchonism, heart block, tachyarrhythmias, prolongation of PR, QRS, QT torsade de pointes, thrombocytopenia, rash, and fever.[26,61,84]

Dosing Adjustments and Precautions

Caution in patients with pre-existing intraventricular conduction defects, digitalis toxicity, electrolyte, and acid/base imbalances. Monitor carefully in severe renal disease, congestive heart failure, and in presence of alkalotic urine as elimination is decreased. Control ventricular rate of atrial flutter/fibrillation with digitalis before adding quinidine.[61,62,102]

Nursing Implications and Methods of Administration

IV form is usually reserved for emergency situations. IM is painful. Monitor blood pressure, heart rate, ECG (50% increase in width of QRS complex is related to toxicity). Hemodialysis may be of value in quinidine toxicity.[8,61]

Interactions

Quinidine + cimetidine → enhanced quinidine effect; quinidine + digoxin → enhanced digoxin level; quinidine + neuromuscular blockers → enhanced paralysis.[21,43]

RANITIDINE (ZANTAC)

Ranitidine is a H_2 receptor antagonist similar in efficacy to cimetidine in the treatment of peptic ulcer disease. Because it is more potent than cimetidine, it can be dosed twice daily when given orally. Ranitidine 150 mg po is equivalent to 800 mg of cimetidine (see cimetidine).[13,103]

Dosage

po: 150 mg bid. IV: 50 mg q6–8h.[13,31]

Pharmacokinetics and Biopharmaceutics

Bioavailability: 50%. Peak (po): 1–3 hours. Duration: 8–12 hours; duration of effect with IV ranitidine shorter than with po. Protein binding: 15%. T½: 2.0–2.5 hours; renal impairment T½—4.8 hours.[31,82] Vd: 1.5 liter/kg; increased in renal failure. Elimination: hepatically metabolized to three metabolites, approximately 70% excreted unchanged in the urine.

Adverse Effects

Bradycardia, hepatotoxicity, reversible leukopenia, granulocytopenia, thrombocytopenia; rarely mental confusion, agitation, depression, hallucinations.[31]

Dosing Adjustments and Precautions

The dose of ranitidine must be decreased in the presence of renal dysfunction. Ranitidine is removed by hemodialysis, and doses should be given postdialysis. There is no dosage adjustment required in hepatic cirrhosis, although caution is recommended.[31,67]

Nursing Implications and Methods of Administration

Ranitidine may be diluted to 20 ml and given over 2 minutes or administered ADC in 100 ml over 20 minutes. It is compatible with commonly used intravenous solutions and many drugs. Ranitidine is incompatible with Amphotericin B and cephalothin.[31,101]

Interactions

Ranitidine + metoprolol → increased metoprolol T½; ranitidine + procainamide → elevated procainamide serum concentration; ranitidine + theophylline → increased theophylline toxicity (only a few cases reported).[51]

SALBUTAMOL (VENTOLIN)

Salbutamol is a β_2-agonist that is used as a bronchodilator in the treatment of reversible bronchospasm. The drug may also cause vasodilation mediated through vascular beta receptors and reflex tachycardia. When the drug is given by inhalation, adverse effects are minimal.[31,61,76]

Dosage

Inhalation (respirator solution): 0.25–0.5 ml (1.25–2.5 mg) in 2–5 ml NS given over 10–15 minutes. Inhaler (metered dose): 1–2 puffs (100–200 μg) qid. IV (bolus injection): 250 μg over 2–5 minutes, repeat in 15 minutes if necessary; followed by continuous infusion—5 μg/min increased to 10 and 20 μg/min at 15–30 minutes.[26,76]

Pharmacokinetics and Biopharmaceutics

Inhalation: onset—5–15 minutes. Peak: 0.5–2 hours. Duration: 3–4 hours. T½: 3.8 hours. Salbutamol is hepatically metabolized to an inactive metabolite.[61]

Adverse Effects

Tachycardia, arrhythmias, peripheral vasodilation, fine muscular tremor, nervousness, hypokalemia, hyperglycemia.[26,61,76]

Dosing Adjustments and Precautions

Salbutamol should be administered cautiously in patients with cardiovascular disorders, hyperthyroidism, and diabetes mellitus. Admixture of salbutamol infusion in dextrose-containing solutions is not suitable for patients with diabetes due to danger of glucose overload.[76]

Nursing Implications and Methods of Administration

Inhalation salbutamol is the route of choice for most patients. Parenteral drug is indicated for patients who have airway inflammation or mucus plugging after failure to respond to inhaled drug. Salbutamol for infusion is prepared by adding 5 mg to 500 ml of NS/D5W (see precautions). The solution is stable for 24 hours. Monitor glucose, potassium. Patients should have continuous ECG monitoring.[76]

Interactions

Salbutamol + other sympathomimetics → increased toxicity; salbutamol + β-blockers → reversal of salbutamol effect.[31,61]

SODIUM NITROPRUSSIDE (NIPRIDE)

Sodium nitroprusside is a smooth muscle vasodilator that produces a balanced arteriolar dilation and venodilation, reducing preload and afterload and increasing cardiac output. It has no direct effect on the heart, and its effects on coronary perfusion are still under study. A reduction in myocardial oxygen consumption has been shown in heart failure. As an antihypertensive, it may be effective where other compounds have failed and resistance to hypotensive effects and tachyphylaxis are rare. As with other vasodilators, the effect upon hemodynamics is dependent upon pre-existing state.[62]

Dosage

IV infusion: 0.5 μg/kg/min and increase by 0.2 μg/kg/min every 5 minutes; maximum dose is 8 μg/kg/min.[26,97]

Pharmacokinetics and Biopharmaceutics

IV infusion only. Onset: almost immediate. Duration: short. T½: (SNP): short; thiocyanate, 2.7 days (9 days with renal impairment). Fate: sodium nitroprusside (SNP) is rapidly metabolized to cyanide in the blood and extracellular space. Cyanide is converted to thiocyanate by the liver and metabolites of thiocyanate are eliminated by the kidneys. Thiocyanate levels increase dependent on renal function.[88]

Adverse Effects

Hypotension usually occurs with rapid infusion. Resistance to the vasodilating effect of sodium nitroprusside may occur. *Cyanide toxicity* manifests as tachycardia, pronounced base deficits, elevated lactate, and elevated mixed venous blood oxygen content. Increasing tolerance to the hypotensive effects of the drug is an early indication of cyanide toxicity. Doses of >2 μg/kg/min are associated with cyanide accumulation. *Thiocyanate toxicity:* fatigue, weakness, rash, hypothyroidism, mental confusion, tinnitus. Thiocyanate toxicity tends to correlate with levels over 1.7 μm/liter and is dialyzable. Cyanide toxicity may occur as early as 45–60 minutes after initiation of infusion and may be fatal even with usual doses.[61,63,85,88]

Dosing Adjustments and Precautions

Enhanced sensitivity to thiocyanate occurs in patients with hypothyroidism, hypovolemia, and hyponatremia. Caution in patients with renal and hepatic impairment, acidosis, patients with low cyanacobalamin levels, or Leber's optic atrophy.[61]

Nursing Implications and Methods of Administration

IV infusion containing 50 mg/500 ml D5W or NS (100 μg/ml), prepared by dissolving 1 vial containing 50 mg of SNP powder using sterile water without preservative or D5W and further diluting the solution. Protect prepared solution from light, and discard solution after 12 hours or if change in color is observed (freshly prepared solution has slight brownish tinge). No other drugs should be mixed with SNP. Monitor blood pressure, heart rate, and signs of toxicity (see adverse effects).[26,97,101]

Interactions

Sodium nitroprusside + dopamine/dobutamine → more favorable hemodynamic effects than when either agent is administered alone. Sodium nitroprusside lowers hydroxycobalamins and interferes with thyroid function tests.[94,99]

THEOPHYLLINE

Theophylline is an xanthine derivative that causes bronchodilation; it improves diaphragmatic contractility, promotes diuresis, causes cardiac and gastric stimulation, and relaxes smooth muscle by increasing cyclic adenosine monophosphate (cAMP).[9,41]

Dosage

For aminophylline: Adults (loading dose): 6 mg/kg over 30 minutes if not presently taking theophylline-containing products. If there is a history of ingestion of these agents, the loading dose should be substantially reduced. Maintenance dose: by continuous IV infusion may be calculated from the following equation:

Infusion rate (mg/kg/hr) = 0.5 mg/kg/hr × disease factor(s)

Disease state	Factor
Nonsmoker	1.0
Smoker	1.6
Congestive heart failure	0.4
Cirrhosis	0.4
Severe obstruction	0.8

For example, a 50-kg nonsmoker with CHF should receive a maintenance dose of MD = 0.5 mg/kg/hr × 50 kg × 1.0 × 0.4 = 10 mg/hr.[73]

Pharmacokinetics and Biopharmaceutics

Onset (IV): within 15 minutes. T½: 3–9 hours (adults), 1–10 hours (children). Vd: 450 ml/kg. Plasma levels: therapeutic—55–110 μm/liter; toxic—greater than 110 μm/liter. Fate: extensively metabolized by the liver.[20,73]

Adverse Effects

Anorexia, nausea, nervousness, irritability, insomnia, headache, arrhythmias, convulsions, and hypotension.[20]

Dosing Adjustments and Precautions

Dosing adjustments may be required in patients with liver impairment, CHF, and smoking history as above. Chronic barbiturate users may clear drug more rapidly. IM and rectal routes should be avoided. Care must be taken when giving other catecholamines. Theophylline (anhydrous) is available in oral dosage formulation. Aminophylline, which is approximately 80% theophylline, is available in oral, IV, and rectal formulations. Oxtriphylline (Choledyl) is available as an oral formulation containing 64% theophylline.[26,43,61]

Nursing Implications and Methods of Administration

Watch for signs of toxicity as listed above. Serious side effects (i.e., arrhythmias) are not always preceded by the less toxic, bothersome side effects, such as nausea. Aminophylline is a basic solution with a pH 8–9, and therefore alkali-labile drugs, such as epinephrine HCl, norepinephrine bitartrate, isoproterenol HCl, and penicillin G potassium, should be avoided in admixtures. Additionally, aminophylline has been reported to be incompatible with clindamycin, doxapram, erythromycin gluceptate, dopamine, and multivitamin infusion (MVI).[101]

Interactions

Theophylline + erythromycin → increased effect of theophylline; theophylline + sympathomimetics → increased heart rate; theophylline + cimetidine → increased theophylline effect; theophylline + ketamine → reduction in seizure threshold; theophylline + propranolol → increased theophylline levels; theophylline + verapamil → increased theophylline levels.[4,22,27,47,106]

VERAPAMIL (ISOPTIN)

Verapamil is an antiarrthymic agent that acts by blocking slow channel conduction in the atrioventricular (AV) node. This reduces supraventricular tachycardia by inhibiting re-entry mechanisms. Because of verapamil's effects on AV nodal conduction, the ventricular rate in atrial fibrillation and flutter is reduced. The drug should be used with caution in Wolff-Parkinson-White syndrome (WPW) due to risk of increasing ventricular rate. Use may be extended to treatment of hypertension, angina, and variant angina.[69,105]

Dosage

IV (bolus): 5–10 mg over 1 minute and repeated 30 minutes later if needed; in circulatory failure, 75 μg/kg followed by 150 μg/kg in 15 minutes. IV (infusion): 1 mg/min to a total of 10 mg, then 5 μg/kg/min. In patients with severe myocardial disease or receiving β-blockers the infusion is started at a very low dose (0.1 μg/kg/min) and titrated against heart rate.[69,71]

Pharmacokinetics and Biopharmaceutics

Onset (IV): rapid. Peak: 5 minutes. Distribution may be delayed in acute circulatory failure, and onset and peak may be delayed. Duration: up to 6 hours. Verapamil shows a strong affinity for nodal tissues, and hence even with a short plasma T½ of 10–20 minutes following IV administration the duration of effect on nodal tissues is significantly longer. Protein binding: 90%. Fate: metabolized in the liver to *N*-dealkylated and *N*-demethylated metabolites thought to contribute to drug's effect.[69,71,105]

Adverse Effects

Nausea, dizziness, sinus brachycardia and arrest, hypotension, shock, heart block and asystole, especially in patients with impaired AV conduction or impaired sinus node function. Hypotension occurs especially with rapid IV administration in predisposed patients. Elevations of hepatic enzymes have been reported.[17,31,61,69]

Dosing Adjustments and Precautions

Avoid verapamil in patients with sick sinus syndrome, cardiogenic shock, second- or third-degree AV block, and digitalis toxicity. Cautious administration in patients with hypotension or those receiving β-blockers. Dosage as listed above should be used if verapamil is deemed necessary in this setting. Dosage reductions are required in hepatic and circulatory failure. Toxic cardiac effects can be treated with 1–2 gm IV calcium gluconate or 1 mg IV atropine.[69,71,105]

Nursing Implications and Methods of Administration

IV direct dose is given over 2 minutes (3 minutes in older individuals) or IV infusion as above. Compatible in commonly employed large-volume parenterals and with digoxin, lidocaine, procainamide, aminophylline. Incompatible with albumin, Amphotericin B, hydralazine, and sulfas.[28,69,101]

Interactions

Verapamil + digoxin → increased serum digoxin levels; verapamil + propranolol → additive negative inotropic effects and cardiac depressant properties; verapamil + β-adrenergic agonists (e.g., isoproterenol) → opposes action of verapamil.[53,61,69]

References

1. American Hospital Formulary Service: Current drug therapy: cardiac glycosides. *Am J Hosp Pharm* 35:1495–1507, 1978.
2. Anavekar SN: Management of hypertensive crises. *Ration Drug Ther* 8: 11, 1977.
3. Anderson JL, Patterson E, Wagner JG, et al: Clinical pharmacokinetics of intravenous bretylium tosylate in survivors of ventricular tachycardia or fibrillation: clinical application of a new assay for bretylium. *J Cardiovasc Pharmacol* 3:485–499, 1981.
4. Adverse interactions of drugs. *Med Letter* 21:5–12, 1979.
5. Dobutamine. *Med Letter* 21:15–16, 1979.
6. Nitroglycerin in acute myocardial infarction. *Med Letter* 18:457, 1979.
7. Symposium on vasodilator and inotropic therapy of heart failure. *Am J Med* 65:101–126, 1978.
8. Treatment of cardiac arrhythmias. *Med Letter* 20:113–120, 1978.
9. Aubier M, DeTroyer A, Sampson A, et al: Aminophylline improves diaphragmatic contractility. *N Engl J Med* 305:249–252, 1981.
10. Bartle WR, Walker JE, Shapero T: Dose-dependent effect of cimetidine on phenytoin kinetics. *Clin Pharmacol Ther* 33:649–655, 1983.
11. Bennett WM, Aronoff GR, Morrisson G, et al: Drug prescribing in renal failure: dosing guidelines for adults. *Am J Kidney Dis* 3:155–193, 1983.
12. Berotti JR, Grossman W, Braunwald E, et al: Effects of amrinone on myocardial energy metabolism and hemodynamics in patients with severe CHF due to CAD. *Circulation* 62:28–34, 1980.
13. Berner BD, Connor CS, Sawyer DR, et al: Ranitidine—A new histamine H_2 receptor antagonist. *Clin Pharm* 1:499–509, 1981.
14. Bivins BA, et al: Dopamine-phenytoin interaction. *Arch Surg* 113:245–249, 1978.
15. Borgstrom L, Johansan CG, Larson H, et al: Pharmacokinetics of propranolol. *J Pharmacokin Biopharmaceutics* 9:419–428, 1981.
16. Bottorff MB, Rutledge DR, Piper JA: Evaluation of intravenous amrinone: the first of a new class of positive inotropic agents with vasodilator properties. *Pharmacotherapy* 5:227–237, 1985.
17. Bradsky SJ, et al: Hepatotoxicity due to treatment with verapamil. *Ann Intern Med* 94:490–491, 1981.
18. Brogden RN, et al: Cimetidine: a review of its pharmacological properties and therapeutic efficacy in peptic ulcer disease. *Drugs* 15:93–131, 1978.
19. Browne TR: Drug therapy of status epilepticus. *Am J Hosp Pharm* 35:915–922, 1978.
20. Bukowskyi M, Nakatsu K, Munt PW: Theophylline reassessed. *Ann Intern Med* 101:63–73, 1984.
21. Burkle WS, Matzke GR: Effect of quinidine on serum digoxin concentrations. *Am J Hosp Pharm* 36:968–971, 1979.
22. Burnakis TG, Jeldon M, Czaplicki AD: Increased serum theophylline concentration secondary to oral verapamil. *Clin Pharm* 2:458–461, 1982.
23. Castle L: Therapy of ventricular tachycardia. *Am J Cardiol* 54:26A–33A, 1984.
24. Check W: Heparin therapy and thrombocytopenia. *JAMA* 241:1224, 1979.

25. Chernow B, Fletcher JR: Catecholamines, opioid peptides and prostaglandins: implications for critical care medicine. In Shoemaker WC (ed): *Critical Care State of the Art.* Fullerton, CA, Society of Critical Care Medicine. 1983, pp 2–81.
26. *Compendium of Pharmaceuticals and Specialties.* Toronto, Canadian Pharmaceutical Association, 1986.
27. Conrad KA, Nyman DW: Effects of metoprolol and propranolol on theophylline elimination. *Clin Pharmacol Ther* 28:463–467, 1980.
28. Cutie MR: Compatibility of verapamil hydrochloride with other additives. *Am J Hosp Pharm* 38:231, 1981.
29. Cutter RE, Forrey AW: Pharmacokinetics of furosemide in normal subjects and functionally anephric patients. *Clin Pharmacol Ther* 15:588–596, 1974.
30. deCarvalho JDR, et al: Treatment of hypertensive emergencies. *Drug Ther* 3:9, 1979.
31. *Drugdex Micromedex Inc.* Englewood, CO, Drug and Poison Information Services, 1986.
32. Edelson J, LeJemtel TH, Alousi AA, et al: Relationship between amrinone plasma concentration and cardiac index. *Clin Pharmacol Ther* 29:723–728, 1981.
33. Feely J, Wilkinson GR, Wood AJJ: Reduction of liver blood flow and propranolol metabolism by cimetidine. *N Engl J Med* 304:692–695, 1981.
34. Feretis CB, Contou TL, Paoutis GC, et al: The effect of preoperative treatment with cimetidine on post-operative wound sepsis. *Am Surg* 50:594–598, 1984.
35. Fitchen HJ, Koeffler HP: Cimetidine in granulopoiesis: bone marrow culture studies in normal man with cimetidine-associated neutropenia. *Br J Hematol* 46:361–366, 1980.
36. Foster CA, Aston SI: Propranolol-epinephrine interaction: a potential disaster. *Plast Reconstruct Surg* 72:74–78, 1983.
37. Fredrick DS, et al: Lidocaine infusions—effect of duration and method of discontinuation on recurrence of arrhythmia and pharmacokinetic variables. *Am J Hosp Pharm* 36:778–781, 1979.
38. Jarrett BN, Kaplah NM: Efficacy of slow infusion of diazoxide in the treatment of severe hypertension without organ hypoperfusion. *Am Heart J* 103:390–394, 1982.
39. Gledhill T, Buck M, Hunt RH: Effect of no treatment, cimetidine 1 g/day, cimetidine 2 g/day and cimetidine combined with atropine on normal gastric secretion in cimetidine non-responders. *Gut* 25:1211–1216, 1984.
40. Goldberg L, Yen Yau H: Clinical uses of dopamine. *Ration Drug Ther* 11:11, 1979.
41. Goodman L, Gillman A: *The Pharmacological Basis of Therapeutics.* New York, Macmillan, 1975.
42. Graham CF, Turner WM, Jones JK: Lidocaine-propranolol interactions. *N Engl J Med* 304:1301, 1981.
43. Hansten PD: *Drug Interactions.* Philadelphia, Lea & Febiger, 1976.
44. Haley RJ, Licht JH: Metoprolol, atenolol, propranolol: a comparison of equivalent doses in the treatment of hypertension. *Curr Ther Res* 36:993–1003, 1984.
45. Herling IM: Intravenous nitroglycerin: clinical pharmacology and therapeutic considerations. *Am Heart J* 108:141–149, 1984.
46. Higbee MD, Wood JS, Mead RA: Procainamide-cimetidine interaction: a potential toxic interaction in the elderly. *J Am Geriatr Soc* 32:162–164, 1984.
47. Hirshman CA, Kreiger W, Littlejohn G, et al: Ketamine-aminophylline induced decrease of the seizure threshold. *Anesthesiology* 56:464–467, 1982.
48. Johnson CE, Wiener JS, Wagner DS, et al: Effect of H_1 and H_2 receptor blockade on the inhibition of immediate cutaneous reactions. *Clin Pharm* 3:60–63, 1984.
49. Johnston GD, McDevitt DG: Is maintenance digoxin necessary in patients with sinus rhythm? *Lancet* 1:567, 1979.
50. Kaplan KJ, Taber M, Teagarden R, et al: Association of methemmaglobinemia and intravenous nitroglycerin administration. *Am J Cardiol* 55:181–183, 1985.
51. Kirch W, Janisch WD: Interactions and non-interactions with ranitidine. *Clin Pharmacokin* 9:493–510, 1984.
52. Kirch W, Kohler H, Spahn, et al: Interaction of cimetidine with metoprolol, propranolol or atenolol. *Lancet* 2:531–532, 1981.
53. Klein HO, et al: Verapamil-digoxin interaction. *N Engl J Med* 303:160, 1980.
54. Klinken WP, Gilbert JAL: Diazoxide in primary pulmonary hypertension. *N Engl J Med* 302:91–92, 1980.
55. Klotz U, Reimann I: Elevation of steady state diazepam levels by cimetidine. *Clin Pharmacol Ther* 30:513–517, 1981.
56. Knapp AB, Maguire W, Keren G, et al: The cimetidine-lidocaine interaction. *Ann Intern Med* 98:174–177, 1983.
57. Kotter V, et al: Comparison of hemodynamic effects of phentolamine, sodium nitroprusside, and glyceryl trinitrate in acute myocardial infarction. *Br Heart J* 39: 1196–1204, 1977.
58. Lima J, et al: Safety and efficacy of procainamide infusions. *Am J Cardiol* 43:98–105, 1979.
59. Marquis JF, et al: Phenytoin-theophylline interaction. *N Engl J Med* 307:1189, 1982.
60. Martyn JAJ, Greenblatt DJ, Abernathy DR: Increased cimetidine clearance in burn patients. *JAMA* 253:1288–1291, 1985.
61. McEvoy GK, McQuarrie GM (eds): *American Hospital Formulary Service: Drug Information 86.* Bethesda MD, American Society of Hospital Pharmacists, 1986.
62. Melmon KL, Moreilli HF. *Clinical Pharmacology: Basic Principles in Therapeutics.* New York, Macmillan, 1972.
63. Montoliu J, et al: Fatal hypotension after an average dose of IV sodium nitroprusside. *Am Heart J* 97:541, 1979.
64. Mroczek WJ, et al: The importance of rapid administration of diazoxide in accelerated hypertension. *N Engl J Med* 285:603, 1971.
65. Nissenson AR, et al: Mannitol. *West J Med* 131:277–284, 1979.
66. Ochs HR, Carstens G, Greenblatt DJ: Reduction of lidocaine clearance during continuous infusion by co-administration of propranolol. *N Eng J Med* 303:373–377, 1980.
67. Okolicsanyi C, Venuti M, Strazzabasco M, et al: Oral and intravenous pharmacokinetics of ranitidine in patients with liver cirrhosis. *Int J Clin Pharmacol Ther Toxicol* 22:329–332, 1984.
68. Olson LG, Hensley MJ, Saunders NA: Ventilatory responsiveness to hypercapnia during dopamine infusion in humans. *Am Rev Resp Dis* 126:783–787, 1982.
69. Opie LH: Drugs and the heart. III Calcium antagonists. *Lancet* 1:806–810, 1980.
70. O'Reilly RA: Therapy with anticoagulant drugs. *Ration Drug Ther* 6:8, 1974.
71. Pentel P, Benowitz N: Pharmacokinetic and pharmacodynamic considerations in drug therapy of cardiac emergencies. *Clin Pharmcokin* 9:273–308, 1984.
72. Potter PH, Westby RG: Interstitial nephritis after cimetidine but not ranitidine. *JAMA* 249:351, 1983.
73. Powell HR, Jackson JE: Counterpoint discussion: theophylline. In Evan WE, Schentag JJ, Jasko WJ (eds): *Applied Pharmacokinetics: Principles of Therapeutic Drug Monitoring.* San Francisco, Applied Therapeutics, 1980, pp 139–166.
74. *Product Information: Intropin (Dopamine).* Montreal, Desbergers Ltd, 1977.
75. *Product Information: Tridil (Nitroglycerine)* Mississauga, Ontario, AHS Division, GTN, McGaw Supply Ltd, 1982.
76. *Product Information: Ventolin Injections.* Toronto, Allan and Hanburys/Glaxo, 1983.
77. *Product Monograph: Dobutamine.* Indianapolis, Eli Lilly & Company, 1978.
78 Rachel CL: Endotracheal drug therapy in cardiopulmonary resuscitation. *Clin Pharm* 5:572–579, 1986.
79. Ram CV, Kaplan NM: Individual titration of diazoxide dosage in the treatment of severe hypertension. *Am J Cardiol* 43:627–630, 1979.
80. Ramanathan KB, et al: Contrasting effects of nitroprusside and phentolamine in experimental myocardial infarction. *Am J Cardiol* 39: 994–999, 1977.
81. Rapaport WG: Clinical pharmacokinetics of bretylium. *Clin Pharmacokin* 10:248–256, 1985.
82. Roberts CJC: Clinical pharmacokinetics of ranitidine. *Clin Pharmacokin* 9:211–221, 1984.

83. Roizer MF, Freely TW: Pancuronium bromide. *Ann Intern Med* 88:64–68, 1978.
84. Romankiewicz JA, et al: The noninterference of aluminum hydroxide gel with quinidine sulfate absorption: an approach to control quinidine-induced diarrhea. *Am Heart J* 94:518–519, 1978.
85. Rouby JJ, Gory G, Bourrelli B, et al: Resistance to sodium nitroprusside in hypertensive patients. *Crit Care Med* 10:301–304, 1982.
86. Sawyer D, et al: Cimetidine: adverse reactions and acute toxicity. *Am J Hosp Pharm* 38:188–197, 1981.
87. Schentag JJ, et al: Pharmacokinetic and clinical studies in patients with cimetidine-associated mental confusion. *Lancet* 1:177, 1979.
88. Schulz V: Clinical pharmacokinetics of nitroprusside, cyanide, thiosulfate and thiocyanate. *Clin Pharmcokin* 9:239–251, 1984.
89. Shand DG: Propranolol: resolving problems of usage. *Drug Ther* 3:52–60, 1978.
90. Shearer CA: Rational digoxin dosing by total body stores—a review. *Can J Hosp Pharm* 30:49–51, 1977.
91. Silver BA, Bell WR: Cimetidine-warfarin interaction. *Ann Intern Med* 90:348, 1979.
92. Shook TL, Kirshenbaum JM, Hundley R, et al: Ethanol intoxication complicating intravenous nitroglycerin therapy. *Ann Intern Med* 101:498, 1984.
93. Small RE, Marshall JH: Quinidine-digoxin interaction. *Drug Intell Clin Pharm* 13:286–289, 1979.
94. Sonnenblick EH, et al: Dobutamine: a new synthetic cardiactive sympathetic amine. *N Engl J Med* 300:17–22, 1979.
95. Storstein O: Slow pulse rate as a sign of digitalis toxicity. *Lancet* 1:445, 1979.
96. Tarazi RC: Sympathomimetic agents in the treatment of shock. *Ann Intern Med* 81:364–371, 1974.
97. Tinker JH, Michenfelder JD: Sodium nitroprusside: pharmacology, toxicology, and therapeutics. *Anesthesiology* 45:340–354, 1976.
98. Tishler M, Abramov AL: Cimetidine-induced eosinophilea. *Drug Intell Clin Pharm* 19:377, 1985.
99. Tourville J: Sodium nitroprusside. *Drug Intell Clin Pharm* 9:361–364, 1975.
100. Treadway G: Clinical safety of intravenous amrinone—a review. *Am J Cardiol* 56:39B–40B.
101. Trissel LA: *Handbook of Injectable Drugs,* ed 4. Washington, DC, American Society of Hospital Pharmacists, 1986.
102. Ueda CT, et al: Disposition kinetics of quinidine. *Clin Pharmacol Ther* 19:30–36, 1975.
103. Walt RP, Price D, Hunt RH, et al: The potency and duration of action of ranitidine and cimetidine on meal stimulated acid output. *Gastroenterology* 30:1311, 1981.
104. Ward A, Brogden RN, Heel RG, Speight TM, Avery GS: Amrinone. *Drugs* 26:468–502, 1983.
105. Waxman HL, et al: Verapamil for control of ventricular rate in paroxysmal supraventricular tachycardia and atrial fibrillation and flutter. *Ann Intern Med* 94:1–6, 1981.
106. Weinberger MM, et al: Decreased theophylline clearance due to cimetidine. *N Engl J Med* 304:672, 1981.
107. Wilkinson ML, O'Driscoll R, Kiernan TJ: Cimetidine and pancreatitis. *Lancet* 1:610–611, 1981.
108. Wyman MG, Staughter RL, Farolino DA, et al: Multiple bolus technique for lidocaine administration in acute ischemic heart disease: II Treatment of refractory ventricular arrhythmias and the pharmacokinetic significance of severe left ventricular failure. *J Am Coll Pharmacol* 7:764–769, 1983.

Index

Page numbers in *italics* denote figures; those followed by "t" denote tables.